CORE TEXT OF NEUROANATOMY

THIRD EDITION

CORE TEXT OF

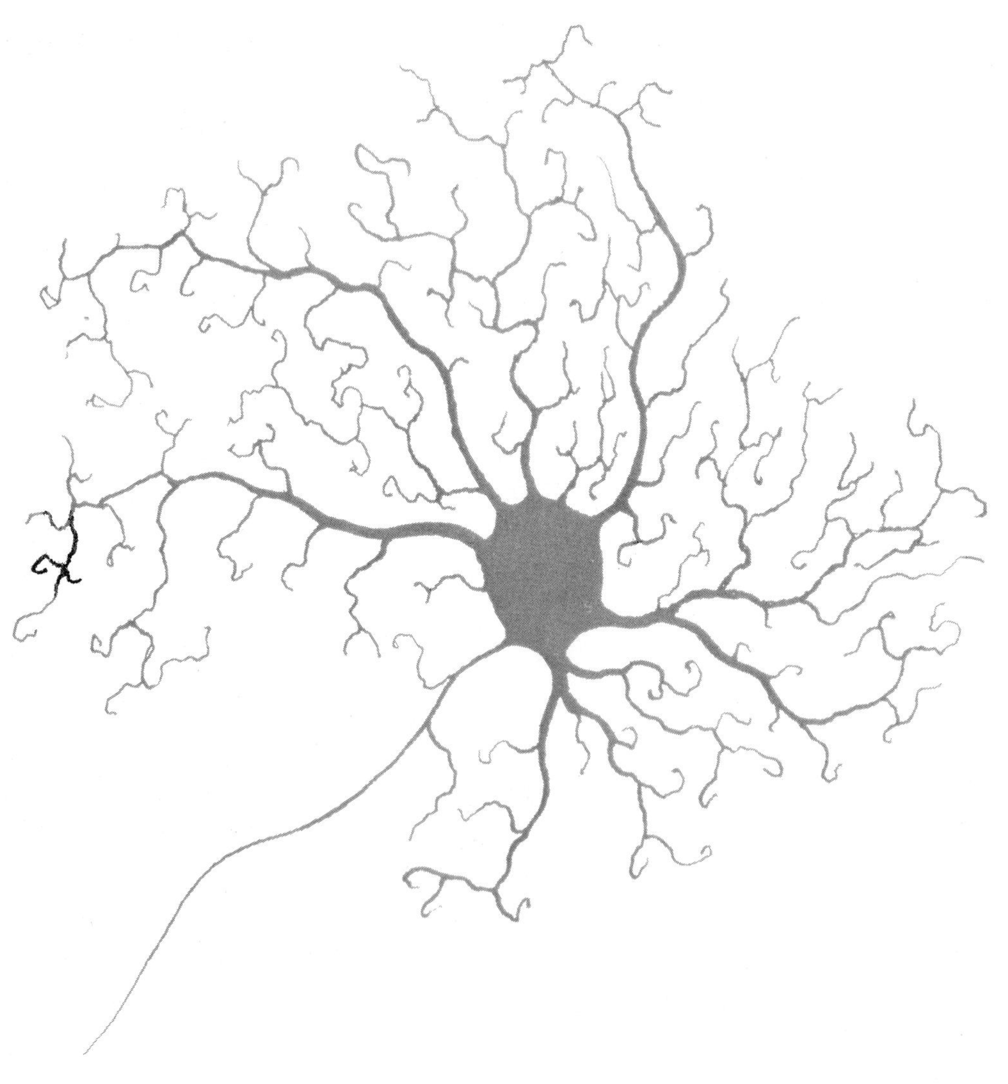

NEUROANATOMY

THIRD EDITION

MALCOLM B. CARPENTER, A.B., M.D.

Professor of Anatomy
F. Edward Hébert School of Medicine
Uniformed Services University of the Health Sciences
Bethesda, Maryland

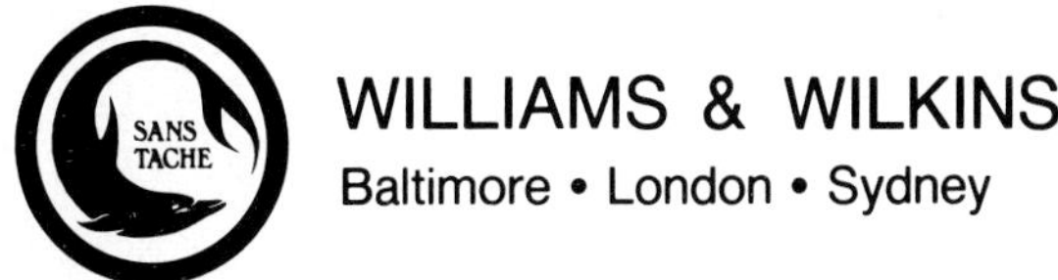

WILLIAMS & WILKINS
Baltimore • London • Sydney

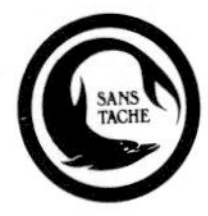

Editor: Toni M. Tracy
Associate Editor: Victoria M. Vaughn
Copy Editor: William Vinck
Design: JoAnne Janowiak
Illustration Planning: Wayne Hubbel
Production: Raymond E. Reter

Made in the United States of America

First Edition, 1972
Reprinted 1972, 1973, 1974, 1975, 1976
Second Edition, 1978
Reprinted 1978, 1979, 1980, 1981, 1982, 1983, 1984

Italian edition, 1976
Portuguese edition, 1979
Spanish edition, 1981
Japanese edition, 1982

Library of Congress Cataloging in Publication Data

Carpenter, Malcolm B.
Core text of neuroanatomy.
Bibliography: p.
Includes index.
1. Neuroanatomy. I. Title. [DNLM: 1. Nervous System—anatomy & histology. WL 101 C296c]
QM451.C37 1985 611′.8 84-15375
ISBN 0-683-01455-2

Composed and printed at the
Waverly Press, Inc.

Preface to the Third Edition

The tremendous expansion of knowledge in the neurosciences continues and its ramifications extend broadly into all basic sciences and into a variety of clinical disciplines. The challenge remains the same: to present a synthesis of modern concepts of the structure and function of the central nervous system within the time allotted. The objective of this text from the beginning has been to present and explain the organization of the central nervous system in a lucid, meaningful fashion that will serve the needs of the student now and in the future. The suggestion that the text be expanded to include other pertinent and related subjects has been resisted. Instead a little more depth has been added in those areas where progress has changed or clarified basic concepts. Attempts have been made not to duplicate material considered in other anatomical areas. The text represents a reasonable treatment of the central nervous system and should meet the requirements of a broad spectrum of medical students.

The third edition of the *Core Text of Neuroanatomy*, like previous editions, is based upon part of the material appearing in Carpenter and Sutin's *Human Neuroanatomy* (eighth edition). While the organization of the book follows a format similar to that used in the larger work and shares many of the same illustrations, the text has been rewritten in a more concise fashion. Most chapters have been revised and brought up-to-date; all have benefited by the clarity that characterizes hindsight. Considerable new material has been added to chapters on the mesencephalon, diencephalon, corpus striatum, and cerebral cortex. Attempts have been made to balance factual material and its interpretation. Over 90 new or revised illustrations have been added, many in the form of teaching diagrams which students find especially helpful. Each chapter contains sections entitled "Functional Considerations" which address special problems and attempt to elucidate major relationships and clinical applications.

The author is grateful to colleagues and associates for their constructive criticisms and generous comments relative to the text as a teaching guide. Particular thanks goes to my mentor, the late Professor Fred A. Mettler of the College of Physicians and Surgeons of Columbia University, whose contributions to my understanding of the nervous system spanned a forty-year period. Permission to use the superb illustrations from Mettler's *Neuroanatomy* (1948) have greatly enhanced the quality of this text. The artistic skills of Robert J. Demarest, Director of the Audiovisual Department of the College of Physicians and Surgeons of Columbia University, is evident throughout the text and each of his illustrations displays his rare talent and insight. Martin Nau of the Department of Anatomy, Uniformed Services University, also contributed his artistic skill to many drawings, for which the author is grateful. The author is pleased to acknowledge the continued expert assistance of Antonio B. Periera. The strong support of Dean Jay P. Sanford deserves special thanks for creating the academic environment conducive to scholarly pursuit. My teaching colleagues at the Uniformed Services University, Drs. Rosemary C. Borke, Rita P. C. Liu, and Donald B. Newman, contributed in many ways during our teaching experience. Mrs. Doris Lineweaver provided superb secretarial and editorial assistance which the author considered invaluable. The author is grateful to the Publishers, especially Toni M. Tracy, Vice President and Editor-in-Chief, for numerous courtesies and helpful suggestions which made this endeavor a pleasure.

MALCOLM B. CARPENTER

Preface to the First Edition

At a time when many American medical schools have shifted to the new core curriculum, or are considering doing so, it is apparent that few of the standard textbooks are entirely appropriate. If the basic medical sciences are to be presented in one academic year, more or less, it is necessary to winnow that which is not essential, to reduce duplications and to present the basic concepts and facts so lucidly that their importance is obvious and their assimilation is possible. With these principles in mind, an attempt has been made to present a *Core Text of Neuroanatomy.*

This text is patterned after part of the material appearing in Truex and Carpenter's *Human Neuroanatomy* (6th edition) and utilizes a similar format and many of the same illustrations. Material which properly falls within the provinces of gross anatomy, histology and embryology has been left to those disciplines except where it is germane to the subject under discussion. The text deals primarily with organization of the central nervous system. References have been kept to a minimum. While the labors of my scientific colleagues, past and present, are not always cited, they are acknowledged fully in the text of *Human Neuroanatomy*, and the interested student will have little difficulty in finding the authors who made the original contributions. The Paris Nomina Anatomica (PNA) in its amended form (1965) has been used throughout.

The author is grateful to Professor Raymond C. Truex, of Temple University School of Medicine, for his permission to use materials from Truex and Carpenter's *Human Neuroanatomy* (6th edition) and for his valued advice and encouragement. Professor Fred A. Mettler, at the College of Physicians and Surgeons, Columbia University, generously permitted the use of many superb illustrations from his *Neuroanatomy* (1948), which were made by Ivan Summers. I am indebted to both Dr. Mettler and The C. V. Mosby Company of St. Louis for permission to publish these illustrations. New illustrations were prepared by Mr. Robert J. Demarest, of the Department of Anatomy, College of Physicians and Surgeons, Columbia University. His skill and talent are acknowledged with deep appreciation. Special acknowledgment must go to Mrs. Ruth Gutmann for her excellent secretarial and editorial assistance in preparing the manuscript.

The author is especially grateful to the Publishers for their continued confidence, encouragement and numerous courtesies which have made the preparation of this book a satisfying experience.

MALCOLM B. CARPENTER

Contents

CHAPTER 1

Meninges and Cerebrospinal Fluid

The brain and spinal cord are delicate semisolid structures requiring protection and support. The brain is invested by three membranes, floated in a clear fluid, and encased in a bony vault. Three membranes surround the brain. The most external membrane is a dense connective tissue envelope known as the *dura mater* or *pachymeninx.* The innermost connective tissue membrane is the *pia mater,* a thin, translucent membrane, adherent to the surface of the brain and spinal cord, which accurately follows every contour. Between these membranes is a delicate layer of reticular fibers forming a weblike membrane, the *arachnoid.* The pia mater and arachnoid have a similar structure and collectively are called the *leptomeninges.*

DURA MATER

The cranial dura consists of: (1) an outer *periosteal layer* adherent to the inner surface of the cranium which is rich in blood vessels and nerves and (2) an inner *meningeal layer* lined with flat cells. At certain sites these layers are separated and form large venous sinuses (Figs. 1-1, 1-2, and 1-3). The meningeal layer gives rise to several septa which divide the cranial cavity into compartments. The largest of these is the sickle-shaped *falx cerebri* which extends in the midline from the crista galli to the internal occipital protuberance (Fig. 1-2). Posteriorly this septum is continuous with other transverse dural septa arising from the superior crest of the petrous portion of the temporal bone. These septa form the *tentorium cerebelli* which roofs over the posterior fossa. The free borders of the tentorium form the *tentorial incisure* (Figs. 1-2 and 1-3). Thus these dural reflections divide the cranial cavity into paired lateral compartments for the cerebral hemispheres, and a single posterior compartment for the cerebellum and lower brain stem. The tentorial incisure (notch) forms the only opening between these compartments. The brain stem passes through the tentorial notch (Fig. 1-4). The occipital lobes lie on the superior surface of the tentorium. A small midsagittal septum below the tentorium forms the *falx cerebelli* (Fig. 1-2) which partially separates the cerebellar hemispheres. The *diaphragma sellae* roofs over the pituitary fossa and is perforated by the infundibulum. The dural sinuses are discussed with the cerebral veins in Chapter 14.

The major blood supply for the dura is provided by the middle meningeal artery, a branch of the maxillary artery, which enters the skull via the foramen spinosum (Fig. 1-3). The ophthalmic artery gives rise to anterior meningeal branches and the occipital and vertebral arteries provide posterior meningeal branches. Skull fractures lacerating these meningeal arteries produce

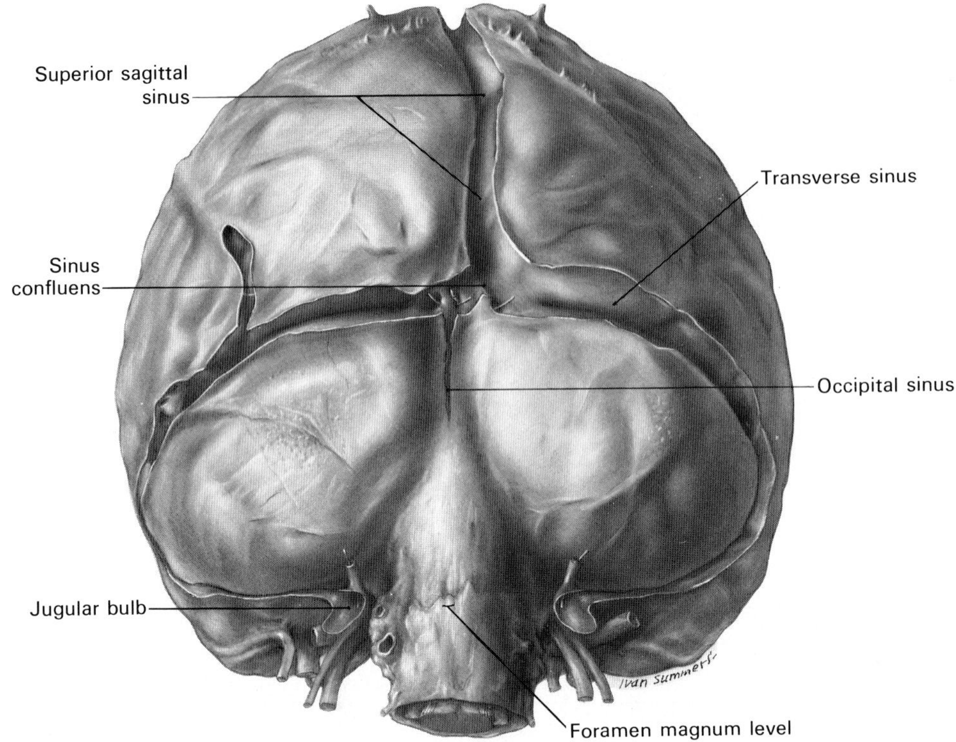

Figure 1-1. Posterior view of the dura surrounding the brain. Prominent dural sinuses have been opened. The periosteal layer of the dura has been cut at the margins of the foramen magnum. (From Mettler's *Neuroanatomy*, 1948; courtesy of The C. V. Mosby Company.)

space occupying epidural hemorrhages between the skull and the dura that require prompt surgical intervention.

The supratentorial dura is innervated by branches of the trigeminal nerve, while the infratentorial dura is supplied by branches of the upper cervical spinal nerves and the vagus nerve.

The *spinal dura* is a continuation of the meningeal layer of the cranial dura (Figs. 1-4, 1-5, and 1-6). The periosteum of the vertebrae corresponds to the outer layer of the cranial dura. Inner and outer surfaces of the spinal dura are covered by a single layer of flat cells, and the dense membrane is separated from the periosteum by the *epidural space*. The spinal epidural space, containing areolar tissue and the internal vertebral venous plexus (Fig. 14-3), is largest at the level of the second lumbar vertebra. This space is used to inject local anesthetics to produce an extensive paravertebral nerve block, known as *epidural anesthesia. Caudal anesthesia*, used in obstetrics, is a form of epidural anesthesia in which the anesthetic agent is injected into the epidural space via the sacral canal.

The spinal dura extends as a closed tube from the margins of the foramen magnum to the level of the second sacral vertebra (Fig. 1-7). The caudal termination of the dural sac invests the filum terminale to form a thin fibrous cord, the *coccygeal ligament* (Fig. 1-7). This ligament extends caudally to the coccyx where it becomes continuous with the periosteum. The spinal cord ends at the lower border of the first lumbar vertebra. Extensions of the dura passing laterally around the spinal nerve roots form dural root sleeves (Figs. 1-5 and 1-6).

PIA MATER

This vascular membrane is composed of: (1) an inner membraneous layer, the *intima pia*, and (2) a more superficial *epipial layer*. The intima pia, adherent to underlying ner-

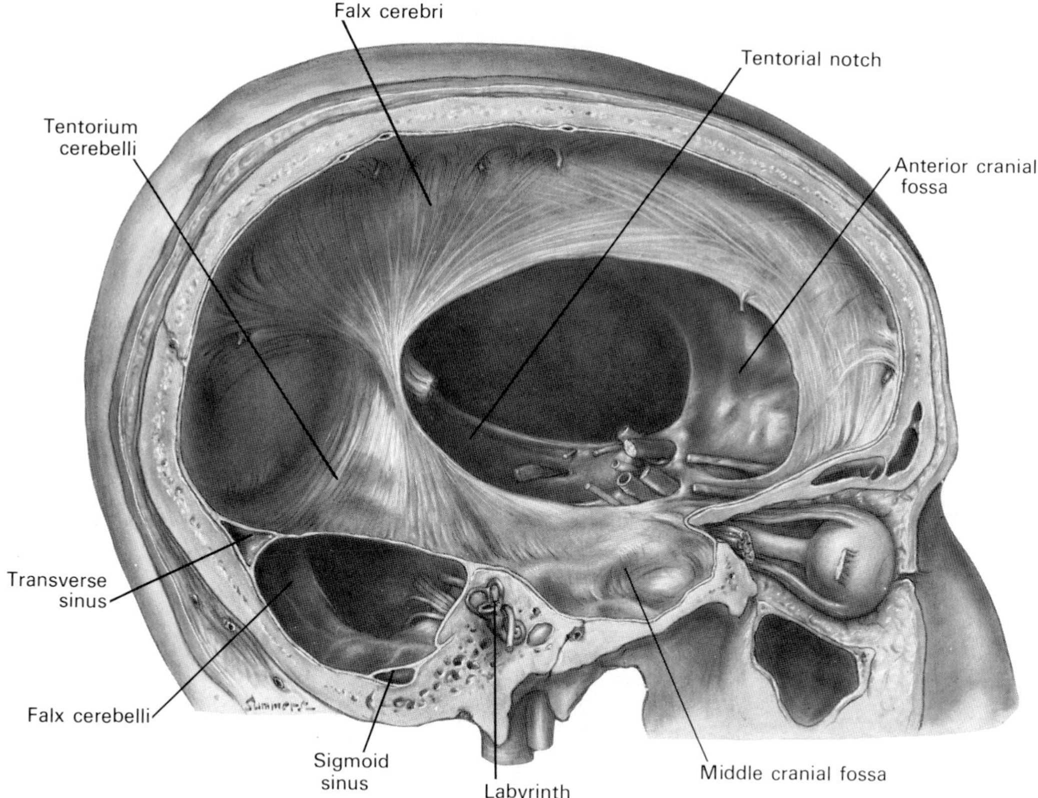

Figure 1-2. Sagittal section of the head showing the falx cerebri, the tentorium cerebelli and the falx cerebelli. (From Mettler's *Neuroanatomy*, 1948; courtesy of The C. V. Mosby Company.)

vous tissue, follows its contours closely and is composed of the fine reticular and elastic fibers. Where blood vessels enter and leave the central nervous system, the intima pia is invaginated forming a perivascular space (Fig. 1-12). The intima pia is avascular and derives its nutrients from the cerebrospinal fluid and underlying neural tissue. The epipial layer is formed by a meshwork of collagenous fiber bundles continuous with the arachnoid trabeculae. The blood vessels of the spinal cord lie within the epipial layer. Cerebral vessels lie on the surface of the intima pia within the subarachnoid space (Fig. 1-8).

The spinal cord is attached to the dura mater by a series of lateral flattened bands of epipial tissue known as the *denticulate ligaments* (Figs. 1-4 and 1-5). Each triangular-shaped dendiculate ligament is attached medially to the lateral surface of the spinal cord midway between the dorsal and ventral roots. The bases of these ligaments arise in the pia mater, and apices are firmly attached to the arachnoid and the inner surface of the dura. The denticulate ligaments anchor the spinal cord to the dura and are present throughout the length of the spinal cord. In the region of the conus medullaris epipial tissue forms a covering of the filum terminale (Fig. 1-7).

The more fibrous intima pia is firmly attached to the surface of the spinal cord by the superficial glial membrane. The latter is composed of fine processes of more deeply located fibrous astrocytes.

ARACHNOID

The arachnoid is a delicate nonvascular membrane between the dura and the pia mater which passes over the sulci without following their contours (Figs. 1-5 and 1-8). This membrane also extends along the roots of the cranial and spinal nerves. Arachnoid trabeculae extend from the

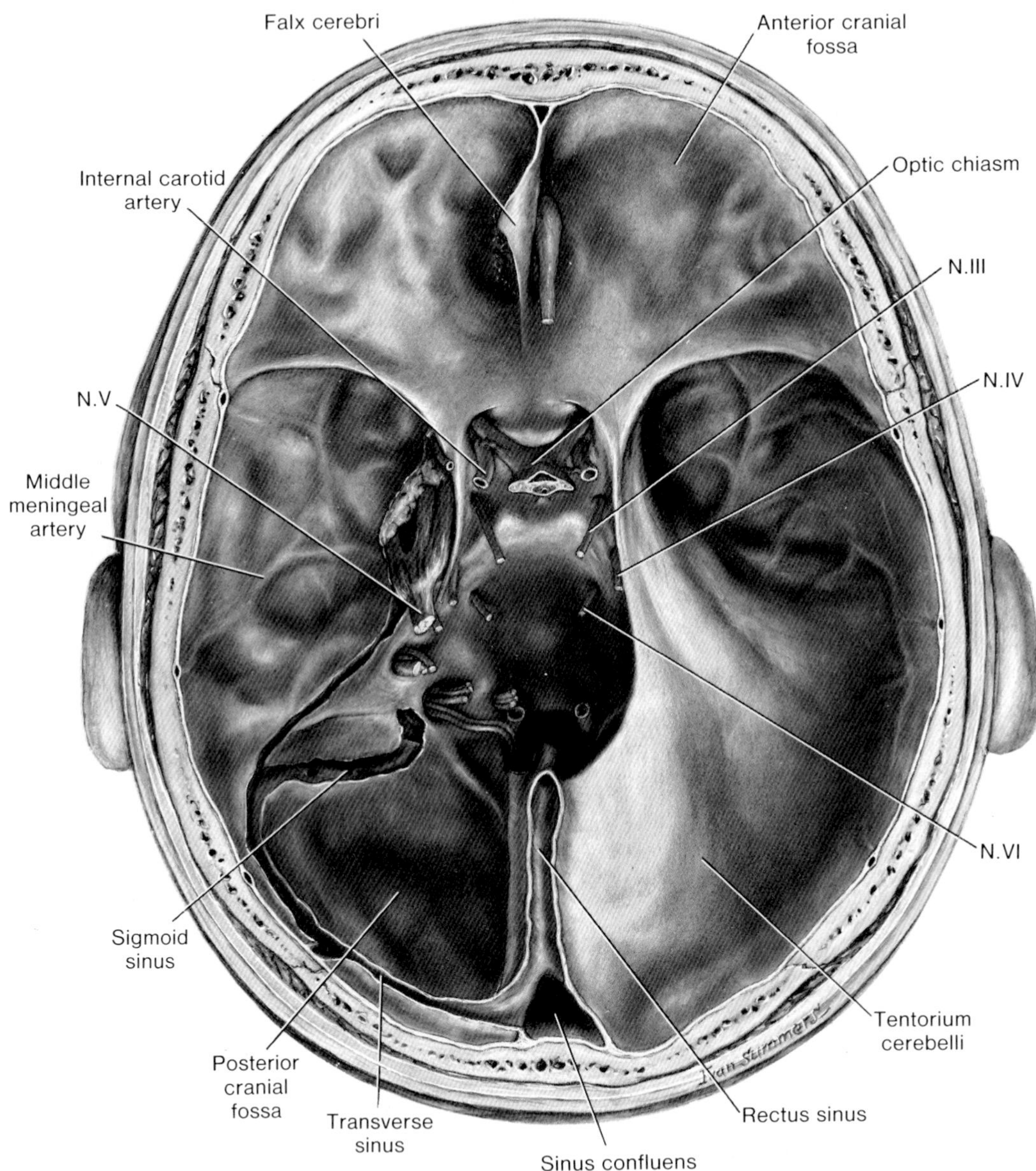

Figure 1-3. View of the base of the skull with dura mater. The falx cerebri has been removed and the tentorium cerebelli has been cut away on the left to expose the posterior fossa. (From Mettler's *Neuroanatomy*, 1948; courtesy of The C. V. Mosby Company.)

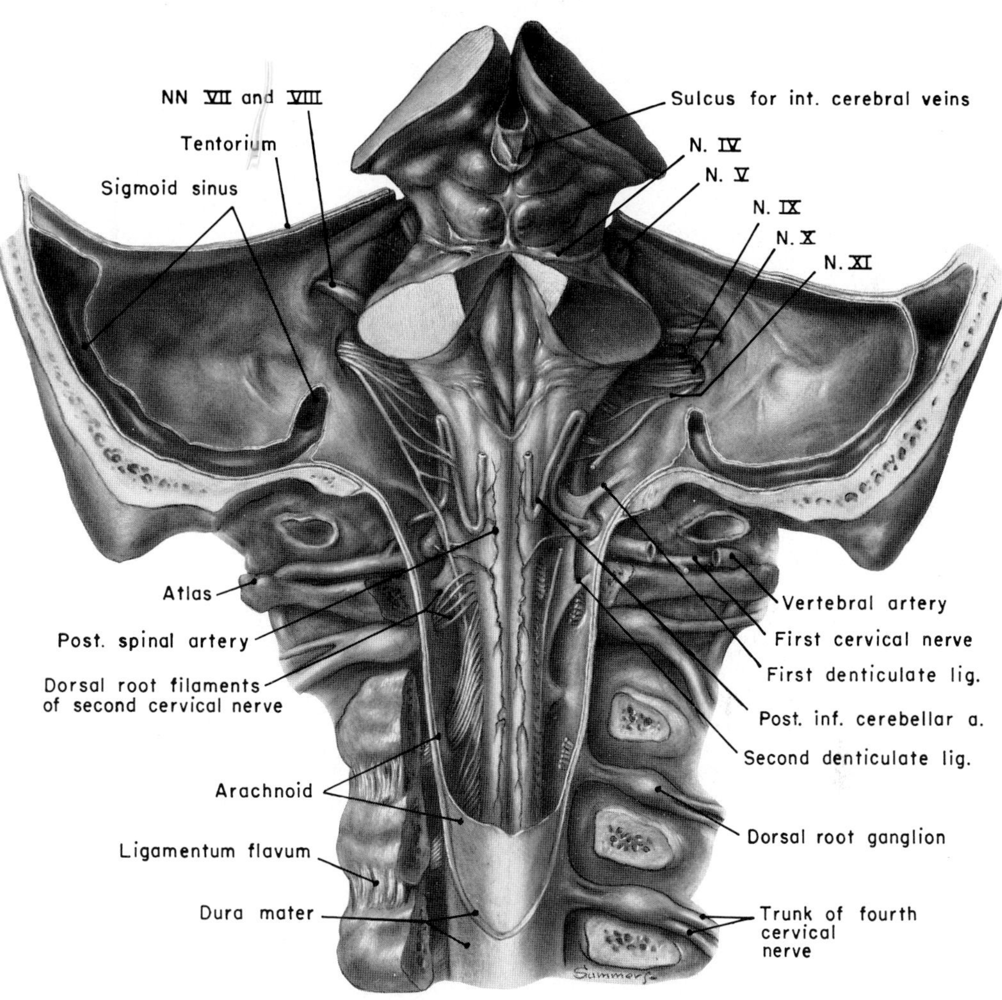

Figure 1-4. Posterior view of the brain stem, upper cervical spinal cord and meninges. (From Mettler's *Neuroanatomy*, 1948; courtesy of The C. V. Mosby Company.)

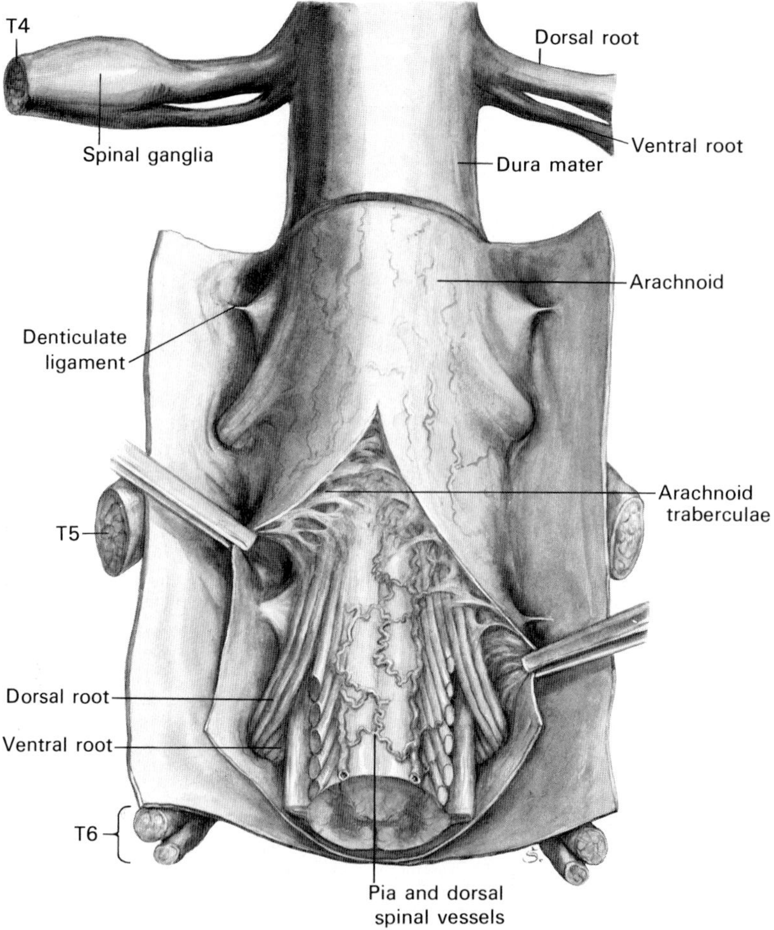

Figure 1-5. Posterior view of part of the upper thoracic spinal cord. The dura and arachnoid have been split at the midline to expose the spinal cord and pial vessels. Above the intact dura covers the spinal cord and spinal nerve roots. (From Mettler's *Neuroanatomy*, 1948; courtesy of The C. V. Mosby Company.)

arachnoid to the pia (Figs. 1-11 and 1-12). The space between the arachnoid and the pia mater, filled with cerebrospinal fluid, is called the *subarachnoid space* (Fig. 1-9). The extent of the subarachnoid space surrounding the brain shows local variations. Over the convexity of the cerebral hemisphere this space is narrow, except in the depths of the sulci. At the base of the brain and around the brain stem the pia and the arachnoid often are widely separated, creating what are called *subarachnoid cisterna* (Figs. 1-8 and 1-9). The largest cistern, found between the medulla and the cerebellum is called the *cerebellomedullary cistern* (cisterna magna) (Figs. 1-8, 1-9, and 1-10). Cerebrospinal fluid from the fourth ventricle passes into the cerebellomedullary cistern via the median *foramen of Magendie* and the two lateral foramina of Luschka (Figs. 1-9 and 1-10). Other cisterns of considerable size are the *pontine cistern*, the *interpeduncular cistern*, the *chiasmatic cistern*, and the *superior cistern* (Figs. 1-8 and 1-9). The superior cistern, surrounding the posterior, superior, and lateral surfaces of the midbrain, is referred to clinically as the *cisterna ambiens*. This cistern is of importance because it contains the great vein of Galen, and the posterior cerebral and superior cerebellar arteries. Most of these cisterns can be visualized in pneumoencephalograms and computerized tomograms.

The *lumbar cistern* extends from the conus medullaris (lower border of the first

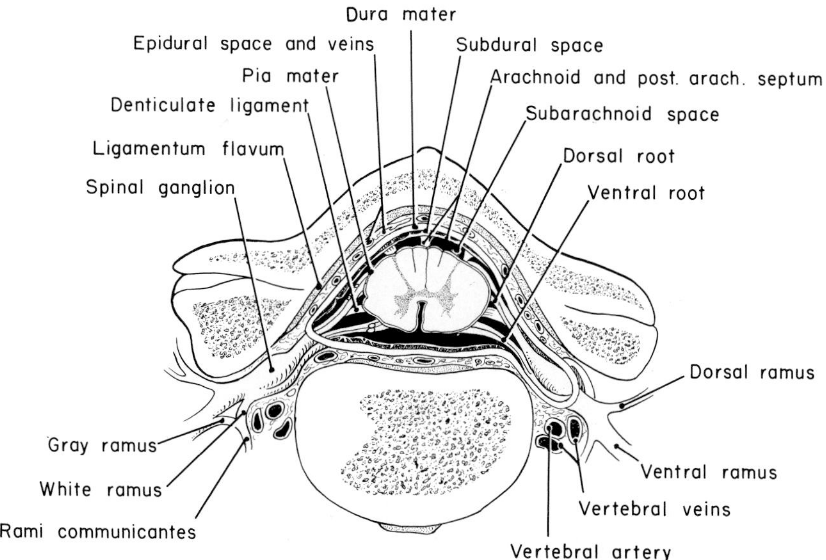

Figure 1-6. Spinal cord and its meningeal coverings in cross section. Note the continuities of the pia mater with the denticulate ligament, and of the dura mater with the epineurium of the spinal nerves. (Modified from Corning, '22; from Carpenter and Sutin, *Human Neuroanatomy*, 1983; courtesy of Williams & Wilkins.)

lumbar vertebra) to about the level of the second sacral vertebra (Fig. 1-7). It contains the filum terminale and nerve roots of the cauda equina. It is from this cistern that cerebrospinal fluid is withdrawn in a lumbar spinal tap.

ARACHNOID GRANULATIONS

In regions adjacent to the superior sagittal sinus the cerebral pia-arachnoid gives rise to tufted prolongations which protrude through the meningeal layer of the dura into the superior sagittal sinus (Fig. 1-11). These granulations are variable in number and location and each consists of numerous arachnoid villi. These villi have a thin outer limiting membrane beneath which are bundles of collagenous and elastic fibers. Cells similar to those of the pia-arachnoid are scattered among the fibers, and small oval epithelial cells cap the surface of the villi. Arachnoid granulations frequently are surrounded by a venous lacuna along the margin of the superior sagittal sinus. At advanced age the arachnoid granulations are larger, more numerous, and tend to become calcified.

Arachnoid villi and granulations are considered to be a major site of transfer of cerebrospinal fluid from the subarachnoid space to the venous system. The hydrostatic pressure of cerebrospinal fluid is greater than that in the dural venous sinuses, so fluid moves from the subarachnoid space into the venous system. The arachnoid granulations appear to function as pressure-dependent, passive one-way valves whose membranes are readily permeable.These valves are spongy tissue containing a series of interconnecting tubules. Tubules remain open only when the cerebrospinal fluid (CSF) pressure exceeds venous pressure in the dural sinuses (Jayatilaka, '65, '65a; Gomez et al., '74; '74a). When the pressure of venous blood exceeds that of the CSF, the tubules collapse (Welch and Friedman, '60). In the absence of pressure differences between the CSF and venous blood, the membranes of these cells are folded and have numerous microvilli. Bulk volume flow of CSF occurs through the arachnoid tubular system and between the stretched endothelial cells. Flow of CSF into the venous sinuses is proportional to the increase in CSF pressure but does not begin until it exceeds venous pressure by 3 to 6 cm of water. Even large molecular-weight substances such as plasma proteins and serum albumin can

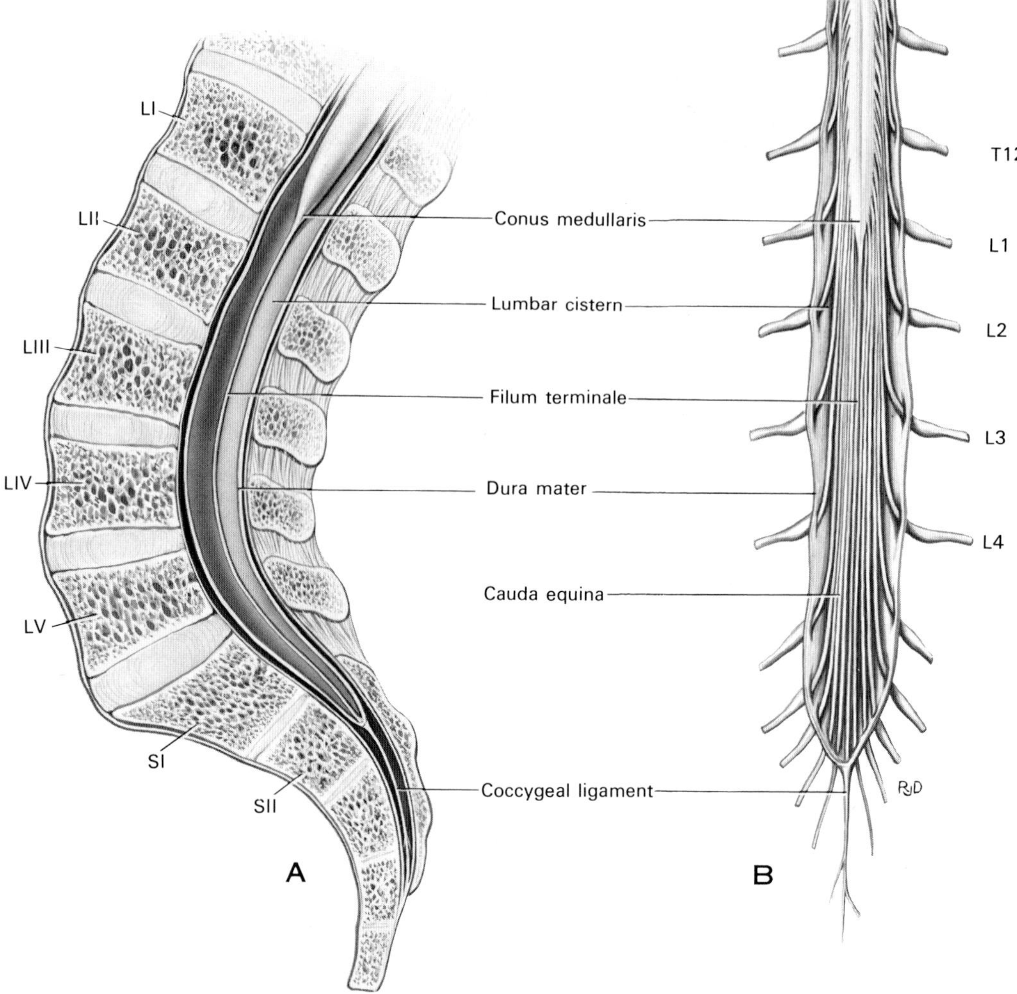

Figure 1-7. Diagrammatic representation of the caudal part of the spinal cord and lumbar cistern. *A* is a sagittal view of the conus medullaris, lumbar cistern and lumbosacral vertebrae. *B* is a posterior view of the cauda equina and nerve roots.

pass from the CSF to venous blood via the arachnoid granulations.

PIA-GLIA AND PERIVASCULAR SPACES

The intima pia or pia-glia is regarded as the external limiting membrane of the central nervous system (CNS). Both the intima pia and the arachnoid are considered to be of ectodermal origin (Miller and Woollam, '61; Pease and Schultze, '58; Davson, '67). Thus the parenchyma of the CNS, the glia, the ependyma and the leptomeninges arise from ectoderm, while the blood vascular system and the dura mater are of mesodermal origin. As blood vessels enter and leave nervous tissue, they carry with them arachnoid and pia-glia which form a cuff around each vessel called the Virchow-Robins space (Fig. 1-12). It has been suggested that spaces might permit flow of CSF into the depths of the tissue. Electron microscopic studies indicate that these two layers ultimately become continuous and there is no real space between them (Maynard et al., '57). At levels of the smallest veins and capillaries no adventitial elements are found, although processes of astrocytes surround the basement membranes of the capillary endothelium.

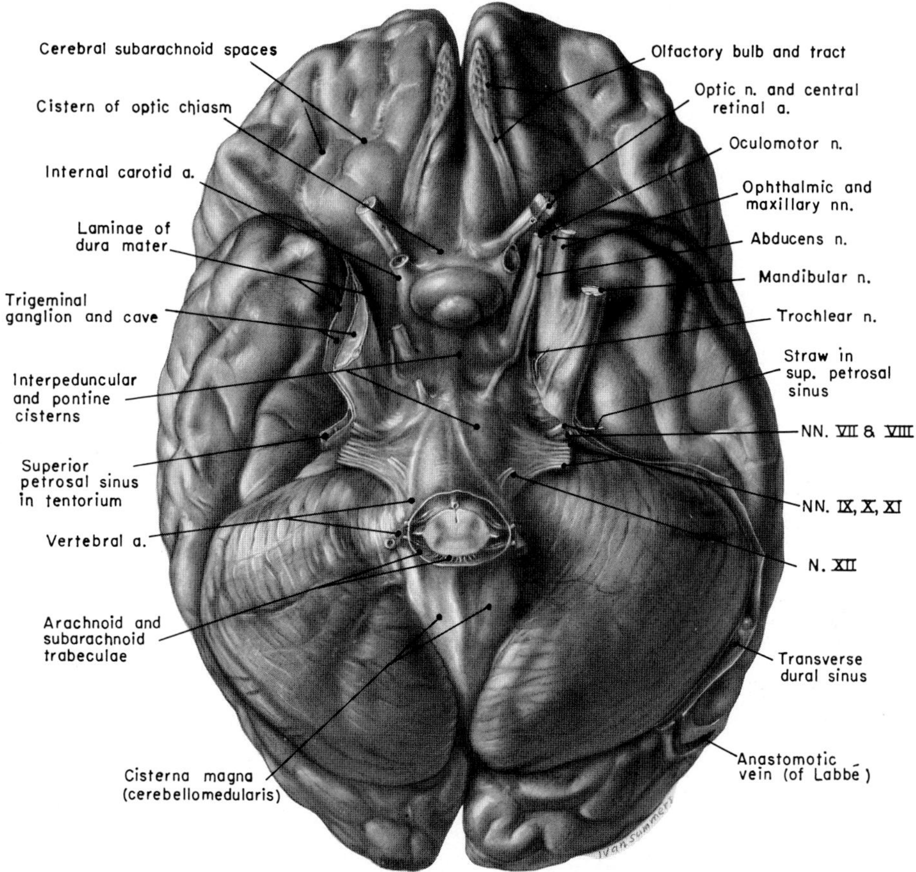

Figure 1-8. Inferior view of brain, cranial nerves and meninges showing locations of subarachnoid cisterns. (From Mettler's *Neuroanatomy*, 1948; courtesy of The C. V. Mosby Company.)

CEREBROSPINAL FLUID

The CSF is a clear, colorless liquid containing small amounts of protein, glucose and potassium and relatively large amounts of sodium chloride. There are no substances normally found in CSF which are not also found in blood plasma. There is no cellular component in CSF, although 1 to 5 cells per cubic millimeter maybe considered to be within normal limits. The CSF serves to support and cushion the CNS against trauma. The buoyancy of CSF is indicated by the fact that a brain weighing 1500 g in air weighs only 50 g when immersed in CSF (Livingston, '65). This buoyancy serves to reduce the momentum and acceleration of the brain when the cranium is suddenly displaced, thereby reducing concussive damage. The CSF removes waste products of metabolism, drugs, and other substances which diffuse into the brain from the blood. As the CSF flows over the ventricular and pial surfaces of the brain it carries away solutes which pass into venous blood via the arachnoid villi. Certain drugs (penicillin) and neurotransmitters (serotonin and norepinephrine) are rapidly removed from the CSF by the choroid plexus (Bárány, '72). In addition CSF plays an important role in integrating brain and peripheral endocrine functions in that hormones, or hormone-releasing factors, from the hypothalamus are secreted into the extracellular space or directly into the CSF. These hormones, which include hormone-releasing hormones are carried via the CSF to the median eminence in the floor of the third ventricle; from this site they are transported by ependymal cells (i.e., tanycytes)

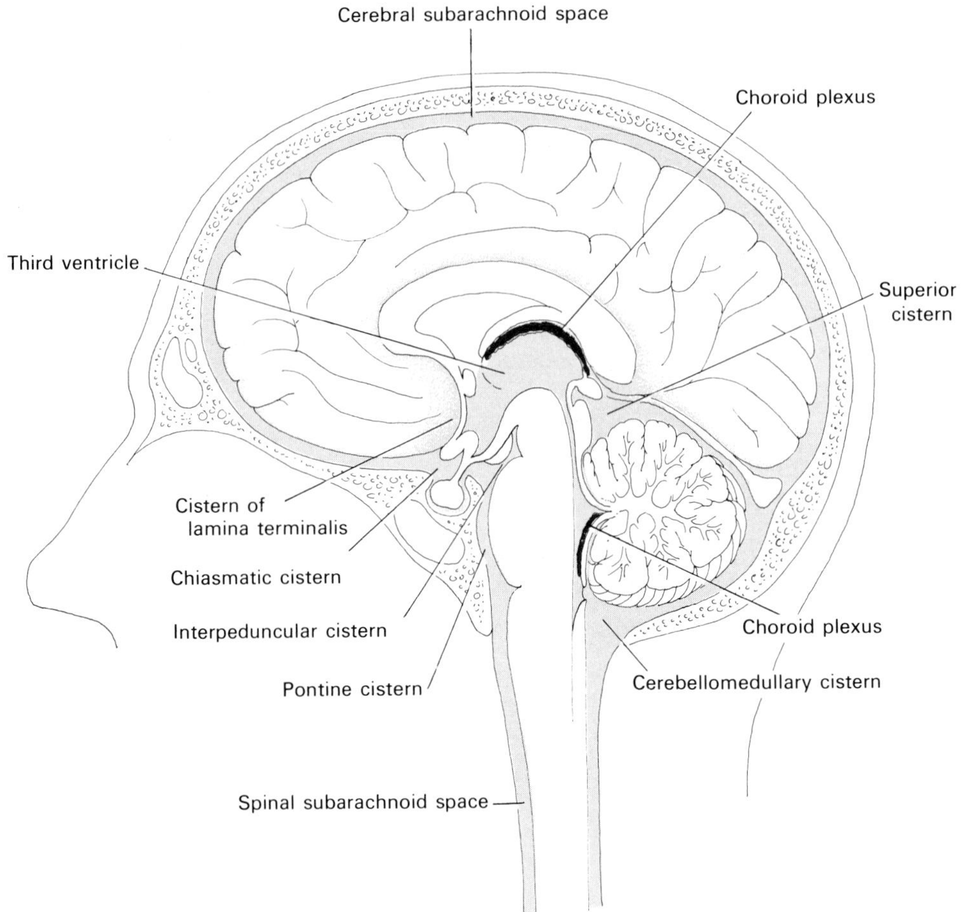

Figure 1-9. Diagram of the subarachnoid cisterns as seen in a midsagittal view. The superior cistern is referred to clinically as the cisterna ambiens. The choroid plexus in the roof of the third and fourth ventricles is shown in *red*. (From Carpenter and Sutin, *Human Neuroanatomy*, 1983; courtesy of Williams & Wilkins.)

into the hypophysial portal system (Figs. 10-12 and 10-13). The CSF also influences the microenvironment of neurons and glial cells because there is no diffusion barrier between the CSF and the brain at either the ependymal lining of the ventricles or the pia-glial membrane (Rapoport, '76). Changes in the ionic concentrations of calcium, potassium, and magnesium in the CSF may affect blood pressure, heart rate, vasomotor reflexes, respiration, muscle tone, and the emotional state (Leusen, '72).

The CSF has been regarded as an ultrafiltrate of the blood plasma because of their resemblance, except for differences in protein concentration (plasma, 6500 mg/100 g; CSF, 25 mg/100 g). The characteristic distribution of ions and nonelectrolytes in CSF and plasma, however, is such that the CSF cannot be described as a simple filtrate, or dialysate, of the blood plasma. In general the CSF has higher Na^+, Cl^- and Mg^{2+} concentrations and lower K^+, Ca^{2+} and glucose concentrations than would be expected in a plasma dialysate. In addition the osmotic pressure relationships are not sufficient to produce a virtually protein-free fluid from the blood plasma (Davson, '67). For these reasons, current evidence supports the theory that the CSF is a secretory product involving active transport mechanisms and the expenditure of energy. Approximately 70% of the CSF is secreted by the choroid plexus located in the lateral ventricles and in the roof of the third and fourth ventricles (Figs. 1-9, 1-10, and 2-8).

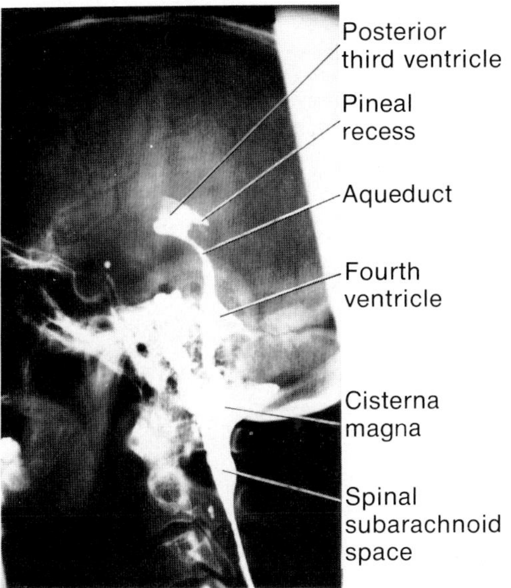

Figure 1-10. Positive contrast ventriculogram clearly outlining the posterior part of the third ventricle, the cerebral aqueduct, the fourth ventricle, and part of the cisterna magna. In this lateral view some radiopaque material also is seen in the basal cisterns and the spinal subarachnoid space.

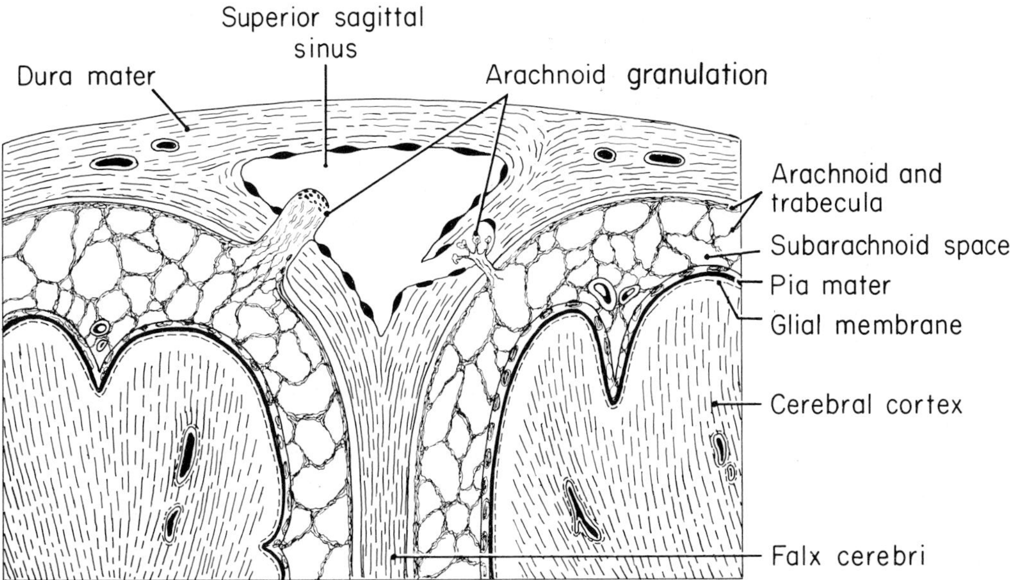

Figure 1-11. Diagram of meningeal-cortical relationships. Arachnoid granulations may penetrate dural sinus or terminate in a lateral lacuna of a sinus. The pia is firmly anchored to cortex by the glial membrane. (From Carpenter and Sutin, *Human Neuroanatomy*, 1983; courtesy of Williams & Wilkins.)

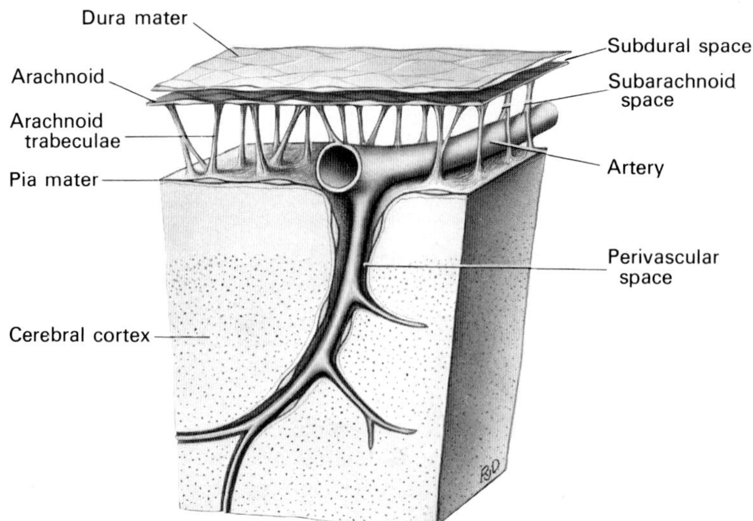

Figure 1-12. Diagram of the meninges showing relationships of the membranes to the subarachnoid and perivascular spaces. (From Carpenter and Sutin, *Human Neuroanatomy*, 1983; courtesy of Williams & Wilkins.)

The remaining 30% of the CSF is derived from metabolic water production (Sahar, '72; Rapoport, '76). Estimates of metabolic water production, based upon the assumption of complete oxidation of glucose, suggest a net contribution of about 12% to the CSF. Extrachoroidal sources produce the remaining 18% of the CSF, largely as a capillary ultrafiltrate. The CSF is formed under a hydrostatic pressure head of 15 ml of H_2O which is sufficient to drive it through the ventricular system and into the subarachnoid space (Davson, '67). Pulsations of the choroid plexus also contribute to the movement of CSF within the ventricular system. The total volume of the CSF in man has been estimated to be about 140 ml of which about 25 ml are contained within the ventricles. Net production of CSF in man has been estimated to be about 0.35 ml per minute, which indicates the formation of over 400 ml per day (Davson, '67; Rapoport, '76).

The choroid plexus is a villous structure extending from the ventricular surface into the CSF. This plexus consists of a single layer of cuboidal epithelium with basal infoldings resting on a basement membrane enclosing an extensive capillary network embedded in a connective tissue stroma (Fig. 1-15). Apical microvilli of the epithelial cells are in contact with the CSF. Capillaries in the connective tissue stroma have endothelial fenestrations, but tight junctions surrounding apical regions of the epithelial cells (Fig. 1-15) form a barrier to the passive exchange of proteins and hydrophilic solutes between the blood and the CSF. Blood-borne horseradish peroxidase (HRP) passes through capillary fenestrations and diffuses into the connective tissue stroma, but does not go beyond the tight junctions of epithelial cells (Brightman et al., '70). The choroid plexus regulates the production and composition of the CSF. A Na^+-K^+ exchange pump, catalyzed by Na^+-K^+-ATPase, drives Na^+ toward the ventricular surface of the plexus and K^+ in the opposite direction. Thus K^+ is transported out of the CSF, while Na^+ is actively transported into it (Miner and Reed, '72). The choroid plexus also plays a role in the regulation of Mg^{2+} and Ca^{2+} in the CSF. CSF secreted by the choroid plexus contains a higher concentration of Mg^{2+} and a lower concentration of Ca^{2+} than an ultrafiltrate of the plasma. The manner in which water, the largest constituent of the CSF, moves across the choroidal epithelium is controversial. According to one theory, modifications of choroidal blood flow can increase or decrease the rate of CSF secretion (Welch, '63). Approximately 25% of the volume of blood flowing to the choroid plexus normally is secreted as CSF. Other data suggest that water moves across the choroidal epithelium under a standing osmotic gradient established by the active transport of Na^+. This hypothesis indicates that movement of water into the CSF is coupled to the active transport of Na^+ by the choroid plexus (Vates et al., '64).

CSF formed in the lateral and third ventricles passes via the cerebral aqueduct into the fourth ventricle. The fluid enters the cerebellomedullary cistern via the median and lateral apertures of the fourth ventricle (Figs. 1-8, 1-9, 1-10, and 2-18). From this site the fluid circulates in the subarachnoid spaces surrounding both the brain and the spinal cord. The bulk of the CSF is passively returned to the venous system via the arachnoid villi (Fig. 1-11). The hydrodynamic permeability of the arachnoid villi is large compared with that of peripheral capillaries. Large protein molecules leave the CSF by passage through the arachnoid villi at roughly the same rate as smaller molecules. The rate of exit of CSF via the arachnoid villi is pressure dependent and begins when the CSF pressure exceeds venous pressure by 3 to 6 ml of water. The arachnoid villi serve as one-way valves. If the CSF pressure is greater than venous pressure, the tubelike valves open and CSF enters the dural sinuses. When venous pressure exceeds CSF pressure, the valves close and blood cannot enter the CSF. Small amounts of CSF may be taken up by the ependyma, arachnoid capillaries, and lymphatics of the meninges and perivascular tissues.

In the recumbent position, the CSF pressure measured at the lumbar cistern normally is about 100 to 150 mm of H_2O; in the sitting position the pressure measured at the same site varies between 200 and 300 mm of H_2O. Because the brain is nearly incompressible within the cranium, the combined volumes of brain, CSF, and blood must be maintained at a constant level. A volume increase in any one of these components can only be at the expense of one or both of the others. Thus a space-occupying lesion, such as a tumor or hematoma, usually results in an increase in CSF pressure.

An excessive amount of CSF produces an elevated pressure and in infants can cause hydrocephalus with enlargement of the ventricles, damage to neural tissue, and changes in the neural cranium. Such increases in CSF may result from an overproduction of fluid, an obstruction to its flow, or inadequate absorption. In most instances hydrocephalus results from obstruction within the ventricular system. Removal of the choroid plexus from one lateral ventricle usually causes that ventricle to collapse, while obstruction of one interventricular foramen causes dilatation of the ipsilateral lateral ventricle.

An extensive plexuses of serotonin axons exists in supra- and subependymal systems in the walls of the ventricles and in the arachnoid sheath around major cerebral blood vessels (Chan-Palay, '76). The raphe nuclei in the pons are considered to be the source of axons forming these plexuses. It has been suggested that serotonergic axons in ventricular and pial surfaces may be important modifiers of local CSF composition and that subarachnoid plexuses around major cerebral blood vessels may influence local vasomotor activity and thus affect cerebral blood flow.

BRAIN BARRIERS

The functioning of all neurons of the central nervous system is dependent upon the maintenance of a physical and chemical milieu within certain narrow limits. The system which regulates the exchange of water and solutes between the plasma, the CSF, and the brain involves membranes with selective permeability. This multicompartmental "barrier" arrangement regulates the transport of chemical substances between the arterial blood, the CSF, and the brain. The "barrier" system regulates and stabilizes the physical and chemical milieu of the CNS. This system maintains the physiochemical composition of the microenvironment of neurons, axons, and glia within the narrow limits required for neuronal survival. The blood-brain barrier separates the two major compartments of the CNS, the brain and the CSF, from the third compartment, the blood. The sites of the barrier are the interfaces between the blood and these two compartments of the CNS. Two separate barriers, a "blood-CSF barrier" and a "blood-brain barrier" have been recognized in order to explain why intravascular substances enter the CSF and the brain at different rates (Davson, '67). The intravascular injection of substances, such as glucose and urea diffuse rapidly into most tissues and come to equilibrium promptly with extracellularly and intracellular fluids. The transport of substances from the blood to the CSF requires hours instead of minutes. Injections of certain dyes into the blood, such as trypan blue, quickly stain most body tissues, but do not enter the CSF. Early studies, indicating important differences between the CSF and the interstitial fluid of most body tissues, established that this barrier is not absolute, but selectively permeable. The kinetic aspects of the passage of substances from the blood into brain are included under the term blood-brain barrier and by analogy with the blood-CSF barrier. The concept of the restricted passage of dissolved substances from the blood to the brain was based upon observations that intravenous injection of many vital dyes stained practically all body tissues except the brain (Ehrlich, 1885). These two barriers differ greatly in surface area; the surface area of the blood-brain barrier is estimated to be 5000 times greater than that of the blood-CSF barrier (Pardridge et al., '81). The brain barriers are considered to develop at an early stage when the blood vessels invade the brain.

The ependyma surfaces of the cerebral ventricles and the pia-glial membrane on the brain surface do not impede the exchange of substances between the CSF and the brain. Thus the brain-CSF interface does not constitute a sub-barrier (Rapoport, '76). Ependymal cells of the ventricles are not connected by tight junctions and do not hinder macromolecular exchange between the CSF and the brain (Brightman, '65). Drugs injected into the cerebral ventricles easily cross the ependymal lining and produce prompt pharmacological and behavioral effects. A schematic diagram of relationships between the blood-brain barrier, the blood-CSF barrier, and the brain-CSF interface is shown in Fig. 1-13. There are striking differences in the concentration of various substances in the CSF and plasma and there are differences in the rates of transfer of these substances from plasma to CSF and to neurons.

Blood-Brain Barrier. The pia and subjacent glial membrane blend with the vessel wall before it penetrates the substance of the brain or spinal cord (Fig. 1-12). Smaller arterial branches have only thin neuroglial investments which persist to the capillary level. The capillary endothelium, a continuous homogeneous basement membrane, and numerous astrocytic processes are all that separate the plasma from the extracellular space (i.e., interstitial) within the CNS. These structures usually are equated with the *blood-brain barrier* (Fig. 1-13).

In all parts of the body exchanges between blood and tissue take place in the capillary bed. This generalization applies to the brain, but with some significant differences. The wall of a capillary consists only of flattened endothelial cells resting on a basement membrane surrounded by a thin adventitial layer. Capillaries within the CNS contain a continuous inner layer of endothelial cells connected by tight junctions and are considered to be derived totally or partially from neuroectoderm (Olsson and Reese, '71; Hamilton and Mossman, '72). The tight junctions between endothelial cells of brain capillaries restrict intercellular diffuse of solutes and in essence form a continuous cell layer with the permeability properties of a plasma membrane (Fig. 1-14). The basement membrane surrounding the endothelial cells has approximately 85% of its surface covered by glial cells (Maynard et al., '57). The tight junctions between endothelial cells prevent the transfer of microperoxidase, HRP, and ferritin (Reese and Karnovsky, '67; Brightman and Reese, '69; Brightman et al., '70). One gram of brain has about 240 cm^2 of capillary surface (Crone, '63). Cerebral blood vessels have neither a well-developed small pore system nor a vesicular transport system. Pinocytotic vesicles are rare in endothelial cells of cerebral capillaries. In the CNS capillary endothelial cells are metabolically active with respect to both oxidative and hydrolytic enzymes. Enzymes within these cells regulate and transport amines and amino acids (Fig. 1-14). An example of this regulation is seen in Parkinson's disease (paralysis agitans) in which there is a deficiency of dopamine.

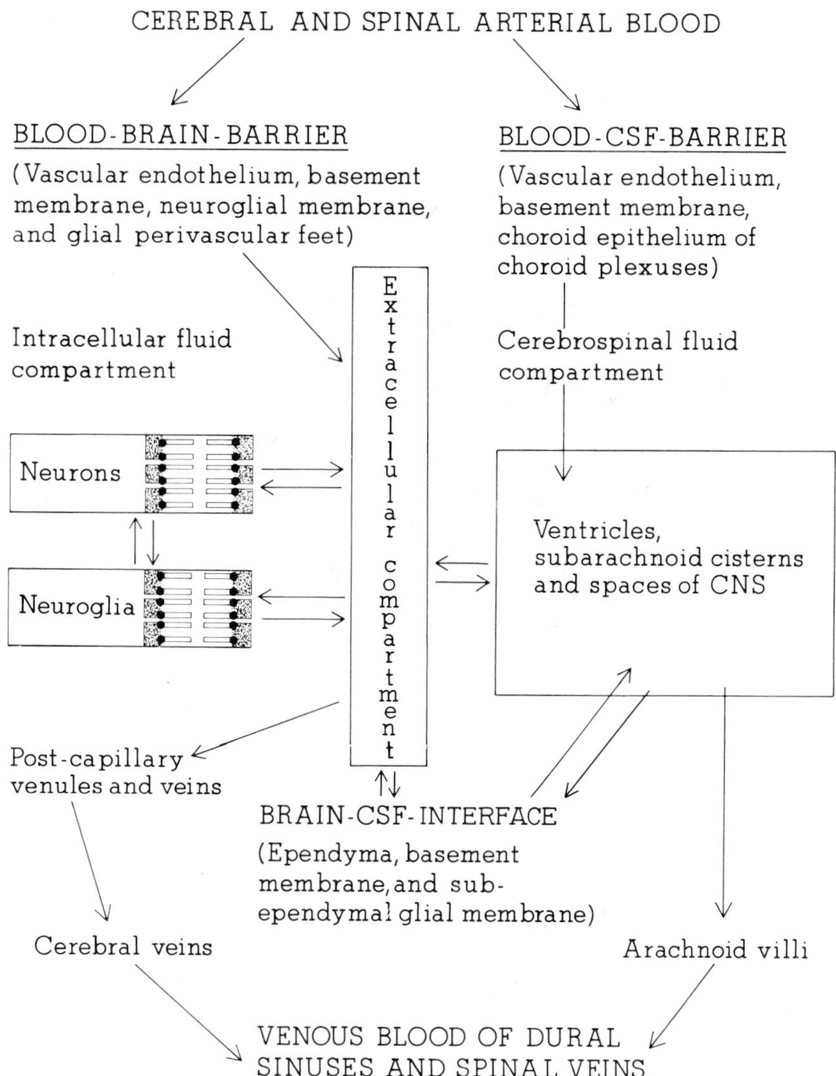

Figure 1-13. Schematic diagram of the blood-brain barrier, the blood-CSF barrier, and the brain-CSF interface that separate the brain and cerebrospinal fluid from the cerebral vascular compartment. The blood-brain barrier is a series of interfaces between arterial blood, cerebrospinal fluid and neural tissue that regulate the transport of chemical substances. Tight junctions between endothelial cells (see Fig. 1-14) of cerebral capillaries (the blood-brain barrier) and a paucity of pinocytosis restrict the passage of solutes from the blood into the extracellular compartment (i.e., interstitial fluid). The blood-CSF barrier is formed by tight junctions surrounding apical regions of the cuboidal epithelium of the choroid plexus (see Fig. 1-15). The brain-CSF interface, consisting of the ependymal lining of the cerebral ventricles and the pia-glial membrane on the external surface of the brain, does not impede the exchange of solutes between the CSF and the brain. The extracellular compartment has been estimated to constitute about 18% of wet brain weight (Fenstermacher and Rall, '73). (From Carpenter and Sutin, *Human Neuroanatomy*, 1983; courtesy of Williams & Wilkins.)

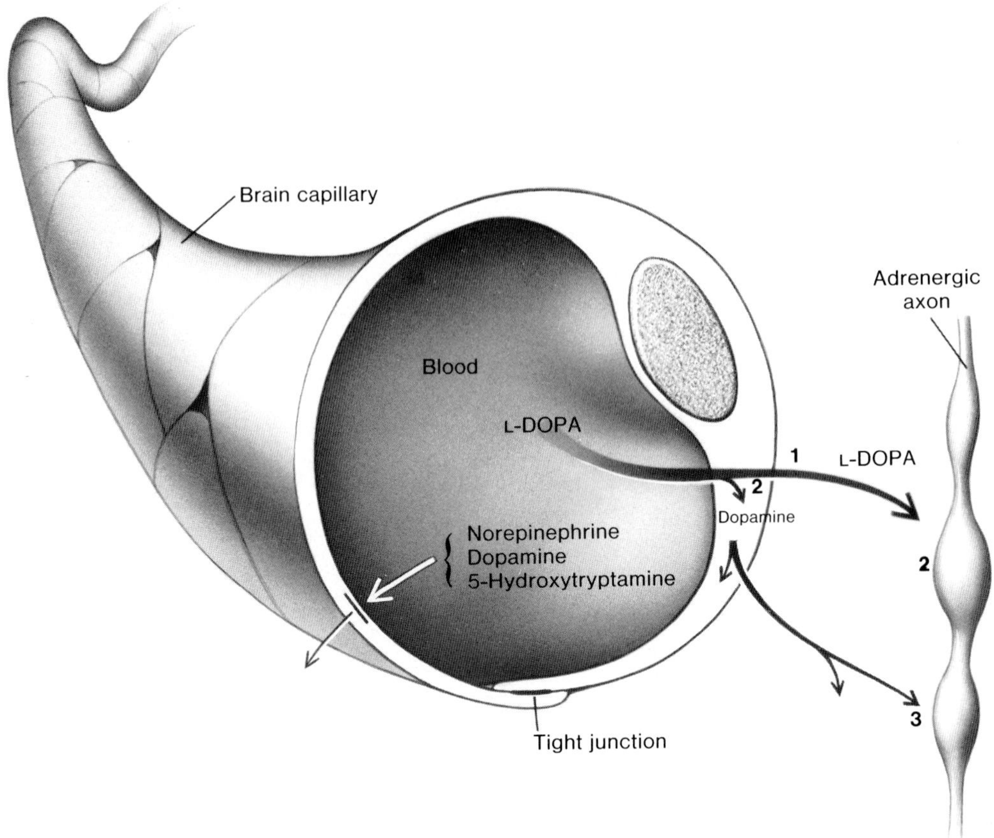

Figure 1-14. Diagrammatic drawing of a brain capillary demonstrating a tight junction between endothelial cells that constitute the blood-brain barrier. Endothelial cells of brain capillaries contain enzymes that regulate the specific transport of biogenic amines (norepinephrine, dopamine, and 5-hydroxytryptamine) and amino acids. L-dopa passes the blood-brain barrier (*1*), is decarboxylated to dopamine in the capillary endothelium (*2*), and enters neural tissue (*3*), where it is degraded by monamine oxidase. Decarboxylation of L-dopa to dopamine (*2*) also takes place after its incorporation into axonal varicosities of aminergic neurons (Rapoport, '76). (From Carpenter and Sutin, *Human Neuroanatomy*, 1983; courtesy of Williams and Wilkins.)

Because dopamine cannot cross the blood-brain barrier, L-dopa is given to correct this metabolic defect. L-dopa crosses the blood-brain barrier and is decarboxylated in the capillary endothelium to dopamine, a therapeutically effective biogenic amine (Figs. 1-14, 1-15, and 11-10).

In contrast to cerebral capillaries, capillaries in skeletal muscle contain endothelial cells separated by 10-nm clefts, have abundant pinocytotic vesicles for transport of macromolecules and contain contractile protein. Although occasional tight junctions between endothelial cells are seen in muscle capillaries, they are almost uniformly not present as in brain capillaries. The blood-brain carrier in the CNS is not everywhere complete. In certain regions of the brain capillary endothelia with tight junctions is replaced by capillaries with fenestrated endothelia. Regions of the brain devoid of a blood-brain barrier included the pineal body, the subfornical organ, the organum vasculosum of the lamina terminalis (or supraoptic crest), the median eminence of the hypothalamus, the neurohypophysis and the area postrema (Fig. 1-16). These structures are known as the *circumventricular organs* and all except the area postrema bear relationships to the diencephalon. In the regions of the circumventricular organs, capillary fenestrations provide specific sites for the transfer of proteins and solutes, irrespective of molec-

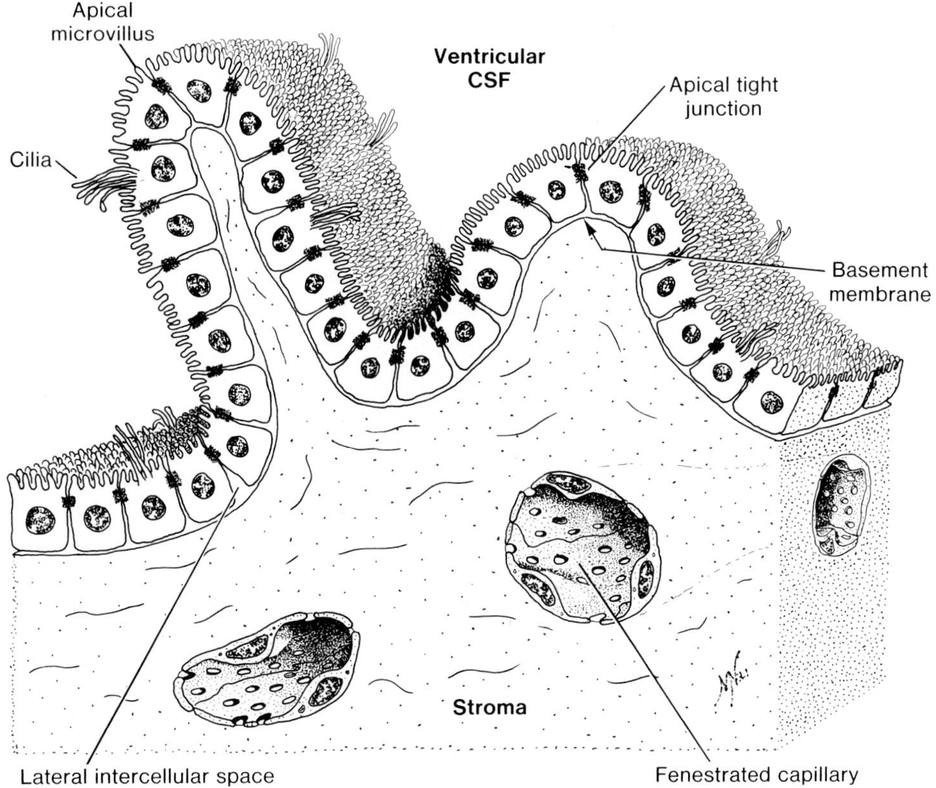

Figure 1-15. Diagram of a choroid plexus villus covered by a single layer of cuboidal epithelium with apical microvilli protruding into the ventricular CSF. Epithelial cells rest upon a basement membrane and have tight junctions connecting apical regions which constitute the blood-CSF barrier. The underlying connective tissue stroma contains capillaries with fenestrations. (From Carpenter and Sutin, *Human Neuroanatomy*, 1983; courtesy of Williams & Wilkins.)

ular size and lipid solubility. Thus the blood-brain barrier, except in the special regions noted, functions as a differential filter that permits the selective exchange of only certain substances from the blood to the brain. This barrier is impermeable to many substances, particularly vital dyes.

Neurons and neuroglial comprise the *intracellular fluid compartment* of the brain (Fig. 1-13). Passage of solutes into, and out of, neurons and glial takes place from the *extracellular space* (i.e., interstitial space) through the cell membranes. Estimates of the total extracellular space vary widely as determined by different methods. Ultrastructural studies suggest that neurons, neuroglia, and their processes take up most of the available space, except for a fairly constant 20-nm cleft between adjacent cellular elements (estimate 4%). Neurochemical data, based on the assumption that the chloride ion is distributed mainly in extracellular space, suggest the extracellular space ranges from 25 to 40% (Elliott and Jasper, '49; Woodbury, '58). More recent data indicates that the extracellular space equals approximately 18% of wet brain weight (Fenstermacher and Rall, '73).

The water content of the rhesus monkey brain progressively diminishes during fetal development and postpartum maturation (Selzer et al., '72). The developing and immature brain have an expanded extracellular space, although tight junctions surrounding epithelial cells of the choroid plexus at early developmental stages do not differ qualitatively from the adult (Pappas and Tennyson, '62). The increased extracellular space appears to account for the observation that trypan blue given intravenously stains the brains of immature animals. Although the dye enters the brain

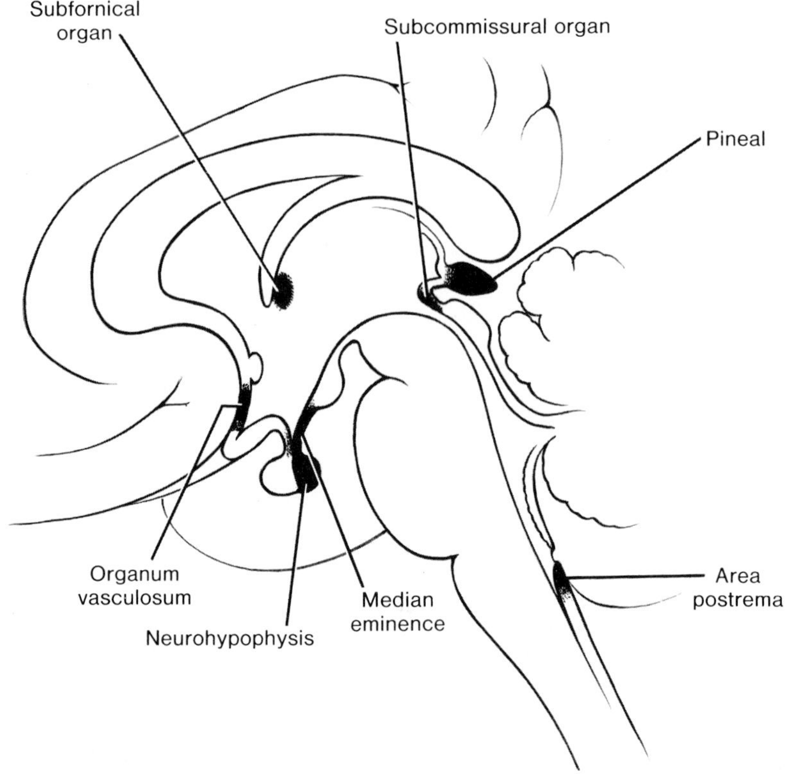

Figure 1-16. Drawing of a midsagittal section of the human brain indicating the locations of the circumventricular organs. All of these structures, except the *area postrema*, are unpaired, situated in the midline, and related to diencephalic structures. All, except the *subcommissural organ*, are highly vascularized and lack a blood-brain barrier. Neuropeptides have limited transport across the blood-brain barrier but can enter and leave the brain, via the CSF, in regions of the circumventricular organs. The *organum vasculosum of the lamina terminalis* (OVLT) resembles the median eminence but its function has not yet been clarified; this structure, particularly prominent in rodents, is also designated as the supraoptic crest. The *median eminence* serves as a neuroendocrine transducer and the final common pathway by which releasing hormones are discharged into the hypophysial portal system (modified from Weindl and Safroniew, '81). (From Carpenter and Sutin, *Human Neuroanatomy*, 1983; courtesy of Williams & Wilkins.)

only at nonbarrier sites, it extends further into the extracellular space than it does in the mature brain.

Blood-Cerebrospinal Fluid Barrier. The epithelium and adnexa of the choroid plexus in the lateral, third, and fourth ventricles actively secrete CSF which has higher concentrations of Na^+, Cl^-, and Mg^{2+} and lower concentrations of K^+, Ca^+, glucose, and protein than the plasma. The barrier to passive exchange of protein and solutes between blood and CSF is not at the choroidal capillaries which have fenestrated endothelial cells. The blood-CSF barrier is located at tight junctions which surround and connect apical regions of cuboidal epithelial cells on the surface of the choroid plexus (Fig. 1-15). Protein tracers and HRP injected intravascularly stain the stroma of the choroid plexus by passing through pores in the choroidal capillaries, but they do not pass beyond the tight junctions of the epithelial cells and they do not enter the CSF (Brightman et al., '70). The surface area of the blood-CSF barrier is only about 0.02% of the surface area of the blood-brain barrier (Bindslev et al., '74). In spite of great quantitative differences in surface area, some circulating substances probably enter the brain via the blood-CSF barrier (Pardridge et al., '81). Some circulating peptides (insulin) and plasma proteins may be selectively transported into the CSF via the blood-CSF barrier. The ependymal lining of the ventricles and the pia-glial membrane on the surface of the brain do not impede exchanges between the CSF and the brain.

Circumventricular Organs. Specialized tissues located at strategic positions in the midline ventricular system which lack a blood-brain barrier collectively are referred to as the circumventricular organs (Fig. 1-16). Included under this designation are: (1) the pineal body, (2) the subcommissural organ, (3) the subfornical organ, (4) the organum vasculosum of the lamina terminalis (supraoptic crest), (5) the median eminence, (6) the neurohypophysis, and (7) the area postrema (Akert et al., '61; Mestres, '78; Weindl and Sofroniew, '81). With the exception of the area postrema, located bilaterally along the caudal margins of the fourth ventricle (Figs. 1-10 and 5-7), all of these structures are unpaired and occupying midline positions related to portions of the diencephalon. All of these structures, except the subcommissural organ, contain fenestrated capillaries and are excluded from the blood-brain barrier (Broadwell and Brightman, '76). The *neurohypophysis* receives fibers from magnocellular hypothalamic nuclei (i.e., paraventricular and supraoptic nuclei) which terminate around fenestrated capillaries. These terminal fibers contain a carrier protein, neurophysin, and vasopressin and oxytocin which are stored and released into the general circulation from the neural lobe of the hypophysis. The *organum vasculosum of the lamina terminalis* (OVLT) may also serve as a neurohemal outlet for hypothalamic peptides. In addition it may serve a neurohemal function in which certain peptides, amines, and proteins in the blood are sensed by neurons with receptor properties. The *median eminence* serves as a neuroendocrine transducer (Scott and Krobisch-Dudley, '75). The final common pathway for neuroendocrine control of the anterior pituitary by the hypothalamus is provided by neurosecretory neurons whose axons discharge hormone-releasing factors into the hypophysial portal system (Fig. 10-12) (Knigge and Silverman, '74). The *subfornical organ*, located between the interventricular foramina, has connections with the choroid plexus and may serve to regulate body fluids (Weindl and Sofroniew, '81). The *pineal body*, containing pinealocytes, produces melatonin in animals deprived of photic stimuli and has been viewed as a biological clock which regulates circadian rhythms. The *subcommissural organ* is located beneath the posterior commissure at the junction of the third ventricle and cerebral aqueduct. The function of this structure is unknown. The *area postrema*, the only pair circumventricular organ, is located along the caudal margins of the fourth ventricle (Fig. 5-7) and has a structure similar to that of the subfornical organ. The area postrema is considered a chemoreceptor that triggers vomiting in response to circulating emetic substances, such as digitalis glycosides and apomorphine (Borison and Wang, '49, '53).

The widespread distribution of peptides in the CNS suggests that the CSF may be a conduit by which peptides modulate neuronal function in different regions of the brain (Jackson, '81). Neural peptides have limited access to the CNS across the blood-brain barrier, but have been detected in high concentrations in the circumventricular organs. Peptides identified in the CSF include: (1) thyroid-releasing hormone, (2) luteinizing hormone-releasing hormone, (3) somatostatin, (4) opioid peptides, (5) cholecystokinin, (6) angiotensin II, (7) substance P, (8) adenohypophysial hormones, and (9) neurohypophysial hormones. It is possible that if neural peptides could be accurately measured in the CSF, they might serve as a sensitive "marker" for anatomical localization of pathological processes in the CNS (Jackson, '81).

CHAPTER 2

Gross Anatomy of the Brain

The nervous system is composed of two parts, the central nervous system and the peripheral nervous system. The *peripheral nervous system* consists of the spinal and cranial nerves, while the *central nervous system* is represented by the brain and spinal cord. The autonomic nervous system, often considered as a separate functional entity, is part central and part peripheral.

The human brain is a relatively small structure weighing about 1400 g and constituting about 2% of the total body weight. The brain commonly is regarded as the organ solely concerned with thought, memory, and consciousness. While these are some of its most complex functions, there are many others. All information we have concerning the world about us is conveyed centrally to the brain by an elaborate sensory system. Receptors of many kinds act as transducers which change physical and chemical stimuli in our environment into nerve impulses which the brain can read and give meaning to. The ability to discriminate between stimuli of the same and different types forms one of the bases for learning. Attention, consciousness, emotional experience, and sleep are all central neural functions. Such higher neural functions as memory, imagination, thought, and creative ability are poorly understood but must be related to complex neuronal activity. The brain also is concerned with all kinds of motor activity, with the regulation of visceral, endocrine and somatic functions, and with the receptive and expressive use of symbols and signs that underlie communication. While the gross features of the human brain are not especially impressive, its versatility, potential capabilities, efficiency, and self-programming nature put it in a class beyond any "electronic brain."

The brain consists of three basic subdi-

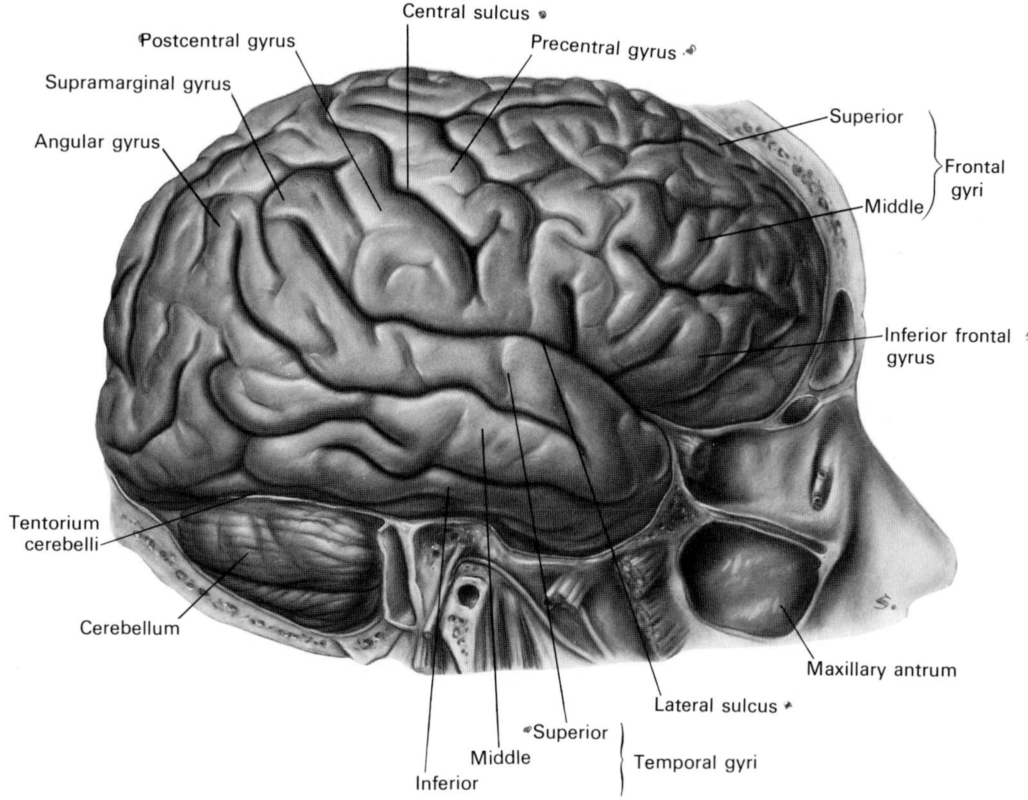

Figure 2-1. Lateral view of the brain exposed in the skull to show topographical relationships. (From Mettler's *Neuroanatomy*, 1948; courtesy of The C. V. Mosby Company.)

visions, the cerebral hemispheres, the brain stem, and the cerebellum. The massive paired *cerebral hemispheres* are derived from the *telencephalon*, the most rostral cerebral vesicle. The brain stem consists of four distinct parts: (1) the *diencephalon*, (2) the *mesencephalon*, (3) the *metencephalon*, and (4) the *myelencephalon*. The diencephalon, the most rostral brain stem segment, is the part of the brain stem most intimately related to the forebrain (i.e., telencephalon). The mesencephalon, or midbrain, is the smallest and least differentiated division of the brain stem. The metencephalon (pons) and myelencephalon (medulla) together constitute the *rhombencephalon* or hindbrain. The cerebellum is a derivative of the metencephalon that develops from ectodermal thickenings about the rostral borders of the fourth ventricle, known as the rhombic lip.

CEREBRAL HEMISPHERES

The paired cerebral hemispheres are mirror image duplicates consisting of a highly convoluted gray cortex, (pallium), an underlying white matter of considerable magnitude, and a collection of deeply located neuronal masses, known as the basal ganglia. The cerebral hemispheres are partially separated from each other by the *longitudinal fissure*. This fissure in situ contains the falx cerebri (Fig. 1-2). In frontal and occipital regions the separation of the hemispheres is complete, but in the central region the fissure extends only to fibers of the broad interhemispheric commissure, the corpus callosum (Fig. 2-6). Each cerebral hemisphere is subdivided into lobes by various sulci (Figs. 2-1 and 2-2). The major lobes of the brain are named for the bones of the skull which overlie them. Although

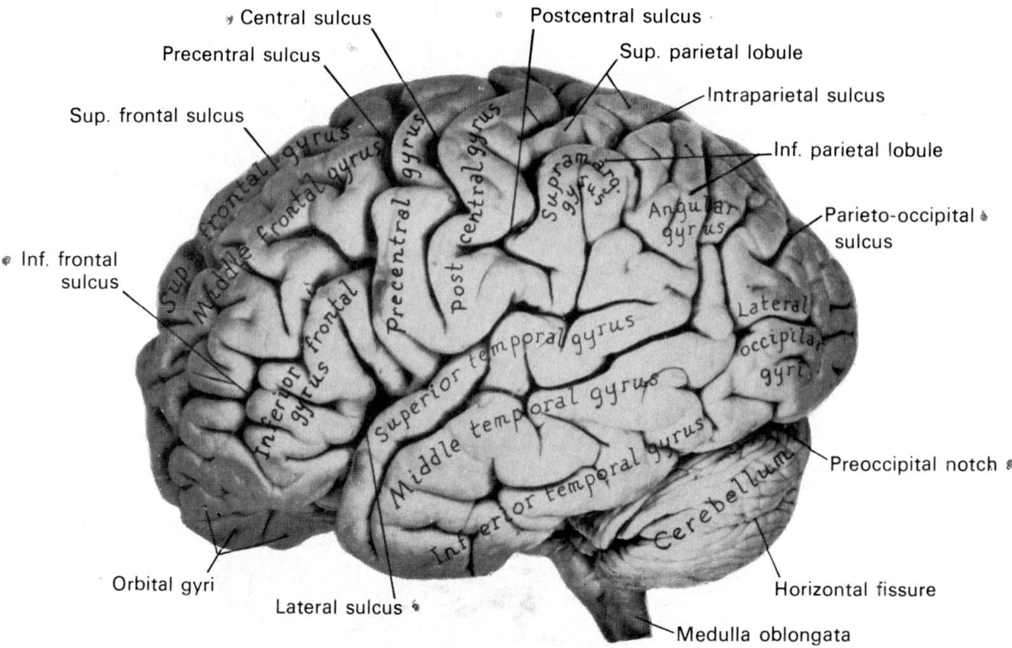

Figure 2-2. Photograph of the lateral surface of the brain. (From Carpenter and Sutin, *Human Neuroanatomy*, 1983; courtesy of Williams & Wilkins.)

the boundaries of the various lobes as seen in the gross specimen are somewhat arbitrary, multiple cortical areas in each lobe are histologically distinctive. The gray cellular mantle of the cerebral cortex in man is highly convoluted. The crest of a single convolution is referred to as a *gyrus*; *sulci* separate the various gyri, producing a pattern with more or less constant features. On the basis of the more constant sulci and gyri, the cerebrum is divided into six so-called lobes: (1) frontal, (2) temporal, (3) parietal, (4) occipital, (5) insular, and (6) limbic. Neither the insular nor limbic lobe is a true lobe. The insular cortex lies buried in the depths of the lateral sulcus. The limbic lobe is a synthetic lobe on the medial aspects of the hemisphere consisting of marginal portions of the frontal, parietal, occipital, and temporal lobes which are in continuity. This cortex, which partially encircles the rostral brain stem, appears concerned particularly with visceral and behavioral functions.

Lateral Surface

The two most important sulci for topographical orientation on the lateral convexity of the hemisphere are the lateral and central sulci (Figs. 2-1 and 2-2). The *lateral sulcus* begins inferiorly in the Sylvian fossa and extends posteriorly, separating the frontal and temporal lobes. Caudally this sulcus separates portions of the parietal and temporal lobes. The terminal ascending ramus of the sulcus extends into the inferior part of the parietal lobe. Portions of the frontal, parietal and temporal lobes, adjacent to the lateral sulcus, which overlie the insular region are referred to as the *opercular portions* of these lobes (Fig. 2-4). The *central sulcus* is a prominent sulcus running from the superior margin of the hemisphere downward and forward toward the lateral sulcus (Figs. 2-1 and 2-2). Usually this sulcus is bowed in two locations and superiorly it does not extend onto the medial surface of the hemisphere for any distance. The depths of the sulcus constitute the boundary between the frontal and parietal lobes.

Frontal Lobe. This, the largest of all the lobes of the brain, comprises about one-third of hemispheric surface. The frontal lobe extends rostrally from the central sulcus to the frontal pole (Fig. 2-3); its inferior

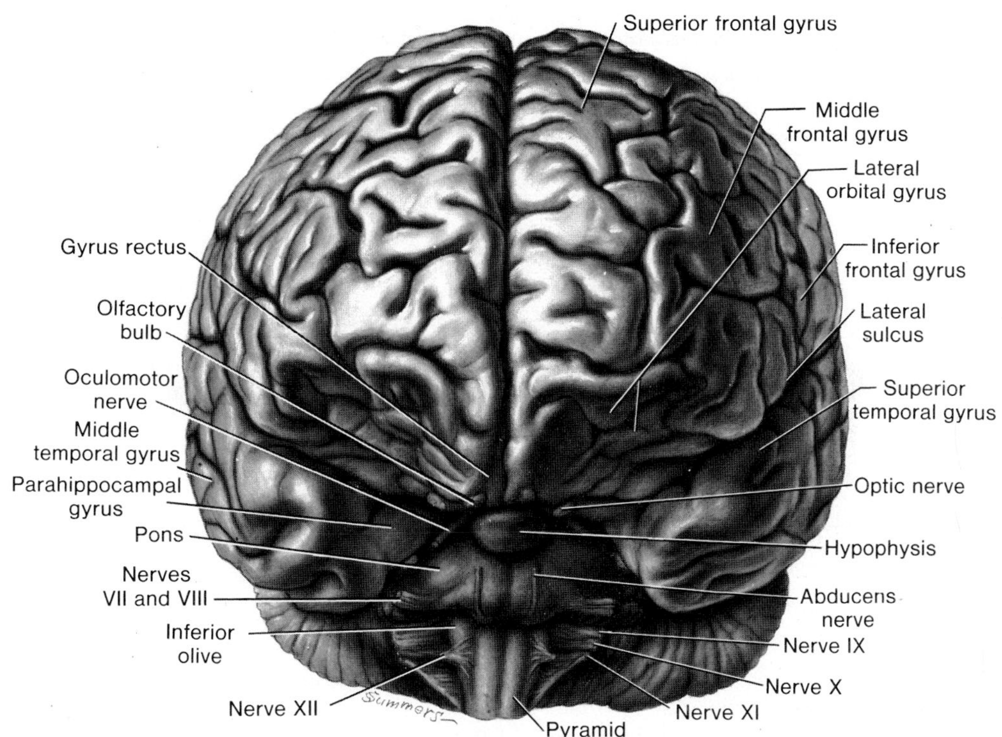

Figure 2-3. The rostral aspect of the brain. (From Mettler's Neuroanatomy, 1948; courtesy of The C. V. Mosby Company.)

boundary is the lateral sulcus. The convexity of the frontal lobe has four principal convolutions: (1) a *precentral* gyrus that parallels the central sulcus, and (2) three horizontally oriented convolutions, the *superior*, *middle*, and *inferior frontal gyri* (Figs. 2-1 and 2-2). The anterior boundary of the precentral gyrus is the *precentral sulcus* which extends onto the medial surface of the hemisphere. The precentral gyrus and the anterior bank of the central sulcus comprise the primary motor area where all parts of the body are represented in a distorted but topographical manner (Fig. 13-7). Regions of the frontal lobe rostral to the primary motor area are referred to as *premotor* and *prefrontal* areas. The broad middle frontal gyrus often is divided by a shallow horizontal sulcus into upper and lower tiers (Figs. 2-1 and 2-2). The inferior frontal gyrus is divided by anterior ascending rami of the lateral sulcus into three parts: (1) *pars orbitale*, (2) *pars triangularis*, and (3) *pars opercularis*. The pars triangularis and opercularis in the dominant hemisphere (usually the left in right-handed individuals) are referred to as *Broca's speech area*, a region concerned with the motor mechanisms of speech formulation. The inferior surface of the frontal lobe lies on the superior surface of the orbital part of the frontal bone and is slightly concave (Fig. 2-3).

Parietal Lobe. The boundaries of the parietal lobe are less precise, except for its anterior border on the lateral convexity formed by the central sulcus (Fig. 2-2). Its best defined border lies on the medial aspect of the hemisphere (*parieto-occipital sulcus*) (Fig. 2-6). On the convexity of the hemisphere the posterior boundary is arbitrarily considered as an extrapolated line projected from the superior limit of the parieto-occipital sulcus to the small indentation on the inferior surface known as the *preoccipital notch* (Fig. 2-2). Three parts of the parietal lobe are distinguished: (1) a *postcentral gyrus* running parallel and caudal to the central sulcus, (2) a *superior parietal lobule*, and (3) an *inferior parietal*

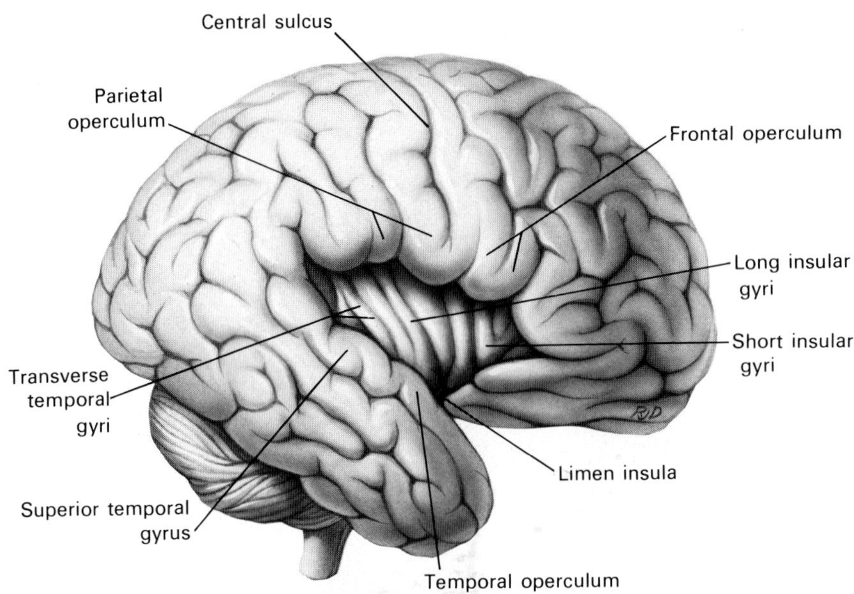

Figure 2-4. View of the right cerebral hemisphere with the banks of the lateral sulcus drawn apart to expose the insula.

lobule. The postcentral gyrus, usually not continuous, but broken up into superior and inferior segments, lies between the central and postcentral sulci. The *postcentral sulcus* extends over the superior margin of the hemisphere and demarcates the caudal limit of the paracentral lobule (Fig. 2-6). The posterior bank of the central sulcus and the postcentral gyrus constitute the *primary somesthetic area*, the cortical region where impulses concerned with tactile and kinesthetic sense from superficial and deep receptors converge and are somatotopically represented. The majority of cortical neurons in the postcentral gyrus are concerned with fixed receptive fields on the contralateral side of the body that are place specific, modality specific and related to discriminative aspects of sensation.

The *intraparietal sulcus*, a horizontally oriented sulcus, divides portions of the parietal lobe caudal to the postcentral gyrus into superior and inferior parietal lobules (Fig. 2-2). The *inferior parietal lobule* consists of two gyri, the *supramarginal*, about both banks of an ascending ramus of the lateral sulcus, and the *angular*, which surrounds the ascending terminal part of the superior temporal sulcus (Figs. 2-1 and 2-2). The inferior parietal lobule represents a cortical association area where multisensory perceptions of a higher order from adjacent parietal, temporal, and occipital regions overlap. This region is especially concerned with mnemonic constellations that form the basis for understanding and interpreting sensory signals. This is one region of the cortex where strikingly different disturbances occur as a consequence of lesions in the dominant and nondominant hemispheres.

Temporal Lobe. This large lobe lies ventral to the lateral sulcus and on its lateral surface displays three obliquely oriented convolutions, the *superior*, *middle*, and *inferior temporal gyri* (Figs. 2-1 and 2-2). The *superior temporal sulcus* courses parallel with the lateral sulcus and its ascending ramus terminates in the angular gyrus. On the inner bank of the lateral sulcus several short, oblique convolutions form the transverse gyri of Heschl; these gyri constitute the *primary auditory cortex* in man (Figs. 2-4 and 2-9). The inferior surface of the temporal lobe which lies in the middle fossa of the skull reveals part of the *inferior temporal gyrus*, the broad *occipitotemporal gyrus*, and the *parahippocampal gyrus* (Figs. 2-7 and 2-8). The parahippocampal gyrus and its most medial protrusion, the *uncus*, are separated from the occipitotemporal gyrus by the collateral

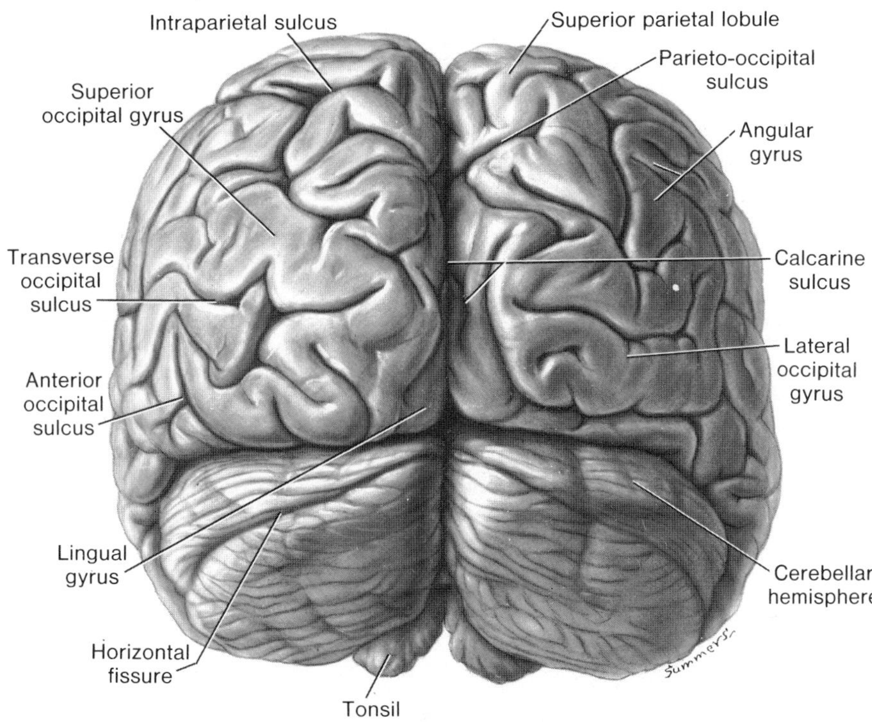

Figure 2-5. Posterior view of the cerebral hemispheres and cerebellum. (From Mettler's *Neuroanatomy*, 1948; courtesy of The C. V. Mosby Company.)

sulcus. The rostral part of the parahippocampal gyrus, the uncus, and the lateral olfactory stria constitute the pyriform lobe, parts of which constitute the *primary olfactory cortex* (Figs. 2-7 and 2-8).

Occipital Lobe. The small occipital lobe rests on the tentorium cerebelli and constitutes the occipital pole of the hemisphere (Figs. 2-1 and 2-5); its rostral boundary is the parieto-occipital sulcus, present on the medial aspect of the hemisphere (Fig. 2-6). The lateral surface of the occipital lobe is poorly delimited from the parietal lobe and is composed of a number of irregular lateral *occipital gyri* which are separated into groups by a more constant *lateral occipital sulcus* (Fig. 2-2). On the medial aspect of the hemisphere the occipital lobe is divided by the *calcarine sulcus* into the cuneus and the *lingual gyrus* (Figs. 2-6 and 2-8). The calcarine sulcus joins the parieto-occipital sulcus rostrally in a Y-shaped formation. The cortex on both banks of the calcarine sulcus represents the *primary visual cortex* (i.e., striate). The visual cortex in each hemisphere receives impulses from the temporal half of the ipsilateral retina and the nasal half of the contralateral retina and is concerned with perception from the contralateral half of the visual field. Binocular fusion occurs in layers of the visual cortex even though fibers of the visual radiation conducting impulses from each eye terminate in alternate areas in the principal receptive layer of the cortex. Central (macular) vision is represented nearest the occipital pole (Fig. 2–5). Fibers conveying impulses from the upper halves of the retinae terminate on the superior bank of the calcarine sulcus while the inferior bank of the sulcus receives impulses from the lower halves of the retinae.

Insula. This invaginated cortical area lies buried in the depths of the lateral sulcus and can be seen only when the temporal and frontal lobes are separated. This so-called lobe is a triangular cortical area, the apex of which is directed forward and downward to open into the lateral fossa (Figs. 2-4 and 2-9). The surface is covered by the *gyri breves* and *longus* which course nearly parallel to the lateral sulcus. The

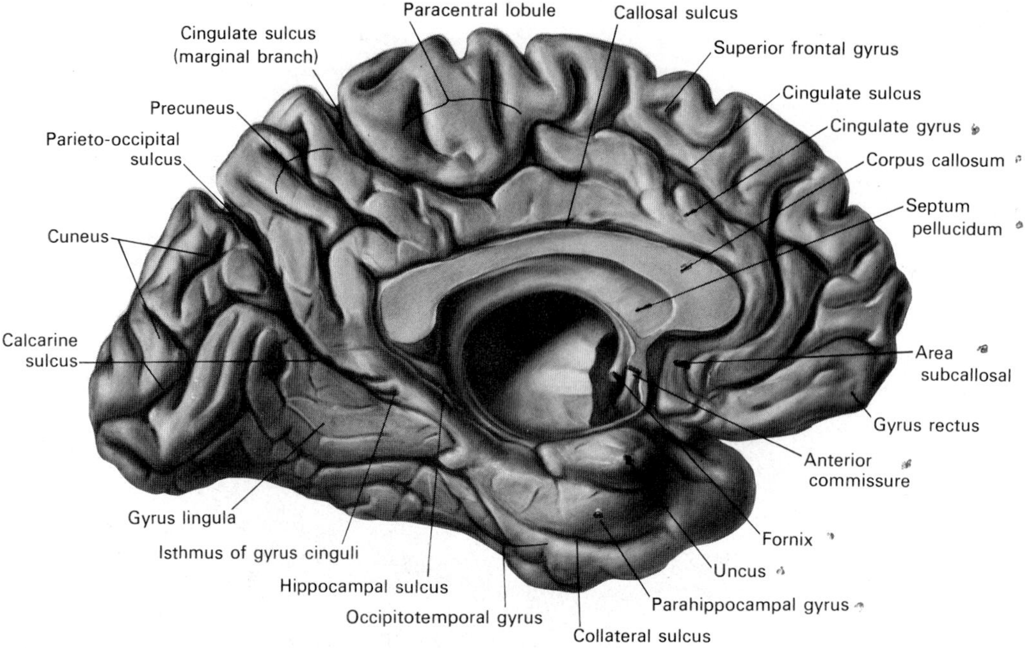

Figure 2-6. Medial surface of the cerebral hemisphere with diencephalic structures removed. (From Mettler's *Neuroanatomy*, 1948; courtesy of The C. V. Mosby Company.)

relationships of this region can be appreciated in transverse sections of the hemisphere (Figs. 2-16 and 2-17). The opening leading to the insular region is called the *limen insula.* The temporal, frontal and parietal opercular regions cover the insula.

Medial Surface

In a hemisected brain convolutions on the medial surface can be studied. The convolutions on the medial surface of the cerebral hemisphere are somewhat flatter than those on the convexity. The most prominent structure on the medial surface is the massive interhemispheric commissure, the *corpus callosum* (Fig. 2-6). This structure, composed of myelinated fibers, reciprocally interconnects nearly all cortical regions of the two hemispheres. Different parts of the corpus callosum are referred to as the *rostrum*, *genu*, *body*, and *splenium* (Figs. 2-9 and 2-15). Fibers in this structure spread out as a mass of radiations to nearly all parts of the cortex. Callosal fibers, projecting to parts of the frontal and occipital lobes, form the so-called *anterior* and *posterior forceps*, which are best appreciated in horizontal sections of the brain (Figs. 2-9 and 2-11). The corpus callosum forms the floor of the longitudinal fissure, as well as part of the roof of the lateral ventricle. The corpus callosum plays an important role in interhemispheric transfer of learned discriminations, sensory experience, and memory. Complete surgical section of the corpus callosum does not result in obvious neurological deficits, but these patients show a striking functional independence of the two hemispheres with respect to perceptual, cognitive, mnemonic, learned, and volitional activities. The activities of the separated hemispheres are not known to each other and information perceived exclusively by, or generated in, the nondominant (right) hemisphere cannot be communicated in speech or writing. No impairment of linguistic expression is noted in information processed by the dominant (left) hemisphere (Gazzaniga and Sperry, '67). These studies indicate that linguistic expression and analytic functions are organized almost exclusively in the dominant hemisphere. The nondominant hemisphere is concerned with spatial concepts, recognition of faces, and some elements of music.

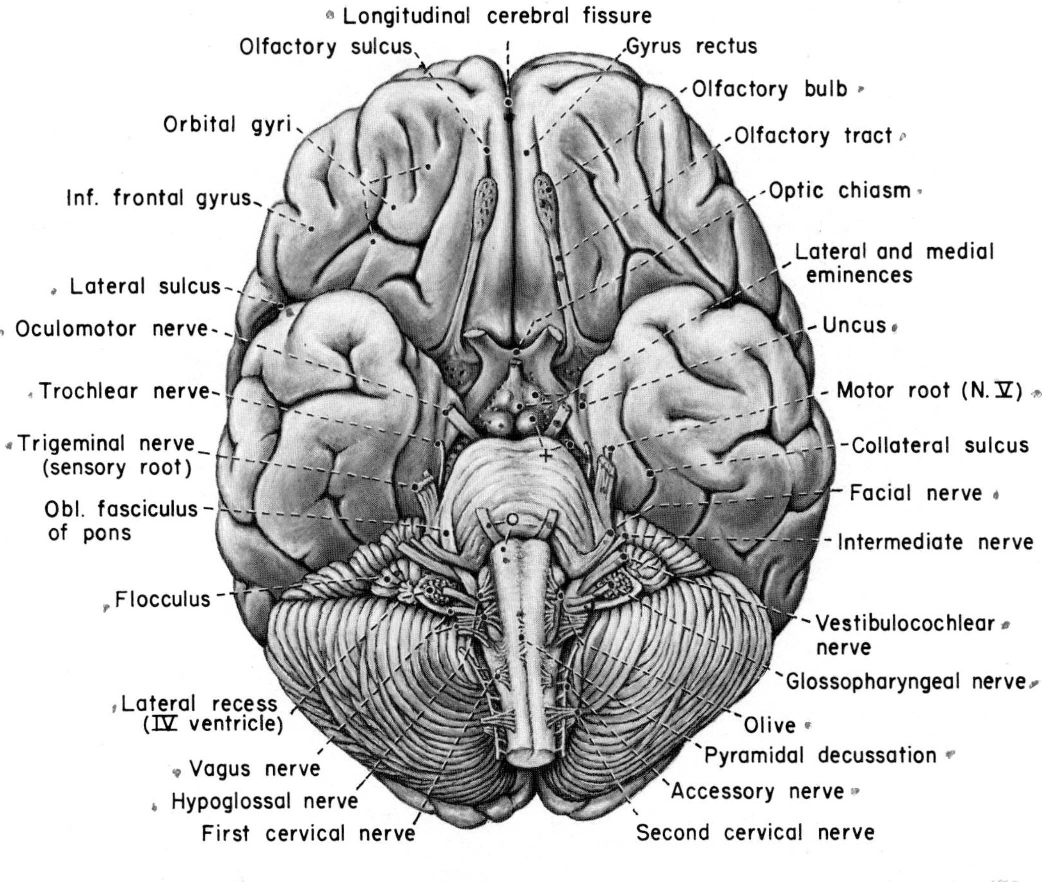

Figure 2-7. Inferior surface of the brain showing the cranial nerves. (From Truex and Kellner's *Detailed Atlas of the Head and Neck*, 1958; courtesy of Oxford University Press.)

The *callosal sulcus* separates the corpus callosum from the cingulate gyrus; posteriorly this sulcus curves around the splenium to be continued into the temporal lobe as the *hippocampal sulcus* (Fig. 2-6). The *cingulate gyrus*, dorsal to the callosal sulcus, encircles the corpus callosum and consists of two tiers. The *cingulate sulcus*, superior to the cingulate gyrus, runs parallel to the callosal sulcus, but near the splenium turns dorsally as the *marginal sulcus*. The rostral portion of cortex superior to the cingulate gyrus is the medial surface of the superior frontal gyrus. The *paracentral lobule* is formed by the precentral and postcentral gyri which extend onto the medial surface of the hemisphere, and is notched by the central sulcus (Fig. 2-6). The *paracentral sulcus*, continuous with the precentral sulcus, forms the rostral border of this lobule, while the *marginal sulcus*, continuous with the postcentral gyrus, forms the caudal border. (Fig. 2-6) The portion of the parietal lobe caudal to the paracentral lobule is known as the *precuneus* (Fig. 2–6); this lobule lies rostral to the parieto-occipital sulcus.

Limbic Lobe. This is a synthetic lobe, consisting of the most medial margins (i.e., the limbus) of the frontal, parietal, and temporal lobes which closely surround the interhemispheric commissure (Fig. 12-17). The limbic lobe (Broca, 1878) includes the *subcallosal*, *cingulate*, and *parahippocampal gyri*, as well as primitive cortical derivatives, the *hippocampal formation* and the

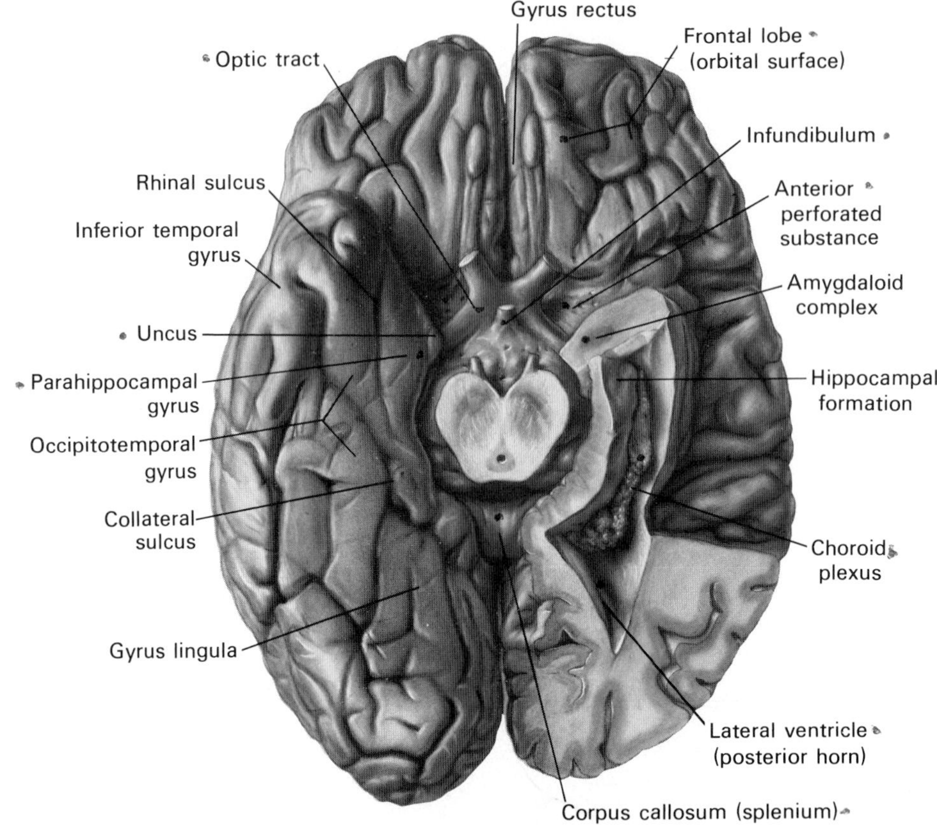

Figure 2-8. View of the inferior surface of the brain following transection of the midbrain. The inferior and posterior horns of the left lateral ventricle have been opened and portions of the temporal and occipital lobes have been removed. (From Mettler's *Neuroanatomy*, 1948; courtesy of The C.V. Mosby Company.)

dentate gyrus, which in the course of development have become invaginated within the temporal lobe (Fig. 2-8). The parahippocampal gyrus is directly continuous with the cingulate gyrus by a narrow strip of cortex, posterior and inferior to the splenium of the corpus callosum, known as the *isthmus of the cingulate gyrus* (Fig. 2-6). The parahippocampal gyrus, the most medial convolution of the temporal lobe, is bounded laterally by the *rhinal* and *collateral sulci* and superiorly and medially by the *hippocampal sulcus* (Figs. 2-6, 2-7, and 2-8). Rostrally the parahippocampal gyrus hooks around the hippocampal sulcus to form a medially protruding convolution, the *uncus* (Figs. 2-7 and 2-8). The proximity of the uncus to the cerebral peduncle is of clinical importance and should be noted.

There are differences of opinion concerning what should be grouped together as the so-called "limbic lobe" (Brodal, '81). While all structures composing the limbic lobe appear early in phylogenesis, physiological evidence suggests functional differences between various components, although most are related to visceral and behavioral activities.

Inferior Surface

The inferior surface of the hemisphere consists of two parts: (1) a larger posterior portion, representing the inferior surfaces of the temporal and occipital lobes, and (2) the orbital surface of the frontal lobe (Figs. 2-7 and 2-8). The inferior surface of the occipital lobe and the posterior part of the temporal lobe lie on the tentorium cerebelli (Figs. 1-2 and 2-1), while rostral parts of the temporal lobe lie in the middle cranial fossa. Gyri present in this posterior part include: (1) the lingual gyrus, (2) the extensive occipitotemporal gyrus, and (3) the

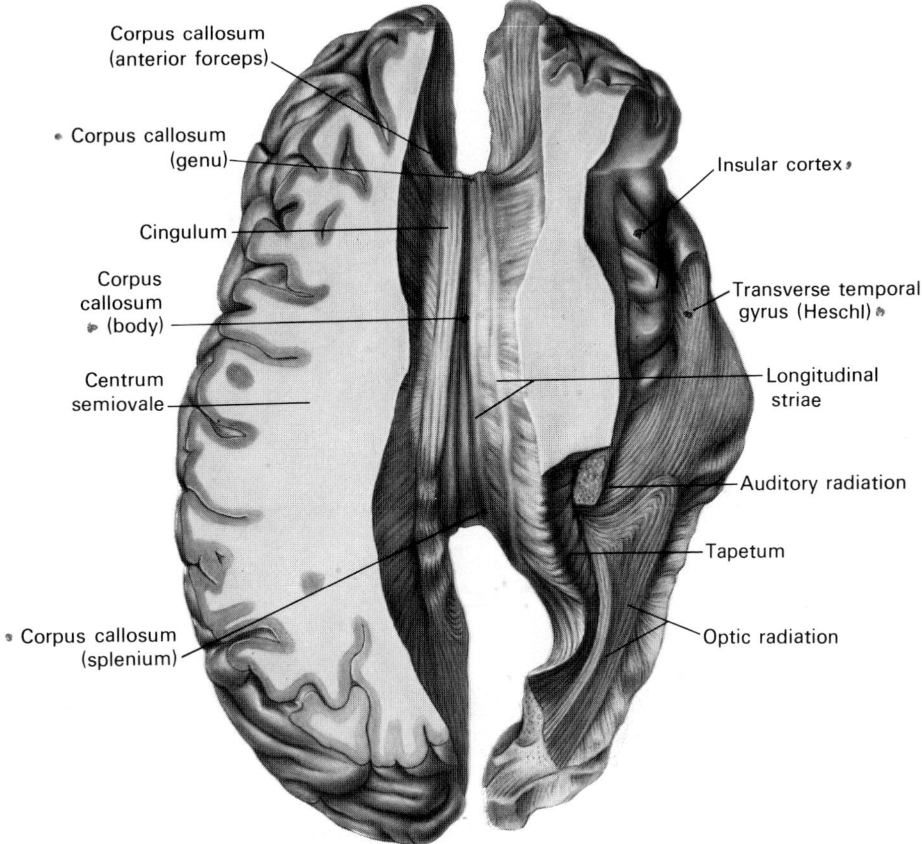

Figure 2-9. Dissection of the superior surface of the hemispheres exposing the corpus callosum, cingulum, longitudinal striae and the optic and auditory radiations. (From Mettler's *Neuroanatomy*, 1948; courtesy of The C. V. Mosby Company.)

parahippocampal gyrus and uncus (Fig. 2-8). Part of the inferior temporal gyrus may be seen lateral to the occipito-temporal gyrus. A small part of the isthmus lies medially posterior to the splenium of the corpus callosum.

The orbital surface of the frontal lobe has a deep straight sulcus medially, the olfactory sulcus, which contains both the olfactory bulb and tract (Figs. 2-3, 2-7, and 2-8). The *gyrus rectus* lies along the ventromedial margin of the frontal lobe medial to the olfactory sulcus. The region lateral to the olfactory sulcus contains the orbital gyri whose convolutional patterns are variable. Posteriorly the olfactory tract divides into medial and *lateral olfactory striae* (Fig. 12-2). Caudal to this is the olfactory trigone and the *anterior perforated substance*, a region studded with small openings through which numerous small arteries (lateral striate) pass to subcortical structures (Figs. 2-7, 2-8, 2-19 and 14-8).

White Matter

The massive white matter of the cerebral hemisphere, which forms the medullary core of cortical convolutions and separates the cortex from the subcortical nuclei, contains three types of fibers in large numbers. Fibers within the white matter are classified as: (1) *projection fibers* that convey impulses either from the cortex to distant loci, or from distant loci to the cortex; (2) *association fibers* that interconnect various cortical regions of the same hemisphere; and (3) *commissural fibers* that interconnect corresponding cortical regions of the two hemispheres. The white matter extends from the cortex to the subcortical nuclei

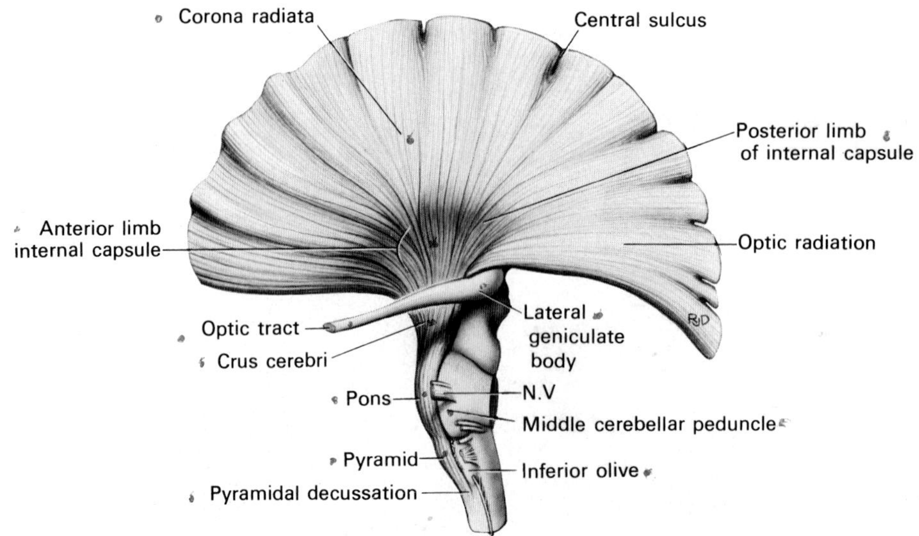

Figure 2-10. Drawing of a dissection demonstrating the continuity and relationships of the corona radiata, the internal capsule, the crus cerebri, and the medullary pyramids.

and the ventricular system (Figs. 2-9, 2-16 and 2-17). The common central mass of white matter, containing commissural, association and projection fibers, has an oval appearance in horizontal sections of the brain and is termed the *semioval center* (Fig. 2-9).

Projection Fibers. Afferent and efferent fibers conveying impulses to and from the entire cerebral cortex enter the white matter in radially arranged bundles that converge toward the brain stem (Fig. 2-10). These radiating projection fibers form the *corona radiata.* Near the rostral part of the brain stem these fibers form a compact band of fibers known as the *internal capsule,* which is flanked medially and laterally by nuclear masses (Figs. 2-11 and 2-12). Two distinct parts of the internal capsule are evident in horizontal sections of the hemispheres: (1) an anterior limb and (2) a posterior limb (Fig. 2-11).

The *anterior limb of the internal capsule* partially separates two of the largest components of the corpus striatum, the caudate nucleus and the putamen. Fibers in the anterior limb of the internal capsule are directed horizontally, obliquely laterally and upward toward the frontal lobe, and in horizontal sections of the hemisphere appear to be cut in the longitudinal axis of the fiber bundles (Figs. 2-10, 2-11 and 2-12). In horizontal sections of the hemisphere, the anterior and posterior limbs of the internal capsule meet at an obtuse angle with the apex directed medially. The region of junction between the anterior and posterior limbs of the internal capsule is referred to as the *genu* (Fig. 9-21).

The *posterior limb of the internal capsule* is flanked medially by the diencephalon (thalamus) and laterally by a part of the corpus striatum known as the lentiform nucleus. Fibers in the posterior limb of the internal capsule course in nearly a vertical plane toward the brain stem, and in horizontal sections fibers are cut transversely (Fig. 2-11). The most posterior component of the posterior limb of the internal capsule contains fibers radiating toward the calcarine sulcus, known as the *optic radiation* (Figs. 2-8, 2-9, and 9-24). Afferent fibers in the internal capsule arise mainly from the thalamus and project to nearly all regions of the cortex; such fibers are referred to as the *thalamocortical radiations.* Efferent fibers in the internal capsule arise from cells in deep layers of various regions of the cerebral cortex and project to specific nuclear masses in the brain stem and spinal cord. These corticofugal fibers are categorized as corticostriate, corticothalamic, corticopontine, corticobulbar, and corticospinal.

Association Fibers. Fibers interconnecting various cortical regions within the

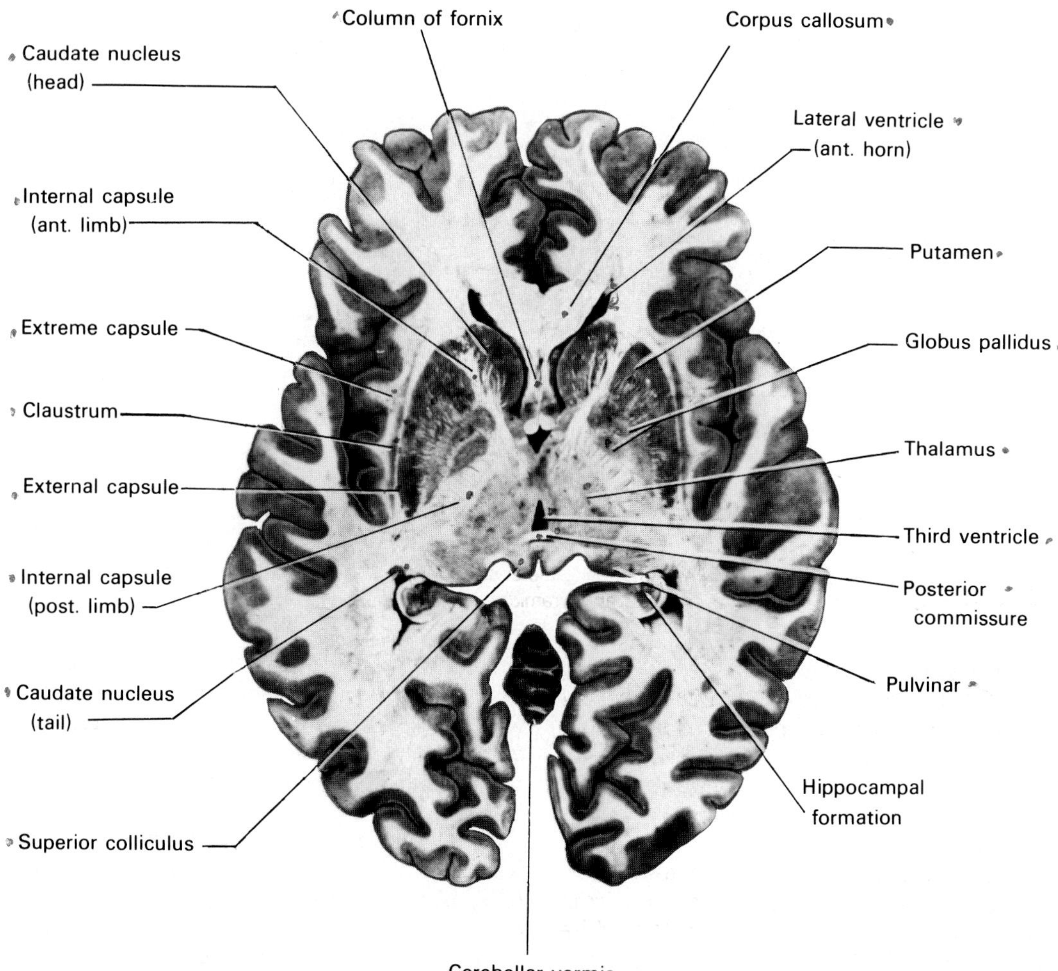

Figure 2-11. Photograph of a horizontal section through the cerebral hemispheres showing relationships of internal structures to the internal capsule. (From Carpenter and Sutin, *Human Neuroanatomy*, 1983; courtesy of Williams & Wilkins.)

same hemisphere are divided into long and short groups (Fig. 2-13). *Short association fibers* arch through the floor of each sulcus to connect cells in adjacent convolutions; these fibers course transversely to the long axis of the sulci. *Long association fibers,* interconnecting cortical regions in different lobes within the same hemisphere, form three main bundles: (1) the uncinate fasciculus, (2) the arcuate fasciculus, and (3) the cingulum. The *uncinate fasciculus* is a compact bundle beneath the limen insula which connects the orbital frontal gyri with anterior portions of the temporal lobe (Fig. 2-14). A deeply placed part of this fasciculus is thought to connect the frontal and occipital lobes (i.e., inferior occipitofrontal fasciculus). The *arcuate fasciculus* sweeps around the insular region and its fan-shaped ends connect the superior and middle frontal gyri with parts of the temporal lobe. A group of superiorly situated fibers in this bundle extends caudally into portions of the parietal and occipital lobe, and is known as the *superior longitudinal fasciculus* (Fig. 2-14).

The principal association bundle on the medial aspect of the hemisphere lies in the white matter of the cingulate gyrus. This bundle, known as the *cingulum,* contains fibers of variable length which connect regions of the frontal and parietal lobes with parahippocampal and adjacent temporal cortical regions (Figs. 2-9 and 2-15).

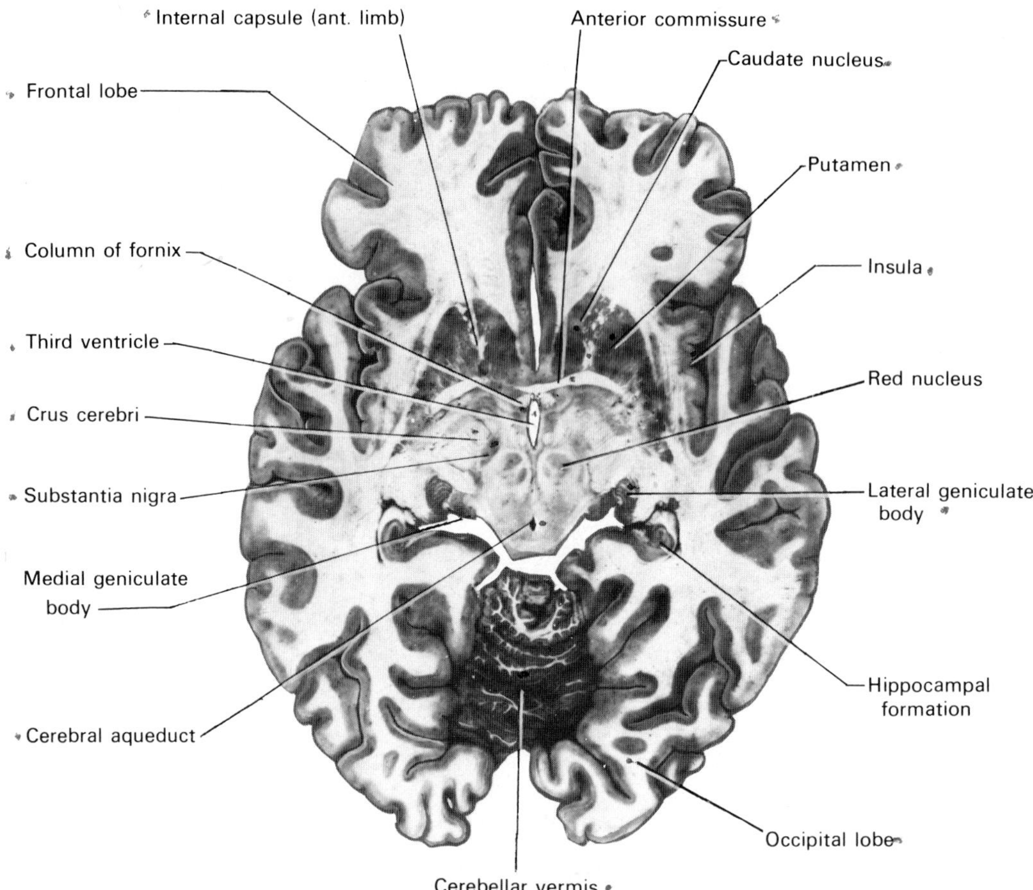

Figure 2-12. Photograph of a horizontal section through the cerebral hemispheres passing through the anterior commissure and the crus cerebri. (From Carpenter and Sutin, *Human Neuroanatomy*, 1983; courtesy of Williams & Wilkins.)

The cortical area deep to the insula contains association fibers in the *extreme* and *external capsules* (Figs. 2-11, 2-16 and 2-17). These thin capsules composed of white matter are separated by a sheet of gray matter, known as the *claustrum.* All three of these structures lie lateral to the components of the corpus striatum.

Commissural Fibers. Fibers interconnecting corresponding cortical regions of the two hemispheres are represented by two structures: (1) the corpus callosum and (2) the anterior commissure. The *corpus callosum* is a broad thick plate of dense myelinated fibers that reciprocally interconnect broad regions of the cortex in all lobes with corresponding regions of the opposite hemisphere (Figs. 2-6, 2-9, and 2-15). These fibers traverse the floor of the hemispheric fissure, form most of the roof of the lateral ventricles and fan out in a massive callosal radiation as they are distributed to various cortical regions. The parts of the corpus callosum are designated as: (1) rostrum, (2) genu, (3) body, and (4) splenium. The genu contains fibers interconnecting anterior parts of the frontal lobes; fibers from the remaining parts of the frontal lobe and the parietal lobe traverse the body of the corpus callosum. Fibers traversing the splenium relate regions of the temporal and occipital lobes. Fibers in the splenium of the corpus callosum, which sweep inferiorly along the lateral margin of the posterior horn of the lateral ventricle and separate the ventricle from the optic radiation, form the *tapetum* (Fig. 2.9).

The *anterior commissure* is a small compact bundle which crosses the midline rostral to the columns of the fornix (Figs. 2-6,

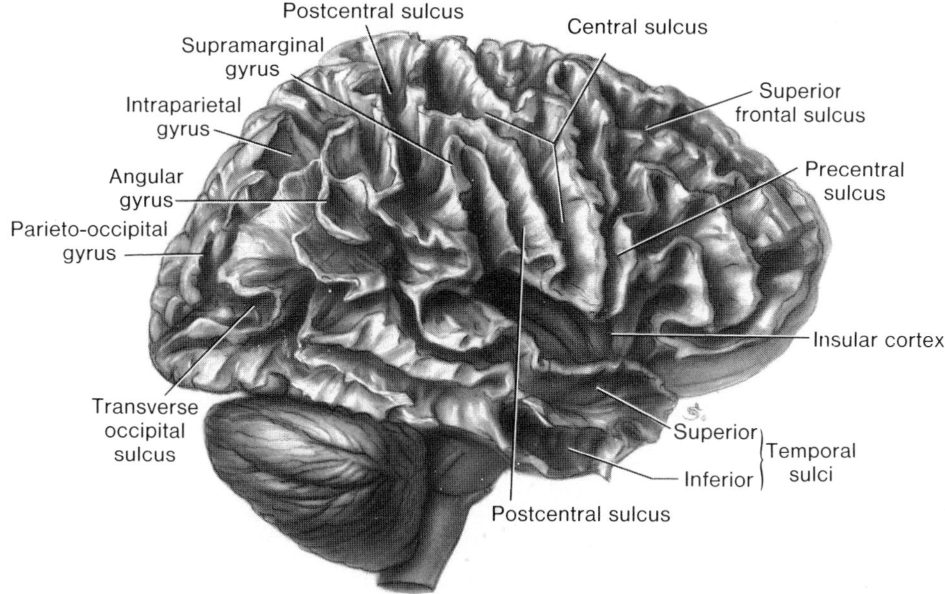

Figure 2-13. Lateral view of the brain after removal of the cortical gray matter from the right hemisphere. The medullary laminae and short association fibers of major gyri are indicated. (From Mettler's *Neuroanatomy*, 1948; courtesy of The C. V. Mosby Company.)

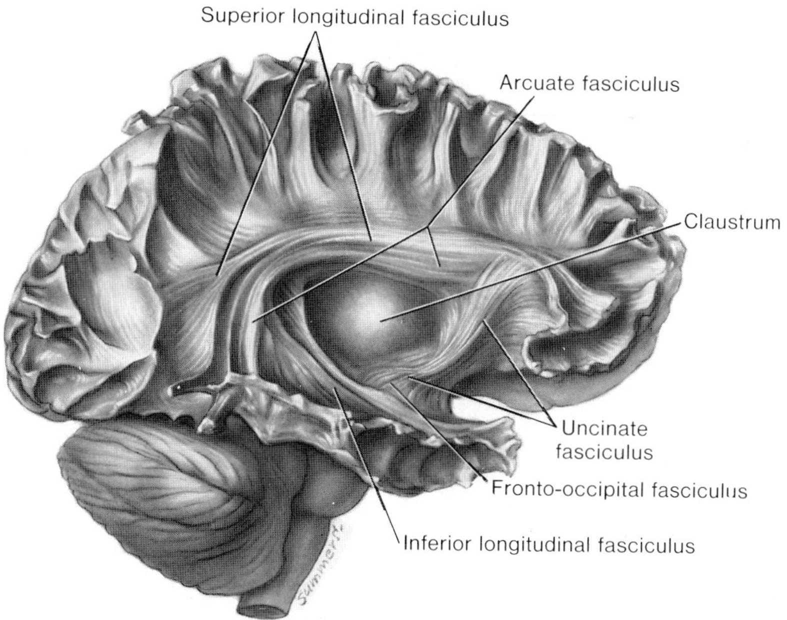

Figure 2-14. Dissection of the lateral surface of the left hemisphere revealing the long association fibers interconnecting cortical regions in different lobes. (From Mettler's *Neuroanatomy*, 1948; courtesy of The C. V. Mosby Company.)

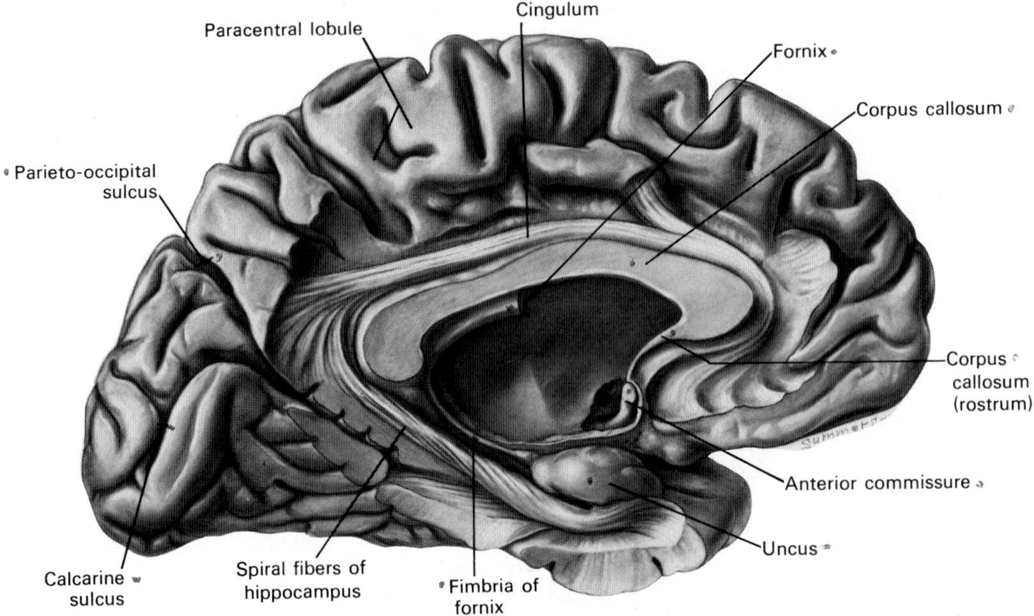

Figure 2-15. Dissection of the medial surface of the left cerebral hemisphere exposing the cingulum. The diencephalon has been removed. (From Mettler's *Neuroanatomy*, 1948; courtesy of the C. V. Mosby Company.)

2-12, 2-15 and 2-16). This commissure has a general shape not unlike bicycle handlebars and consists of two parts that cannot be distinguished in the gross specimen. A small anterior part of the commissure (not evident on gross inspection) interconnects the olfactory bulbs on the two sides (Fig. 12-3); the larger posterior part mainly interconnects regions of the middle and inferior temporal gyri (Whitlock and Nauta; 56).

BASAL GANGLIA

The basal ganglia are subcortical nuclear masses derived from the telencephalon (Figs. 2-11, 2-12, 2-16, and 2-17). Structures composing the basal ganglia are the *caudate nucleus*, the *putamen*, the *globus pallidus* and the *amygdaloid nuclear complex*. The caudate nucleus, putamen and globus pallidus constitute the *corpus striatum*.

The term *lentiform nucleus* refers to the putamen and the globus pallidus. The lentiform nucleus, with the size and shape of a Brazil nut, in transverse sections appears as a wedge with the apex directed medially. This nuclear mass lies between the internal and the external capsules. A slightly curved vertical lamina of white matter divides the lentiform nucleus into an outer portion, the putamen, and an inner portion, the globus pallidus.

Putamen. This is the largest and most lateral part of the corpus striatum; it lies between the lateral medullary lamina of the globus pallidus and the external capsule (Figs. 2-11, 2-16, and 2-17). It is traversed by numerous fascicles of myelinated fibers directed ventromedially towards the globus pallidus, but these are seen clearly only in stained sections. The rostral part of the putamen is continuous ventromedially with the head of the caudate nucleus.

Caudate Nucleus. This nucleus is an elongated arched gray cellular mass related throughout its extent to the lateral cerebral ventricle (Figs. 2-11 and 11-3). It consists of an enlarged rostral part, called the head of the caudate nucleus, which protrudes into the anterior horn of the lateral ventricle, and a narrower body and tail. The body of the caudate nucleus lies dorsolateral to the thalamus near the lateral wall of the lateral ventricle. The tail of the caudate nucleus follows the curvature of the inferior horn of the lateral ventricle and enters the temporal lobe. The tail of the caudate nucleus terminates in the region of the amygdaloid nuclear complex (Fig. 11-3).

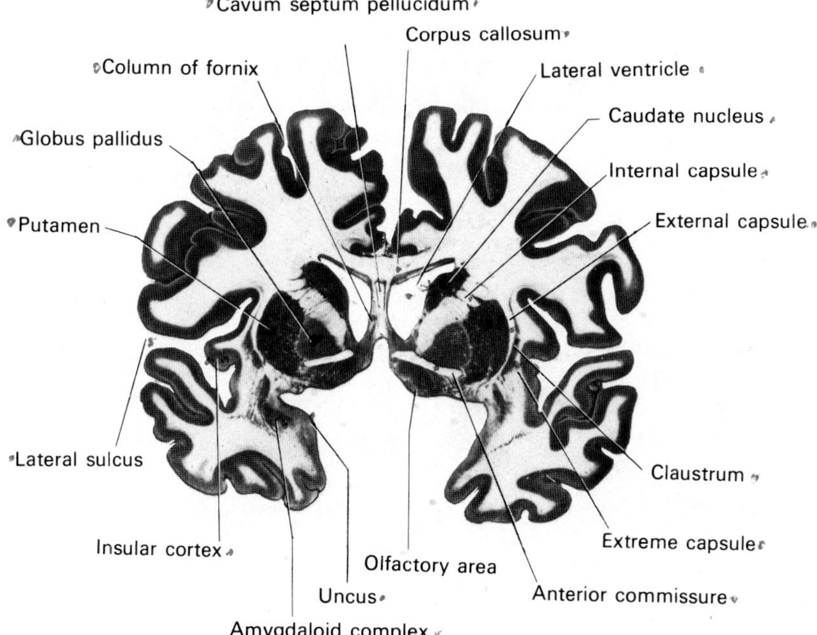

Figure 2-16. Photograph of a frontal section of the brain passing through the columns of the fornix and the anterior commissure. (From Carpenter and Sutin, *Human Neuroanatomy*, 1983; courtesy of Williams & Wilkins.)

Globus Pallidus. The most medial part of the lentiform nucleus, consisting of two parallel segments separated by the medial medullary lamina, is the globus pallidus (Figs. 2-11, 2-16, and 2-17). The globus pallidus appears pale and homogeneous in freshly sectioned brains. Its medial border is formed by the fibers of the posterior limb of the internal capsule.

Amygdaolid Nuclear Complex. This is a gray mass in the dorsomedial part of the temporal lobe which underlies the uncus (Figs. 2-8, 2-16, and 2-17). This complex lies dorsal to the hippocampal formation and rostral to the tip of the inferior horn of the lateral ventricle. The amygdaloid complex gives rise to fibers of the *stria terminalis*, which arch along the entire medial border of the caudate nucleus and are especially evident near the junction of the caudate nucleus and thalamus (Figs. 2-20 and 2-25). The terminal vein lies near the stria terminalis.

LATERAL VENTRICLES

The ependymal-lined cavities of the cerebral hemisphere constitute the lateral ventricles. The arch-shaped lateral ventricles contain cerebrospinal fluid and conform to the general shape of the hemispheres (Fig. 2-18). The paired lateral ventricles can be divided into five parts: (1) the anterior (frontal) horn, (2) the ventricular body, (3) the collateral (atrium) trigone, (4) the inferior (temporal) horn, and (5) the posterior (occipital) horn. Each lateral ventricle communicates with the slit-shaped, midline third ventricle by two short channels, known as the interventricular foramina (Munro). These foramina serve as a basic reference point and are of great importance in radiographic studies.

Anterior (Frontal) Horn of the Lateral Ventricle. This part of the lateral ventricle lies rostral to the interventricular foramen, has a triangular shape in frontal section and extends forward, laterally and ventrally to end in a rounded termination in the substance of the frontal pole (Figs. 2-11 and 2-16). The roof and rostral wall of this horn are formed by the corpus callosum, while its medial boundary is the *septum pellucidum* which rostrally separates the ventricles of the two hemispheres (Figs. 2-6 and 2-25). The lateral wall of the ventricle is formed by the head of the caudate nucleus whose convex surface bulges

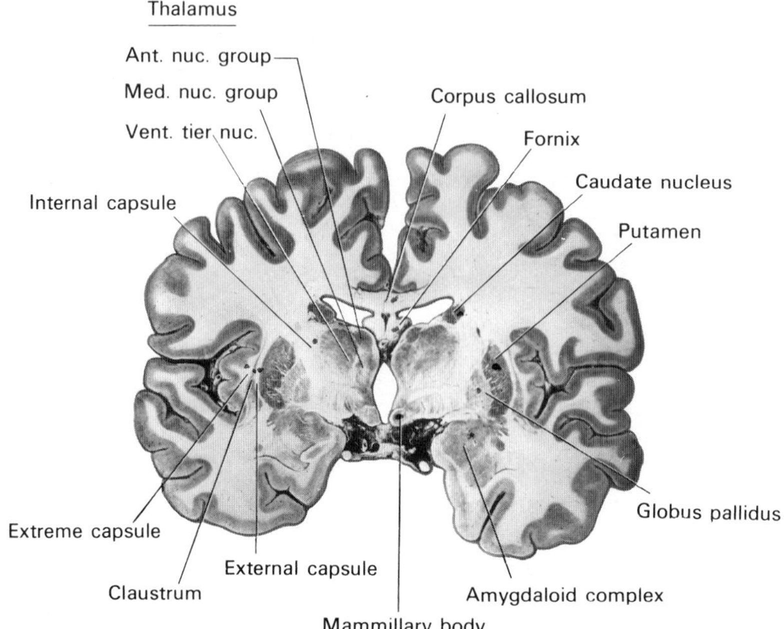

Figure 2-17. Photograph of a frontal section of the brain at the level of the mammillary bodies. In this section the main nuclear groups of the thalamus are identified and portions of all conponents of the basal ganglia are present. The amygdaloid nuclear complex lies in the temporal lobe internal to the uncus and ventral to the lentiform nucleus (i.e., putamen and globus pallidus). (From Carpenter and Sutin, *Human Neuroanatomy*, 1983; courtesy of Williams & Wilkins.)

into the cavity (Figs. 2-11, 2-12, 2-16, and 2-24).

Body of the Lateral Ventricle. This part of the lateral ventricle extends caudally from the interventricular foramen to an ill-defined point near the splenium of the corpus callosum. This narrower arched part of the ventricle continues until the ventricle begins to widen into the collateral trigone (referred to by neuroradiologists as the atrium). The *collateral trigone* comprises that part of the lateral ventricle near the splenium of the corpus callosum where the body of the lateral ventricle is confluent with the temporal and occipital horns (Fig. 2-18).

Inferior (Temporal) Horn of the Lateral Ventricle. This horn of the ventricle curves downward and forward around the caudal aspect of the thalamus, and extends rostrally into the medial part of the temporal lobe to end approximately 3 cm from the temporal pole (Fig. 2-18). The roof and lateral wall of the horn are formed by the tapetum (Fig. 2-9) and the optic radiation; the floor contains the *collateral eminence* caused by the deep collateral sulcus (Fig. 2-7). The inferior horn of the lateral ventricle contains the *hippocampal formation* in its medial wall which extends from the region of the splenium to the tip of the ventricle (Figs. 2-8, 2-11 and 2-12). The hippocampal formation, representing the phylogenetically oldest type of cortex, has become folded into the ventricle along the hippocampal sulcus. Along the superior and medial surfaces of the hippocampus is a flattened band of fibers, known as the fimbria, which extends from the region of the uncus towards the splenium of the corpus callosum. The fimbria extends under the corpus callosum and becomes the fornix (Figs. 2-15 and 2-25).

Posterior (Occipital) Horn of the Lateral Ventricle. This horn of the lateral ventricle extends from the collateral trigone into the occipital lobe. The horn exhibits a high degree of variability in appearance and is often rudimentary (Fig. 2-18). Often the occipital horn has the appearance of a small finger-like projection with a rounded tip. The roof and lateral

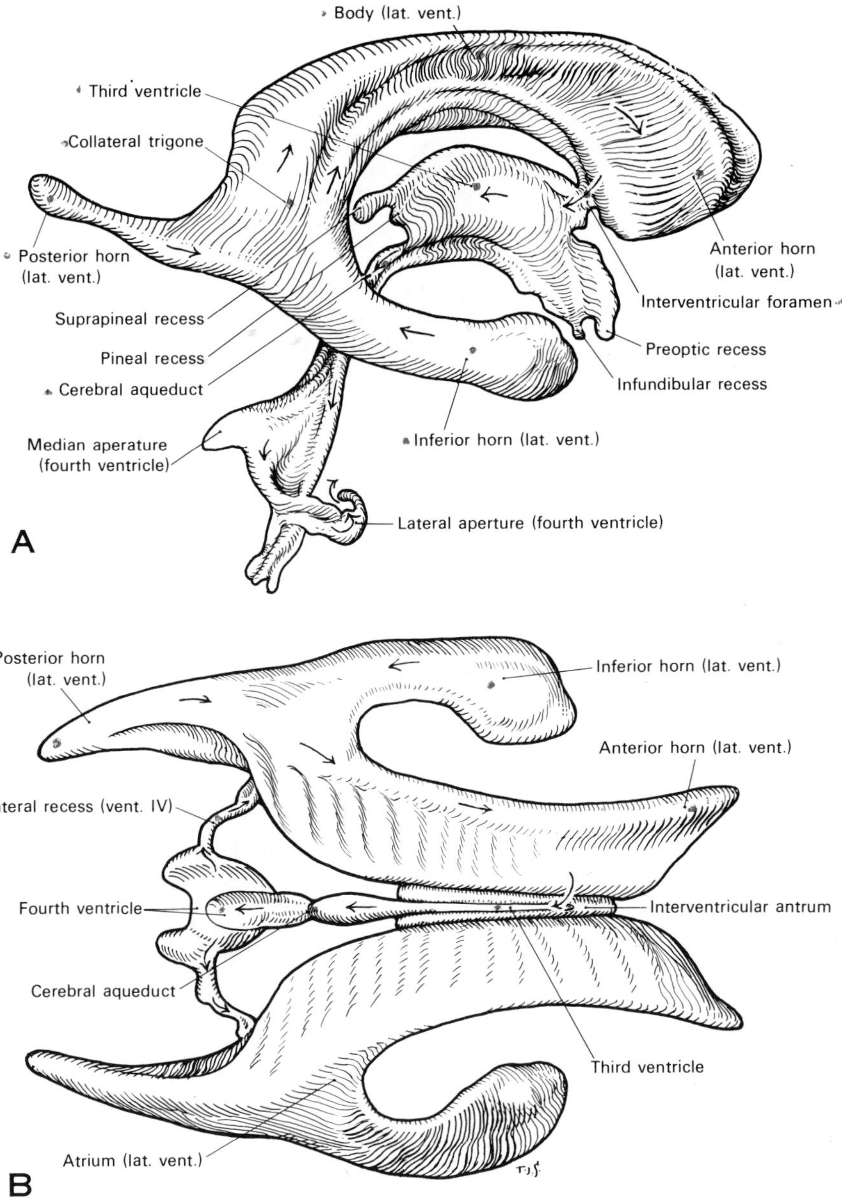

Figure 2-18. Diagrams of the ventricular system in lateral (*A*) and superior (*B*) views. (After Bailey, '48.)

wall of this horn are formed by tapetal fibers of the corpus callosum, while its floor is the white matter of the occipital lobe. The *calcar avis*, a longitudinal prominence, is produced by the deep indentation of the calcarine sulcus.

Portions of the lateral ventricles contain *choroid plexus* which is formed by the invagination of the ependymal roof plate into the ventricular cavities. Choroid plexus develops at sites where ependyma and pia mater containing blood vessels come together. This plexus is present in the body, the collateral trigone, and in the inferior horn of the lateral ventricle, and extends through the interventricular foramen to lie in the roof of the third ventricle (Figs. 1-9 and 2-24).

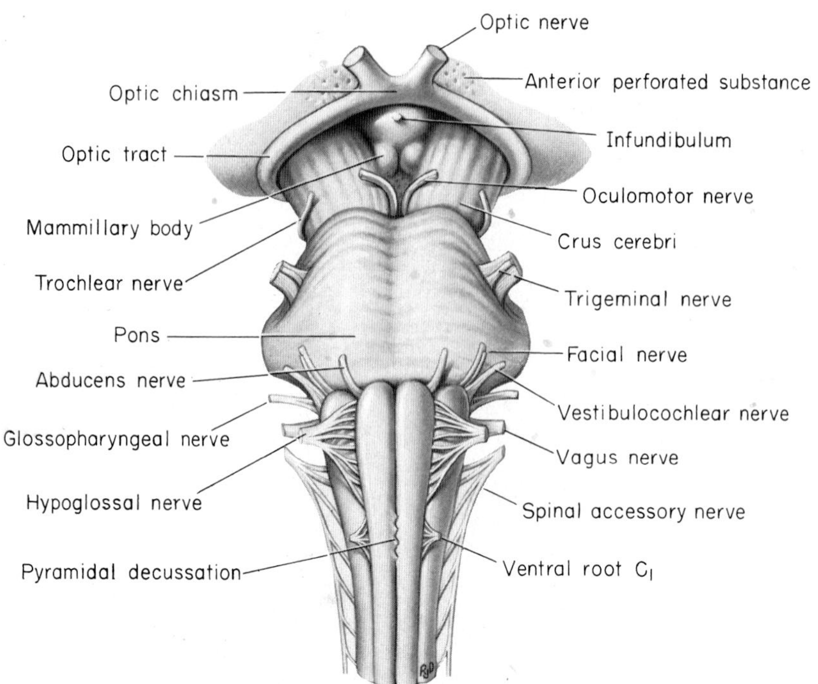

Figure 2-19. Drawing of the anterior surface of the medulla, pons, and midbrain. (From Carpenter and Sutin, *Human Neuroanatomy*, 1983; courtesy of Williams & Wilkins.)

BRAIN STEM

In the intact brain only the anterior, or ventral, surface of the brain stem can be seen throughout its extent, because the cerebral hemispheres and cerebellum overlap the lateral and posterior surfaces. On the anterior surface of the brain stem the medulla, pons, midbrain and part of the *hypothalamus* (diencephalon) can be identified (Figs. 2-7 and 2-19). The most rostral portion of the brain stem, the diencephalon, is surrounded by hemispheric structures on all sides except for a small region between the *optic chiasm* and the *mammillary bodies.* The midbrain appears very small, but root fibers of the oculomotor nerve can be seen emerging between two massive fiber bundles, the *crura cerebri* (Figs. 2-7, 2-12, 2-19 and 2-21). The ventral surface of the pons produces a convex protrusion covered by transversely oriented fiber bundles which course laterally in the substance of the cerebellum. The medulla, caudal to the pons, reveals the *medullary pyramids* medially and the oval *olivary eminences* dorsolaterally (Fig. 2-21). The transition from medulla to spinal cord is characterized by the disappearance of the medullary pyramids, the development of the anterior median fissure of the spinal cord, a conspicuous reduction in size, and the appearance of paired spinal nerves.

Removal of the cerebral hemispheres and cerebellum reveals the posterior and lateral surfaces of the brain stem (Figs. 2-20 and 2-21). The expanded diencephalon appears as two paired oval nuclear masses on each side of a vertical slitlike third ventricle (Fig. 2-20). The *thalamus* and *epithalamus*, seen in a posterior view of the brain stem, lie between the fibers of the internal capsule and are flanked dorsolaterally by the body and tail of the caudate nucleus and the *stria terminalis*. Along the dorsomedial margin of the thalamus is the *stria medullaris*, a band of fibers coursing posteriorly toward the base of the pineal gland (Fig. 2-20). The most caudal part of the thalamus, the pulvinar, overlies part of the midbrain.

The posterior aspect of the midbrain reveals the *superior* and *inferior colliculi* and their *brachia*, which relate these structures to particular parts of the thalamus. The

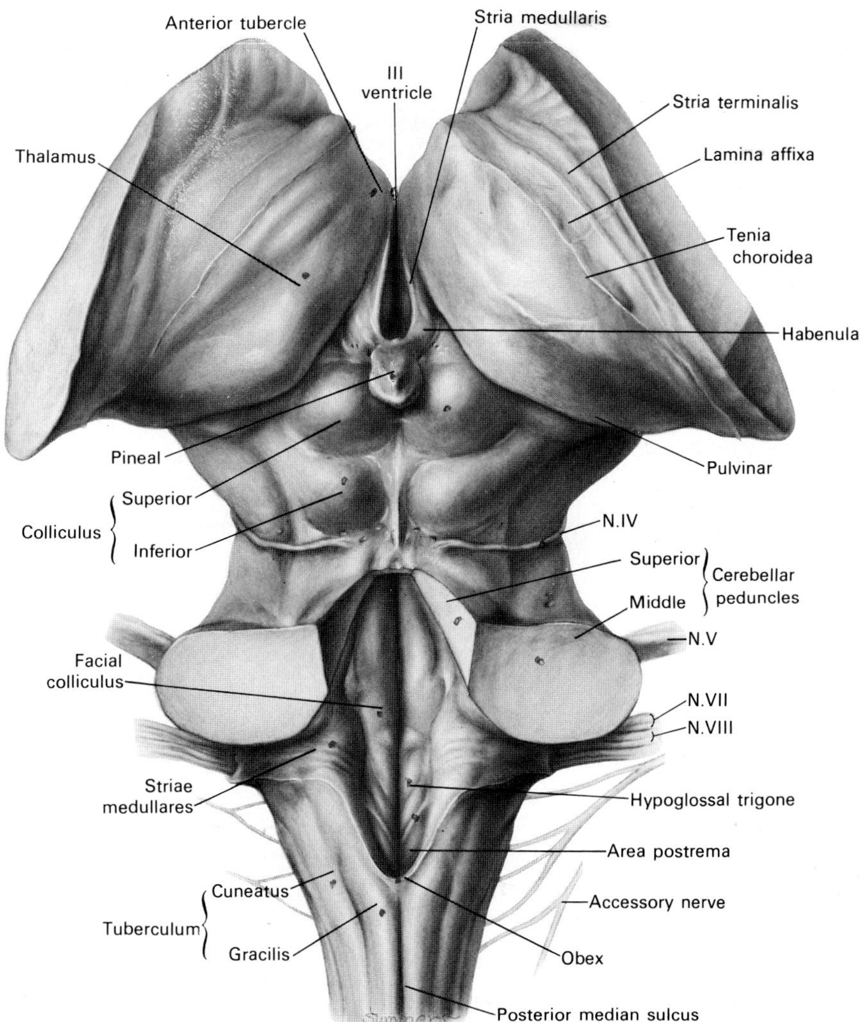

Figure 2-20. Posterior aspect of the brain stem with the cerebellum removed. (From Mettler's *Neuroanatomy*, 1948; courtesy of The C. V. Mosby Company.)

crossed trochlear nerves emerge from the dorsal part of the midbrain caudal to the inferior colliculus (Fig. 2-20).

The posterior aspects of the hindbrain, revealed by removing the cerebellum (Figs. 2-20 and 2-21), disclose the rhomboid fossa, an unpaired symmetrical ventricle that overlies the pons and medulla. The rhomboid-shaped fourth ventricle is surrounded by three paired cerebellar peduncles, which relate the three lowest brain stem segments to the cerebellum (Fig. 2-20). The fourth ventricle contains several eminences which overlie nuclear masses in the pons and medulla, the most evident of which are the *facial colliculus* and the *hypoglossal eminence* or trigone (Fig. 2-20). Caudal to the fourth ventricle on the posterior surface of the medulla are nuclear masses related to ascending spinal systems, namely, the *cuneate* and *gracilis tubercles*.

Structurally the midbrain and hindbrain consist of three distinctive parts: (1) a roof plate superior to the ventricular system, (2) a central core of cells and fibers beneath the ventricular system known as the tegmentum, and (3) a massive collection of ventrally located fibers derived from cells of the cerebral cortex (Figs. 2-22 and 2-23). The *roof plate* of the midbrain is represented by the tectum or *quadrigeminal plate*, consisting of the superior and inferior

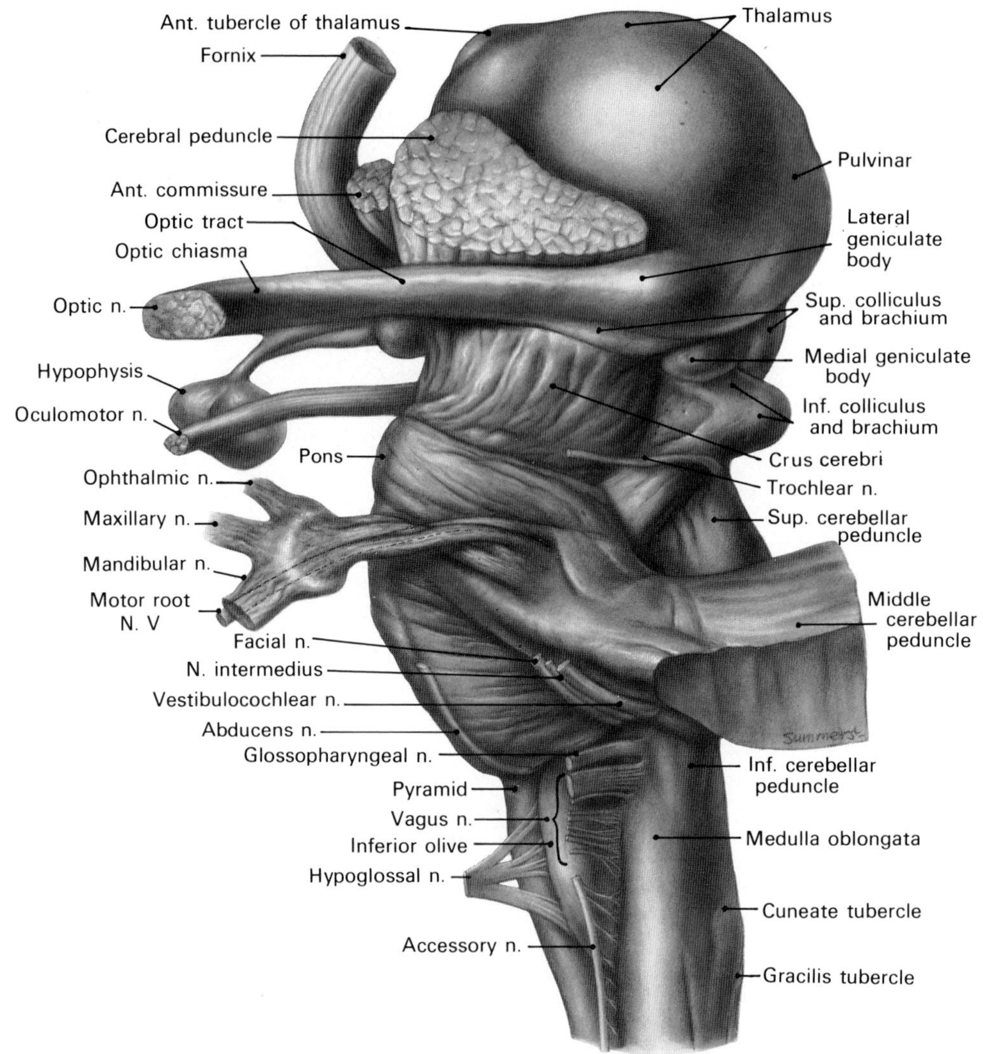

Figure 2-21. Lateral view of the brain stem with the cerebellum removed showing the sites of emergence and entrance of most of the cranial nerves. (From Mettler's *Neuroanatomy*, 1948; courtesy of The C. V. Mosby Company.)

colliculi; in the hindbrain the roof plate is represented by the *cerebellum* and the *tela choroidea.* The *tegmentum* of the midbrain, pons and medulla represents the brain stem *reticular formation,* a large collection of cells and intermingled fibers that subserve multiple functions. The *cortically derived ventral fiber system* forms the *crus cerebri* at midbrain levels, one of the principal constituents of the *ventral* or *basilar part of the pons,* and the *medullary pyramids* of the medulla (Figs. 2-20 and 2-21). Both the reticular formation and the cortically derived ventral fiber system are continuous within the brain stem, but undergo change and modification at various levels (Fig. 2–10).

Medulla

The medulla (myelencephalon), the most caudal basic subdivision of the brain stem, extends from the level of the foramen magnum to the caudal border of the pons. The transition from spinal cord to medulla is gradual and characterized by: (1) the obliteration of the anterior median fissure ventrally and the decussation of the medullary

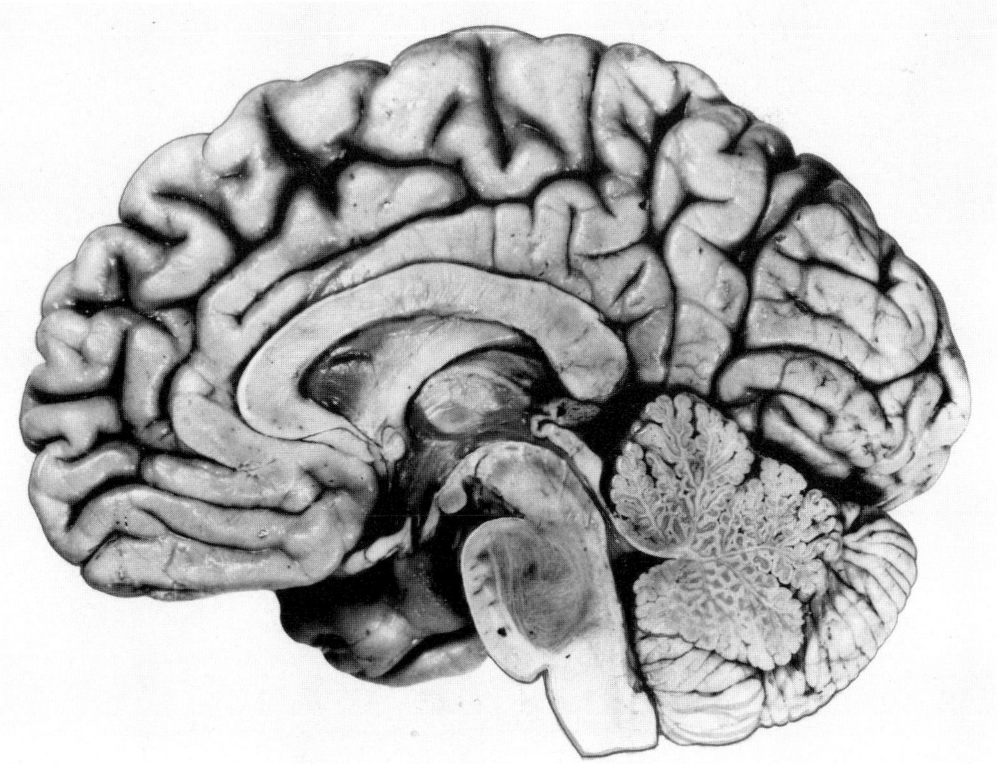

Figure 2-22. Photograph of a midsagittal section of the brain. Brain stem structures are identified in Figure 2-23. (From Carpenter and Sutin, *Human Neuroanatomy*, 1983; courtesy of Williams & Wilkins.)

pyramids, (2) the appearance of the gracilis and cuneate tubercles dorsally, (3) the disappearance of spinal nerves, (4) the appearance of cranial nerves, and (5) the development of the fourth ventricle (Figs. 2-18, 2-20, 2-22, and 2-23). The full development of the medullary pyramids, the appearance of the eminence of the inferior olivary complex, the widening of the fourth ventricle and the gradual increase in size of the inferior cerebellar peduncle give the medulla its characteristic configuration. Cranial nerves associated with the medulla are: (1) the hypoglossal (N. XII) whose fibers emerge ventrolaterally between the pyramid and the inferior olivary complex, (2) the accessory (N. XI), the vagus (N. X) and the glossopharyngeal (N. IX) whose fibers emerge from the postolivary sulcus, and (3) the vestibulocochlear nerve (N. VIII) whose separate components enter the brain stem at the cerebellopontine angle, formed by the junction of the pons, medulla and cerebellum (Figs. 2-19, 2-20, and 2-21). Auditory fibers are most dorsal and caudal and partially arch over the lateral aspect of the inferior cerebellar peduncle.

Fourth Ventricle

The fourth ventricle is a broad shallow rhomboid-shaped cavity overlying the pons and medulla that extends from the central canal of the upper cervical spinal cord to the cerebral aqueduct of the midbrain (Figs. 2-18 and 2-20). Its roof is formed by the *superior* and *inferior medullary veli*, which extend toward an apex within the cerebellum known as the *fastigium* (Figs. 2-22, 2-23, 2-28, and 2-29). The superior medullary velum forms the roof of the pontine part of the ventricle, while the inferior medullary velum and the *tela choroidea* roof over the medullary part of this ventricle. A *choroid plexus* from the tela choroidea in the caudal part of the ventricle passes into the lateral recess on each side (Fig. 2-18). The widest part of the fourth ventricle is immediately

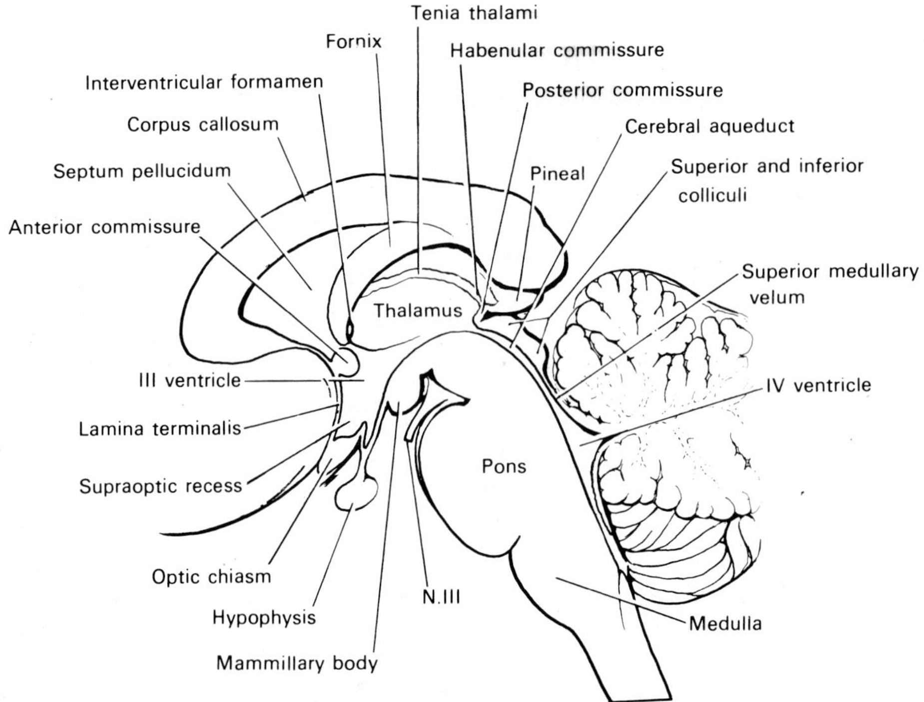

Figure 2-23. Outline drawing of a midsagittal section of the brain stem identifying structures shown in Figure 2-22. (From Carpenter and Sutin, *Human Neuroanatomy*, 1983; courtesy of Williams & Wilkins.)

caudal to the *middle cerebellar peduncles.* In this region a *lateral recess* on each side extends over the surface of the inferior cerebellar peduncle to open into the *cerebellomedullary* (magna) *cistern* (Figs. 1-8 and 1-9). These small lateral recesses contain choroid plexus that protrudes through the *foramina of Luschka* into the subarachnoid space (Figs. 2-7 and 2-18). A small median aperture in the caudal part of the ventricle is known as the *foramen of Magendie.* Through these three apertures cerebrospinal fluid flows from the ventricular system into the subarachnoid spaces.

The *rhomboid fossa* which forms the floor of the fourth ventricle is divided by the *median sulcus* into symmetrical halves. The sulcus limitans divides each half into a *medial eminence* and a lateral region known as the *vestibular area* (Fig. 5-2). The vestibular nuclei lie beneath the vestibular area. The *facial colliculus* and the *hypoglossal trigone* lie within the medial eminence, with the latter near the caudal border of the ventricle. Transversely coursing fibers of the *striae medullares* run from the region of the lateral recess towards the midline and disappear in the median sulcus (Fig. 2.20); these strands of myelinated fibers lie rostral to the hypoglossal trigone. The *vagal trigone* lies lateral to the hypoglossal trigone. The most caudal end of the rhomboid fossa resembles a pen and is called the *calamus scriptorius.* The point of caudal junction of the walls of the fourth ventricle is known as the *obex* (Fig. 2-20). Immediately rostral to the obex on each side of the fourth ventricle is a slightly rounded eminence, the *area postrema,* one of the so-called circumventricular organs (Figs. 1-16 and 5-7).

Pons

The pons (metencephalon), represents the rostral part of the hindbrain and is well delimited on the anterior surface of the brain stem (Figs. 2-19, 2-21, 2-22, and 2-23). The massive pontine protruberance is covered ventrally by broad bands of transversely oriented fibers and is separated from: (1) the midbrain by the superior pontine sulcus and (2) the medulla by the inferior pontine sulcus (Fig. 2-19). The predominantly transverse fibers in the ventral part of the pons form the *middle cerebellar peduncle*. An anterior median depression, the *basilar sulcus*, indicates the position occupied by the basilar artery (Figs. 2-19 and 14-4).

Transverse sections of the pons reveal the basic organization (Fig. 6-1). The pons consists of a massive *ventral part* composed of: (1) longitudinal descending fiber bundles, (2) pontine nuclei, and (3) transversely oriented fibers projecting to the cerebellum, and a smaller dorsal part, known as the *tegmentum*. The tegmental portion contains aggregations of cells and fibers which form a central core known as the reticular formation. The pontine tegmentum is continuous with the reticular formation of the medulla and midbrain. Cranial nerve nuclei, ascending sensory systems and older descending motor pathways arising from brain stem nuclei are found within the tegmentum. Cranial nerves associated with the pons are the trigeminal (N. V), abducens (N. VI), facial (N. VII), and the two components of the vestibulocochlear nerve (N. VIII). The *abducens nucleus* lies in the floor of the fourth ventricle and is partially encircled by fibers of the facial nerve. Facial nerve fibers and cells of the abducens nucleus underlie the *facial colliculus* in the floor of the fourth ventricle (Fig. 2-20). Fibers of the abducens nerve emerge from the ventral surface of the brain stem at the junction of the pons and medulla. The facial and vestibulocochlear nerves emerge and enter the lateral surface of the pons at the *cerebellopontine angle*, formed by the junction of pons, medulla and cerebellum. The trigeminal nerve, consisting of motor and sensory fibers, traverses rostrolateral parts of the middle cerebellar peduncle to reach nuclei in the dorsolateral pontine tegmentum (Fig. 2-19).

The *middle cerebellar peduncle* consists of a massive collection of crossed fibers, arising from the pontine nuclei, which project to the opposite cerebellar hemisphere; this is the largest of the three cerebellar peduncles (Figs. 2-20 and 2-21).

Midbrain

The midbrain (mesencephalon) is the smallest and least differentiated brain stem segment (Figs. 2-19, 2-20, 2-21, and 2-22). It consists of: (1) the *tectum*, represented by the superior and inferior colliculi, (2) the *tegmentum*, ventral to the cerebral aqueduct, and (3) the massive *crura cerebri* (Figs. 2-10, 2-12, 2-19 and 2-21). The tegmentum and *crura cerebri* are separated by a large pigmented nuclear mass, the *substantia nigra*. The cells of the substantia nigra contain melanin pigment, synthesize dopamine, and can be readily identified in fresh cut sections of the midbrain. The superior colliculus and a region immediately rostral to it, known as the *pretectum*, are important structures which receive inputs from fibers of the optic tract; these structures are involved in relays that mediate visual reflexes. The inferior colliculus relays auditory impulses to thalamic nuclei that in turn project to specific cortical areas.

Two cranial nerves are associated with the midbrain, the oculomotor (N. III) and the trochlear (N. IV). The oculomotor nerve emerges from the *interpeduncular fossa*, between the massive crura cerebri (Figs. 2-7 and 2-19). The slender trochlear nerve exits from the posterior surface of the brain stem, caudal to the inferior colliculus; fibers of this nerve cross in the superior medullary velum (Fig. 2-20). The fibers of the *superior cerebellar peduncle*, seen on each side of the upper part of the fourth ventricle (Fig. 2-20), constitute the largest efferent system to emerge from the deep nuclei of the cerebellum. Fibers in this peduncle decussate completely in the caudal midbrain tegmentum. Crossed fibers of this peduncle traverse and surround cells in a discrete nuclear mass in the midbrain tegmentum called the *red nucleus*. A large proportion of these crossed fibers ascend to terminations in diencephalic (thalamic) nuclei.

Crus Cerebri. On the ventral surface of the midbrain are collections of fibers originating from broad areas of the cerebral cortex that pass through the internal capsule (Figs. 2-10 and 2-19). Fibers forming the crus cerebri project to: (1) spinal cord (i.e., corticospinal); (2) pontine nuclei (i.e., corticopontine); and (3) specific regions of the lower brain stem (i.e., corticobulbar). A large part of the so-called corticobulbar fibers project to portions of the reticular formation.

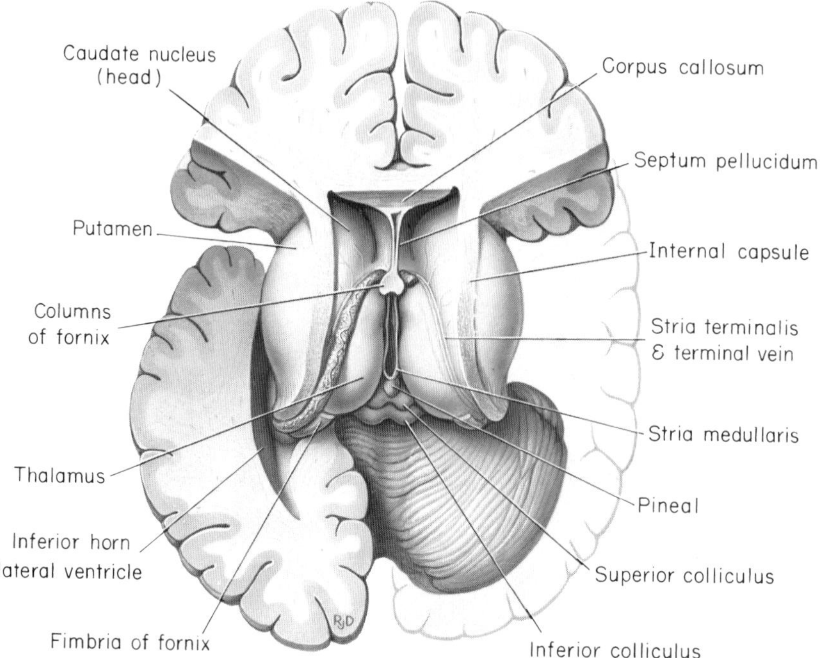

Figure 2-24. Drawing of a brain stem dissection showing the gross relationships of the thalamus, internal capsule, corpus striatum and the ventricular system. (From Carpenter and Sutin, *Human Neuroanatomy*, 1983; courtesy of Williams & Wilkins.)

The pigmented *substantia nigra*, situated along the superior border of the crus cerebri, is the largest single nuclear mass in the midbrain. This nucleus has connections with parts of the corpus striatum and thalamus and is considered to subserve a motor function (Figs. 2-12 and 7-1).

Diencephalon

The diencephalon, the most rostral part of the brain stem, is a paired structure on each side of the third ventricle (Figs. 2-20, 2-21, 2-22, 2-23, and 2-24). The lateral ventricles, corpus callosum, fornix and velum interpositum lie superior to the diencephalon. Fibers of the posterior limb of the internal capsule and the body and tail of the caudate nucleus lie along its lateral border. Caudally the diencephalon appears continuous with the tegmentum of the midbrain; the posterior commissure demarcates as the junctional zone between the diencephalon and mesencephalon (Fig. 2-23). The rostral boundary of the diencephalon is near the interventricular foramen, but portions of the hypothalamus extend almost to the *lamina terminalis* (Figs. 2-22 and 2-23). This nuclear complex consists of four subdividions: (1) the epithalamus, (2) the thalamus, (3) the hypothalamus and (4) the subthalamus (Figs. 2-20, 2-21, 2-22, 2-23, and 2-25).

The epithalamus, evident on the superior surface of the diencephalon, consists of: (1) the pineal body, (2) the habenular nuclei, (3) the striae medullares and the tenia thalami (Figs. 2-23 and 2-24).

Thalamus

The largest diencephalic subdivision is an oblique egg-shaped nuclear mass at the rostral end of the brain stem (Figs. 2-20, 2-21, 2-23, and 2-24). This nuclear complex lies between the interventricular foramen and the posterior commissure and extends from the third ventricle to the medial border of the posterior limb of the internal capsule. The thalamus lies dorsal to the hypothalamic sulcus, a shallow groove on the lateral wall of the third ventricle (Figs. 2-25 and 9-5). The lateral and caudal parts of the thalamus are enlarged and overlie

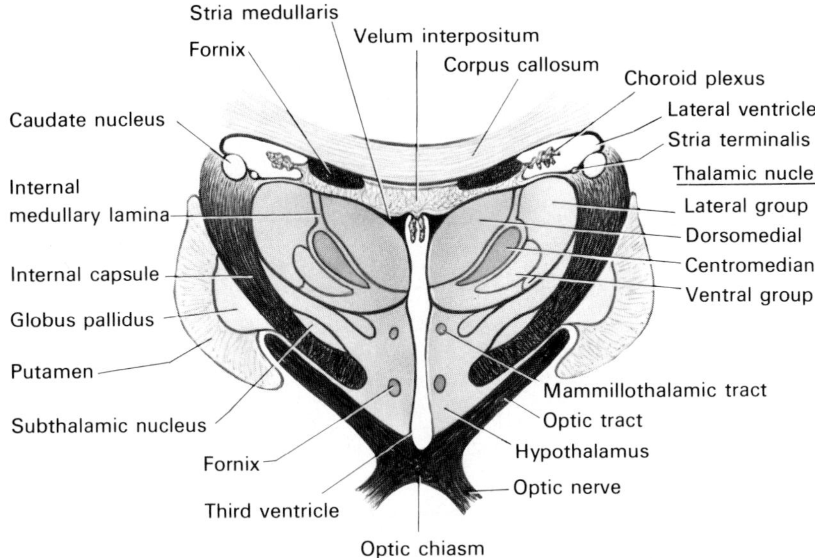

Figure 2-25. Schematic drawing of a frontal section through the diencephalon (see Fig. 9-5) and adjacent structures indicating some of the major nuclear groups of the thalamus. The hypothalamus lies below the hypothalamic sulcus on both sides of the third ventricle and is continuous across the floor of this ventricle. The subthalamic regions lie lateral and caudal to the hypothalamus..(From Carpenter and Sutin, *Human Neuroanatomy*, 1983; courtesy of Williams & Wilkins.)

midbrain structures. The superior surface of the thalamus is covered by a thin layer of fibers known as the *stratum zonale* (Fig. 9-5). A narrow lateral strip on the superior surface, adjacent to the body and tail of the caudate nucleus, is covered by ependyma and forms part of the floor of the lateral ventricle. This strip is called the *lamina affixa* (Fig. 2-20). The *stria terminalis* and the terminal vein are present dorsally at the junction of thalamus and caudate nucleus. The *stria medullaris* extends along the dorsomedial margin of the thalamus near the roof of the third ventricle (Fig. 2-24). The medial surfaces of thalami on each side of the third ventricle are partially fused in about 80% of human brains. This place of fusion is called the *interthalamic adhesion* or *massa intermedia.*

Although most subdivisions of the thalamus are not evident in gross specimens, the *anterior tubercle* of the thalamus is discernible rostrally as a distinct swelling. The expanded posterior part of the thalamus that overhangs part of the midbrain is known as the *pulvinar* (Figs. 2-11 and 2-20). The *medial* and *lateral geniculate bodies*, important relay nuclei concerned with audition and vision, lie ventral to the pulvinar. Together these structures are referred to as the *metathalamus.* The thalamus is divided into anterior, lateral, medial and ventral nuclear groups by a thin layer of myelinated fibers, known as the *internal medullary lamina* of the thalamus, which can be seen grossly in some transverse sections of the brain (Figs. 2-11 and 2-17). Nuclear groups within the internal medullary lamina are collectively referred to as the *intralaminar thalamic nuclei* (Fig. 2-25).

The thalamus is the neural structure whose relationships with other parts of the neuraxis provide the key to understanding the organization of the central nervous system. Like most keys it is small but of great importance. This small part of the diencephalon is concerned with: (1) distributing most of the afferent input to the cerebral cortex, (2) the control of the electrocortical activity of the cerebral cortex, and (3) the integration of motor functions by providing the relays through which impulses from the corpus striatum and cerebellum can reach the motor cortex. The functions of the thalamus are much more complex and elaborate than that of a simple relay station. The

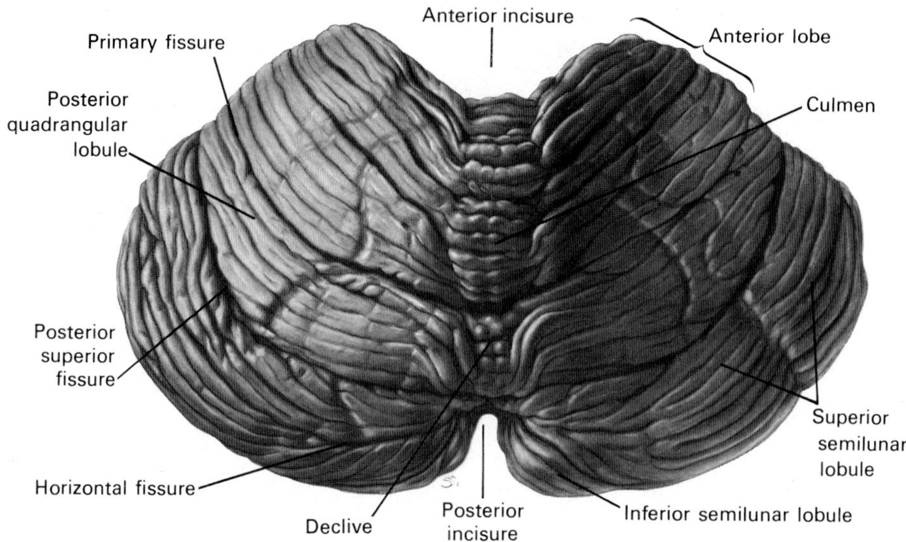

Figure 2-26. Superior surface of cerebellum. (From Mettler's *Neuroanatomy*, 1948; courtesy of The C. V. Mosby Company.)

thalamus is concerned with input selection, output tuning, high fidelity impulse transmission, synchronization and desynchronization of cortical activities, parallel processing of sensory signals, and the integration of inputs that modify motor activities (Purpura, '70). This structure plays a dominant role in the maintenance and regulation of states of consciousness, alertness, and attention. The thalamus may be regarded as the chief integrating and tuning mechanism of the neuraxis.

Hypothalamus

This structure lies ventral to the hypothalamic sulcus and forms the floor and lateral walls of the third ventricle (Figs. 2-22, 2-23, 2-25, 9-5, and 10-1). This subdivision of the diencephalon extends from the region of the optic chiasm to the caudal border of the mammillary bodies. The gross structures visible on the ventral surface include the *optic chiasm*, *infundibulum*, *tuber cinereum*, and *mammillary bodies* (Fig. 2-8). The hypothalamus is divided into medial and lateral nuclear groups by fibers of the fornix most of which end in the mammillary body. Three rostrocaudal regions of the hyothalamus are recognized: (1) a supraoptic, dorsal to the optic chiasm, (2) a tuberal region centrally, and (3) a mammillary region caudally (Fig. 10-1). The zone forming the floor of the third ventricle is called the *median eminence*; portions of this eminence lie both rostral and caudal to the infundibular stem. The median eminence is the anatomical site of the interface between central neural pathways and the anterior pituitary (Knigge and Silverman, '74).

The hypothalamus has a rostrocaudal extent of about 10 mm. This subdivision of the diencephalon is concerned with visceral, endocrine and metabolic activity, as well as with temperature regulation, sleep, and emotion.

Subthalamus

This transitional diencephalon zone lies ventral to the thalamus and lateral to the hypothalamus. It is bounded by the thalamus above, the hypothalamus medially, and the internal capsule laterally (Figs. 2-7 and 2-25). The largest discrete nuclear mass is the *subthalamic nucleus*, a lens-shaped structure on the inner aspect of the internal capsule. (Fig. 9-5). This region is traversed by many important fiber systems in their projection to thalamic nuclei. A small, relatively clear area dorsal and rostral to the subthalamic nuclear, known as the *zona incerta*, serves as an important landmark

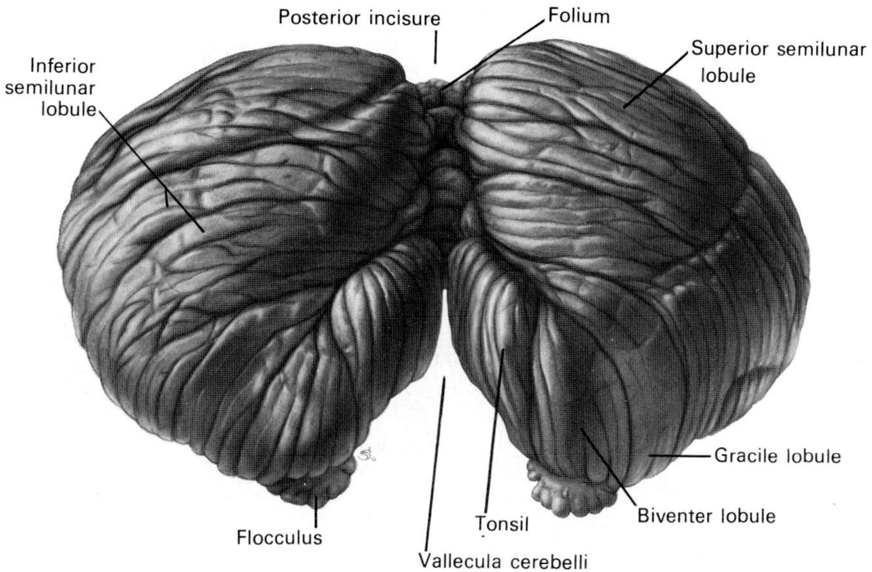

Figure 2-27. Posteroinferior view of the cerebellum. (From Mettler's *Neuroanatomy*, 1948; courtesy of the C. V. Mosby Company.)

in distinguishing fiber bundles with specific origins and trajectories. The subthalamic nucleus and pathways traversing this region are concerned with somatic motor function.

CEREBELLUM

The cerebellum overlies the posterior aspect of the pons and medulla and extends laterally under the tentorium to fill the greater part of the posterior fossa (Fig. 2-1). The superior surface is somewhat flattened, while the inferior surface is convex. A shallow *anterior cerebellar incisure* is present superiorly. A deeper and narrower *posterior cerebellar incisure* contains a fold of dura mater, the *falx cerebelli* (Fig. 1-2).

The cerebellum consists of a midline portion, the *vermis*, and two lateral lobes or *hemispheres*. This structure is essentially wedge-shaped, having a superior surface which is covered by the tentorium, a posterior surface in the suboccipital region, and an inferior surface which overlies the fourth ventricle. On the superior surface the distinction between vermis and hemispheres is not sharp (Fig. 2-26). On the inferior surface two deep sulci clearly separate the vermis from the hemispheres. Inferiorly a deep median fossa, the *vallecula cerebelli*, is continuous with the posterior incisure. The floor of this fossa is formed by the inferior vermis (Fig. 2-27).

Structurally the cerebellum consists of a gray cortical mantle, the cerebellar cortex, a medullary core of white matter and four pairs of intrinsic nuclei. Three paired cerebellar peduncles connect the cerebellum with the three lower segments of the brain stem (Figs. 2-20 and 2-28).

The cerebellar cortex consists of a large number of narrow leaflike laminae known as cerebellar folia. Surface cerebellar folia are nearly parallel with each other and for the most part are transversely oriented. Each lamina contains several secondary and tertiary folia.

Five transversely oriented fissures divide the cerebellum into lobes and lobules (Fig. 8-1). These fissures and the various lobular subdivisions can be identified on the isolation cerebellum or in midsagittal section (Fig. 2-29). On the superior surface of the cerebellum two fissures can be identified: (1) the *primary* and (2) the *posterior superior* (Fig. 2-26). The primary fissure is the deepest of all cerebellar fissures. The *horizontal fissure*, one of the most distinctive, roughly divides the cerebellum into supe-

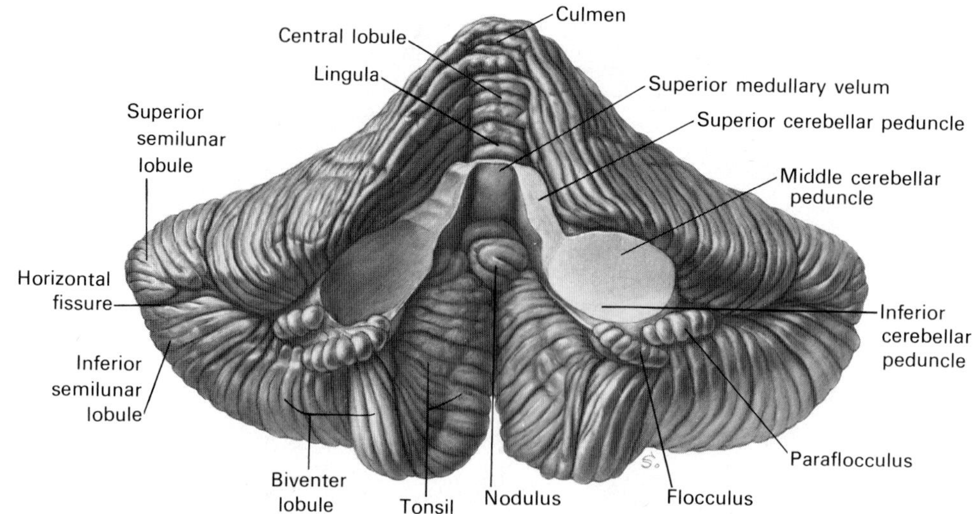

Figure 2-28. Inferior surface of cerebellum removed from brain stem by transection of cerebellar peduncles. (From Mettler's *Neuroanatomy*, 1948; courtesy of the C. V. Mosby Company.)

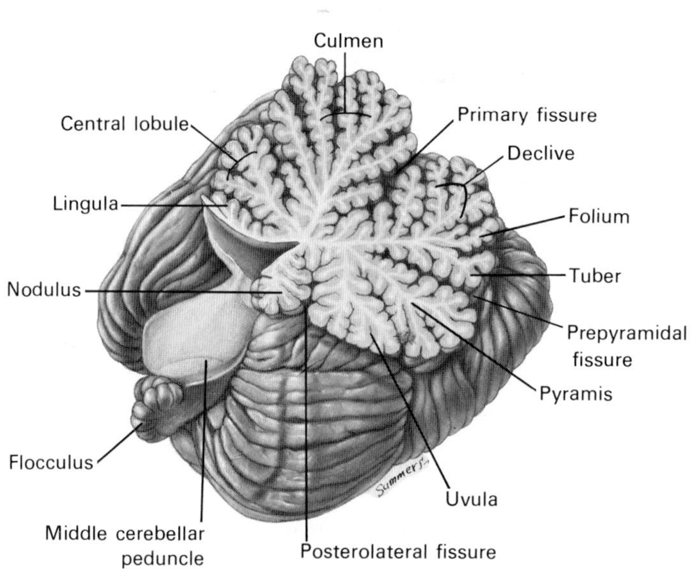

Figure 2-29. Sagittal view of the sectioned cerebellum showing the lobules of the cerebellar vermis. The primary fissure is the deepest of all cerebellar fissures. (From Mettler's *Neuroanatomy*, 1948; courtesy of the C. V. Mosby Company.)

rior and inferior halves. On the inferior surface the *prepyramidal* and *posterolateral fissures* are found (Fig. 2-29). The prepyramidal fissure lies between the *tuber* and the pyramidal-shaped *pyramis* in the cerebellar vermis (Figs. 2-29 and 8-1). In the cerebellar hemisphere this fissure separates gracile and biventer lobules which constitute parts of the *paramedian lobule.* The posterolateral fissure separates the *nodulus,* which lies in the roof of the fourth ventricle, from the rest of the cerebellar vermis.

The cerebellar vermis is the key to un-

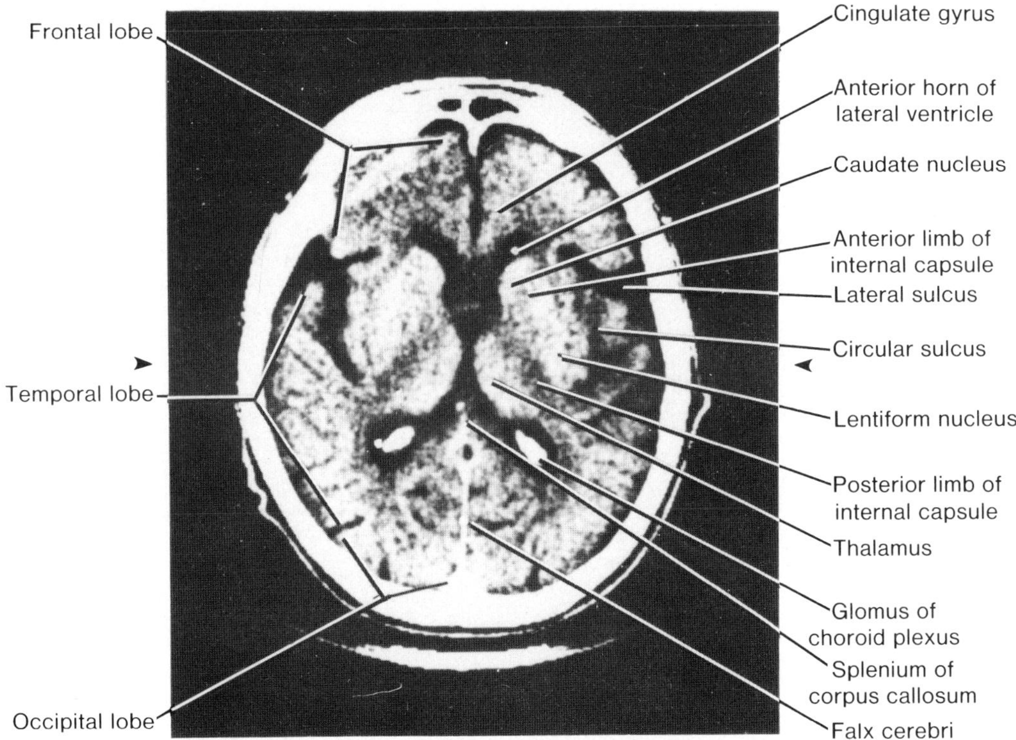

Figure 2-30. Computerized tomogram of the head taken in a plane parallel to the base line of Reid and passing through the corpus striatum, internal capsule and thalamus. (From Hanaway et al., '80; courtesy of Dr. J. Hanaway and Warren H. Green, II, Inc., St. Louis.)

derstanding the gross organization of the cerebellum, but in this part there is no median raphe and the midline is difficult to establish (Madigan and Carpenter, '71). Portions of the cerebellum rostral to the primary fissure constitute the *anterior lobe of the cerebellum* (Figs. 2-26 and 8-1). In the vermis the lobules consist of the lingula, the central lobule and the culmen (Fig. 2-29); in the hemisphere the lingula has no corresponding part, but the *alar central lobule* and the *anterior quadrangular lobule* correspond to the central lobule and the culmen.

The *posterior lobe* of the cerebellum lies between the primary and posterolateral fissures and represents the largest subdivision of the cerebellum (Figs. 2-29 and 8-1). Vermal parts of the posterior lobe in sequence are the *declive*, *folium*, *tuber*, *pyramis*, and *uvula* (Fig. 2-29). The *simple lobule*, between the primary and posterior superior fissure, corresponds to the declive of the vermis (Fig. 8-1). The *ansiform lobule* is that part of the cerebellar hemisphere between the posterior superior fissure and the *gracile lobule*. The horizontal fissure divides the ansiform lobule into the *superior semilunar lobule* (crus I) and the *inferior semilunar lobule* (crus II). The vermal counterparts of the ansiform lobule are the folium and tuber. Between the prepyramidal and posterolateral fissures are the *pyramis* and *uvula* in the vermis and the *biventer lobule* and the *cerebellar tonsil* in the hemisphere (Figs. 2-28 and 2-29).

The *flocculonodular lobule* lies rostral to the posterolateral fissure and consists of the vermal nodulus and the paired flocculi (Fig. 2-28). The *nodulus* lies immediately caudal to the inferior medullary velum (Fig. 2-29).

In midsagittal section the relationships of the cerebellum to the brain stem are

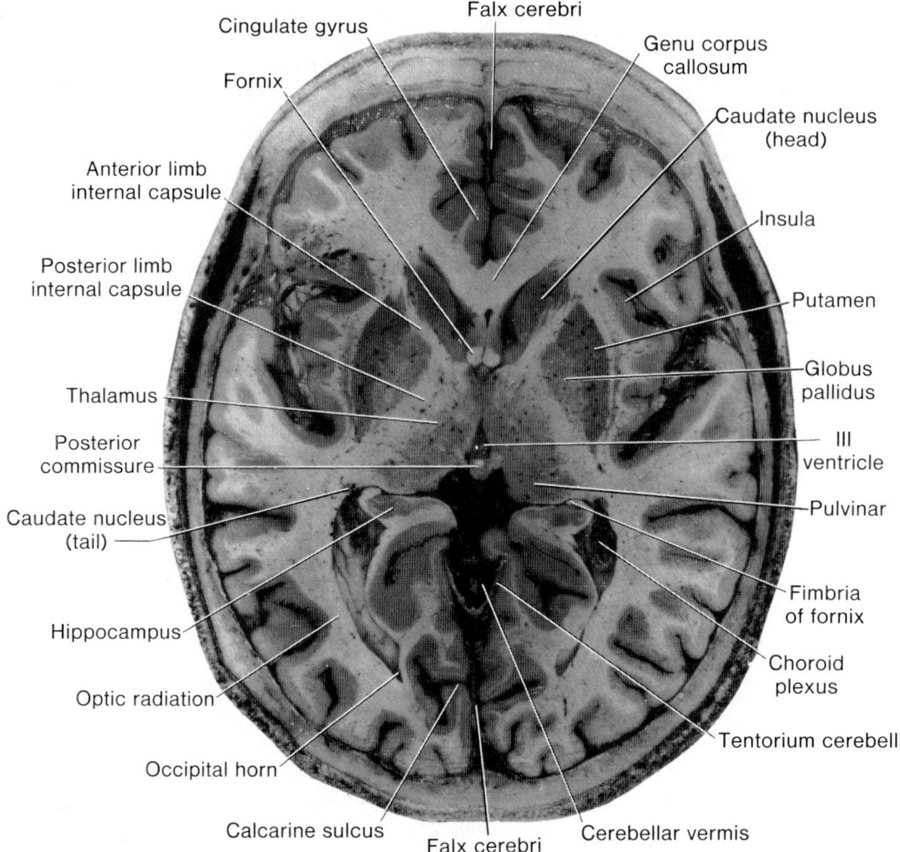

Figure 2-31. Section of the head and brain cut in a horizontal plane corresponding to that of the computerized tomogram in Figure 2-30. (From Hanaway et al., '80; courtesy of Dr. J. Hanaway and Warren H. Green, II, Inc., St. Louis.)

evident (Fig. 2-23). The complex branching of the medullary core and the treelike appearance of the laminae and folia have given rise to the descriptive term, *arbor vitae* (Figs. 2-22 and 2-29). The intrinsic deep nuclei of the cerebellum can be seen only in sections. These nuclei are the dentate (most lateral), the emboliform, the globose and the fastigial (Fig. 6-20). The fastigial nuclei, commonly called the roof nuclei, lie in the roof of the fourth ventricle.

Although the cerebellum is derived from the metencephalon, this portion of the neuraxis functions in a suprasegmental manner. It is concerned primarily with coordination of somatic motor function, the control of muscle tone and the maintenance of equilibrium. Sensory signals generated in nearly every kind of receptor are projected to the cerebellum, but none of these give rise to conscious sensory perceptions. The cerebellum functions as a special kind of computer that processes, organizes, and integrates sensory inputs and provides an output that contributes to the smooth and effective control of somatic motor function. Output systems of the cerebellum arise largely from the deep cerebellar nuclei and exert their major influences upon brain stem nuclei at multiple levels.

COMPUTERIZED TOMOGRAPHY

Several roentgenographic technics have been used to visualize structures in and around the brain. These technics have involved introduction of air or contrast media into the ventricles or subarachnoid space (i.e., ventriculography and pneumoencephalography) or injection of a water-soluble contrast media into the common carotid or the vertebral arteries (cerebral angiography; see Figs. 14-7, 14-12, and 14-13). Plain films of the head do not reveal images of the brain because of its homogeneous radiodensity. Computerized tomography, a technic capable of presenting an image of a cross section of the brain or body, uses scintillation counters rather than x-ray film and feeds data into a computer capable of direct imaging. This method uses photon detectors accurately aligned with a thin x-ray beam to provide a detailed plot of the x-ray absorption coefficients in a scanned section of the body. The scanning unit and the detectors rotate so that 180 scans are taken, each 1 degree apart. An example of a computerized tomogram in a horizontal plane and a corresponding section of the head and brain in the same plane are shown in Figures 2-30 and 2-31. In order to visualize the largest number of intracranial structures, including those in the posterior fossa, computerized tomograms often are taken in parallel planes at angles of 15 to 25° with reference to the base line of Reid (a plane established by the external auditory meati and the inferior margin of the orbit).

Computerized tomography provides a cross sectional image of the intracranial contents and the brain at multiple levels which cannot be obtained by any other technic. The method is noninvasive and has the capacity to reveal differential densities in the structural components of the brain (Taveras and Wood, '76). Because of differing absorption coefficients, the scanner can distinguish between gray and white matter.

CHAPTER 3

Spinal Cord: Gross Anatomy and Internal Structure

The spinal cord is the least modified portion of the embryonic neural tube and the only part of the adult nervous system in which the primitive segmental arrangement clearly is preserved.

GROSS ANATOMY

The spinal cord is a long cylindrical structure, invested by meninges, which lies in the vertebral canal. It extends from the foramen magnum (Fig. 1-4), where it is continuous with the medulla, to the lower border of the first lumbar vertebra (Fig. 1-7). Two enlargements of the spinal cord are recognized, cervical and lumbar, each associated with nerve roots which innervate, respectively, the upper and lower extremities (Fig. 3-1). Caudal to the lumbar enlargement, the spinal cord has a conical termination, the *conus medullaris* (Figs. 1-7 and 3-1). A condensation of pia mater, extending caudally from the conus medullaris, forms the *filum terminale*; the latter structure penetrates the dural tube at levels of the second sacral vertebra, becomes invested by dura, and continues as the coccygeal ligament to the posterior surface of the coccyx (Fig. 1-7).

While the spinal cord is a continuous unsegmented structure, the 31 pairs of spinal nerves associated with localized regions produce an external segmentation. On the basis of this external segmentation, the spinal cord is considered to consist of 31 segments, each of which receives and furnishes paired dorsal and ventral root filaments (Fig. 3-1). The spinal cord is divided into the following segments: 8 cervical, 12 thoracic, 5 lumbar, 5 sacral and 1 coccygeal. Up to the third month of fetal life the spinal cord occupies the entire length of the vertebral canal, but after that time the differential rate of growth of the vertebral column exceeds that of the spinal cord. At birth the conus medullaris is located near the L3 vertebra; in the adult it is between the L1 and L2 vertebrae, and occupies only the upper two-thirds of the vertebral canal. The sites of emergence of the spinal nerves do not change, but there is a lengthening of root filaments between the intervertebral foramina and the spinal cord which is most marked for the lumbar and sacral spinal roots (Fig. 3-2). These roots descend for a considerable distance within the dural sac before reaching their respective intervertebral foramina. Collectively lumbosacral roots surrounding the filum terminale are known as the *cauda equina* (Fig. 1-7). Spinal nerves emerge from the vertebral canal via the intervertebral foramina. The first cervical nerve emerges between the atlas and the occiput (Fig. 1-4). The eighth cervical root emerges from the intervertebral foramen between C7 and T1; all other spinal nerves emerge from the intervertebral foramina beneath the vertebrae of their same number (Fig. 3-2). Dorsal root fibers usually are absent in the first cervical and the coccygeal roots, and there are no corresponding dermatomes for these segments.

The spinal cord, like the entire central nervous system, is derived from the embryonic neural tube. The central canal, lined by ependymal cells, represents the vestigial lumen.

Topography. On the anterior surface a deep *anterior median fissure* penetrates the spinal cord almost to the gray commissure (Figs. 3-3 and 3-4). On the posterior surface of the spinal cord, is a small *posterior median sulcus*, continuous with a delicate glial partition, the *posterior median septum*, which extends to the spinal gray. Lateral to the midline posteriorly are two *posterolateral sulci* located near the dorsal root entry zones. Ascending and descending fibers occupying particular regions of the white matter are organized into more or less distinct bundles. Fiber bundles having the same, or similar, origin, course and termination are known as *tracts* or *fasciculi*. The white matter of the spinal cord is divided into three paired *funiculi*: posterior, lateral, and anterior. The *posterior funiculus* lies between the posterior horn and the posterior median septum. In upper thoracic and cervical regions a smaller, less definite *posterior intermediate septum* divides each posterior funiculus into two white columns (Figs. 3-3 and 3-4). The *lateral funiculus* lies between the dorsal root entry zone and the site where ventral root fibers emerge from the spinal cord. The anterior lateral sulcus marks the site at which ventral root fibers emerge (Fig. 3-4). The *anterior funiculus* lies between the anterior median fissure and the emerging ventral root filaments. The posterior funiculus is the largest and is composed almost exclusively of long ascending and short descending fibers

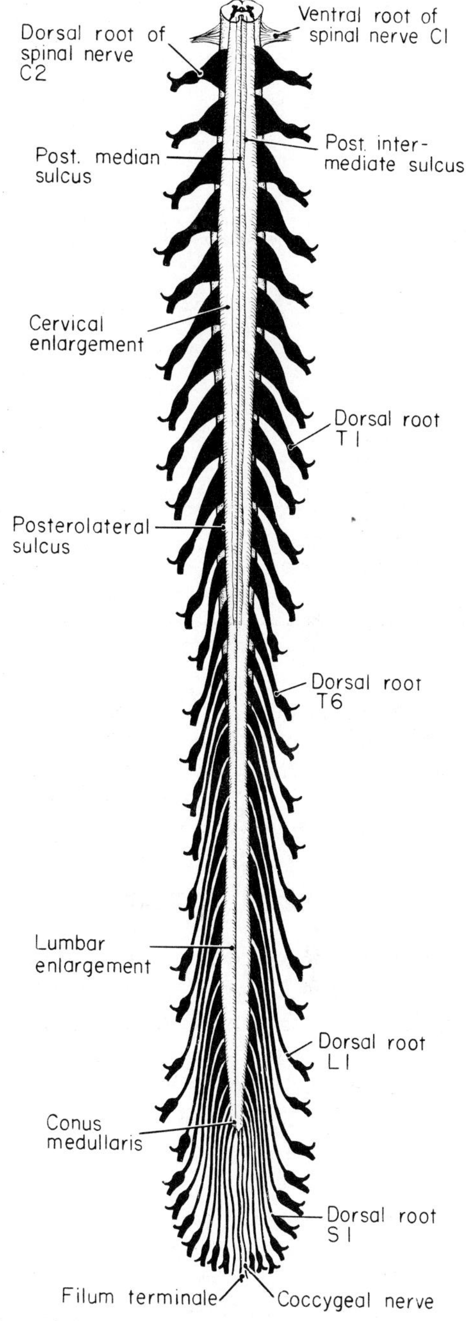

Figure 3-1. Posterior view of spinal cord showing attached dorsal root filaments and spinal ganglia. *Letters* and *numbers* indicate corresponding spinal nerves. (From Carpenter and Sutin, *Human Neuroanatomy*, 1983; courtesy of Williams & Wilkins.)

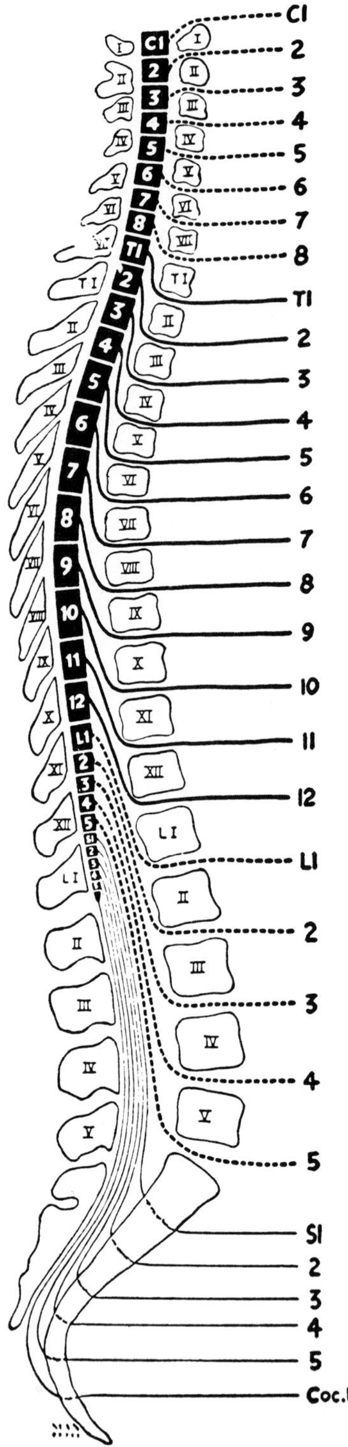

Figure 3-2. Diagram of the position of the spinal cord segments with reference to the bodies and spinous processes of the vertebrae (Haymaker and Woodhall, '45). (From Carpenter and Sutin, *Human Neuoroanatomy*, 1983; courtesy of Williams & Wilkins.)

that arise from cells in the spinal ganglia. Tracts composing the lateral and anterior funiculi are both ascending and descending. These ascending tracts arise from cells within the spinal gray, while long descending tracts arise from nuclei in the brain stem and the cerebral cortex.

The *cervical enlargement*, consisting of the four lowest cervical segments and the first thoracic segment, gives rise to nerve roots which form the *brachial plexus* (Fig. 3-1). The *lumbar enlargement* gives rise to fibers that form the *lumbar plexus* (L1 to L4) and the *sacral plexus* (L4 to S2).

Although the spinal cord constitutes only 2% of the central nervous system, its functions are of great importance since it contains: (1) afferent pathways which conduct sensory impulses from most of the body, (2) the descending pathways which mediate voluntary motor function, and (3) fiber systems and neurons which provide autonomic innervation for most of the viscera.

INTERNAL STRUCTURE

In transverse section the spinal cord consists of: (1) a butterfly-shaped central gray substance composed of collections of cell bodies and their processes, and (2) a surrounding mantle of white matter composed of bundles of myelinated fibers which are either ascending or descending in the three paired funiculi (Figs. 3-3 and 3-4). The symmetrical butterfly-shaped gray consists of cell columns which extend the length of the spinal cord and vary in configuration at different levels. Each half of the spinal cord has a *posterior gray column* or *posterior horn* which extends posterolaterally almost to the surface. An *anterior gray column* or *anterior horn* extends anteriorly but does not reach the surface. In thoracic spinal segments a small, pointed *lateral horn* is evident near the base of the anterior horn (Figs. 1-6 and 3-5). A *gray commissure*, connecting the gray substance of the two sides, encompasses the central canal.

The gray and white matter of the spinal cord are composed of neural elements sup-

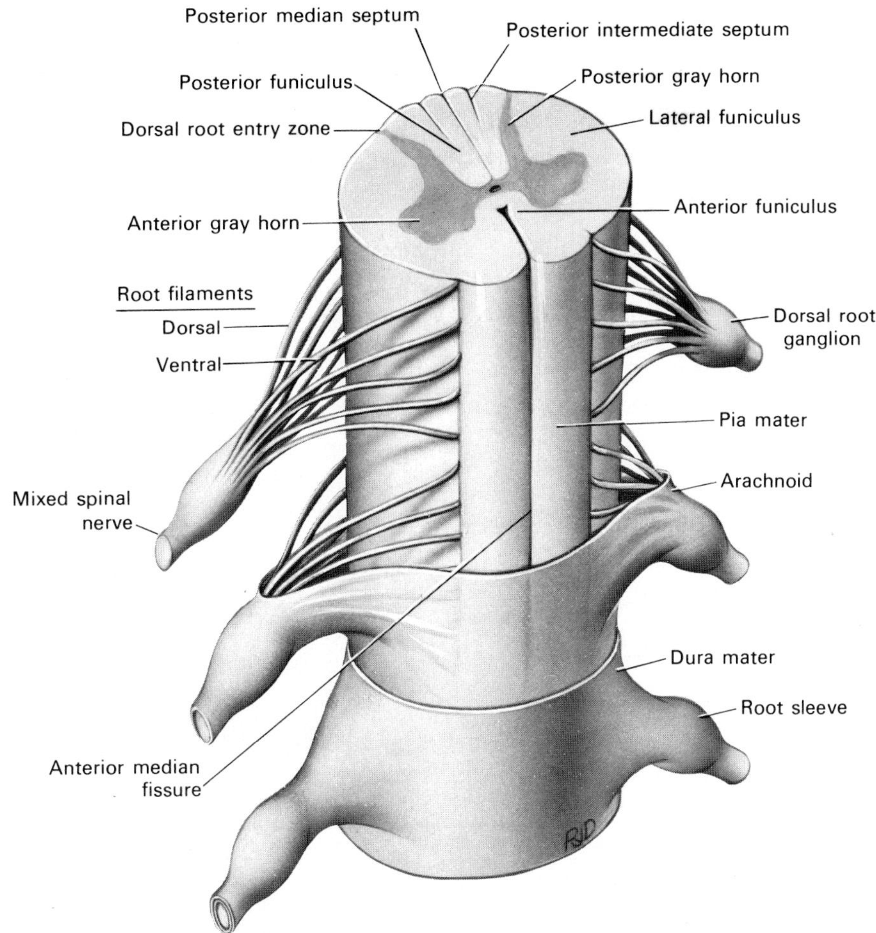

Figure 3-3. Drawing of the spinal cord, nerve roots and meninges. The blood supply and venous drainage of the spinal cord are shown in Figures 14-1 and 14-2.

ported by a neuroglial framework. Sections stained with hematoxylin and eosin, thionin, or cresyl violet reveal the cellular elements of the gray matter, but leave the fibrous elements of the neuropil unstained. Only neuronal perikarya, glia, and endothelial nuclei are stained (Figs. 3-10 and 3-12). Myelin sheath stains such as the Weigert method, Marchi method, and Luxol fast blue reveal the bundles of myelinated fibers that compose the white matter and enter and leave the gray matter (Figs. 3-8 and 3-9). Golgi silver technics reveal cell bodies and their processes in minute detail in successful preparations. Information concerning the internal structure and organization of the spinal cord has been based upon the above classic histological technics, as well as upon silver impregnation methods (Nauta and Gygax, '54; Fink and Heimer, '67). Methods utilizing the physiological property of axoplasmic transport and radioactive amino acids, the enzyme horseradish peroxidase (HRP) and a variety of fluorescent dyes have further expanded knowledge of the organization of the nervous system (Cowan and Cuénod, '75; Kooy et al, '78).

Spinal Cord Levels. Different levels of the spinal cord vary: (1) in size and shape, (2) in the relative amounts of gray and white matter, and (3) in the disposition and configuration of the gray matter (Fig. 3-5). Cervical spinal segments contain the larg-

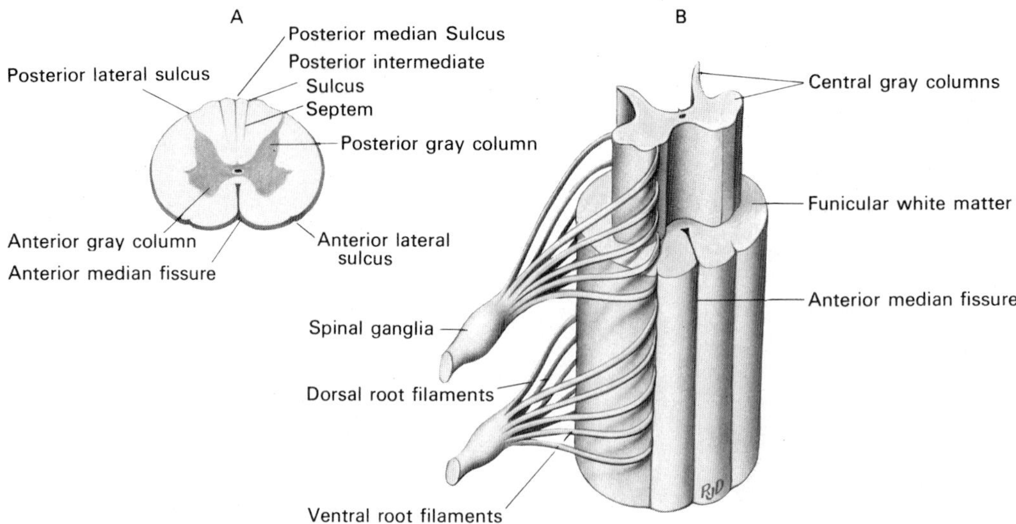

Figure 3-4. (*A*) External and internal topography of cervical spinal cord. (*B*) Diagram showing internal arrangement of gray and white matter of the spinal cord. (From Carpenter and Sutin, *Human Neuroanatomy*, 1983; courtesy of Williams & Wilkins.)

est number of fibers in the white matter because: (1) descending fiber systems have not yet contributed fibers to lower segmental levels, and (2) ascending fiber systems, augmented at each successively rostral segment, reach their maximum. The gray columns are maximal in the cervical and lumbar enlargements which are associated with the larger nerves that innervate the extremities. Lumbosacral segments contain large amounts of gray matter, relative to both the size of the cord segments and the amount of white matter.

Cervical Segments. These segments are characterized by their relatively large size, relatively large amounts of white matter, and an oval shape (Figs. 3-5 and 3-6). The transverse diameter exceeds the anteroposterior diameter at nearly all levels (Figs. 3-8 and 3-9). The posterior funiculus on each side is divided by a prominent posterior intermediate septum into a *fasciculus gracilis* (medial) and a *fasciculus cuneatus* (lateral) (Figs. 3-3, 3-4 and 3-5). In the lower cervical segments (C5 and below) the posterior horns are enlarged, and well-developed anterior horns extend into the lateral funiculi. Near the neck of the posterior horn is a serrated cellular area known as the reticular process, present throughout all cervical segments. In upper cervical segments (C1 and C2) the posterior horn is enlarged, but the anterior horn is relatively small (Fig. 3-8).

Thoracic Segments. At different levels these segments show considerable variation in size. The small diameter of thoracic segments is due primarily to a marked reduction in gray matter (Fig. 3-5). Both the fasciculi gracilis and cuneatus are present in upper thoracic segments (T1 to T6) while only the fasciculus gracilis is seen at more caudal levels (Figs. 3-11 and 3-13). The anterior and posterior horns generally are small and somewhat tapered; the first thoracic segment is an exception in that it forms the lowest segment of the cervical enlargement. A small lateral horn is present at all thoracic levels and contains the intermediolateral cell column which gives rise to preganglionic sympathetic efferent fibers (Figs. 3-11 and 3-12). At the base of the medial aspect of the posterior horn is a rounded collection of large cells, the *dorsal nucleus of Clarke* or *nucleus thoracicus* (Fig. 3-11). While this nucleus is present in all thoracic segments, it is particularly well developed at T10 through L2 (Fig. 3-13).

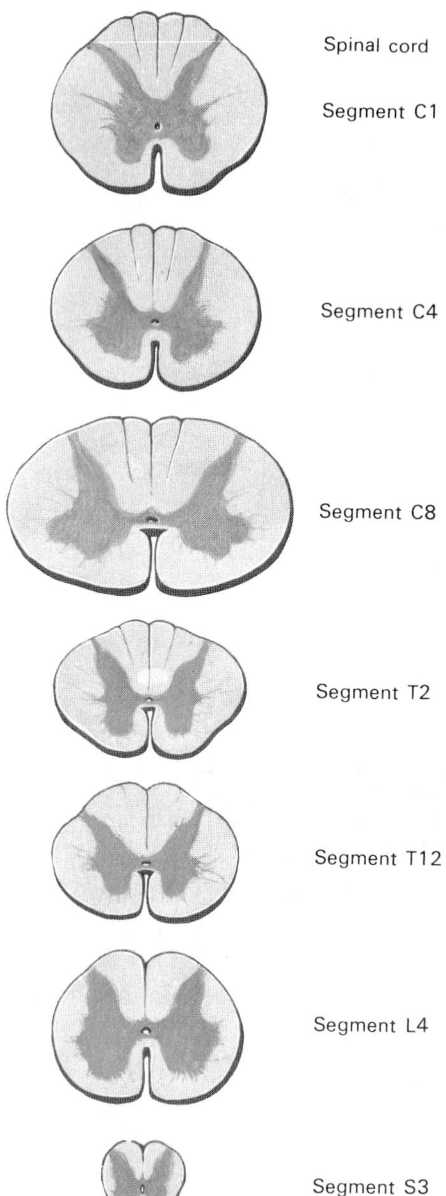

Figure 3-5. Diagram of selected spinal cord segments at different levels showing the variations in size, shape and the topography of gray and white matter.

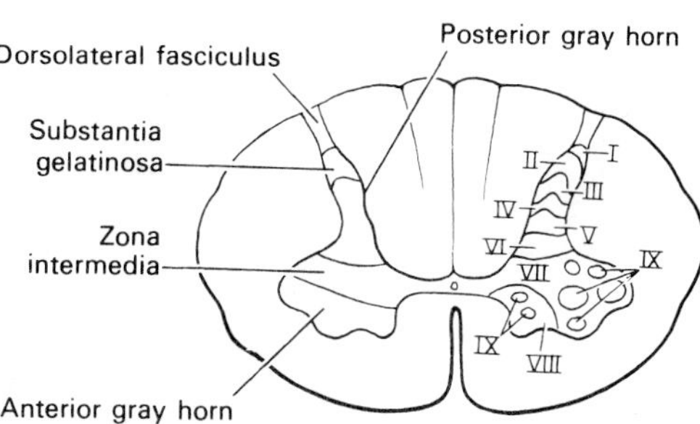

Figure 3-6. Schematic drawing through the eighth cervical spinal segment with the laminae of Rexed ('52, '54) on the *right* and more general divisions of the spinal gray indicated on the left (Carpenter, 1971; courtesy of W. B. Saunders Company).

Lumbar Segments. These segments are nearly circular in transverse section, have massive anterior and posterior horns, and contain relatively and absolutely less white matter than cervical segments (Fig. 3-5). The fasciculi gracilis which compose the posterior funiculus are not as broad as at higher levels, especially near the gray commissure, and have a highly characteristic configuration (Fig. 3-14). The well-developed anterior horns have a blunt process that extends into the lateral funiculi; motor cells in this process in segments L3 through L5 innervate large muscle groups in the lower extremities. Upper lumbar levels (L1 and L2) resemble lower thoracic spinal segments in that they contain a large well-developed nucleus thoracicus and intermediolateral cell column.

Sacral Segments. These segments are characterized by their small size, relatively large amounts of gray matter, relatively small amounts of white matter, and a short, thick gray commissure (Fig. 3-5). The anterior and posterior horns are large and thick, but the anterior horn is not bayed out laterally as in lumbar spinal segments. In caudal sequence sacral segments conspicuously diminish in overall diameter but retain relatively large proportions of gray matter (Figs. 3-16 and 3-17). Coccygeal segments resemble lower sacral spinal segments but are greatly reduced in size (Fig. 3-18). The posterior columns are not so deep and tend to spread laterally over an enlarged posterior horn.

Nuclei and Cell Groups. The butterfly-shaped gray matter of the spinal cord contains an enormous number of neurons of varying size and shape. Basically these cells can be classified as root cells and column cells. *Root cells* lie in the anterior

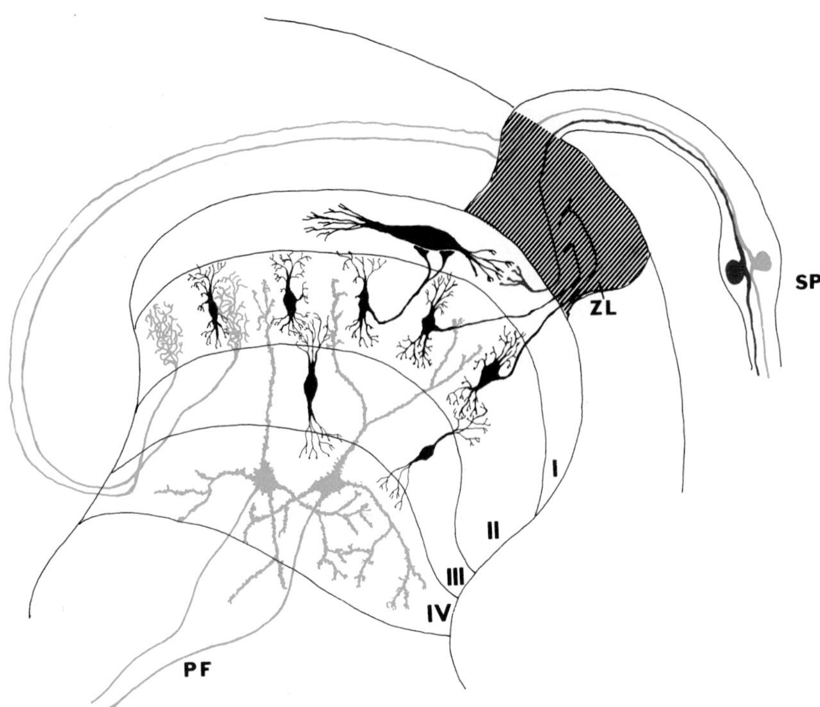

Figure 3-7. Schematic diagram of cutaneous input into the posterior gray horn. *I*, *II*, *III*, and *IV* represent laminae of Rexed; *SP* is the spinal ganglion and *ZL* (*shaded area*) is the zone of Lissauer. Primary nociceptive afferents (*red*) enter lateral parts of the root entry zone, traverse the zone of Lissauer and synapse upon distal dendrites of larger cells in the posteromarginal nucleus (lamina I). Gelatinosa neurons in lamina II provide axons, or axon collaterals, that synapse on the soma of cells in lamina I and longer axons that ascend or descend in the zone of Lissauer to ultimately return to lamina II at other levels. Non-nociceptive primary afferents (*blue*) enters as part of the medial division of root fibers by either passing medial to, or through the superficial gray laminae. These larger caliber fibers enter lamina II from its ventral aspect and end in terminal arbors near gelatinosa neurons and in relation to dendrites of large cells of the proper sensory nucleus in lamina IV. Large cells in lamina IV give rise to projection fibers (*PF*) some of which cross in the anterior white commissure and project to the thalamus. Some cells in laminae I and V also give rise to projections that reach the thalamus. (From Carpenter and Sutin, *Human Neuroanatomy*, 1983; courtesy of Williams & Wilkins.)

and lateral horns and give rise to axons which exit via the ventral root to innervate somatic or visceral effectors.

Column cells are neurons whose peripheral processes are confined within the central nervous system. On the basis of the length, course, and synaptic articulations of axons, these cells can be classified as *central*, *internuncial*, *commissural*, or *association neurons*. A relatively large number of column cells give rise to fibers that enter the white matter, bifurcate, and ascend or descend for variable distances. Some of these fibers form part of an intersegmental fiber system. Other fibers have long processes which ascend to higher levels of the neuraxis and transmit impulses related to specific sensory modalities. Nerve cells are organized in the gray matter into more or less definite groups which extend longitudinally and are referred to as cell columns or nuclei. In the neuroanatomical sense, a nucleus consists of a collection of cells with common cytological characteristics, which give rise to fibers that follow a common path, have a common termination, and subserve the same function. Most of our information concerning the structural organization of the central nervous system is centered around this concept. The spinal gray also contains Golgi type II cells whose short unmyelinated axons may be commissural,

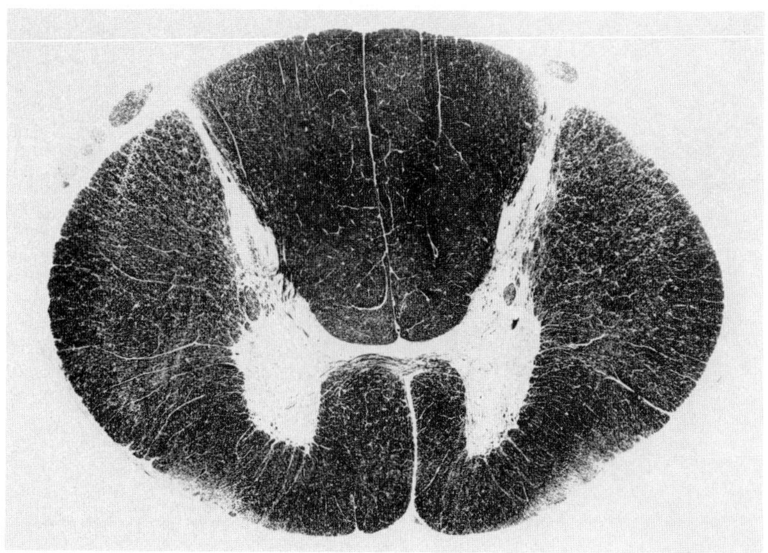

Figure 3-8. Photomicrograph of a transverse section through the second cervical segment of the adult human spinal cord. Note the narrowness of the anterior and posterior gray horns and the abundant white matter. Weigert's myelin stain. (From Carpenter and Sutin, *Human Neuroanatomy*, 1983; courtesy of Williams & Wilkins.)

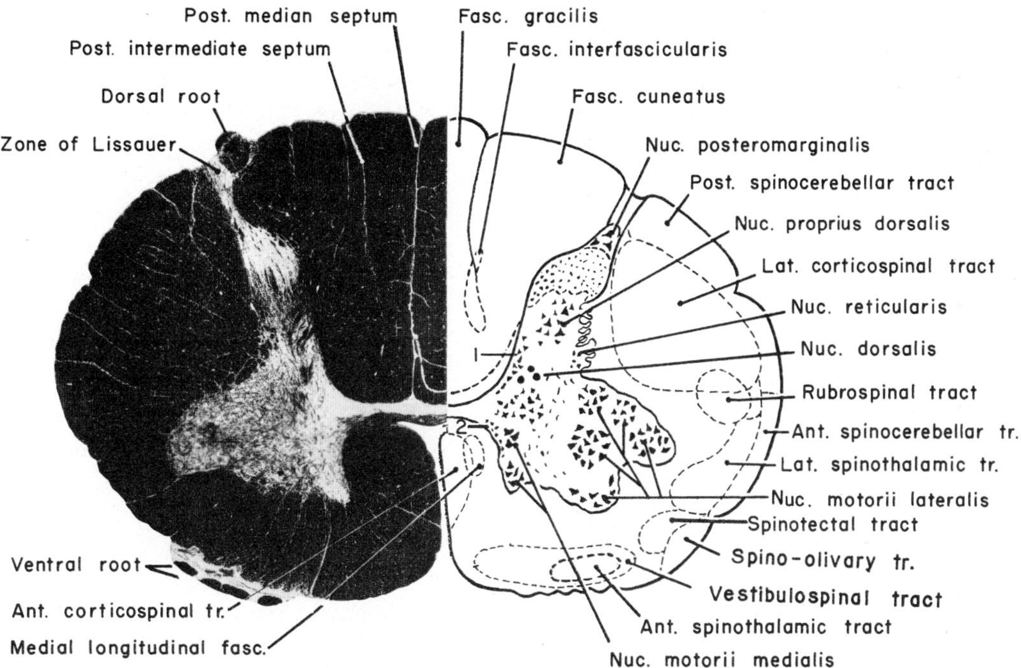

Figure 3-9. Section through eighth cervical segment of adult human spinal cord. The important cell groups and fiber tracts are identified. *1,* Nucleus cornucommissuralis posterior; *2,* nucleus cornucommissuralis anterior. (Weigert's myelin stain; photograph.) (From Carpenter and Sutin, *Human Neuroanatomy*, 1983; courtesy of Williams & Wilkins.)

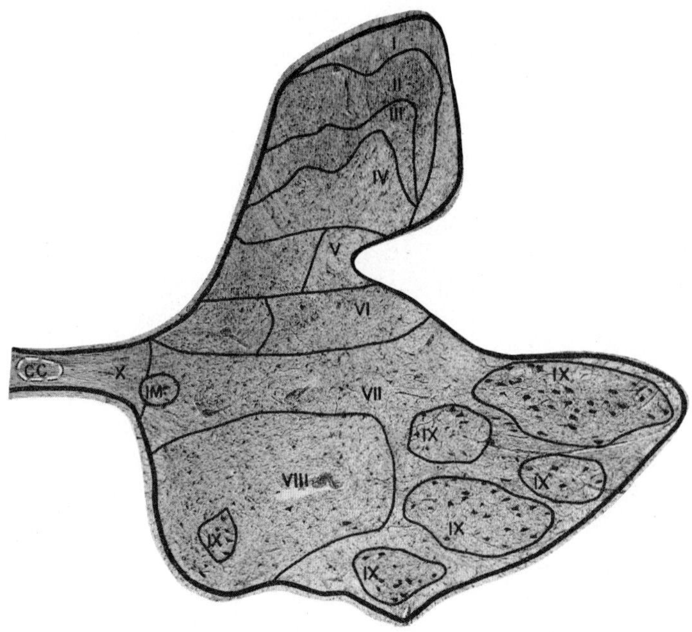

Figure 3-10. Cytoarchitectural lamination of the gray matter of the C6 segment indicated on a thick section of the human spinal cord. The central canal (*CC*) and intermediomedial nucleus (*IM*) are identified. Compare with Figure 3-9. (Thionin stain; photograph; ×9.) (From Carpenter and Sutin, *Human Neuroanatomy*, 1983; courtesy of Williams & Wilkins.)

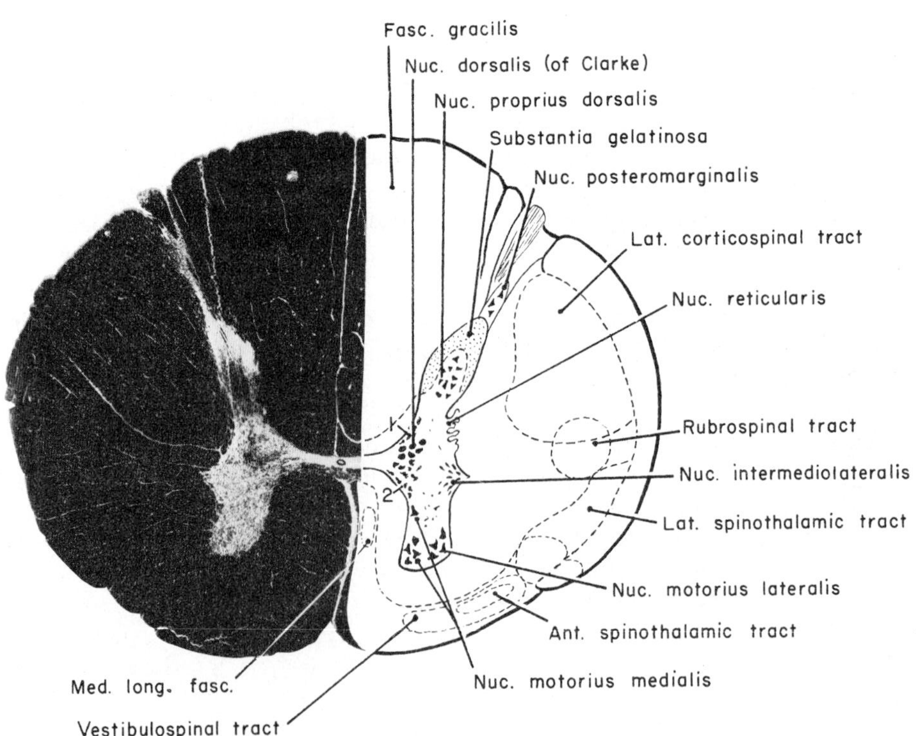

Figure 3-11. Section through fifth thoracic segment of adult human spinal cord. Important cell groups and fiber tracts are identified. *1*, Nucleus cornucommissuralis posterior; *2*, nucleus cornucomissuralis anterior. (Weigert's myelin stain; photograph.) (From Carpenter and Sutin, *Human Neuroanatomy*, 1983; courtesy of Williams & Wilkins.)

intersegmental, or terminate close to their origin.

Cytoarchitectural Lamination. A variety of inconsistent terminologies and eponyms based upon cytological features and topographical location has been used to define the nuclear groups within the spinal gray. This rather imprecise terminology largely has been replaced by a terminology based upon cytoarchitectural lamination of the spinal gray evident in thick sections (80 to 100 μm) stained with cresyl violet (Fig. 3-6). Although Rexed ('52, '54, '64) described this neuronal lamination in the cat spinal cord, it is generally accepted that a similar lamination exists in the spinal gray in all mammals. A comparable cytoarchitectural lamination of the spinal gray has been described in the human (Truex and Taylor, '68) and examples have been used to illustrate this chapter (Figs. 3-10, 3-12, 3-15, and 3-17).

Studies of the *cytoarchitectonic organization* of the spinal cord indicate nine distinct cellular laminae identified by Roman numerals and an area X, representing the gray surrounding the central canal (Figs. 3-6 and 3-10). There are differences in configuration of laminae at various segmental levels of the spinal cord. These laminae constitute regions with characteristic cytological features, but their boundaries are zones of transition where changes may occur either gradually or abruptly. While most laminae are present in some form at all spinal levels, lamina VI represents an exception in that it is absent between T4 and L2 (Fig. 3-12). Lamina VII occupies a large heterogeneous region extending across the central part of the spinal gray with boundaries that vary at different levels. In the spinal enlargements lamina VII extends ventrally into the anterior gray horn (Figs. 3-6 and 3-10), while in thoracic segments it occupies a zone between the anterior and posterior horns (Fig. 3-12), referred to as the *zona intermedia* (intermediate gray). Only the principal features of the individual lamina are described here. Some of the laminae, or cell aggregations within specific lamina, correspond to recognized cell columns or nuclei, while others are regional admixtures of cells.

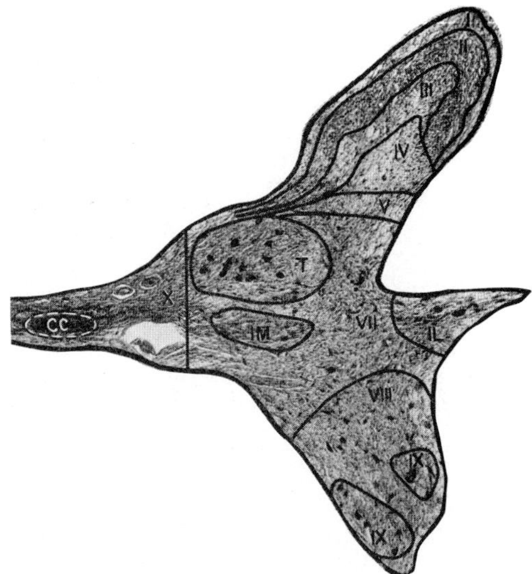

Figure 3-12. Cytoarchitectural lamination of the gray matter of the T10 segment indicated on a thick section of the human spinal cord. The central canal (*CC*), intermediomedial nucleus (*IM*) and the nucleus thoracicus (*T*) are identified. Compare with Figure 3-11. (Thionin stain; photograph; ×14.) (From Carpenter and Sutin, *Human Neuroanatomy*, 1983; courtesy of Williams & Wilkins.)

Lamina I is a thin veil of gray substance that caps the surface of the posterior horn and bends around its margins (Figs. 3-7, 3-10, and 3-12). It contains small and medium-sized cells and scattered fairly large spindle-shaped cells oriented parallel to convex surface of the posterior horn. Complex arrays of nonmyelinated axons, small dendrites, and synaptic knobs lie within this lamina which corresponds to the *posteromarginal nucleus* (Figs. 3-14 and 3-15). Axons from neurons in lamina II end axosomatically upon cells in lamina I, while primary afferent fibers terminate axodendritically upon the same cell population (Fig. 3-7) (Narotsky and Kerr, '78). A large proportion of axons from both of these sources reach lamina I via the *dorsolateral fasciculus of Lissauer* (Figs. 3-7 and 3-14). Evidence from all sources indicate that cells in lamina I respond specifically to noxious

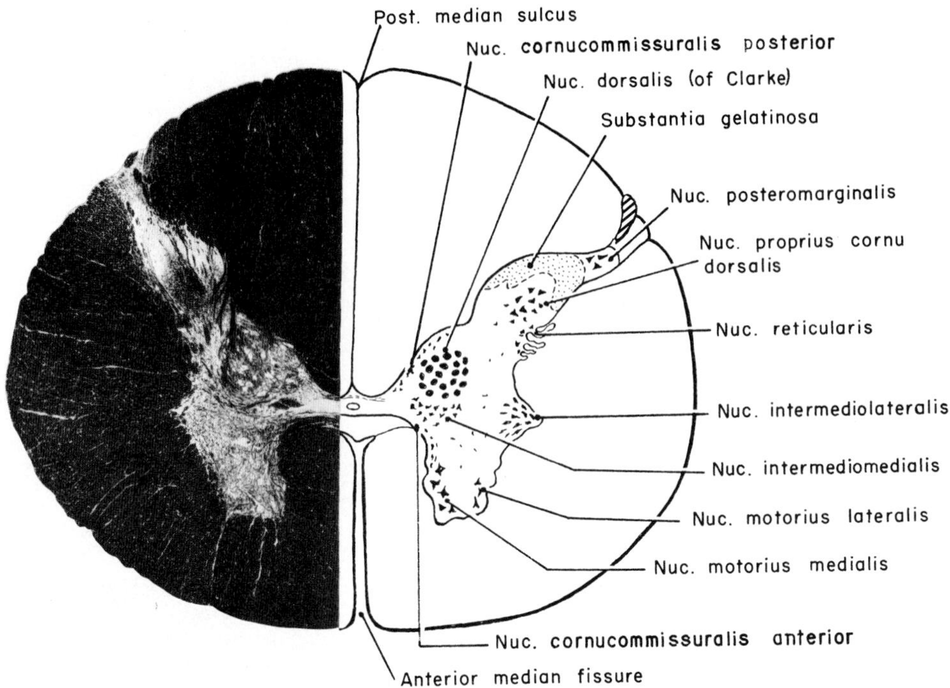

Figure 3-13. Section through the twelfth thoracic segment of the adult human spinal cord. Important cell groups are identified on the right. (Weigert's myelin stain; photograph.) (From Carpenter and Sutin, *Human Neuroanatomy*, 1983; courtesy of Williams & Wilkins.)

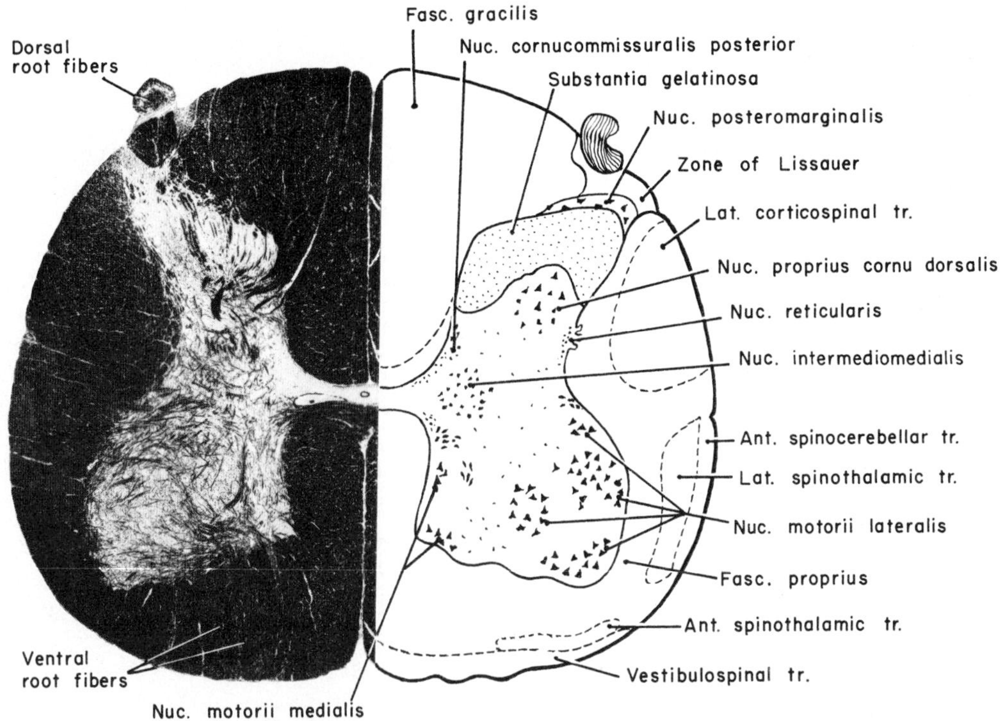

Figure 3-14. Section through the fourth lumbar segment of adult human spinal cord. The important cell groups and fiber tracts are identified. (Weigert's myelin stain; photograph.) (From Carpenter and Sutin, *Human Neuroanatomy*, 1983; courtesy of Williams & Wilkins.)

and thermal stimuli and contribute fibers to the contralateral spinothalamic tract (Willis et al., '74, '78; Kumazawa et al., '75; Trevino and Carstens, '75; Light and Perl, '79, '79a). Some cells, or dichotomizing axons of cells, in lamina I descending to other spinal segments may influence neurons involved in withdrawal reflexes.

Lamina II forms a well-delineated, fairly broad band around the apex of the posterior horn which is readily identified in cell and myelin sheath stains (Figs. 3-7, 3-9, 3-10, 3-14, and 3-15). This highly cellular band is covered dorsolaterally by lamina I, but its medial border is the posterior funiculus (Fig. 3-9). Lamina II, composed of tightly packed small cells, corresponds to the *substantia gelatinosa* of the older terminology and is found at all spinal levels. Two zones are recognized within lamina II: (1) a narrower *outer zone* was slightly smaller cells and (2) a somewhat broader *inner zone*. In both zones neurons are round or elliptical with their long axes oriented radially to the surface (Fig. 3-7). Spindle-shaped cell bodies, hardly larger than the nucleus, give rise to rich dendritic trees from one or both poles (Szentágothai, '64). The absence of discrete Nissl bodies in light microscopy is correlated with a paucity of granular endoplasmic reticulum at the ultrastructural level. Numerous bundles of unmyelinated axons in lamina II run parallel to the axis of the spinal cord and perpendicular to that axis, while myelinated axons pass radially through lamina II to deeper regions of the spinal gray.

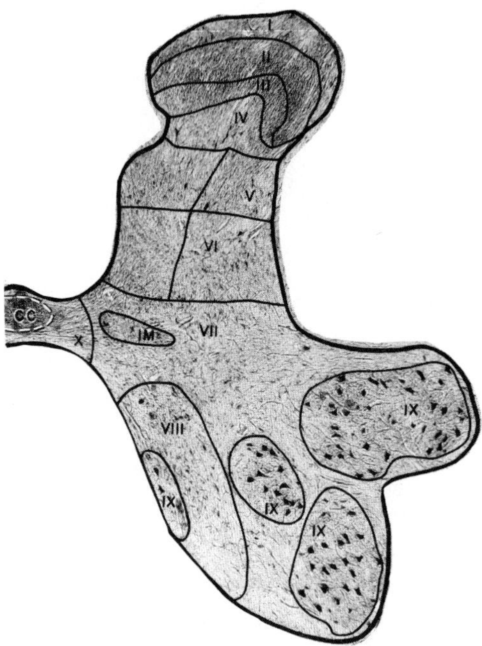

Figure 3-15. Cytoarchitectural lamination of the gray matter of the L5 segment indicated on a thick section of the human spinal cord. The central canal (*CC*) and the intermediomedial nucleus (*IM*) are identified. Compare with Figure 3-14. (Thionin stain; photograph; ×7.5.) (From Carpenter and Sutin, *Human Neuroanatomy*, 1983; courtesy of Williams & Wilkins.)

As central processes of spinal ganglion cells approach the dorsal root entry zone small, fine fibers shift to lateral portions of the rootlets while larger fibers are segregated medially. Upon entering the spinal cord root fibers bifurcate into ascending and descending branches (Fig. 3-22). Small fibers in the lateral division (Fig. 3-20), unmyelinated and poorly myelinated, contribute to the dorsolateral fasciculus of Lissauer (Fig. 3-14). These fibers occupy positions both medial and lateral to the entering rootlets. Afferent fibers to lamina II are derived from: (1) the dorsolateral fasciculus, (2) the posterior funiculus, and (3) adjacent parts of the lateral funiculus. Collateral fibers from these sources enter lamina II in a radial fashion forming flame-shaped terminal arborizations which make synaptic contacts with large numbers of neurons (Fig. 3-7). Terminal arborizations within lamina II have a columnar arrangement with little overlap. The very finest afferent fibers terminate in the outer zone of lamina II, while fine and small myelinated fibers end in the inner zone. Physiological observations on morphologically identified cells indicate that cell bodies of nociceptive and thermoreceptive neurons tend to be located in lamina I and the outer zone of lamina II, while neurons responding to innocuous mechanoreceptive stimuli are located in the inner zone of lamina II (Light et al., '79).

The majority of neurons in lamina II send axons into the dorsolateral fasciculus or the fasciculus proprius, but some form

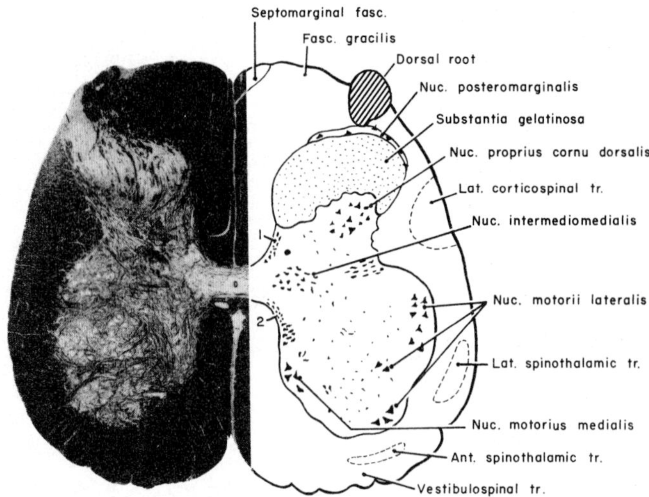

Figure 3-16. Section through third sacral segment of adult human spinal cord. The important cell groups and fiber tracts are identified. *1*, Nucleus cornucommissuralis posterior; *2*, nucleus cornucommissuralis anterior. (Weigert's myelin stain; photograph.) (From Carpenter and Sutin, *Human Neuroanatomy*, 1983; courtesy of Williams & Wilkins.)

axonal plexuses within this lamina (Fig. 3-7). Axons from cells in lamina II also have been traced into this same lamina at other spinal levels. None of the axons from cells in this lamina have been traced into other structures which could relay impulses into recognized ascending sensory pathways. Lamina II has been regarded as a "closed system," although it can influence larger neurons in deeper layers whose dendrites extend into lamina II (Fig. 3-7). Because neurons in lamina II appear organized to exert influences upon larger cells in laminae III and IV, it has been postulated that it plays a modulating role in the transmission of sensory information (Szentágothai, '64; Wall, '78).

Laminae I and II contain high concentrations of substance P (Fig. 3-21), an undecapeptide synthesized in spinal ganglia and transported to terminals of dorsal root fibers (Hökfelt et al., '75; Takahashi and Otsuka, '75). This peptide, selectively distributed in the central nervous system, has especially high concentrations in areas receiving sensory afferents. Substance P is considered to have an excitatory role in the central transmission of impulses associated with pain (Jessel and Iversen, '77). Opiate receptors which mediate all pharmacological effects of opiates are highly concentrated in laminae I and II. Unilateral section of multiple dorsal roots has demonstrated a 50% loss of opiate receptor binding sites in spinal segments on the side of the dorsal rhizotomies (La Motte et al., '76). The distribution of enkephalin, an endogenous opioid peptide, appears to parallel the distribution of opiate receptor binding sites in the primate brain (Simantov et al., '76). Thus opiate receptors and their natural ligand compose an endogenous "pain suppression system."

Lamina III forms a band across the posterior horn parallel with laminae I and II. Cells in this lamina show more variation in cell size and cells in general are larger than those in lamina II. Most of the cells are oriented vertically and their dendritic arborization extend dorsally into laminae I and II (Fig. 3-7). Axons of these neurons bifurcate a number of times and form a dense plexus in laminae III and IV. Thus, most of the cells in lamina III are anatomically organized to function as interneurons.

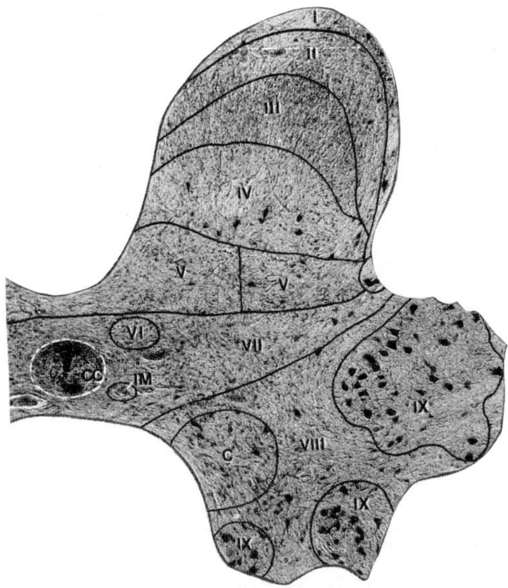

Figure 3-17. Cytoarchitectural lamination of the gray matter of the S4 segment of a thick section of the human spinal cord. Structures identified are the commissural nucleus (*C*), the central canal (*CC*) and the intermediomedial nucleus (*IM*). Compare with Figure 3-16. (Thionin stain; photograph; ×15.) (From Carpenter and Sutin, *Human Neuroanatomy*, 1983; courtesy of Williams & Wilkins.)

Lamina IV is the thickest of the first four laminae of the posterior horn. It extends across the width of the posterior horn and is composed of round, triangular or star-shaped neurons, a few of which are quite large (Figs. 3-7 and 3-9). Dendrites of neurons in lamina IV radiate upward into lamina II in a candelabra fashion parallel to primary sensory fibers and intrinsic neurons of that lamina (Szentágothai, '64). Cells in laminae III and IV correspond to *proper sensory nucleus* of the older terminology (Figs. 3-9, 3-11, and 3-13). Neurons of lamina IV respond to low intensity stimuli, such as light touch. Physiological and axoplasmic transport studies indicate that axons of some cells in this lamina cross at spinal levels and ascend to the thalamus (Trevino et al., '73; Trevino and Carstens, '75).

Lamina V is a broad zone extending across the neck of the posterior horn, which is divided into medial and lateral parts,

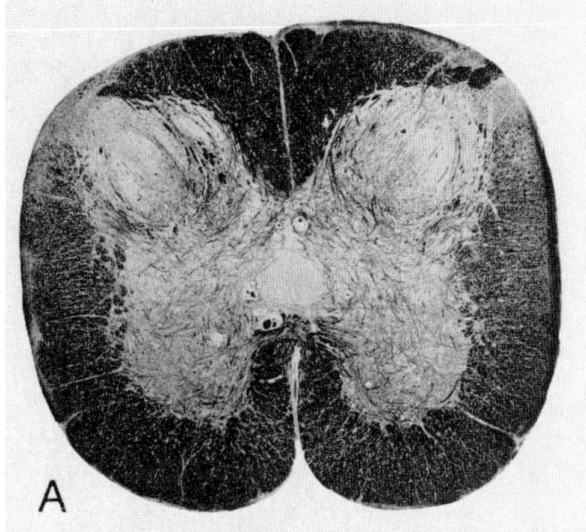

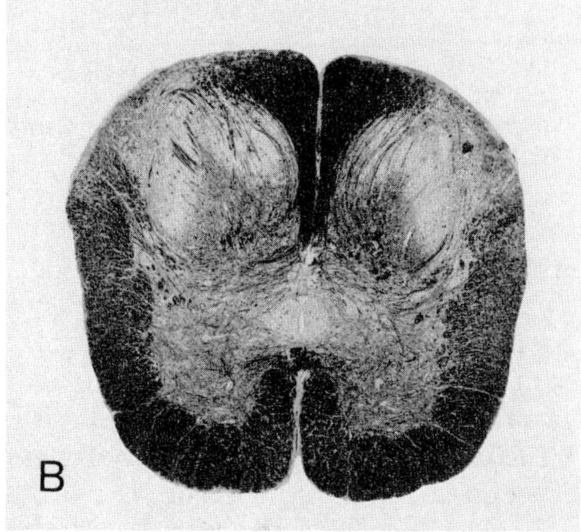

Figure 3-18. Photomicrographs of transverse sections through the fifth sacral (*A*) and first coccygeal (*B*) spinal segments of the adult human spinal cord. Note the abundance of spinal gray in the anterior and posterior horns, the thickness of the gray commissures, the size of the gray surrounding the central canal and the configuration of fasciculus gracilis. (Weigert's myelin stain.) (From Carpenter and Sutin, *Human Neuroanatomy*, 1983; courtesy of Williams & Wilkins.)

except in thoracic segments (Figs. 3-10 and 3-13). The lateral part of lamina V gives rise to the reticular process, prominent at cervical levels (Fig. 3-9). Neurons of lamina V are variable in size and shape and dendrites of some cells extend upward into lamina II where they are contacted by dorsal root fibers.

Lamina VI extends across the base of the posterior horn and is present only in the cord enlargements. This lamina is divided

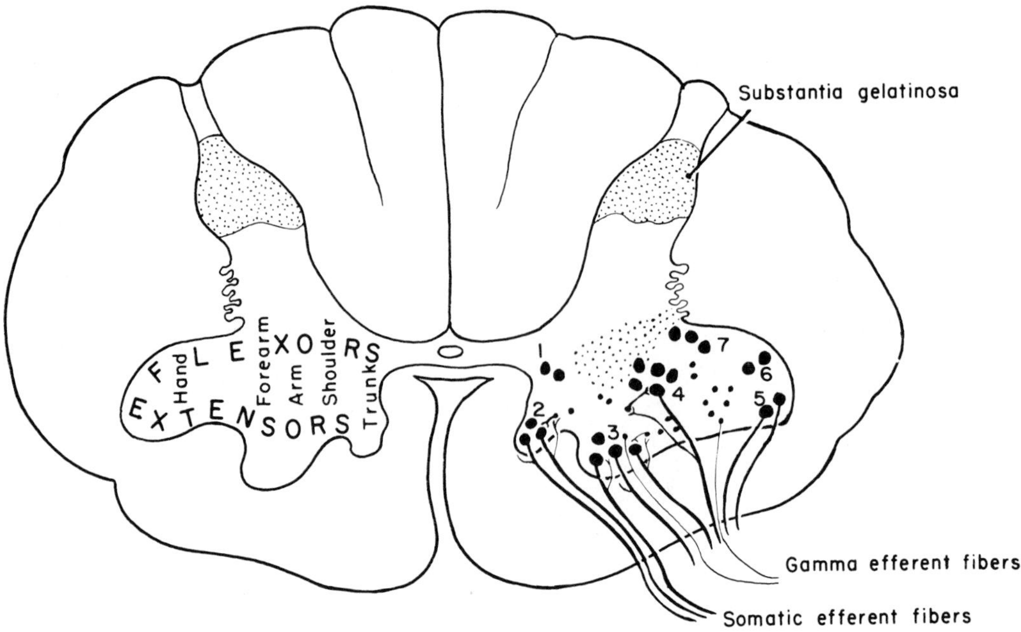

Figure 3-19. Diagram of motor nuclei in anterior gray horn of a lower cervical spinal segment. On the *left* the general location of anterior horn cells innervating the muscle groups of the upper extremity are shown. Groups of motor nuclei indicated on the *right* are: *1*, posteromedial; *2*, anteromedial; *3*, anterior; *4*, central; *5*, anterolateral; *6*, posterolateral; *7*, retroposterolateral. Smaller anterior horn cells (γ neurons) supply the intrafusal muscle fibers of neuromuscular spindle (Fig. 3-23). Note the collaterals from somatic efferent axons that return to gray matter and synapse on small medially placed "Renshaw cells." Smaller cells represented as dots in the intermediate gray (lamina VII) indicate the area of the internuncial neurons. (From Carpenter and Sutin, *Human Neuroanatomy*, 1983; courtesy of Williams & Wilkins.)

into medial and lateral regions; group I muscle afferents terminate in the medial zone, while descending spinal pathways project to the lateral zone. A cell group within lamina VI in the cervical enlargement, known as the *nucleus centrobasalis*, gives rise to an uncrossed cerebellar projection, considered by some to be the rostral spinocerebellar tract (Petras and Cummings, '77; Matsushita et al., '79).

Lamina VII, also known as the *zona intermedia*, lies between the anterior and posterior horns. The boundaries of this lamina vary at different levels; in the spinal enlargements lamina VII extends ventrally into the anterior horn (Fig. 3-6), but at other levels it forms a narrower band across the spinal gray and includes the lateral horn (Fig. 3-12). Light-staining neurons, a large number of which are internuncial, are evenly distributed in this lamina, but in particular regions well-defined cell columns are evident. Cell columns that extend for some length include the dorsal, the intermediolateral, and the intermediomedial nuclei.

The *dorsal nucleus of Clarke* (nucleus thoracicus) forms a prominent round or oval cell column in the medial part of lamina VII that extends from C8 to L2 (Figs. 3-12 and 3-13). Cells of this nucleus are multipolar or oval with large coarse Nissl granules and have characteristic eccentric nuclei. Collaterals of dorsal root afferents establish secure synapses upon cells of this nucleus at multiple levels with extensive overlap. The large cells of the dorsal nucleus give rise to uncrossed fibers of the *posterior spinocerebellar tract*. Cells in lamina VII and adjacent parts of laminae V

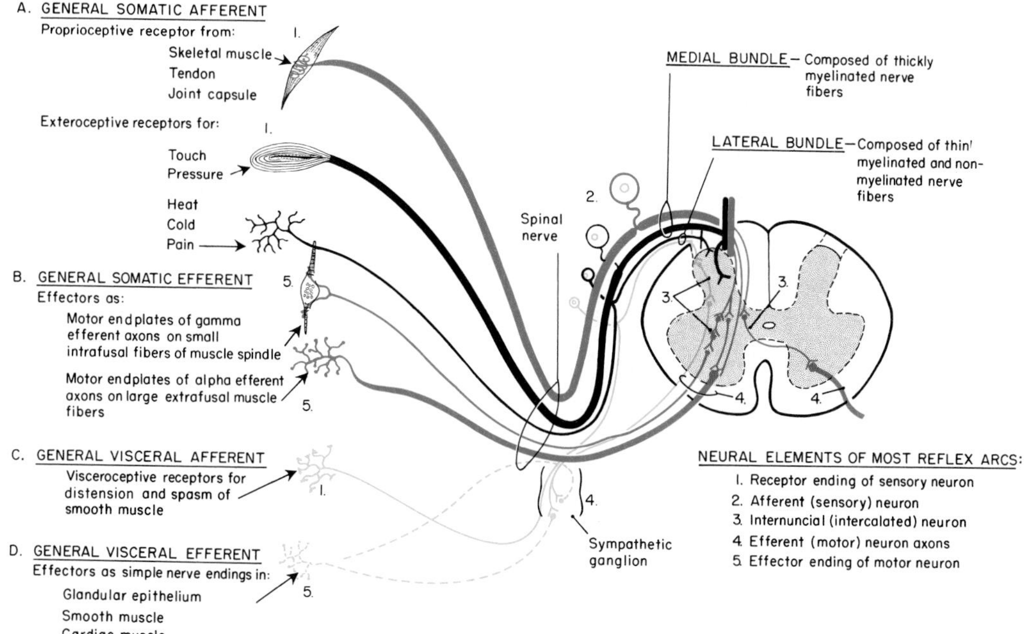

Figure 3-20. Diagram of functional components of a thoracic spinal nerve, and the arrangement of dorsal root fibers as they enter the spinal cord via medial and lateral bundles. Muscle afferent and efferent fibers are indicated in *red.* Visceral afferent and efferent fibers are shown in *blue.* An afferent fiber from a Pacinian corpuscle (*black*) and a thin pain fiber (*black*) also are shown. Numbers in the diagram correspond to neural elements that form reflex arcs. (From Carpenter and Sutin, *Human Neuroanatomy*, 1983; courtesy of Williams & Wilkins.)

and VI, which do not form a discrete nucleus, give rise to crossed fiber that form the *anterior spinocerebellar tract.*

The *intermediolateral nucleus* forms a cell column in the apical region of the lateral horn in thoracic and upper lumbar spinal segments (T1 through L2 or L3). Cells of this nucleus are spindle-shaped and give rise to preganglionic sympathetic fibers that emerge via the ventral roots and reach various sympathetic ganglia via the white rami communicantes (Figs. 3-11 and 3-12). *Sacral autonomic nuclei* occupy corresponding positions in lateral regions of lamina VII in segments S2, S3, and S4, even though no lateral horn is present. These neurons resemble those of the intermediolateral cell column, but give rise to preganglionic parasympathetic fibers which exit via sacral ventral roots and form the "pelvic nerves."

The *intermediomedial nucleus* forms a small cell column in the medial part of lamina VII, lateral to the central canal which extends the length of the spinal cord (Figs. 3-10 and 3-13). This nucleus receives small numbers of dorsal root fibers at all levels, considered to be visceral afferents (Carpenter et al., '68; Shriver et al., '68; Petras and Cummings, '72).

The *central cervical nucleus* forms an interrupted cell column in the upper four cervical spinal segments that extends into the caudal medulla. Fairly large polygonal cells of this nucleus lie lateral to the intermediomedial nucleus. Cells of the central cervical nucleus receive dorsal root fibers and give rise to a cross cerebellar projection (Matsushita and Ikeda, '75; Cummings and Petras, '77).

Lamina VIII is a zone of heterogeneous cells at the base of the anterior horn that

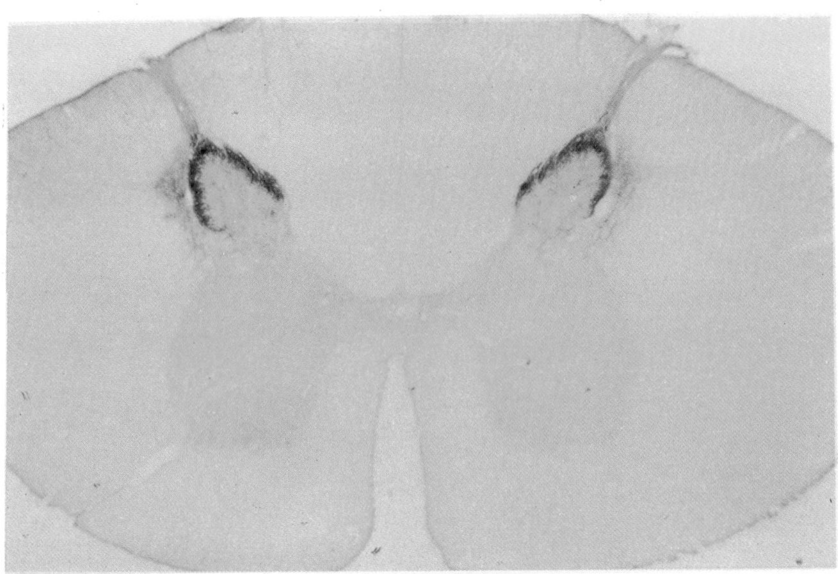

Figure 3-21. Photomicrograph of the monkey spinal cord revealing the localization of substance P in lamina I and parts of lamina II. Tissue has been treated by a immunocytochemical technic that stains substance P, which is present only in laminae of the dorsal horn that receive peripheral pain fibers. The morphine-like peptide enkephalin, also present in lamina I, may regulate the input of painful stimuli by modulating (i.e., inhibiting) the release of substance P (Jessell and Iversen, '77; courtesy of Professor Stephen Hunt, University of Cambridge). (From Carpenter and Sutin, *Human Neuroanatomy*, 1983; courtesy of Williams & Wilkins.)

varies in size and configuration at different levels (Figs. 3-6, 3-10, and 3-12). In the cord enlargements, lamina VIII occupies only the medial part of the anterior horn, but at other levels it extends across the base of the anterior horn ventral to lamina VII. This lamina constitutes a discrete entity, in part, because fibers of a number of specific descending tracts terminate upon cells within its boundaries.

Lamina IX consists of several distinct clusters of large somatic motor neurons which occupy somewhat different positions within the anterior gray horn at various spinal levels (Figs. 3-6, 3-10, 3-12, and 3-15). In thoracic spinal segments smaller islands of motor neurons occupy ventral parts of the anterior horn (Fig. 3-12), but in the cord enlargements increased numbers of motor neurons form larger and more numerous groups (Fig. 3-10). Anterior horn cells of this lamina are large multipolar neurons (30 to 70 μm) with large central nuclei, coarse Nissl granules, multiple dendrites and large axons that exit via the ventral root. Large somatic motor cells of the anterior horn which innervate striate muscle are referred to as alpha (α) motor neurons. Scattered among these large motor cells are smaller gamma (γ) neurons which give rise to efferent fibers that emerge via the ventral root and innervate the contractile elements of the muscle spindle (i.e., intrafusal muscle fibers). Gamma efferent fibers play an essential role in the maintenance of muscle tone and bring the muscle spindle under control of spinal and supraspinal influences (Figs. 3-23 and 3-24).

Anterior horn cells are organized into medial and lateral groups, each with several subdivisions. The *medial nuclear group* extends the entire length of the spinal cord and consists of posteromedial and anteromedial subdivisions (Figs. 3-9 and 3-19). The anteromedial subgroup is larger and most prominent in upper cervical, upper thoracic and in certain lumbosacral segments (L3, S4, S2, and S3). The smaller posteromedial subgroup is most distinct in the cord enlargements. The medial motor

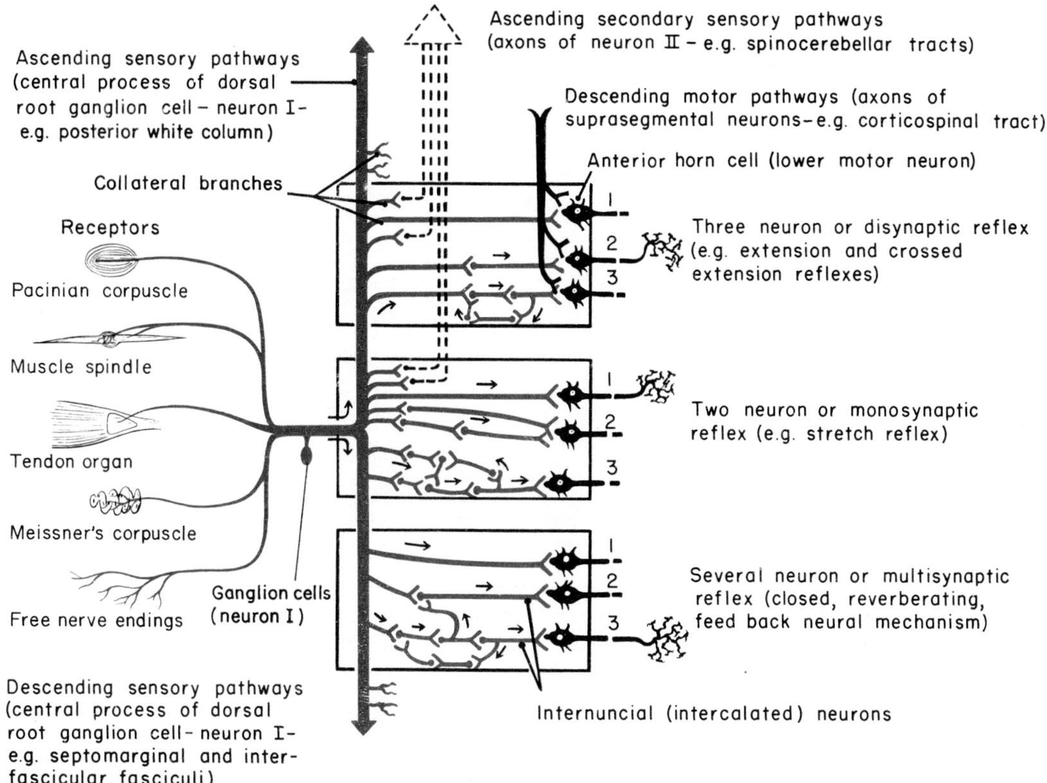

Figure 3-22. Diagram of major branches and collaterals of spinal ganglion cells within three spinal cord segments. On the left are various receptors that generate impulses in response to different kinds of stimuli. Impulses from muscle spindles initiate the myotatic or stretch reflex involving two neurons (monosynaptic reflex). Impulses from tendon organ initiate disynaptic reflex circuits involving inhibitory mechanisms. Other reflex circuits may involve many neurons (multisynaptic). Also indicated are ascending and descending branches of dorsal root fibers in the posterior white column (see Fig. 4-1) and collateral pathways that project fibers to the cerebellum (Fig. 4-5). (From Carpenter and Sutin, *Human Neuroanatomy*, 1983; courtesy of Williams & Wilkins.)

cell column innervates long and short axial muscles. Cells of the *lateral nuclear group* show considerable variations in number and size and innervate the remaining body musculature (Figs. 3-10 and 3-19). In thoracic segments a relatively small number of cells innervate the intercostal and anterolateral trunk muscles (Fig. 3-11). In the cervical and lumbar enlargements the lateral nuclear groups are enlarged and several subgroups can be distinguished. These lateral cell groups innervate the appendicular musculature (Fig. 3-19). In general the more distal muscles are supplied by the more lateral cell groups. Passing from the most medial part of the anterior horn to its lateral periphery, motor neurons successively innervate muscles of the trunk, shoulder and pelvic girdle, proximal arm and leg, and distal arm and leg (Fig. 3-19). The retroposterolateral cell groups supply muscles of the hand and foot.

DORSAL ROOT AFFERENTS

Central processes of cells in the spinal ganglia enter the dorsolateral aspect of the spinal cord in small fascicles over a considerable distance (Fig. 3-3). Peripheral processes of these cells convey impulses centrally from various somatic and visceral receptors (Fig. 3-20). As the central processes of spinal ganglion cells approach the dorsal root entry zone, small fine fibers become segregated in lateral portions of the rootlet. Larger fibers shift medially in the rootlets and enter the posterior columns or

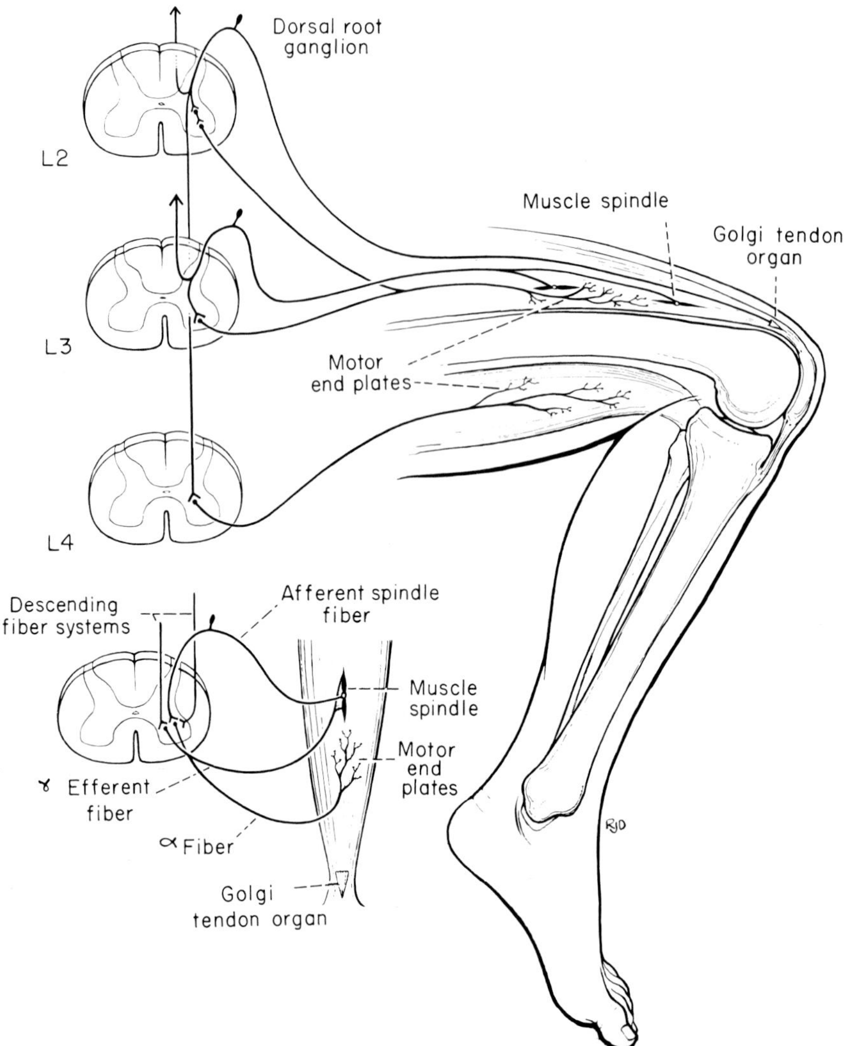

Figure 3.23. Schematic diagram of patellar tendon reflex. Motor and sensory fibers of the femoral nerve associated with spinal segments L2, L3, and L4 mediate this myotatic reflex. The principal receptors are the muscle spindles, which respond to a brisk stretching of the muscle, effected usually by tapping the patellar tendon. Afferent fibers from muscle spindles are shown entering only the L3 spinal segment, while afferent fibers from the Golgi tendon organ are shown entering only the L2 spinal segment. In this monosynaptic reflex, afferent fibers entering spinal segments L2, L3, and L4 and efferent fibers issuing from the anterior horn cells of these levels complete the reflex arc. Motor fibers shown leaving the L4 spinal segment and passing to the hamstring muscles demonstrate the pathway by which inhibitory influences are exerted upon an antagonistic muscle group during the reflex. The *small diagram below* illustrates the gamma (γ) loop. Gamma efferent fibers pass to the polar portions of the muscle spindle. Contractions of the intrafusal fibers in the polar parts of the spindle stretch the nuclear bag region and thus cause an afferent impulse to be conducted centrally. The afferent fibers from the spindle synapse upon an alpha (α) motor neuron, whose peripheral processes pass to extrafusal muscle fibers, thus completing the loop. Both α and γ motor neurons can be influenced by descending fiber systems from supraspinal levels. These are indicated separately. (From Carpenter and Sutin, *Human Neuroanatomy*, 1983; courtesy of Williams & Wilkins.)

traverse medial parts of the posterior horn (Fig. 3-20). Thus root fibers of spinal ganglia become segregated into a medial bundle of thick myelinated fibers and a lateral bundle of thinly myelinated and nonmyelinated fibers. The *medial bundle* of thickly myelinated fibers represents central processes of spinal ganglion cells conveying impulses from encapsulated somatic receptors, such as neuromuscular spindles, Golgi tendon organs, Pacinian corpuscles and Meissner's corpuscles (Fig. 3-20). The *lateral bundle* represents the central processes of smaller ganglion cells related to free nerve endings, tactile, thermal and other somatic and visceral receptors. Upon entering the spinal cord, the central processes of each dorsal root ganglion cell divide into ascending and descending branches which give rise to collateral branches (Fig. 3-22). Most of the collateral branches are given off in the segment of entry; these collaterals either participate in intrasegmental reflexes or relay impulses to other neurons. The long ascending primary branches of the medial bundle enter the ipsilateral posterior funiculus and many, but not all, fibers ascend without synapse as far as the medulla (Figs. 3-20 and 3-22). Most of the primary afferent fibers entering laminae III and IV are intermediate to thick fibers that pass through or around lamina II and after a recurving course in the gray matter approach cells in the proper sensory nucleus from a ventral direction (Fig. 3-7). Primary afferent fibers largely terminate upon dendrites of these neurons. Most neurons in lamina IV respond to low intensity stimuli, such as light touch (Price and Mayer, '74).

One of the principal sites of termination of large myelinated dorsal root fibers is the dorsal nucleus of Clarke (Fig. 3-13). This nucleus receives fibers at different levels from all ipsilateral dorsal roots, except upper cervical roots. There is considerable overlap of afferent fibers from different dorsal roots which reach the nucleus via both ascending and descending collaterals. The greatest number of afferents are related to the hindlimb. Synapses of dorsal root afferents upon the cells of Clarke's nucleus appear uniquely secure. Collateral branches of dorsal root fibers traverse central parts of lamina VII to enter laminae VIII and IX. Dorsal root collaterals from muscle spindle afferents (i.e., group Ia) projecting to lamina IX participate in the monosynaptic myotatic reflex (Figs. 3-22 and 3-23).

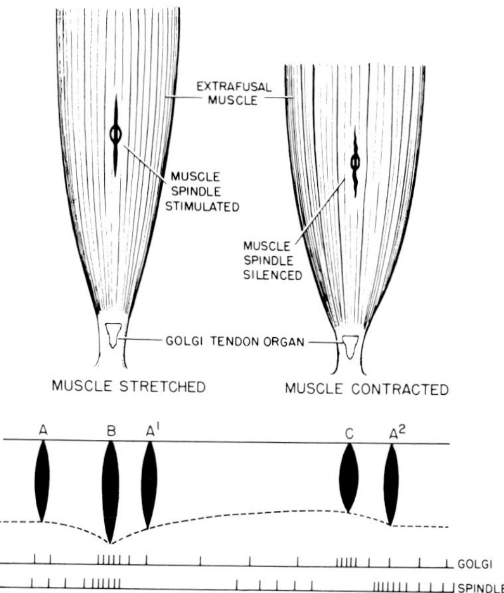

Figure 3-24. Diagram showing the anatomical and functional relationships of the muscle spindle and the Golgi tendon organ to extrafusal muscle fibers. The muscle spindles are arranged in "parallel" with the extrafusal muscle fibers, so that stretching the muscle causes the spindles to discharge. Contraction of the muscle tends to "unload" or "silence" the muscle spindles. The Golgi tendon organs are arranged in "series" with respect to the extrafusal muscle fibers. Thus, the Golgi tendon organs can be discharged by either a stretch of the tendon or a contraction of the muscle. The threshold of the Golgi tendon organ is much higher than that of the muscle spindle. The *lower diagram* summarizes the functional characteristics of the muscle spindle and Golgi tendon in relation to changes in muscle length. At *A*, the muscle is shown at its resting length, and the slow spontaneous discharge of the tendon organ and muscle spindle is indicated. At *B*, the muscle is stretched and both receptors discharge, though the adaptation of the muscle spindle is more rapid. At A^1, the muscle resumes its original length and tension, and there is a temporary reduction in the frequency of spontaneous firing of the muscle spindle. At *C*, where the muscle is contracted and shortened, the muscle spindle is silenced, but the rate of discharge of the tendon organ is increased. At A^2, the muscle is stretched out to its resting length, and the muscle spindles are therefore discharged, while the tendon organs are silenced by the drop in tension (Granit, '55). (From Carpenter and Sutin, *Human Neuroanatomy*, 1983; courtesy of Williams & Wilkins.)

The *zone of Lissauer* (dorsolateral fasciculus) lies dorsolateral to lamina I in the root entry zone and is composed of: (1) fine myelinated and unmyelinated dorsal root fibers and (2) large numbers of endogenous propriospinal fibers which interconnect different levels of the substantia gelatinosa (Ranson, '14; Szentágothai, '64). Fine thinly myelinated and unmyelinated fibers in the lateral bundle of the dorsal root, conveying impulses associated with pain, thermal sense and light tactile sense, enter the medial part of the zone of Lissauer and/or terminate directly in portions of laminae I and II (Light and Perl, '79, '79a) (Figs. 3-7, 3-14, and 3-20). Cells in lamina I and the outer zone of lamina II receive projections from cutaneous nociceptors. Primary afferent fibers terminating in the inner zone of lamina II are related to innocuous mechanoreceptors (Light et al., '79).

PAIN MECHANISMS

Pain of widely varying character and intensity constitutes one of the most common complaints in medicine, yet its nature is unresolved. Pain is a sensory experience evoked by stimuli that injure or threaten to destroy tissue which is defined introspectively by every man (Mountcastle, '74). There are two principal theories concerning pain: (1) the specific theory which considers pain a specific sensory modality and (2) the pattern theory which maintains that the impulse pattern for pain is produced by intense stimulation of nonspecific receptors (Melzack and Wall, '65). The *gate control theory*, proposed to explain neural mechanisms associated with pain, is based on three points: (1) while small diameter fibers respond only to noxious stimuli other fibers also may respond to the same stimulus, (2) spinal neurons excited by noxious stimuli may be influenced by afferents signaling innocuous stimuli, and (3) descending systems may modulate the excitability of neurons responding to noxious stimuli (Wall, '78).

The most important advance in the understanding of pain mechanisms has been the identification of opiate receptor binding sites upon synaptic membranes (Pert et al., '74). These binding sites mediate all pharmacological effects of opiates, the most powerful agents in alleviating pain. In the spinal gray opiate receptor binding sites are especially concentrated in Rexed's laminae I and II (La Motte et al., '76). The central nervous system contains endogenous opoids. Enkephalin whose distribution appears to parallel opiate receptor binding sites and β-endorphin identified from pituitary extracts. Thus opiate receptors and endogenous opiates, compose an intrinsic "pain suppression system" (Pert, '78). Opiate receptor binding sites concentrated in laminae I and II probably represent the first level at which this intrinsic mechanism can modulate pain. Enkephalin may in some fashion inhibit the release of substance P (Fig. 3-21) which is associated with the transmission of impulses related to noxious stimuli (Jessel and Iversen, '77).

SPINAL REFLEXES

Most spinal reflexes require: (1) peripheral receptors, (2) sensory neurons, (3) internuncial neurons, (4) motor neurons, and (5) terminal effectors. The *myotatic* or *stretch reflex* is a monosynaptic reflex dependent upon two neurons, one in the spinal ganglion and one α motor neuron in the anterior horn. Receptor endings in the muscle spindle responding to a brisk stretch of the muscle initiate impulses transmitted centrally to α motor neurons (one synapse involved) that cause these neurons to fire (Fig. 3-23). The result is a reflex contraction of the muscle stretched. In the illustrated example in Figure 3-23, striking the patellar tendon produces a forceful reflex contraction of the quadriceps femoris muscle and brisk extension of the leg at the knee. Afferent volleys in the femoral nerve, transmitted centrally to spinal segments L2, L3, and L4, cause α motor neurons in the same segments to discharge and produce contraction in the muscle stretched. The myotatic reflex is useful in determining the levels of motor integrity of the nervous system, but may also reveal evidence of release of higher control.

The *muscle spindle* consists of several bundles of intrafusal muscle fibers surrounded by a connective tissue capsule. The central part of this specialized structure is a noncontractile nuclear bag region. Stretching the noncontractile nuclear bag region by contraction of the polar intrafusal fibers, or stretching the extrafusal muscle fibers to which spindle fibers are attached, constitutes the mechanical stimulus required to fire the annulospiral or primary afferent fiber (group Ia) of this receptor (Fig. 3-24). Group Ia afferents from the muscle spindle make synaptic contact with the cells of the dorsal nucleus and with

α motor neurons. (Fig. 3-20). Gamma efferent fibers terminating in the polar (contractile) portions of the muscle spindle bring this receptor under the control of spinal and supraspinal influences. (Fig. 3-23).

The *Golgi tendon organs* are located in tendons close to their muscular attachments. This relatively high threshold stretch-receptor, is considered to be in "series" with the extrafusal muscle fibers, in that it can be caused to discharge by either a powerful stretch, or a contraction of the muscle (Fig. 3-24). Afferent fibers from the Golgi tendon organ (group Ib) have a disynaptic inhibitory influence upon α motor neurons. In contrast, the muscle spindle is considered to be arranged in "parallel" with extrafusal muscle fibers, in that stretching of extrafusal muscles causes the spindle to discharge while contraction of the muscle "unloads" or "silences" the spindle (Figs. 3-23 and 3-24). An anterior horn cell (lower motor neuron) may be facilitated, or inhibited, by the sum total of all impulses which impinge upon it via thousands of synaptic terminals. Such synaptic endings may be terminals of incoming sensory fibers, internuncial neurons or fibers of several descending pathways arising from higher levels of the neuraxis.

CHAPTER 4

Tracts of the Spinal Cord

Ascending and descending fibers in the spinal cord are organized into more or less distinct bundles which occupy particular areas and regions in the white matter. Bundles of fibers having the same origin, course and terminations are known as tracts of fasciculi. Since the white matter of the spinal cord is divided into three funiculi, all ascending and descending tracts lie in one or more funiculi (Figs. 3-3 and 3-4). A funiculus may contain several different tracts conducting impulses in different directions. Because fibers of certain spinal tracts are partially intermingled, or overlap fibers in other tracts, special technics must be used to demonstrate these tracts. In general, long tracts tend to be located peripherally in the white matter, while shorter tracts are found near the gray matter.

ASCENDING SPINAL TRACTS

Although dorsal root afferent fibers entering the spinal cord convey impulses from all general types of somatic and visceral receptors, the impulses transmitted rostrally in the spinal cord are segregated so that impulses concerned with pain, thermal sense, touch, and kinesthesis (sense of movement and joint position) from various body segments ascend together in more or less specific tracts, sometimes widely separated from each other. Ascending tracts not only transmit impulses concerned with specific sensory modalities that reach consciousness, but they also transmit impulses from stretch receptors and tactile receptors that project directly, or via relay nuclei to the cerebellum. The cerebellum receives sensory inputs from all types of receptors, but is not concerned with conscious sensory perception. Impulses projected to the cerebellum play an important role in the regulation of muscle tone and the coordination of motor function.

Posterior White Columns. A large proportion of the heavily myelinated fibers of the dorsal root curve medially around the posterior horn and enter the posterior funiculus (Fig. 3-20). These fibers, arising from cells of spinal ganglia at all levels, bifurcate into long ascending and short descending branches. Ascending fibers from caudal segmental levels shift medially and posteriorly as they ascend in the posterior funiculus (Fig. 4-1). Branches of fibers from cervical dorsal roots ascend lateral to those of thoracic roots. This patterned arrangement of ascending fibers produces a crude overlapping laminar arrangement in which longer sacral fibers are most medial and posterior, shorter cervical fibers are most lateral, and lumbar and thoracic fibers occupy intermediate positions. The number of ascending fibers derived from a particular root bears a relationship to the size of the root; dorsal roots of the cervical and lumbar enlargements contribute the greatest number of fibers.

The posterior funiculus on each side is divided by a posterior intermediate septum in the upper thoracic and cervical regions (Figs. 3-3 and 3-4). This septum, which becomes discernible at about T6, separates the *fasciculus gracilis* (medial) from the *fasciculus cuneatus* (lateral). The fasciculus gracilis, present at all spinal levels, contains the long ascending branches of fibers from sacral, lumbar, and the lower six thoracic dorsal roots (Figs. 3-13, 3-14 and 3-16). The fasciculus cuneatus first appears at about T6 and contains long ascending branches of the upper six thoracic and all cervical dorsal roots (Fig. 3-9). Fibers in the fasciculus gracilis and cuneatus ascend ipsilaterally and terminate upon the posterior column medullary relay nuclei, namely, the nucleus gracilis and the nucleus cuneatus. Dorsal root fibers projecting to the nuclei gracilis and cuneatus terminate somatotopically; the degree of overlap in the nucleus cuneatus is moderate, but that in the nucleus gracilis is more extensive (Carpenter et al., '68; Shriver et al., '68). The nuclei gracilis and cuneatus give rise to second order fibers which sweep ventromedially, as *internal arcuate fibers*, decussate, and form a single compact fiber bundle, the *medial lemniscus* (Fig. 4-1). The medial lemniscus ascends through the contralateral half of the brain stem and its fibers terminate in the ventral posterolateral nucleus (VPL) of the thalamus. The central processes of spinal ganglion cells which enter the spinal cord and ascend ipsilaterally in either the fasciculus gracilis or fasciculus cuneatus, depending upon the level of ganglion, constitute the first order neuron (neuron I). Fibers of the first order terminate upon cells in posterior column nuclei (i.e., nuclei gracilis or cuneatus) in the caudal medulla (Fig. 4-1). The posterior column nuclei give rise to fibers that decussate in the medulla, form the medial lemniscus, and ascend to the contralateral thalamus. Neurons in the nuclei gracilis and cuneatus (Fig. 4-1) are of the second order (neuron II).

Ascending fibers in the posterior columns and medial lemniscus convey impulses concerned with touch-pressure and kinesthesis (i.e., sense of position and movement). These fibers constitute parts of a large, highly specific sensory pathway in which single elements are responsive to one, or the other, of these forms of physiological stimuli, but not to both. Fibers of this system are highly specific with respect to place, and endowed with an exquisite capacity for temporal and spatial discrimination. These fibers convey tactile impulses for exact localization and for two point discrimination. Ascending impulses from receptors on joint surfaces and in joint capsules, which are excited by movement, convey information concerning the position of different parts of the body. Rapid successive stimuli perceived on bone or skin by Pacinian corpuscles result in a sense of vibration. "Vibratory sense" is not a specific sensory modality but a temporal modulation of tactile sense; impulses concerned with this form of temporally modulated tactile sense are considered to ascend in both the posterior and lateral funiculi.

The posterior columns also contain group Ia muscle spindle afferents and group Ib Golgi tendon organ afferents. Most of the hindlimb group I afferents ascending in the posterior funiculus project to the dorsal nucleus of Clarke (Fig. 3-13) and do not reach the nucleus gracilis (Rosén and Sjölund, '73; '73a). Muscle spindle afferents (Ia) from the forelimb project to the cuneate nucleus and are relayed via thalamic neurons to the sensory cortex. In addition the cuneate fasciculus receives group Ia and Ib afferent fibers that terminate somatotopically in different portions of the *accessory cuneate nucleus.* The accessory cuneate nucleus has cells which resemble those of Clarke's nucleus and, like that

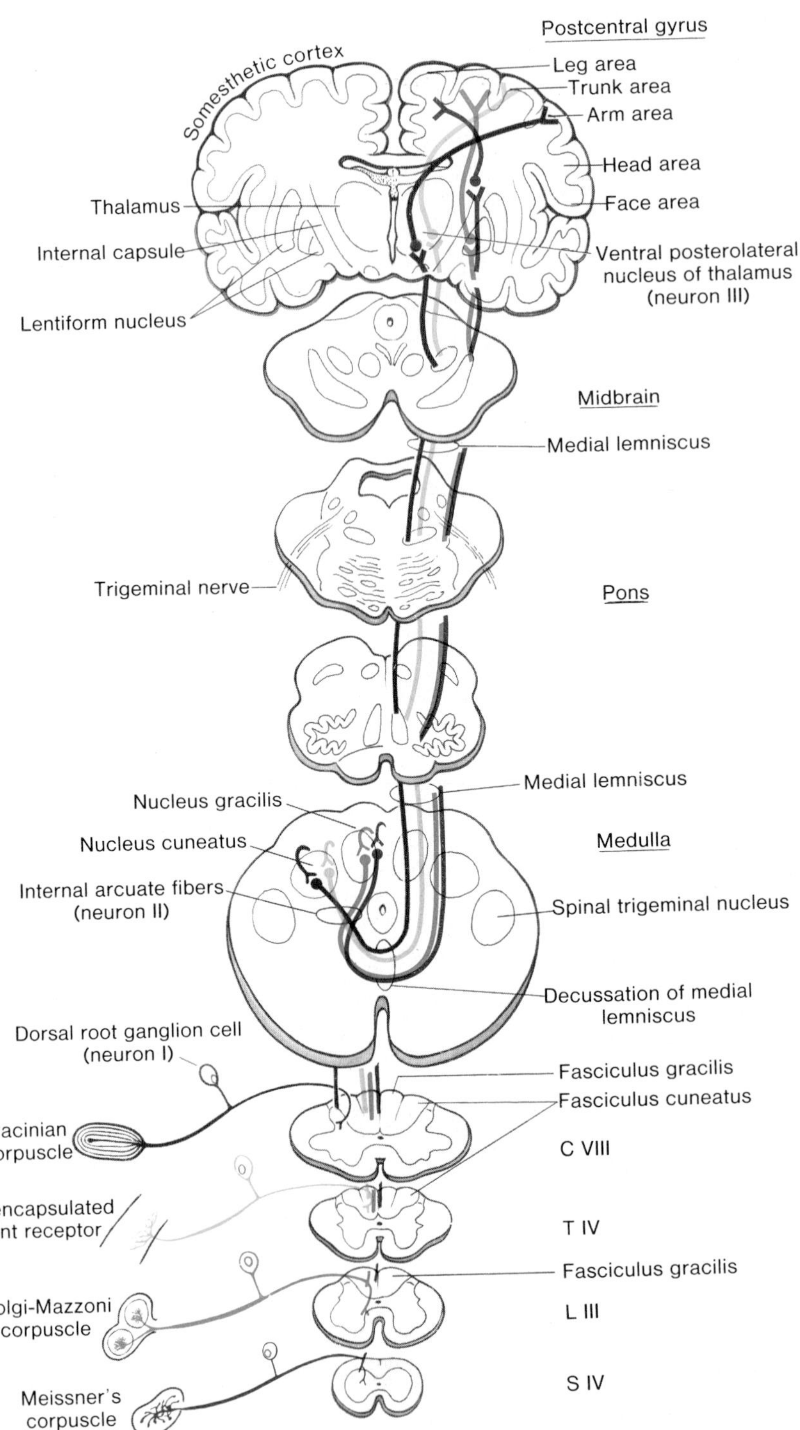

Figure 4-1. Schematic diagram of the formation and course of the posterior white columns in the spinal cord and the medial lemniscus in the brain stem. The posterior white columns are formed from uncrossed ascending and descending branches of spinal ganglion cells. Ascending fibers in the fasciculi gracilis and cuneatus synapse upon cells of the nuclei gracilis and cuneatus. Fibers forming the medial lemniscus arise from cells of the nuclei gracilis and cuneatus, cross in the lower medulla and ascend to the thalamus. Impulses mediated by this pathway largely concern discriminating tactile sense (touch and pressure) and kinesthetic sense (position and movement). Different receptors shown at various spinal levels on the left generate impulses conveyed centrally by this system. Spinal ganglia and afferent fibers entering the spinal cord at different levels (*red*, sacral; *blue*, lumbar; *yellow*, thoracic; *black*, cervical) are color coded. *Letters* and *numbers* indicate segmental levels of the spinal cord. (From Carpenter and Sutin, *Human Neuroanatomy*, 1983; courtesy of Williams & Wilkins.)

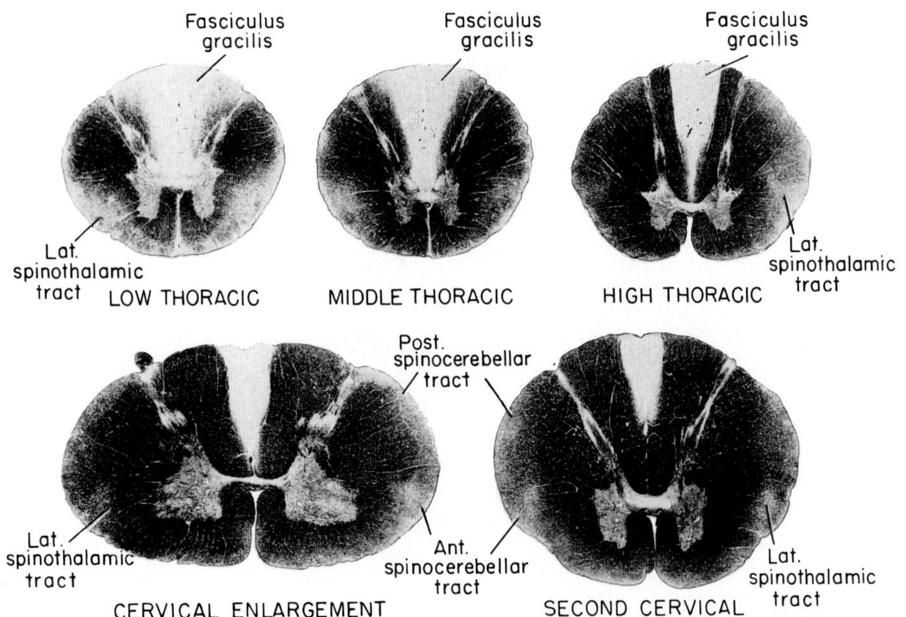

Figure 4-2. Transverse sections of human spinal cord crushed some time previously in the lumbosacral region. In the posterior white columns the progressive diminution of the degenerated area is due to passage into the gray matter of short and medium length ascending branches of lumbosacral dorsal root fibers. The progressive increase in normal fibers adjacent to the posterior horns is due to the addition of ascending branches of dorsal root fibers entering above the level of the injury. (Weigert's myelin stain.) (From Carpenter and Sutin, *Human Neuroanatomy*, 1983; courtesy of Williams & Wilkins.)

nucleus, projects fibers to the cerebellum (Fig. 5-6).

The descending branches of dorsal root fibers in the posterior columns project for variable distances. These fibers appear to terminate upon parts of the dorsal nucleus and cells in medial parts of lamina VI. Bundles of descending fibers in cervical and upper thoracic spinal segments are known as the *fasciculus interfascicularis* and in the lumbar region as the *septomarginal fasciculus* (Fig. 4-16). Cells in the posterior column nuclei also give rise to descending axons in the ipsilateral posterior columns (Burton and Loewy, '77). These fibers, which terminate in parts of laminae IV, V, and possibly I, may regulate ascending transmission of sensory information.

Lesions involving the posterior columns diminish or abolish discriminating tactile sense and kinesthetic sense. These disturbances are most evident in the distal parts of the extremities (i.e., in the digits of the hands and feet). Loss of position sense in the lower extremities, as in tabes dorsalis, greatly impairs the gait in walking (posterior column ataxia). Since a nerve fiber severed from its cell of origin degenerates, injury to fibers of the posterior columns (Fig. 4-2), or to dorsal root fibers proximal to the spinal ganglia (Fig. 4-17), will cause degeneration in the posterior white columns in a specific location depending on the level of the lesion.

Anterior Spinothalamic Tract. The spinothalamic tracts, unlike the fibers in the posterior white columns, arise from neurons within the spinal cord (Figs. 4-3 and 4-4). Although it has long been known that fibers in these tracts cross within the spinal cord and ascend to the thalamus, the cells of origin of these tracts have only recently been established. The cells of origin of the spinothalamic tracts have been identified: (1) physiologically by antidromic stimulation of the specific sensory relay nucleus of the thalamus and recording in the spinal cord (Trevino et al., '73; Albe-Fessard et al., '74) and (2) anatomically by tracing the retrograde transport of the en-

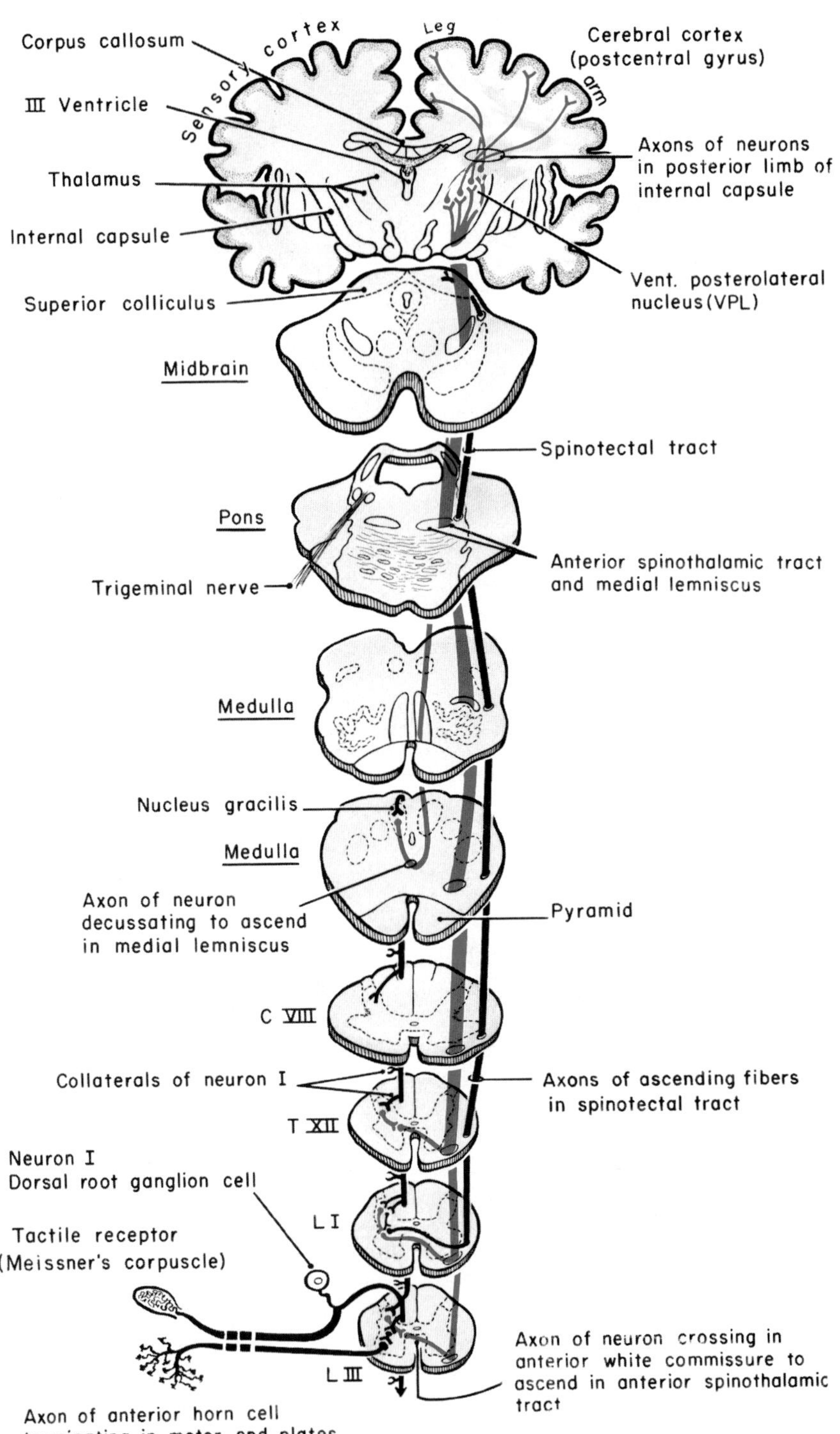

Figure 4-3. Schematic diagram of the anterior spinothalamic (*red*) and the spinotectal (*black*) tracts. These tracts arise from cells in multiple laminae of the spinal gray at all levels. The largest number of spinothalamic fibers appear to arise from cells in laminae I, IV, and V contralaterally. The anterior spinothalamic tract conveys impulses associated with "light touch," the sensation produced by stroking glabrous skin with a wisp of cotton. The spinotectal tract ascends in association with the anterior spinothalamic tract but terminates in deep layers of the contralateral superior colliculus and in parts of the periaquedectal gray; this tract conveys nociceptive impulses. *Letters* and *numbers* indicate segmental spinal levels. (From Carpenter and Sutin, *Human Neuroanatomy*, 1983; courtesy of Williams & Wilkins.)

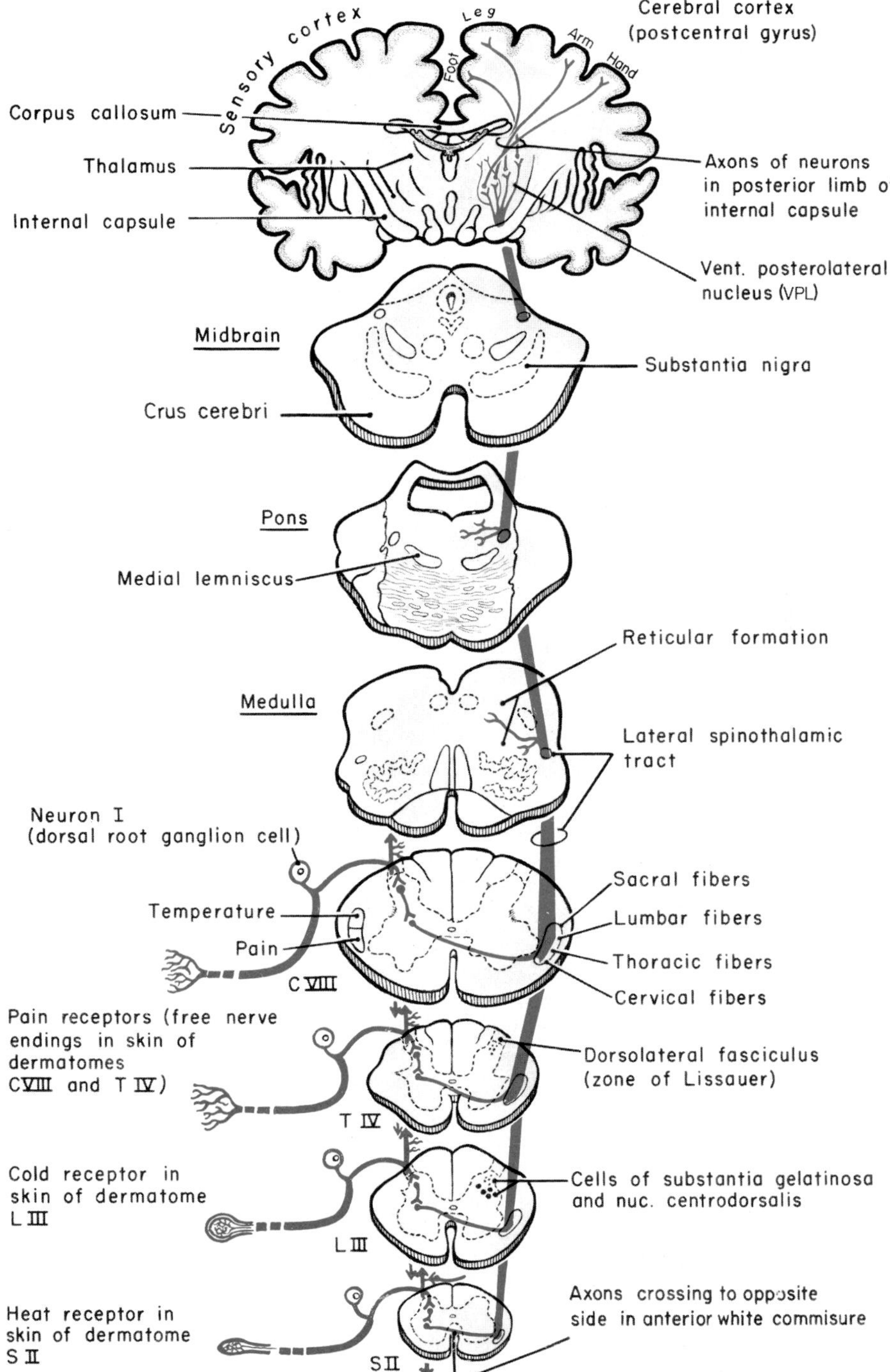

Figure 4-4. Schematic diagram of the lateral spinothalamic tract (*red*). The cells of origin of the lateral spinothalamic tract appear to be largely in laminae I, IV, and V of Rexed. Fibers of this tract cross to the opposite side within one segment in the anterior white commissure. The lateral spinothalamic tract has a more complex termination in the thalamus than indicated here, conveys impulses associated with pain and thermal sense, and has a somatotopic lamination. *Letters* and *numbers* indicate segmental spinal levels. (From Carpenter and Sutin, *Human Neuroanatomy*, 1983; courtesy of Williams & Wilkins.)

zyme horseradish peroxidase (HRP) (Trevino and Carstens, '75). These data agree that fibers of the spinothalamic tracts arise contralaterally in the spinal cord from cells mainly in laminae I, IV, and V (Fig. 3-10). In HRP studies retrogradely labeled cells are more numerous in lumbar spinal segments than in cervical segments. Details concerning the terminations of primary sensory fibers in the posterior gray horn and subsequent synaptic articulations are unclear, but it is presumed that afferent fibers (Fig. 3-7) contact dendrites of cells in laminae III and IV which extend into lamina II (substantia gelatinosa). Spinothalamic fibers cross in the anterior white commissure in a decussation that involves several spinal segments and ascend contralaterally (Fig. 4-3). Fibers forming the anterior spinothalamic tract ascend in the anterior and anterolateral funiculi and are somatotopically arranged, so that those arising from sacral and lumbar segments are most lateral and those from thoracic and cervical segments are most medial (Fig. 4-3). A small number of uncrossed fibers in this tract are not indicated in Figure 4-3.

The anterior spinothalamic tract undergoes a conspicuous reduction in size at medullary levels because some fibers, or collaterals, project to nuclei in the reticular formation. The spinothalamic component of this tract becomes closely associated with the medial lemniscus in the pons and midbrain. At midbrain levels the anterior spinothalamic tract consists of two components. Fibers of the larger lateral component terminate in the posterior thalamic nucleus and in caudal parts of the ventral posterior lateral (VPL) thalamic nucleus (Fig. 4-3). Fibers of the medial component of the tract project into the periaqueductal gray and bilaterally into the intralaminar thalamic nuclei.

Fibers of the anterior spinothalamic tract convey impulses associated with what is called "light touch"; this sensation is provoked by stroking skin, devoid of hair, with a feather or wisp of cotton. Injury to the anterior spinothalamic tract produces little, if any, disturbance because tactile sense also is conveyed by the posterior white columns.

Lateral Spinothalamic Tract. This tract is closely related to the anterior spinothalamic tract but is of much greater clinical importance because it transmits impulses concerned with pain and thermal sense. Fibers of this tract are more concentrated and contain more long fibers that project directly to the thalamus (Kerr, '75). Statements made concerning the cells of origin of the anterior spinothalamic tract apply also to the lateral spinothalamic tract. Cells largely in laminae I, IV, and V give rise to most of the axons that cross in the anterior white commissure and ascend in the contralateral lateral funiculus as the lateral spinothalamic tract (Albe-Fessard et al., '74; Trevino and Carstens, '75) (Fig. 4-4). Fibers of this tract cross obliquely to the opposite side, usually within one spinal segment. This tract is somatotopically organized in a manner similar to that of the anterior spinothalamic tract; the tract lies medial to the anterior spinocerebellar tract. There is an incomplete segregation of fibers concerned with pain and thermal sense; fibers related to thermal sense tend to be posterior to those related to pain. In the brain stem this tract sends branches into the reticular formation while the main fibers terminate in the VPL nucleus of the thalamus.

Anatomical studies of anterolateral cordotomy in the monkey based upon silver impregnation technics indicate that the thalamic projections of the spinothalamic system are far more complex than classic descriptions suggest (Mehler et al., '60). Unilateral anterolateral cordotomy produces: (1) ipsilateral degeneration in the VPL nucleus, (2) bilateral degeneration in certain intralaminar thalamic nuclei, and (3) bilateral degeneration in a posterior thalamic nucleus. In the VPL nucleus of the thalamus: (1) the body surface is represented in an orderly topographic manner, (2) cells of this nucleus are related to small contralateral receptive fields, and (3) most of the cells are not activated by noxious stimuli (Poggio and Mountcastle, '60). In the posterior thalamic nucleus there is a crude topographic representation; cells of this region are activated from large receptive fields, both ipsilaterally and contralaterally, and some cells respond to noxious stimuli.

Unilateral section of the lateral spinothalamic tract produces loss of pain and thermal sense on the opposite side of the body beginning about one segment below the level of the lesion. Even though such lesions concomitantly interrupt fibers of the anterior spinothalamic tract, tactile sense remains intact because it is transmitted centrally also by uncrossed fibers in the posterior funiculus. The position of degenerated fibers in the lateral spinothalamic tracts after a crush of the lumbosacral region of the spinal cord is demonstrated in Figure 4-2.

Spinotectal Tract. Cells of origin of the tectospinal tract are presumed to lie in the posterior horn. Fibers of this crossed tract ascend in the anterolateral part of the spinal cord in close association with the spinothalamic system, but at midbrain levels project into the intermediate and deep layers of the superior colliculus and lateral regions of the central gray substance (Fig. 4-3). The functional significance of this tract is unknown, but certain evidence suggests it may be part of a multisynaptic pathway transmitting nociceptive impulses (Mehler et al., '60). The intermediate and deep layers of the superior colliculus receive multiple sensory inputs while projections to the superficial layer are all related to the visual system (Gordon, '72; Edwards et al., '79).

Posterior Spinocerebellar Tract. This uncrossed tract, which ascends along the posterolateral periphery of the spinal cord, arises from the large cells of the dorsal nucleus of Clarke (Figs. 3-12 and 3-13). Dorsal root afferents reach the dorsal nuclei directly and after ascending and descending in the posterior columns (Fig. 3-22). The large cells of Clarke's nucleus give rise to large fibers which enter the posterolateral part of the lateral funiculus (i.e., lateral to the corticospinal tract) and ascend (Fig. 4-5). In the medulla the fibers of this tract become incorporated in the inferior cerebellar peduncle, enter the cerebellum and terminate ipsilaterally in rostral and caudal portions of the vermis. In the anterior vermis fibers end in Larsell's lobules I to IV; posteriorly fibers terminate mainly in parts of the pyramis and paramedian lobule (Oscarsson, '65).

Since the dorsal nucleus is not present caudal to L3, some dorsal root impulses from more caudal segments are conveyed by fibers in the posterior columns to upper lumbar segments and then discharged upon cells of the dorsal nucleus (Carpenter et al., '68; Shriver et al., '68). Impulses relayed to the cerebellum via the posterior spinocerebellar tract arise from muscle spindles, Golgi tendon organs, and from touch and pressure receptors. Neurons of Clarke's nucleus receive monosynaptic excitation mainly via group Ia, Ib, and group II afferent fibers. The synaptic linkage between group I afferents and the dorsal nucleus allows transmission of impulses at high frequencies. Exteroceptive impulses, also transmitted via the posterior spinocerebellar tract, are related to touch and pressure receptors in skin and slowly adapting pressure receptors in foot pads. The posterior spinocerebellar tract is somatotopically organized at spinal levels and in its cerebellar terminations. None of the impulses conveyed by this tract reaches conscious levels. Impulses transmitted by these tracts are utilized in the fine coordination of posture and movement of individual limb muscles.

Anterior Spinocerebellar Tract. This tract ascends along the lateral periphery of the spinal cord anterior to the posterior spinocerebellar tract (Fig. 4-5). The tract makes its first appearance at lower lumbar levels, and the cells of origin do not constitute a discrete entity such as the dorsal nucleus of Clarke. Fibers of the anterior spinocerebellar tract arise from cells in the base and neck of the posterior horn and lateral parts of the intermediate zone (i.e., parts of laminae V, VI, and VII) (Hubbard and Oscarsson, '62). In the cat, cells giving rise to this tract form a column extending from coccygeal and sacral spinal segments as far rostrally as the L1 segment (Grant, '62; Ha and Liu, '68). Fibers of the anterior spinocerebellar tract are less numerous than those of the posterior spinocerebellar tract, are uniformly large and are virtually all crossed. Like the posterior spinocerebellar tract, it is concerned with the transmission of impulses mainly from the lower extremity. Cells which give rise to the anterior spinocerebellar tract receive monosynaptic excitation from group Ib afferents from Golgi tendon organs whose receptive fields often include one synergic muscle group at each joint of the lower limb.

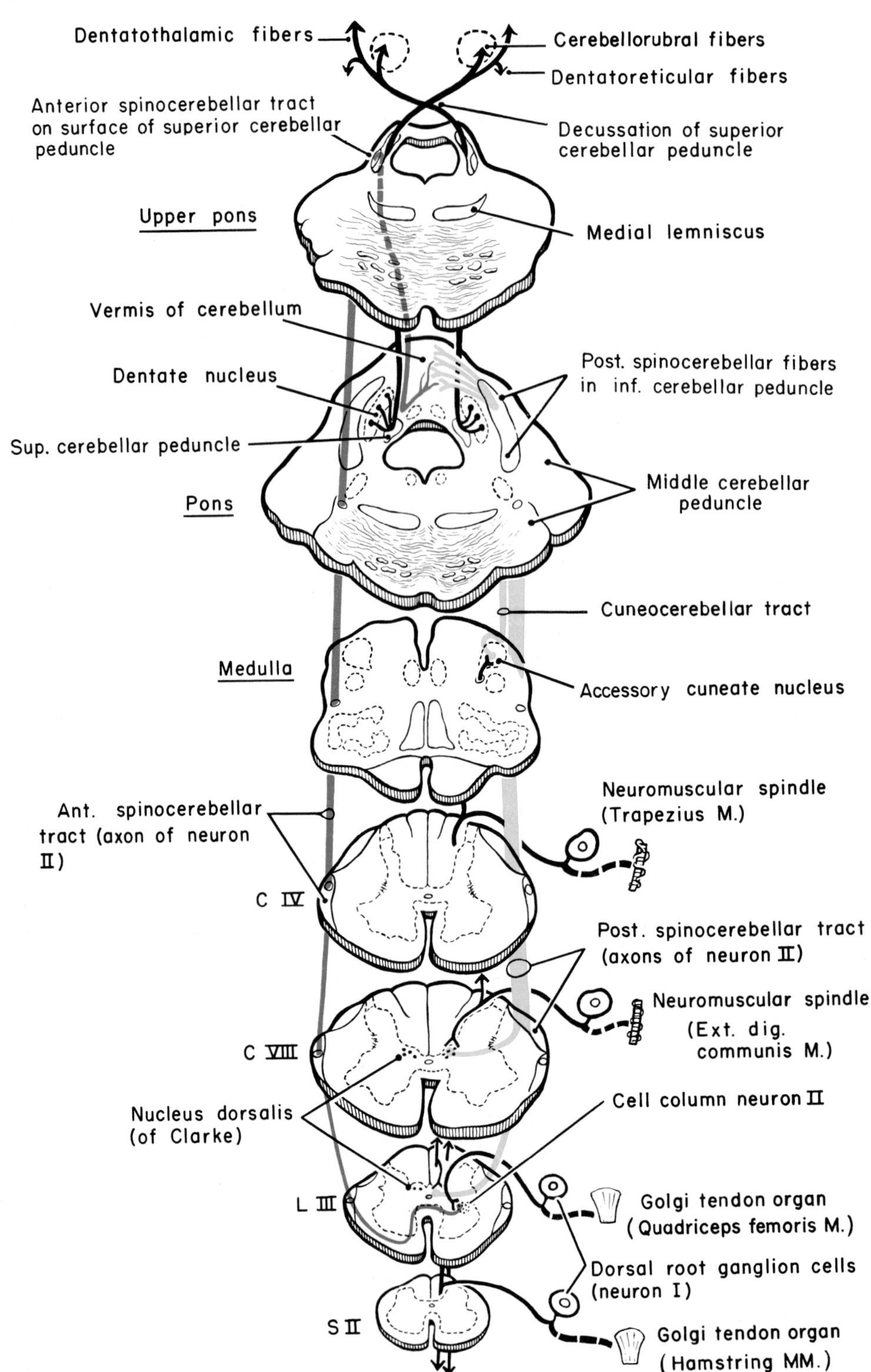

Figure 4-5. Schematic diagram of the anterior (*red*) and posterior (*blue*) spinocerebellar tracts and the cuneocerebellar tract (*blue*). The posterior spinocerebellar tract arises from cells of the dorsal nucleus of Clarke (nucleus thoracicus) and is uncrossed; it conveys impulses arising from muscle spindles and Golgi tendon organs. Fibers of the anterior spinocerebellar tract are crossed and arise from cells in parts of laminae V, VI, and VIII; fibers of this tract are activated by impulses from Golgi tendon organs. The cuneocerebellar tract, arising from cells of the accessory cuneate nucleus in the medulla, is considered the upper limb equivalent of the posterior spinocerebellar tract; this tract is uncrossed. An uncrossed rostral spinocerebellar tract (not shown) is considered the upper limb equivalent of the anterior spinocerebellar tract in the cat. *Letters* and *numbers* indicate spinal levels. (From Carpenter and Sutin, *Human Neuroanatomy*, 1983; courtesy of Williams & Wilkins.)

This pathway to the cerebellum is composed of two neurons: (1) neuron I in the spinal ganglia and (2) neuron II in scattered cell groups at the base of the anterior and posterior horns in lumbar, sacral, and coccygeal spinal segments (Fig. 4-5). Fibers of neuron II cross in the spinal cord and ascend peripheral to fibers of the lateral spinothalamic tract. At upper pontine levels the tract enters the cerebellum by coursing along the dorsal surface of the superior cerebellar peduncle. The majority of the fibers of this tract terminate contralaterally in the anterior cerebellar vermis in lobules I to IV. Fibers of this tract convey impulses concerned with the coordinated movement and posture of the entire lower limb (Oscarsson, '65).

Clinically it is virtually impossible to determine the effects of injury to the spinocerebellar tracts, because other spinal tracts usually are involved. No loss of tactile or kinesthetic sense results from such lesions, since impulses projected to the cerebellum do not enter the conscious sphere.

Cuneocerebellar Tract. Uncrossed dorsal root fibers which ascend in the fasciculus cuneatus convey impulses from muscle afferents (group Ia) and Golgi tendon organ afferents (group Ib); these fibers terminate somatotopically upon cells of the accessory cuneate nucleus (Fig. 5-6). These fibers presumably follow this course because the dorsal nucleus of Clarke is not present above C8. The accessory cuneate nucleus in the dorsolateral part of the medulla is considered to be homologous to the dorsal nucleus. Cells of the accessory cuneate nucleus give rise to *cuneocerebellar fibers* which enter the cerebellum via the inferior cerebellar peduncle (Fig. 4-5). These fibers terminate ipsilaterally in lobule V of the cerebellar cortex (Oscarsson, '65). The cuneocerebellar tract is considered to be the upper limb equivalent of the posterior spinocerebellar tract.

In the cat another spinocerebellar pathway, identified as the *rostral spinocerebellar tract,* is regarded as the forelimb equivalent of the anterior spinocerebellar tract. The cells of origin lie in the cervical spinal cord rostral to the dorsal nucleus of Clarke. The rostral spinocerebellar tract may arise from the large neurons of the centrobasal nucleus in lamina VI of the cervical enlargement (Petras and Cummings, '77; Matsushita and Hosoya, '78). The tract is uncrossed in the spinal cord, reaches the cerebellum via both the inferior and superior cerebellar peduncles, and its fibers terminate mainly ipsilaterally in lobules I to V of the anterior lobe. Another small *crossed cervicospinocerebellar tract* arises from the central cervical nucleus (C1 to C4) and conveys impulses from upper cervical spinal segments to the vestibular nuclei and the cerebellum (Matsushita and Ikeda, '76).

Spino-olivary Pathways. Spino-olivary pathways constitute another component of spinocerebellar circuitry in which impulses from the spinal cord are relayed to the cerebellum via parts of the inferior olive. The two best defined tracts are the posterior and anterior spino-olivary tracts (Oscarsson, '67, '73; Oscarsson and Sjölund, '77). Fibers of the posterior spino-olivary tract ascend in the posterior white columns and synapse upon cells of the nuclei cuneatus and gracilis which relay impulses to the accessory olivary nuclei. Multiple anterior spinocerebellar tracts ascend contralaterally in the anterior funiculus and terminate upon portions of the dorsal and medial accessory olivary nuclei. Fibers contributing to spino-olivary tracts arise at all levels of the spinal cord and are activated by stimulation of cutaneous and group Ib receptors. The accessory olivary nuclei give rise to crossed olivocerebellar fibers which project mainly to the anterior lobe of the cerebellum.

Spinoreticular Fibers. A considerable number of spinoreticular fibers, arising presumably from cells of the posterior horn (Rossi and Brodal, '57), ascend in the anterolateral part of the spinal cord and are distributed to widespread regions of the brain stem reticular formation (Nauta and Kuypers, '58). These fibers are predominantly uncrossed and terminate chiefly upon cells of the nucleus reticularis gigantocellularis of the medulla (Fig. 4-6). Spinoreticular fibers passing to pontine reticular nuclei are distributed bilaterally. A small number of spinoreticular fibers reach the midbrain reticular formation. Functionally, spinoreticular fibers represent a component of a phylogenetically older, polysynaptic

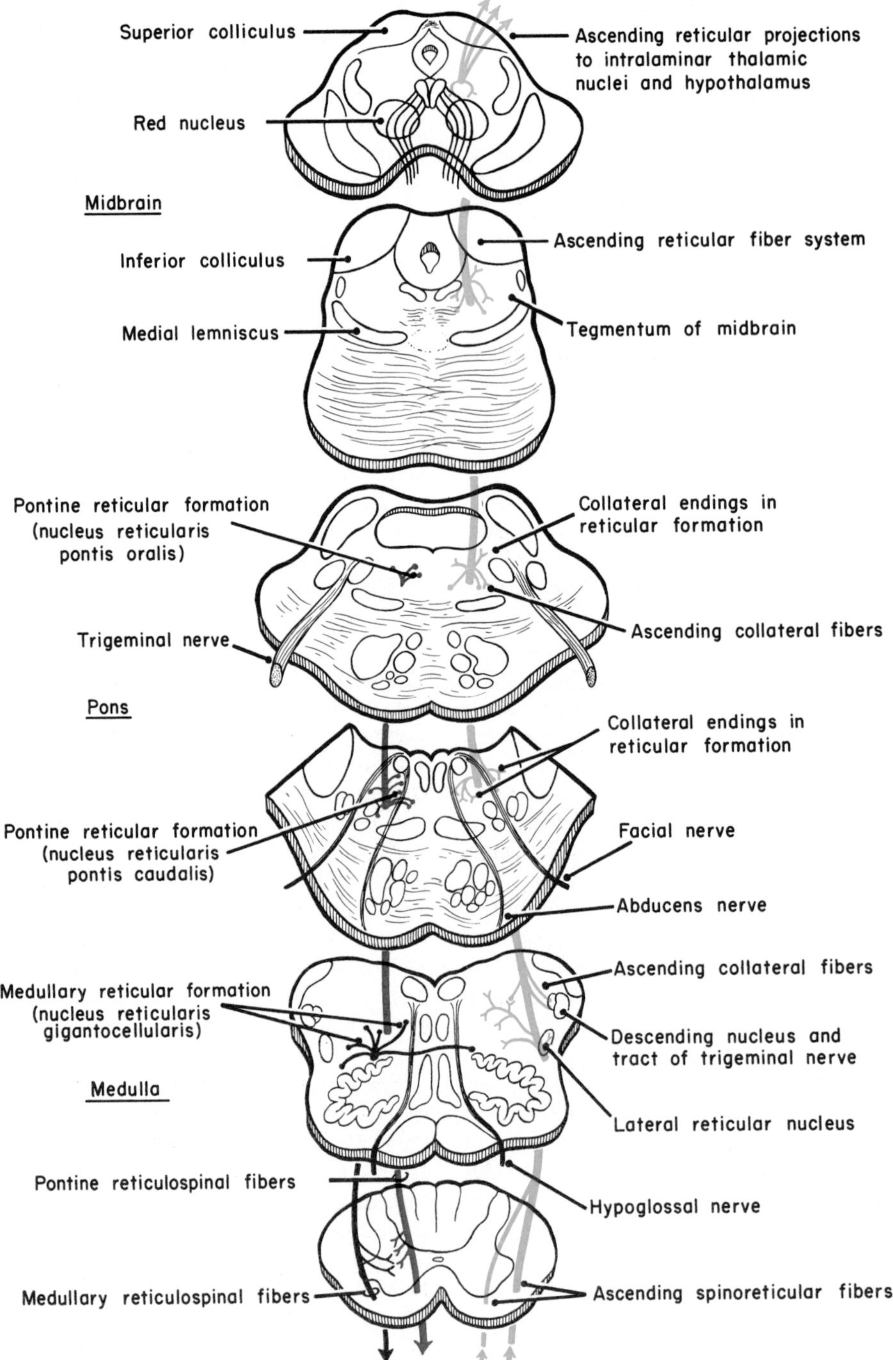

Figure 4-6. Schematic diagram of ascending and descending reticular fiber systems. Ascending spinoreticular projections and collaterals are shown on the *right* (*blue*). In this system collaterals are given off at various brain stem levels and the pathway is augmented by rostrally projecting reticular fibers. Pontine reticulospinal fibers (*red*) are uncrossed and originate largely from the nucleus reticularis pontis caudalis. Medullary reticulospinal fibers (*black*) arise from the nucleus reticularis gigantocellularis and project bilaterally to spinal levels in the anterior part of the lateral funiculi. Descending fibers from these sources are not topographically organized or sharply segregated in the spinal cord. (Based upon Olszewski and Baxter, '54; Brodal, '57; and Nauta and Kuypers, '58). (From Carpenter and Sutin, *Human Neuroanatomy*, 1983; courtesy of Williams & Wilkins.)

system, which plays a significant role in behavioral awareness and in the modulation of electrocortical activities.

Other Ascending Spinal Systems. In addition to the principal ascending spinal tracts, several small ascending spinal pathways have been described. These include (1) a spinopontine tract, (2) a spinovestibular tract, and (3) spino-olivary tracts. The spino-olivary tracts are multiple and constitute part of an indirect spinocerebellar system that conveys sensory information to the cerebellum. The functional significance of the other pathways is unknown.

DESCENDING SPINAL TRACTS

The descending spinal tracts are concerned with somatic movement (motor function), visceral innervation, the modification of muscle tone, segmental reflexes, and central transmission of sensory impulses. The largest and most important of these tracts arises from the cerebral cortex; all other descending spinal tracts arise from localized cell masses in the three lowest segments of the brain stem.

Corticospinal System. These tracts consist of all fibers which (1) arise from cells in the cerebral cortex, (2) pass through the medullary pyramid, and (3) descend into the spinal cord (Figs. 4-7, 4-8, and 4-9). At the medullary level each pyramid consists of about one million fibers; about two-thirds of these fibers have appreciable myelin sheaths. Nearly 90% of these fibers are between 1 and 4 μm in diameter; remaining fibers range from 5 to 22 μm, but only about 3.5% of these are above 20 μm. Fibers of the corticospinal tract arise from cells in the deeper part of lamina V in the precentral motor area (area 4), the premotor area (area 6) and the postcentral gyrus (areas 3a, 3b, 1, 2) and adjacent parietal cortex (area 5) (Coulter et al., '76; Jones and Wise, '77). Cells of origin are arranged in strips of clusters and vary greatly in different cortical areas (Fig. 4-7). The largest fibers arise from the giant pyramidal cells of Betz in the precentral gyrus (Fig. 13-2). These fibers converge in the corona radiata, enter the internal capsule, and descend to form the crus cerebri at midbrain levels (Fig. 2-10). As this tract descends in the ventral part of the infratentorial brain stem, its fibers pass close to the emerging root fibers of the cranial nerves III, VI, and XII. In the medulla the fibers form the massive pyramids (Figs. 5-1 and 5-5). At the junction of medulla and spinal cord, the corticospinal tract undergoes an incomplete decussation (Figs. 4-8 and 5-4) and divides into three separate tracts: (1) the large lateral corticospinal tract (crossed), (2) the small anterior corticospinal tract (uncrossed), and (3) the relatively minute uncrossed anterolateral corticospinal tract (Barnes). Between 75 and 90% of the fibers in the corticospinal tract decussate at caudal medullary levels and enter the posterior part of the lateral funiculus where they form the lateral corticospinal tract (Fig. 4-8). Fibers of this tract lie medial to the posterior spinocerebellar tract and lateral to the fasciculus proprius (Fig. 4-10).

The *lateral corticospinal tract* descends the length of the spinal cord, gives off fibers to the spinal gray at all levels, and progressively diminishes in size at more caudal levels. In lower lumbar and sacral spinal segments, caudal to the posterior spinocerebellar tract, fibers of the lateral corticospinal tract reach the dorsolateral surface of the spinal cord (Fig. 4-13). Fibers of the crossed lateral corticospinal tract enter the spinal gray in the intermediate zone and are distributed to parts of laminae IV, V, VI, and VII. In the monkey a small number of fibers end directly upon anterior horn cells or their processes in lamina IX (Liu and Chambers, '64; Kuypers and Brinkman, '70).

The *anterior corticospinal tract*, formed from a smaller portion of pyramidal fibers, descends uncrossed into the spinal cord and occupies an oval area adjacent to the anterior median fissure. This tract is distinguishable mainly in cervical segments (Figs. 4-7, 4-8, and 4-9). Fibers of this tract cross at upper cervical spinal levels in the anterior white commissure and mostly terminate in lamina VII and centromedial parts of the anterior horn.

Fibers of the *anterolateral corticospinal tract* are uncrossed, of fine caliber, and descend in a more anterior position in the lateral funiculus than those of the crossed lateral corticospinal tract (Fig. 4-8). These fibers remain uncrossed and terminate in the base of the posterior horn, the inter-

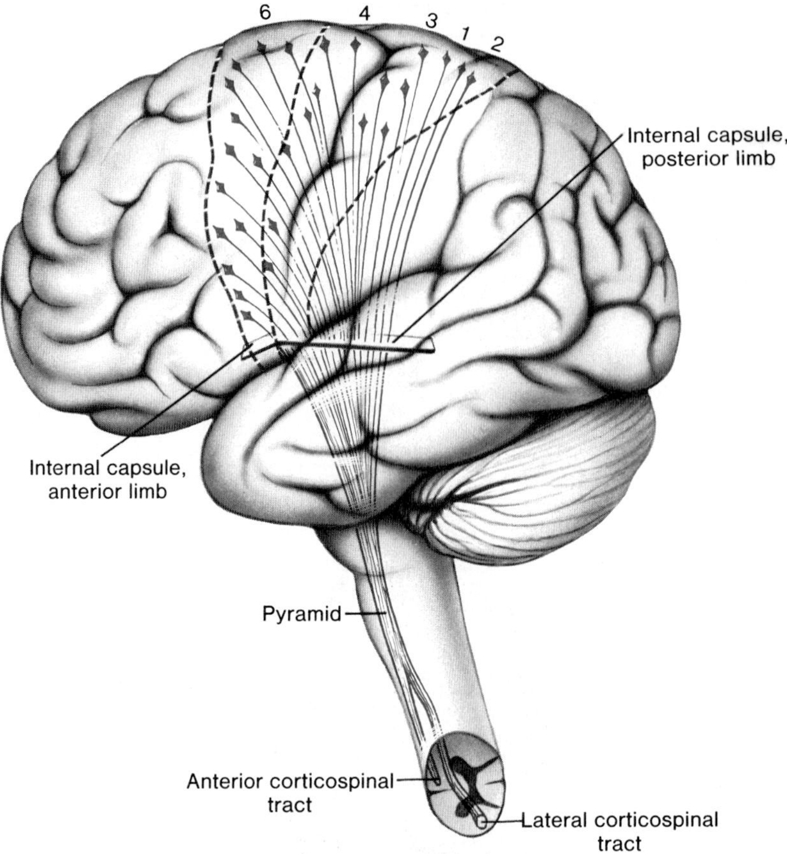

Figure 4-7. Schematic diagram of the lateral and anterior corticospinal tracts (*red*) showing their major regions of origin and the course through the internal capsule, and brain stem to the spinal cord. (From Carpenter and Sutin, *Human Neuroanatomy*, 1983; courtesy of Williams & Wilkins.)

mediate gray and central parts of the anterior horn. Demyelination in the lateral and anterior corticospinal tract can be detected readily in Weigert-stained preparations, but this stain will not reveal demyelination in the anterolateral corticospinal tract (Fig. 4-10).

Autoradiographic studies indicate that fibers from the precentral motor cortex terminate extensively in lamina VII and in dorsolateral parts of lamina IX, while fibers from somatosensory cortex (areas 3, 1, 2, and 5) terminate in overlapping zones in parts of the posterior horn (Coulter and Jones, '77). Although some corticospinal fibers establish synaptic contact with anterior horn cells, the majority terminate on internuncial neurons in lamina VII.

Estimations of percentages of corticospinal fibers ending at different levels are as follows: (1) 55% in cervical spinal segments, (2) 20% in thoracic spinal segments, and (3) 25% in lumbosacral spinal segments. The corticospinal tract is phylogenetically new, is present only in mammals and becomes myelinated in the human after birth. Myelination in the human is complete at the end of the second year.

The corticospinal tract is universally regarded as the descending pathway most concerned with voluntary, discrete, skilled movements. Lesions destroying portions of this tract at any level result in variable degrees of paresis (i.e., paralysis). Such lesions usually are associated with: (1) initial loss of muscle tone, succeeded by gradually

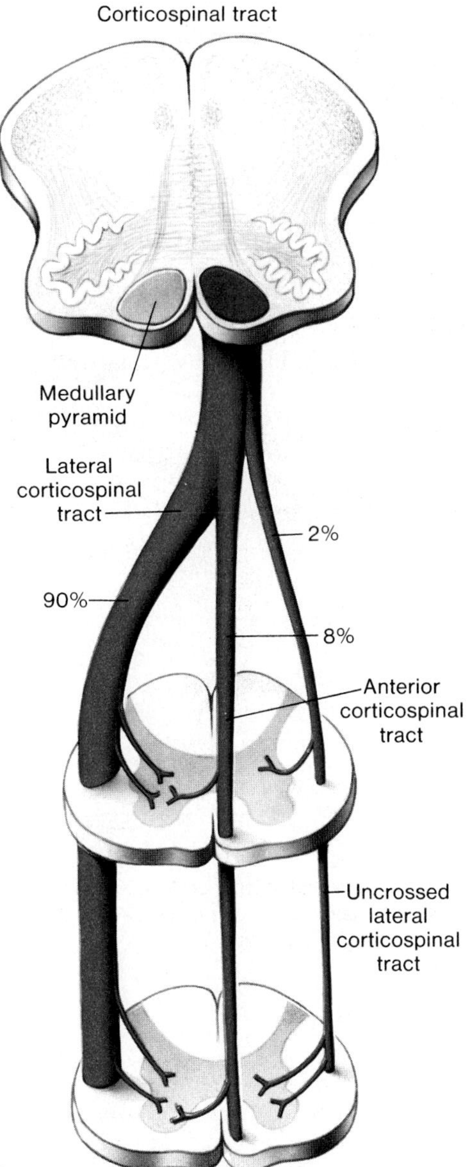

Figure 4-8. Schematic diagram of the decussation of the human corticospinal tract (*red*). Approximately 90% of the corticospinal tract crosses in the lower medulla to form the *lateral corticospinal tract.* Of the fibers which do not decussate in the medulla approximately 8% form the *anterior corticospinal tract* which descends in the anterior funiculus; most of these fibers cross in cervical spinal segments. The small number of fibers in the *uncrossed lateral corticospinal tract* (Barnes, '01) remain uncrossed. (From Carpenter and Sutin, *Human Neuroanatomy*, 1983; courtesy of Williams & Wilkins.)

increased muscle tone in antigravity muscles; (2) hyperactive deep tendon (myotatic) reflexes; (3) loss of superficial abdominal and cremasteric reflexes; and (4) the appearance of an extensor toe response (Babinski sign) on stroking the sole of the foot. The Babinski sign commonly is interpreted to mean injury to the corticospinal system, but it is not an infallible sign, for it can be elicited in the newborn, the sleep-

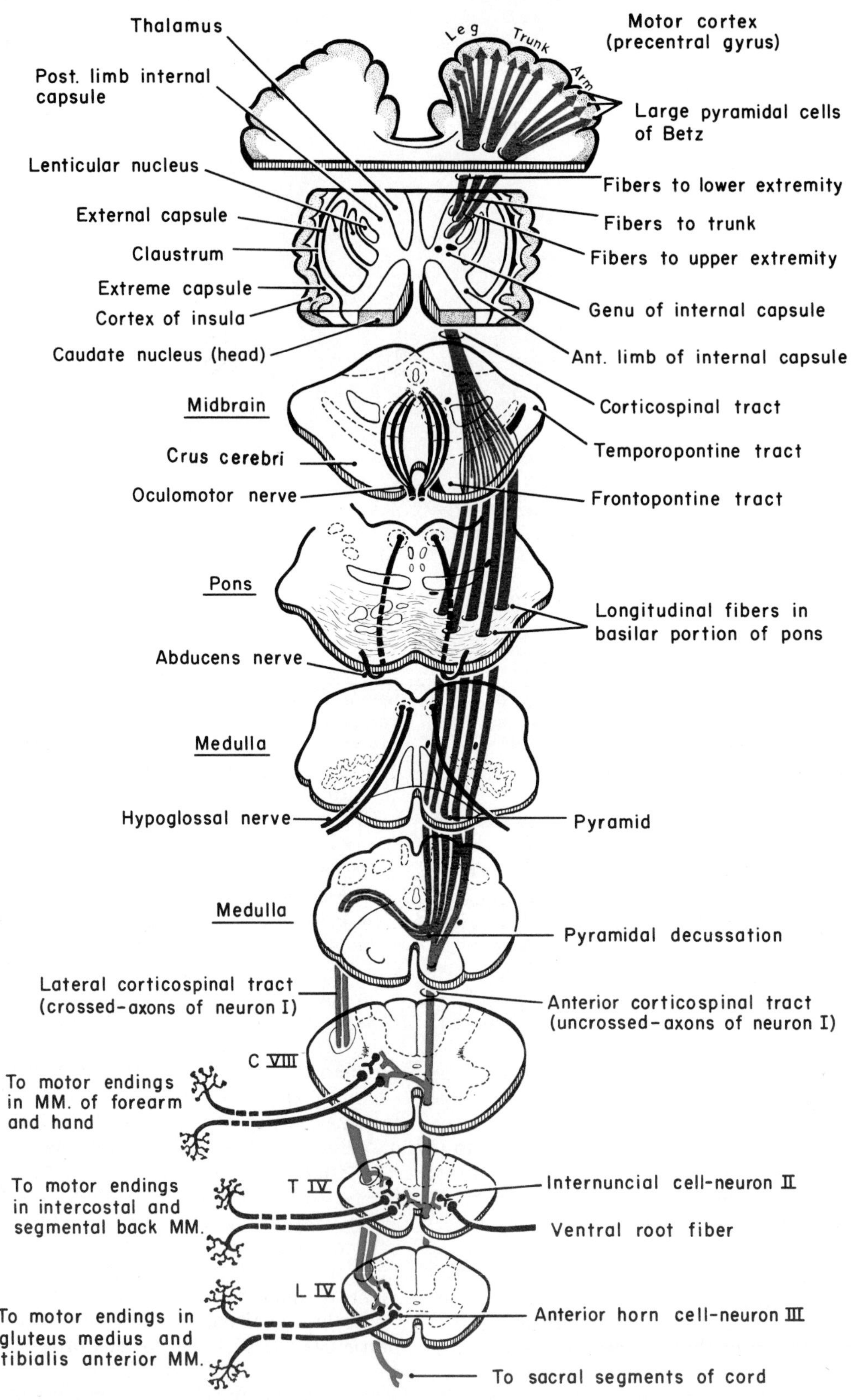

Figure 4-9. Schematic diagram of lateral and anterior corticospinal tracts—the principal descending motor pathway concerned with skilled, voluntary motor activity. The locations of the corticobulbar tracts at each level of the brain stem are indicated by *black areas* (*right side*). *Letters* and *numbers* indicate corresponding segments of the spinal cord. (From Carpenter and Sutin, *Human Neuroanatomy*, 1983; courtesy of Williams & Wilkins.)

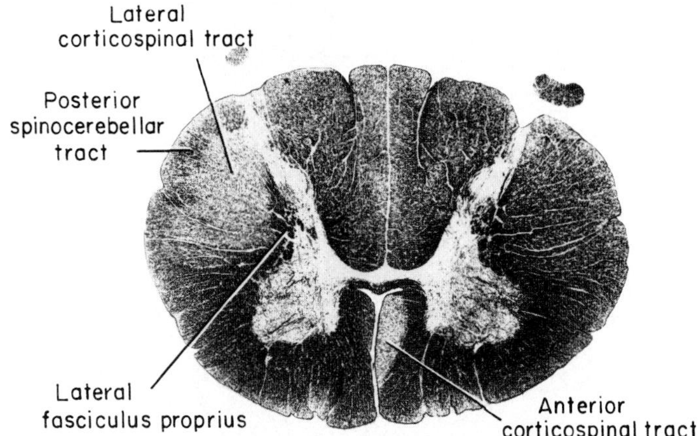

Figure 4-10. Transverse section through the cervical enlargement of an individual sustaining a vascular lesion of one medullary pyramid. The lateral corticospinal tract on the left and the anterior corticospinal tract on the side of the lesion are degenerated and demyelinated. (Weigert's myelin stain; photograph.) (From Carpenter and Sutin, *Human Neuroanatomy*, 1983; courtesy of Williams & Wilkins.)

ing or intoxicated adult, or following a generalized seizure.

Paralysis of both arm and leg on the same side is termed *hemiplegia.* The term *paraplegia* denotes paralysis of both legs, while *quadraplegia* refers to paralysis of all four extremities.

All major descending spinal tracts, other than the corticospinal tract, arise from the brain stem. Three descending spinal tracts arise from the midbrain. These are the tectospinal, interstitiospinal, and rubrospinal tracts.

Tectospinal Tract. Fibers of this tract arise from cells in the deeper layers of the superior colliculus, sweep anteromedially about the periaqueductal gray, and cross the median raphe anterior to the medial longitudinal fasciculus (Fig. 4-11). These fibers cross in the *dorsal tegmental decussation*, and descend near the median raphe anterior to the medial longitudinal fasciculus. At medullary levels tectospinal fibers become incorporated in the medial longitudinal fasciculus (abbreviated MLF). In the spinal cord tectospinal fibers, located in the most anterior part of the anterior funiculus near the anterior median fissure, descend only through cervical levels (Fig. 4-11). The majority of the fibers terminate in the upper four cervical segments (Altman and Carpenter, '61). Tectospinal fibers enter the ventromedial part of the anterior horn and terminate in laminae VIII, VII, and parts of VI (Nyberg-Hansen, '66). None of these fibers end directly upon alpha motor neurons. It is presumed that the tectospinal tract mediates reflex postural movements in response to visual, and perhaps auditory, stimuli.

Rubrospinal Tract. Fibers of this tract arise from the red nucleus, an oval cell mass in the central part of the midbrain tegmentum (Fig. 4-11). The red nucleus usually is divided into a rostral parvocellular part and a caudal magnocellular part, which vary in size in different animals. In the cat the rubrospinal tract arises from cells of all sizes in the caudal three-fourths of the red nucleus (Pompeiano and Brodal, '57). In the monkey the rubrospinal tract arises from the magnocellular region which occupies the caudal third of the nucleus (Poirier and Bouvier, '66, Kuypers and Lawrence, '67). Rubrospinal fibers cross completely in the *ventral tegmental decussation* and descend to spinal levels where they lie anterior to, and partially intermingled with, fibers of the corticospinal tract (Fig. 4-11). Fibers of the rubrospinal tract are somatotopically organized, meaning that cells in particular parts of the nucleus project selectively to defined spinal levels. Fibers projecting to cervical spinal segments arise from dorsal and dorsomedial parts of the red nucleus, while fibers projecting to lum-

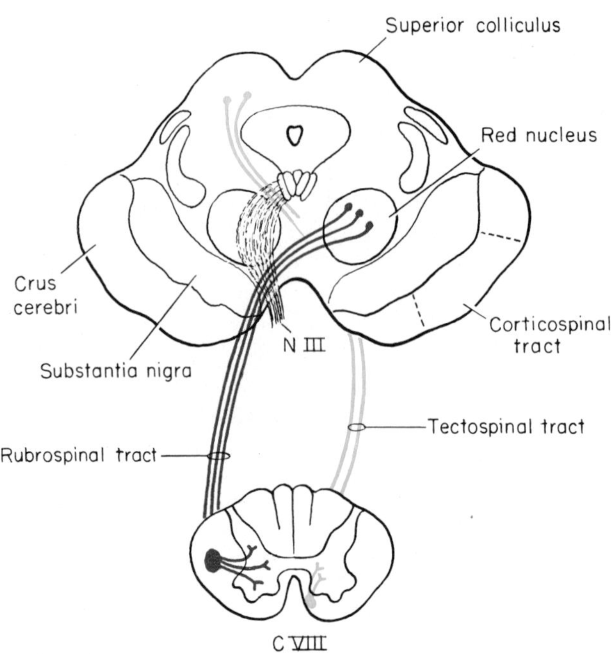

Figure 4-11. Schematic diagram of the rubrospinal (*red*) and the tectospinal (*blue*) tracts. The rubrospinal tract arises somatotopically from cells of the red nucleus, crosses in the ventral tegmental decussation, and descends to spinal levels where fibers terminate in parts of laminae V, VI, and VII. Tectospinal fibers arise from cells in deep layers of the superior colliculus, cross in the dorsal tegmental decussation, and descend in association with the medial longitudinal fasciculus. Fibers of the tectospinal tract are distributed to parts of laminae VIII, VII, and VI only in cervical spinal segments.

bosacral spinal segments arise from ventral and ventrolateral parts of the nucleus (Pompeiano and Brodal, '57). Thoracic spinal segments receive fibers that arise from an intermediate region of the nucleus. Rubrospinal fibers: (1) descend the length of the spinal cord, (2) distribute the greatest number of fibers to cervical spinal segments, and (3) terminate in the lateral half of lamina V, lamina VI, and dorsal and central parts of lamina VII (Nyberg-Hansen and Brodal, '64).

The red nucleus receives fibers from the cerebral cortex and the cerebellum. Corticorubral fibers from the "motor" cortex project bilaterally to the parvicellular part of the red nucleus and ipsilaterally to the magnocellular division (Hartmann-von Monakow, et al., '79). These projections are somatotopically organized with respect to origin and termination. Through this synaptic linkage corticorubral and rubrospinal fibers together constitute a somatotopically organized nonpyramidal pathway between the motor cortex and particular spinal levels. All parts of the red nucleus receive crossed cerebellar efferent fibers via the superior cerebellar peduncle. Fibers from the dentate nucleus project to the rostral third of the red nucleus and those from the anterior interposed nucleus (equivalent to emboliform nucleus in man) relate portions of the cerebellar cortex somatotopically with the caudal two-thirds of the red nucleus (Courville, '66; Massion, '67) (Fig. 8-14). Stimulation of cells in the red nucleus produces excitatory postsynaptic potentials in contralateral flexor alpha (α) motor neurons and inhibitory postsynaptic potentials in extensor alpha motor neurons. The most important function of the rubrospinal tract concerns control of tone in flexor muscle groups.

The *interstitiospinal tract* is uncrossed and forms a component of the descending MLF; it will be discussed with that composite bundle.

Two major descending spinal tracts arise from the pons. These are the vestibulospinal and pontine reticulospinal tracts.

The pontine and medullary reticulospinal tracts will be discussed together.

Vestibulospinal Tract. The vestibular nuclei constitute a cytological complex in the floor of the fourth ventricle in both the pons and medulla. The four major nuclei of this complex receive afferent fibers from the vestibular nerve and the cerebellum which are distributed differentially (Fig. 6-14). The vestibulospinal tract, the principal descending spinal pathway from this complex, arises exclusively from the lateral vestibular nucleus. The lateral vestibular nucleus consists of a fairly discrete collection of giant cells in the lateral part of the complex near the level of entry of the vestibular nerve root. Practically all cells of the lateral vestibular nucleus contribute fibers to the formation of this tract which descends the length of the spinal cord in the anterior part of the lateral funiculus (Figs. 4-12 and 4-13). The vestibulospinal tract, like the rubrospinal tract, is somatotopically organized. Ventral and rostral parts of the nucleus project fibers to cervical spinal segments, while dorsocaudal parts of the nucleus project fibers to lumbosacral spinal segments. Cells in intermediate regions of the nucleus provide fibers passing to thoracic spinal segments (Pompeiano and Brodal, '57a). Fibers of the vestibulospinal tract, entirely uncrossed, are distributed to all parts of lamina VIII and to medial and central parts of lamina VII. Very few, if any, vestibulospinal fibers end directly upon motor neurons of the anterior horn except in thoracic spinal segments.

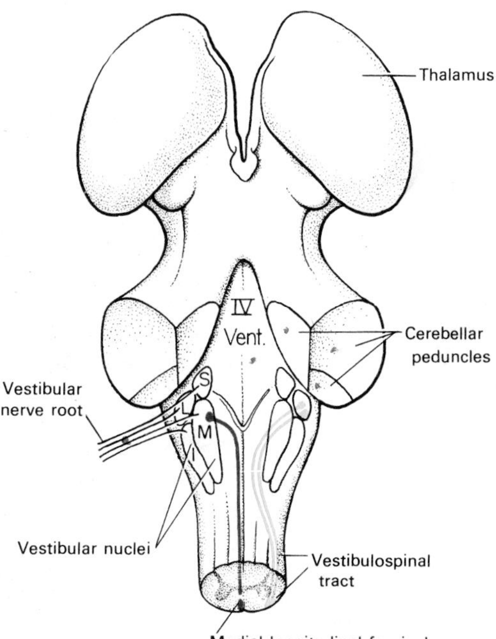

Figure 4-12. Schematic diagram of the spinal projections from the vestibular nuclei. The vestibulospinal tract (*blue*) arises only from cells of the lateral vestibular nucleus. This tract is uncrossed, somatotopically organized, and concerned with the facilitation of extensor muscle tone. Vestibular fibers descending in the medial longitudinal fasciculus (*red*) arise largely from the medial vestibular nucleus and are mainly uncrossed. *S*, indicates superior vestibular nucleus, *L*, indicates the lateral vestibular nucleus, and *I* and *M* indicate the inferior and medial vestibular nuclei.

Vestibular influences, and certain cerebellar influences, upon spinal cord activities are mediated by the vestibulospinal tract. This tract is considered to exert a facilitatory influence upon somatic spinal reflex activity and spinal mechanisms that control muscle tone. Stimulation of the lateral vestibular nucleus in the cat produces excitatory postsynaptic potentials in extensor motor neurons, while no significant changes are seen in flexor motor neurons. These facilitatory effects on extensor α motor neurons are considered to be mediated via interneurons in laminae VII and VIII.

Reticulospinal Tracts. Two relatively large regions of the brain stem reticular formation give rise to fibers that descend to spinal levels. One of these regions is in the pontine tegmentum while the other lies in the medulla, hence it is proper to refer to these as the pontine and medullary reticulospinal tracts (Figs. 4-6 and 4-14).

The *pontine reticulospinal tract* arises from aggregation of cells in the medial pontine tegmentum (Fig. 4-6) referred to as the *nuclei reticularis pontis caudalis* and *oralis* (Olszewski and Baxter, '54). The caudal pontine reticular nucleus begins in the caudal pontine tegmentum and extends rostrally to the level of the motor trigeminal nucleus. This nucleus contains a number of giant cells in addition to various types of smaller cells. The oral pontine reticular nucleus, present in more rostral parts of the medial pontine tegmentum, extends into the caudal mesencephalic reticular formation; giant cells are found only in the

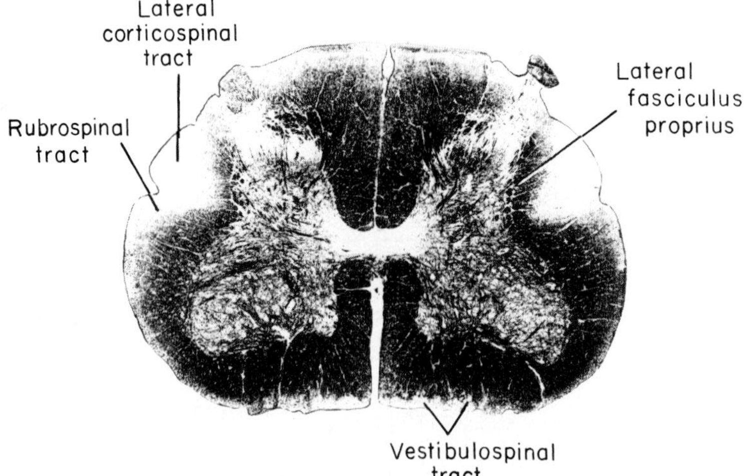

Figure 4-13. Section through fourth lumbar segment of a human spinal cord which had been crushed some time previously in the lower cervical region. The degenerated long descending tracts are unstained. Note that the lateral corticospinal tract reaches the lateral periphery of the spinal cord at this level and the vestibulospinal tract lies on the anterior surface of the cord. (Weigert's myelin stain; photograph). (From Carpenter and Sutin, *Human Neuroanatomy*, 1983; courtesy of Williams & Wilkins.)

more caudal parts of this nucleus. The pontine reticulospinal tract is almost entirely ipsilateral and descends chiefly in the medial part of the anterior funiculus (i.e., sulcomarginal area). In the brain stem and spinal cord these fibers descend in association with the MLF. Pontine reticulospinal fibers are more numerous than those arising in the medulla, descend the entire length of the spinal cord and terminate in lamina VIII and adjacent parts of lamina VII. A few pontine reticulospinal fibers cross at spinal levels in the anterior white commissure. A large proportion of these reticulospinal fibers give off collateral branches to more than one level of the spinal cord, suggesting they may be involved in coordination of activities at different spinal levels (Peterson et al., '75). Electrical stimulation of this reticulospinal pathway evokes both monosynaptic and polysynaptic excitation of motor neurons supplying axial and limb muscles; direct effects are strongest upon axial muscles particularly in the neck (Peterson, '79).

The *medullary reticulospinal tract* arises from the medial two-thirds of the medullary reticular formation (Brodal, '57). The largest number of fibers arise from the *nucleus reticularis gigantocellularis*, lying dorsal to the inferior olivary complex and lateral to the paramedian region (Figs. 4-6 and 4-14). As the name of this nucleus implies, it is composed of characteristic large cells, but large cells are not as conspicuous in man as in lower animals. In addition, this region contains many medium-sized and small cells which give rise to fibers of various sizes. Fibers of the medullary reticulospinal tract project bilateral to spinal levels (crossed and uncrossed) and mainly descend in the anterior part of the lateral funiculi. Fibers crossing to the opposite side do so in the medulla and are less numerous than uncrossed fibers. Some fibers of the medullary reticulospinal tract descend the length of the spinal cord. Reticulospinal fibers from the pons and medulla are not segregated sharply in the spinal cord. Medullary reticulospinal fibers terminate chiefly in lamina VII, but a few fibers terminate in lamina IX. Several components of the medullary reticulospinal tract have been identified physiologically: (1) long projections which provide collaterals to multiple spinal levels and (2) short projections to cervical segments arising mainly from dorsorostral regions of the nucleus reticularis gigantocellularis (Peterson, '79).

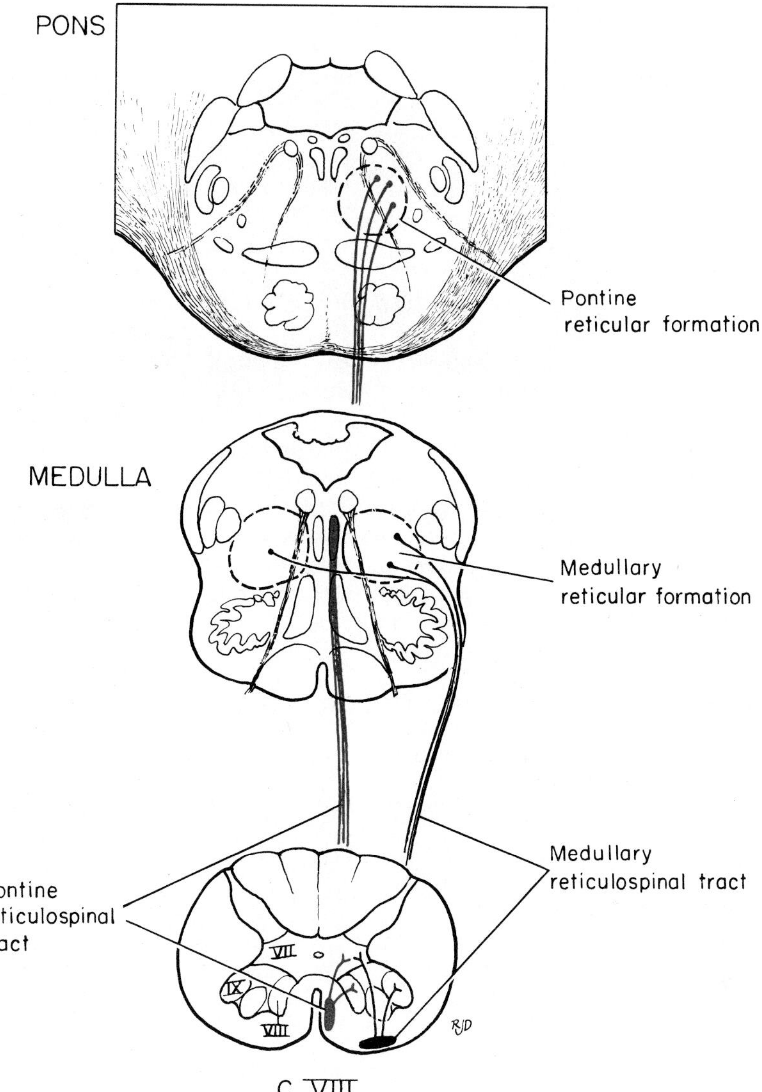

Figure 4-14. Diagram of the reticulospinal tracts indicating regions of origin, course and terminations. Pontine reticulospinal fibers (*red*) descend in the sulcomarginal region of the anterior funiculus, are uncrossed, descend the length of the spinal cord and give off collaterals and terminals at nearly all levels which end in lamina VIII and parts of lamina VII. Medullary reticulospinal fibers (*black*) arise bilaterally, descend in the anterior part of the lateral funiculus and terminate in laminae VII and IX. Neither of these tracts is somatotopically organized.

Reticulospinal fibers, arising in both the pons and medulla, largely terminate upon the somata and dendrites of internuncial neurons, although some end directly upon motor neurons (Schwindt, '81). Most impulses from the reticular formation which influence gamma (γ) motor neurons probably are mediated at segmental levels by internuncial neurons in laminae VII and VIII. Anatomically neither the pontine nor medullary reticulospinal tract is somatotopically organized (Brodal, '57), although physiological data suggest that localized regions of the pontine and rostrodorsal portion of the medullary reticular formation may exert their major influences at particular spinal levels (Peterson, '80). Regions in which pontine reticulospinal fibers terminate are similar to those in which vestibulospinal fibers end; both of these systems are considered to convey facilitatory impulses. Medullary reticulospinal fibers terminate in portions of the gray laminae that also receive fibers from corticospinal and rubrospinal tracts. Autonomic fibers from higher levels descend and traverse portions of the reticular formation which give rise to the reticulospinal tracts.

Experimental studies indicate that stimulation of the brain stem reticular fomation can: (1) facilitate and inhibit voluntary movement, cortically induced movement and reflex activity, (2) influence muscle tone, probably via the gamma system, (3) affect phasic activities associated with respiration, (4) exert pressor and depressor effects upon the circulatory system, and (5) exert facilitating and inhibiting influences upon the central transmission of sensory impulses (Pompeiano, '73). Areas of the medullary reticular formation from which the medullary reticulospinal tract arises correspond to regions from which inhibitory effects are elicited. Facilitatory effects are obtained from far larger regions of the reticular formation rostral to the medulla.

The brain stem reticular formation receives input from many sources, but direct corticoreticular projections seem especially important. Corticoreticular fibers arise from widespread areas of the cortex, although the greatest number originate from the "motor area." These fibers terminate in two fairly restricted regions of the reticular formation, one in the pons and one in the medulla (Rossi and Brodal, '56). In the pons these fibers end mainly in the nucleus reticularis pontis oralis and in the rostral part of the caudal pontine reticular nucleus. In the medulla such fibers terminate in the nucleus reticularis gigantocellularis. Corticoreticular fibers are distributed bilaterally with some crossed preponderance. The regions of termination within the reticular formation correspond to those that give rise to the reticulospinal tracts. Thus, the synaptic linkage of corticoreticular and reticulospinal fibers forms a pathway from the cortex to spinal levels. There is no evidence of a somatotopic linkage within this system (Brodal, '57).

The nuclei of the raphe which have serotonin (5-hydroxytryptamine, 5-HT) as their neurotransmitter give rise to projections distributed extensively in the reticular formation (Bobillier et al., '76). Only the nucleus raphe magnus (medulla) and perhaps nucleus raphe pontis appear to project to spinal levels. Cells of the nucleus raphe magnus give rise to bilateral spinal projections which descend in the dorsolateral funiculus (Fig. 5-11) (Basbaum et al., '78). These fibers terminate most profusely in laminae I and II in the cervical and lumbar enlargements. Stimulation of the nucleus raphe magnus produces an analgesic effect by inhibitory actions upon sensory neurons (Proudfit and Anderson, '75; Basbaum et al., '76).

Medial Longitudinal Fasciculus (MLF). The posterior part of the anterior funiculus contains a composite bundle of descending fibers that originate from different nuclei at various brain stem levels. This composite bundle is known as the MLF. The spinal portion of this bundle represents only a part of the brain stem tract designated by the same name. Descending fibers in the spinal MLF arise from the medial vestibular nucleus, the pontine reticular formation, the superior colliculus (tectospinal) and the interstitial nucleus of Cajal (interstitiospinal) (Figs. 4-11 and 4-12, and 4-14). Fibers of this bundle form a well-defined tract only in cervical spinal segments, but some of the fiber systems descend to sacral levels. Fibers of this bundle arising from the medial vestibular nucleus are predominantly ipsilateral in the spinal cord and terminate in portions of laminae VIII and VII (Fig. 4-12). The largest component of the spinal MLF, the pontine reticulospinal tract, has been described previously. The interstitiospinal tract arises from a small mesencephalic nucleus lateral to the MLF and oculomotor complex. Fibers of this tract are uncrossed and terminate in parts of laminae VIII and VII at all spinal levels (Nyberg-Hansen, '66).

Fastigiospinal Fibers. Although the cerebellum has been considered to exert its influences at segmental levels solely via relay nuclei, one deep cerebellar nucleus has been shown to project directly to spinal levels (Fukushima et al., '77; Batton et al., '77, Matsushita and Hosoya, '78). Fastigiospinal fibers arise from the fastigial nucleus, cross the midline within the cerebellum and descend in the ventral part of the lateral funiculus, partially intermingled with fibers of the vestibulospinal tract. Fibers of this small tract descend only to cervical segments and project into the anterior horn.

Descending Autonomic Pathways. The spinal cord contains descending fibers which convey impulses to visceral cell groups (i.e., intermediolateral cell column and sacral preganglionic cell groups) which innervate smooth muscle, heart muscle, glands and body viscera. Descending autonomic fibers originate from specific nuclei at various brain stem levels. The principal nuclei giving rise to descending autonomic fibers are: (1) nuclei in several regions of the hypothalamus, (2) visceral nuclei of the oculomotor complex, (3) the locus ceruleus, and (4) portions of the nucleus of the solitary tract (Fig. 4-15). In addition some neurons in the reticular formation may be concerned with visceral activities. Hypothalamic neurons projecting to spinal levels include: (1) the paraventricular nucleus and (2) cells in lateral and posterior regions of the hypothalamus (Saper et al., '76). Fibers from these hypothalamic nuclei project to visceral nuclei in the medulla as well as to spinal levels (Fig. 4-15). Direct hypothalamic-spinal fibers descend in the lateral funiculus and terminate upon cells of the intermediolateral cell column in thoracic, lumbar and sacral segments. These fibers are mainly uncrossed and appear to directly influence preganglionic sympathetic and parasympathetic neurons.

Although the visceral nuclei of the oculomotor nuclear complex (Fig. 7-10) classically have been considered to project preganglionic parasympathetic fibers only into third nerve, recent evidence indicates that these neurons also project directly to spinal levels (Saper et al., '76; Loewy et al., '78). Descending fibers from the Edinger-Westphal nucleus contribute fibers to the posterior column nuclei and spinal projections that descend to lumbar levels (Fig. 4-15). In the spinal cord most of these fibers end in lamina I and parts of lamina V.

A small pigmented nucleus in the rostral pons, known as the locus ceruleus (Figs. 4-15, 6-27, and 6-28), has been demonstrated to synthesize, store, and release the neurotransmitter norepinephrine. The locus ceruleus distributes fibers widely in the neuraxis and is regarded as the principal source of norepinephrine in the central nervous system. Spinal projections from this nucleus descend in the anterior and lateral funiculi, are mainly uncrossed and terminate in the anterior horn, intermediate gray and ventral regions of the posterior horn (Nygren and Olson, '77).

Cells in ventrolateral parts of the nucleus of the solitary tract (Figs. 4-15 and 5-19) project to cervical and thoracic spinal segments (Loewy and Burton, '78). Fibers of the solitariospinal tract are predominantly crossed and terminate in the region of phrenic motor neurons at C3–C5 levels and the anterior horn and intermediolateral cell column at thoracic levels. Fibers of this tract are considered to provide excitatory inputs to phrenic and inspiratory motor neurons. Projections to the intermediolateral cell column may be involved in cardiovascular reflexes.

Fasciculi Proprii. Short ascending and descending fiber systems, both crossed and uncrossed, which begin and end within the spinal cord, constitute the fasciculi proprii or spinospinal fasciculi (Fig. 4-16). This intrinsic spinal pathway interconnects various levels and cell groups within the same levels. Descending collaterals of dorsal root fibers in the posterior columns frequently are regarded as part of this system. Fibers of this system participate in intersegmental spinal reflexes. The fasciculi proprii are present in all funiculi adjacent to the spinal gray, but are most numerous in anterolateral regions. These tracts and the major ascending and descending spinal tracts are shown schematically in Figure 4-16.

UPPER AND LOWER MOTOR NEURONS

Lower Motor Neuron. The anterior horn cells and their axons, projecting via the ventral root to striated muscle, constitute an anatomical and physiological unit referred to as the final common pathway or the lower motor neuron. Injury or disease of the anterior horn cells or their projecting axons results in paralysis of the muscles innervated by these fibers, loss of muscle tone and relatively prompt atrophy of the denervated muscle. Myotatic reflexes in the denervated muscle will be abolished be-

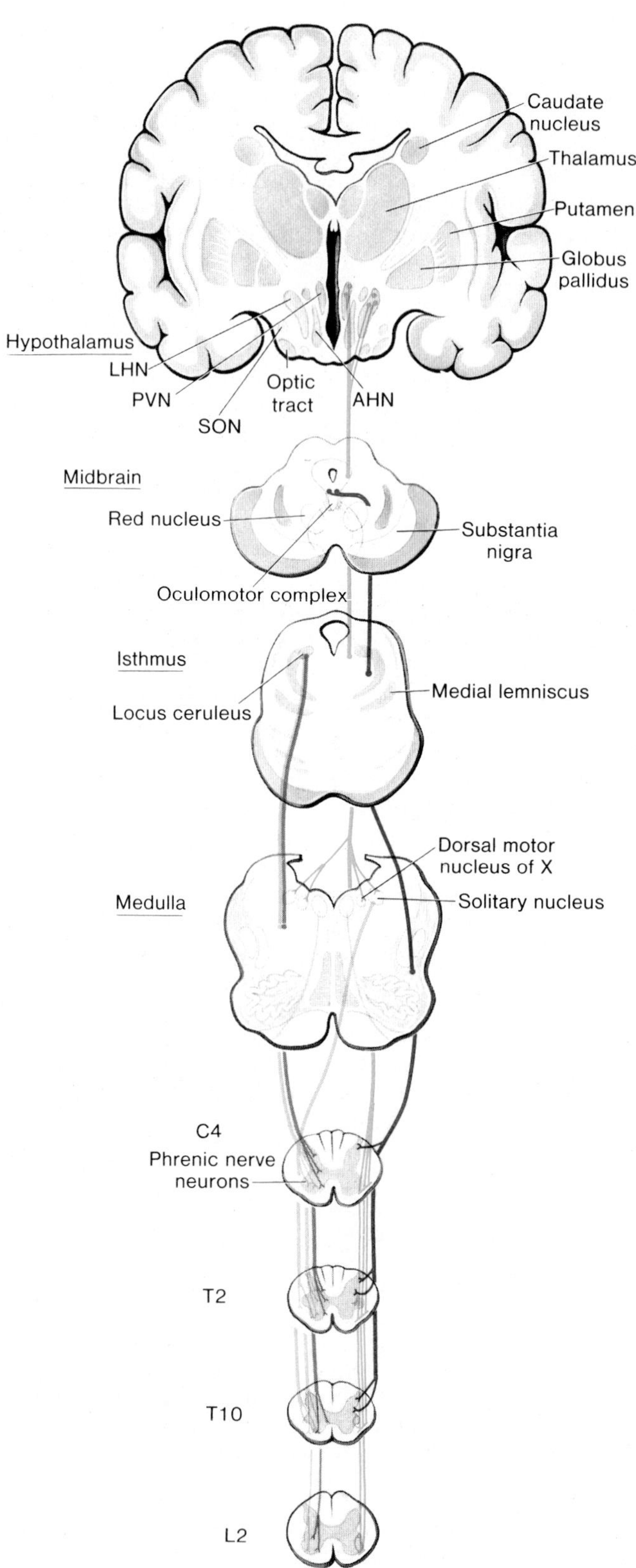
Caudate nucleus
Thalamus
Putamen
Globus pallidus
Hypothalamus
LHN
PVN
SON
Optic tract
AHN
Midbrain
Red nucleus
Substantia nigra
Oculomotor complex
Isthmus
Locus ceruleus
Medial lemniscus
Dorsal motor nucleus of X
Medulla
Solitary nucleus
C4
Phrenic nerve neurons
T2
T10
L2

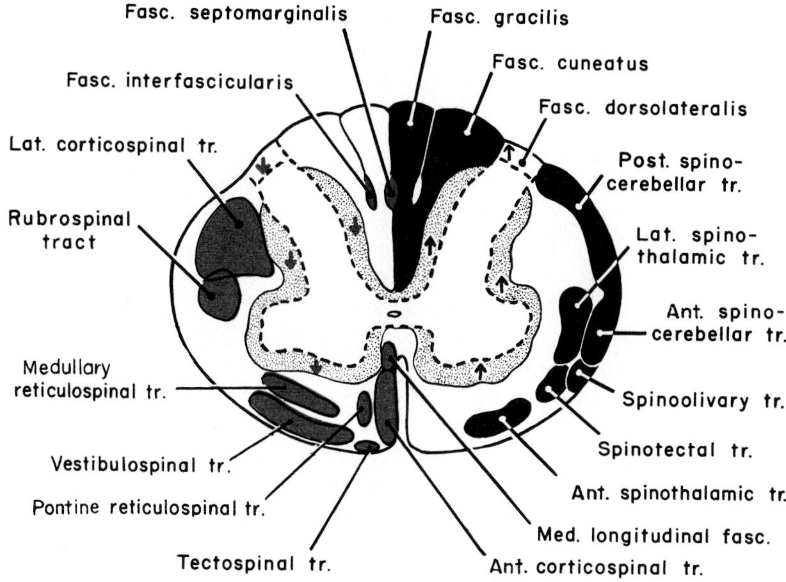

Figure 4-16. Diagram of ascending (*black*) and descending (*red*) pathways of the spinal cord. The fasciculus proprius system (*stippled*) and dorsolateral fasciculus contain both ascending and descending nerve fibers. (From Carpenter and Sutin, *Human Neuroanatomy*, 1983; courtesy of Williams & Wilkins.)

cause the reflex arc is broken. This sequence of events is seen in poliomyelitis, other diseases involving the anterior horn cells and following severance of the ventral roots.

Upper Motor Neuron. The anterior horn cells can be directly and indirectly activated by impulses transmitted by descending fiber systems. Although virtually all of the descending spinal systems influence the activity of the lower motor neuron to some degree, the overwhelming clinical importance of the corticospinal tract has caused it to be equated with the *upper motor neuron.* Lesions of the upper motor neuron are characterized by paresis (i.e., incomplete loss of muscle power) or paralysis, initial loss of muscle tone, followed in time by increased tone in antigravity muscles (i.e., spasticity), hyperactive myotatic reflexes, the Babinski sign, and loss of certain superficial reflexes (i.e., superficial abdominal and cremasteric reflexes). Muscle atrophy is not seen in the early stages, because segmental innervation of striated muscles remains intact; however, with long standing upper motor neuron paralysis, atrophy of disuse becomes evident. The

---

Figure 4-15. Schematic diagram of descending autonomic projections to spinal cord from the hypothalamus, the Edinger-Westphal nucleus, the locus ceruleus and the nucleus of the solitary fasciculus. Direct fibers (*blue*) from the hypothalamus (i.e., paraventricular nucleus, *PVN*; dorsal part of the lateral hypothalamic nucleus (*LHN*) and the posterior hypothalamic area) project to the dorsal motor nucleus of the vagus nerve and the medial nucleus of the solitary fasciculus. This projection is mainly ipsilateral. At spinal levels these fibers terminate largely in the ipsilateral intermediolateral cell column in thoracic and upper lumbar segments. Visceral neurons of the oculomotor complex (Edinger-Westphal nucleus) give rise to descending preganglionic parasympathetic fibers (*red*) distributed to Rexed's laminae I and V. Norepinephrine containing cells in the locus ceruleus and subceruleus project fibers (*purple*) to parts of the anterior horn, the intermediate gray and deep portions of the posterior horn. Cells in the ventrolateral nucleus of the solitary fasciculus project fibers (*light blue*) predominantly contralaterally to phrenic motor neurons (C_3–C_5), to thoracic anterior horn cells and to the intermediolateral cell column. (*AHN*, anterior hypothalamic nucleus; *SON*, supraoptic nucleus). Based upon Saper et al., '76; Loewy et al., '78; Nygren and Olson, '77; Loewy and Burton, '78. (From Carpenter and Sutin, *Human Neuroanatomy*, 1983; courtesy of Williams & Wilkins.)

concepts of the upper and lower motor neuron constitute one of the basic corner stones of clinical neurology and the simple distinctions outlined above must be considered in the neurological examination of every patient.

SPINAL CORD LESIONS

Determination of the origin, course and termination of most spinal pathways from the study of normal Weigert- and Nissl-stained sections is virtually impossible, but such sections provide valuable information concerning spinal cord organization and cytoarchitecture. The most precise data concerning spinal pathways has been derived from anatomical and physiological studies in animals. Secondary degeneration in nerve fibers (severed from cell bodies), studied in sections stained by the Marchi, Nauta, or other silver impregnation technics, provides valuable information concerning the course and termination of fiber bundles. Lesions in nerve fibers also produce alterations of the cell bodies, giving rise to these fibers, which can be detected in Nissl stained sections within a few days. These cell changes, referred to as *retrograde cell changes*, are characterized by swelling and distortion of the perikaryon, eccentric nuclei, and dissolution of Nissl substance. The retrograde technic provides precise data concerning the cells of origin of particular fiber bundles.

More precise information concerning fiber connections in the central nervous system can be obtained using tritiated amino acids and autoradiographic technics (Cowan et al., '72; Rosenquist et al., '74; Cowan and Cuénod, '75). This method is based upon the physiological principle of axoplasmic flow. Since the neuronal soma is the principal site of synthesis of protein and other materials, injection of neurons with radioactive precursors labels substances synthesized in the soma and transported via the axon to the terminals (Figs. 6-13, 6-19, 7-19, 8-15, and 11-19). The enzyme horseradish peroxidase (HRP) is transported by axons in both anterograde and retrograde fashion (Fig. 5-20), HRP taken up at axonal terminals and neuromuscular junctions is transported retrogradely to the cell somata where it is sequestered in lysosomes or in multivesicular bodies. The demonstration of HRP granules in neurons and their processes depends upon the ability of the enzyme to oxidize a chromagen (diaminobenzidine, benzidine dihydrochloride, or tetramethylbenzadine) in the presence of hydrogen peroxide to form a dense precipitate. Tissue reacted with these chromagens and hydrogen peroxide reveals fine spherical granules within retrogradely labeled neurons (Graham and Karnovsky, '66; LaVail, '75; Hardy and Heimer, '77; Mesulam, '78). HRP taken up by neurons or injured axons is transported distally (anterograde) to terminals where it appears as very fine grains in reacted tissue. Reaction product in cells, fibers and terminals can be identified microscopically under bright or dark field illumination. Certain fluorescent compounds also are transported intraaxonally in a retrograde manner similar to HRP (Kooy et al., '78; Bentivoglio et al., '79). Because these compounds fluoresce different colors at different wavelengths, these substances lend themselves to double labeling studies. Fluorescent dyes injected into two separate fields of terminals will double label neurons projecting collaterals to both fields.

The [^{14}C]2-deoxyglucose metabolic method for mapping functional pathways in the central nervous system surmounts the limitations which the synapse imposes upon most anatomical technics (Kennedy et al., '75, '76; Plum et al., '76). Labeled 2-deoxyglucose passes the blood-brain barrier using the same carrier that transports glucose and it competes with glucose for hexokinase, the enzyme that phosphorylates both. Since it competes with glucose at the hexokinase phosphorylation, part of the isotope can be trapped in the neuron after 45 minutes. By autoradiographic technics the preferentially active neurons in functional systems can be identified (Figs. 13-14, 13-15 and 13-16).

Root Lesions. Section of the dorsal roots (dorsal rhizotomy) abolishes all afferent impulses supplied by these roots and interrupts segmental reflex arcs. Because of extensive overlap, section of one dorsal root does not result in readily detectable sensory loss. If multiple dorsal roots are sectioned, for example C5 through T1, cutaneous sensibility will be lost or greatly impaired, in the C6, C7, and C8 dermatomes, but afferent input from stretch receptors entering all five dorsal roots will be abolished. As a consequence muscle tone and myotatic reflexes will be absent in most of the muscles of the upper extremity. Although the muscles can be contracted because the ventral roots remain intact, the deafferented extremity is virtually useless due to loss of cutaneous and kinesthetic sense. Monkeys with such rhizotomies do not use the deafferented limb for walking, climbing or grasping.

Spinal cord degeneration resulting from multiple dorsal rhizotomies (C5 through T1) is distributed most profusely at the level of the sectioned roots to portions of the posterior horn (lamina III and IV), to selected cell groups within lamina VII and to parts of lamina IX (Fig. 3-10). Particularly profuse ascending and descending degeneration is present in the ipsilateral fasciculus cuneatus. No ascending degeneration is present in other ascending spinal tracts, because these arise from cell groups within the spinal cord. In other words, degeneration is limited to the primary afferent fibers and does not involve intrinsic spinal neurons or their processes. A diagrammatic representation of degeneration resulting from section of a single lumbar dorsal root is shown at *1* in Figure 4-17.

Injury or section of the ventral root produces a lower motor neuron paralysis of the muscle units innervated by the particular root (*4*, in Fig. 4-17). If the lesion involves thoracic or upper lumbar ventral roots, preganglionic sympathetic fibers also will be interrupted (*3*, in Fig. 4-17). Secondary (Wallerian) degeneration will result in somatic and visceral efferent fibers; postganglionic neurons and their processes will remain intact. Section of a mixed nerve distal to the sympathetic ganglion in the lower thoracic region (*2* in Fig. 4-17) results in degeneration in motor, sensory and postganglionic sympathetic nerve fibers distal to the lesion.

Spinal Cord Transection. Complete spinal cord transection results in the immediate loss of all neural function below the level of the lesion. There is a complete loss below the level of the lesion of: (1) all somatic sensation, (2) all motor function, (3) all visceral sensation, (4) all reflex activity, (5) all muscle tone, and (6) thermoregulatory control. This complete cessation of all neural function in the isolated spinal cord caudal to the lesion is called *spinal shock* and persists for 1 to 6 weeks (averages 3 weeks) in man. The termination of the period of spinal shock is heralded by the appearance of the Babinski sign (i.e., an extensor toe response to stroking the sole of the foot) and evidence of *minimal reflex responses* to painful stimuli. In time recovery of flexor reflex activity leads to a phase characterized by *flexor muscle spasms.* These spasms, which are bilateral, may result in the *triple flexion response* of Sherrington, characterized by flexion of the lower extremity at the hip and knee and dorsoflexion of the foot. The most extreme form of the triple flexion response is the *mass reflex*, in which repeated discharge in flexor motor units occurs spontaneously or in response to minimal and nonspecific stimuli. Beginning about 4 months after injury there is a slow, gradual and progressive increase in extensor muscle tone. During this period there may be episodes of alternate flexor and extensor muscle spasm. Extensor muscle tone ultimately becomes predominant. Examination of the patient at this time reveals: (1) marked extensor muscle tone, (2) spasticity, (3) hyperactive myotatic reflexes, (4) sustained clonus (a self-perpetuating myotatic reflex activity), (5) bilateral Babinski signs, and (6) loss of all sensation and voluntary motor function below the level of the lesion. Disturbances of bowel and bladder function produce distressing problems in the management of paraplegic patients. Initially there is urinary retention; this is followed by overflow incontinence. This problem usually is handled by a system of tidal drainage which automatically fills and empties the bladder at regular intervals.

Degeneration resulting from complete transection of the spinal cord follows a definite and well established pattern. Above the level of the lesion, ascending tracts will be degenerated, while below the lesion level, they will appear intact. The reverse is seen in the descending tracts.

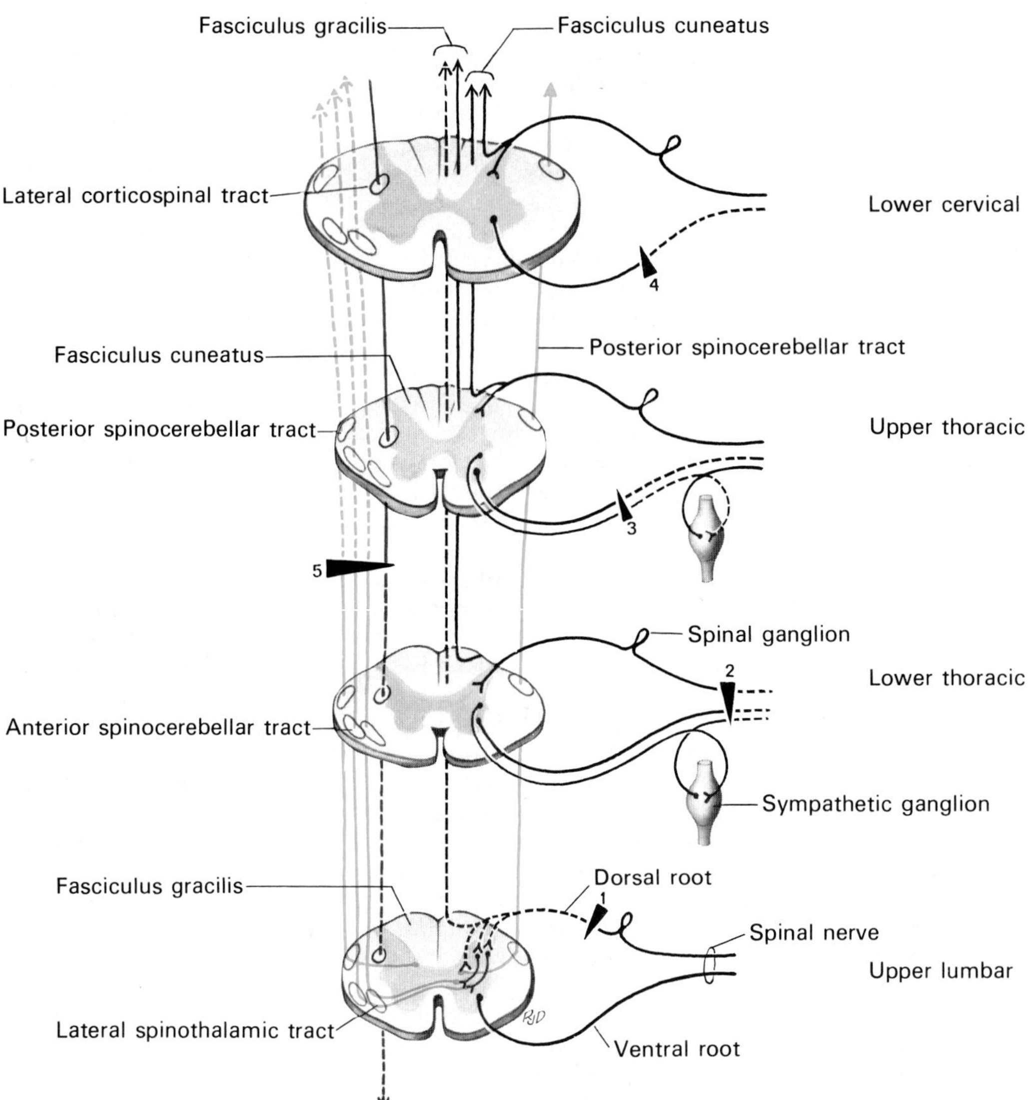

Figure 4-17. Simplified schematic diagram of degeneration resulting from certain lesions of the spinal nerves, spinal roots and spinal cord. Sites of lesions are indicated by black wedges. Dorsal and ventral root fibers, peripheral nerve fibers, fibers in the posterior white columns and short relays are in *black*; ascending spinal tracts are *blue* and the corticospinal tract is *red*. A lesion of the dorsal root, *1* at upper lumbar levels produces degeneration (dashed lines) in the posterior and anterior gray horns (not shown) and in parts of the fasciculus gracilis. No degeneration is present in other ascending spinal tracts because degeneration does not pass beyond the synapse. A lesion of spinal nerve as at *2* produces peripheral degeneration (dashed lines) in somatic motor, sensory and postganglionic sympathetic fibers. A lesion of the ventral root at site *3* produces degeneration in somatic motor and preganglionic sympathetic fibers. A lesion at *4* produces degeneration only in somatic motor fibers distal to the lesion. The lesion at *5* destroys the lateral funiculus and produces ascending degeneration (dashed lines) in the posterior and anterior spinocerebellar tracts (*blue*) and in the spinothalamic tracts (only the lateral spinothalamic tract (*blue*) shown here) above the level of the lesion. This lesion also produces descending degeneration (dashed lines) in the corticospinal tract (*red*) below the level of the lesion. Although other spinal tracts which would degenerate are not indicated, the same principle applies. (From Carpenter and Sutin, *Human Neuroanatomy*, 1983; courtesy of Williams & Wilkins.)

Thus by studying spinal cord sections above and below the level of the lesion, it is possible to predict fairly closely the level of the lesion (Fig. 4-2).

Spinal Cord Hemisection. While spinal cord hemisection is less common than complete cord transection, it presents a highly characteristic syndrome (Brown-Séquard) and is instructive for teaching purposes. This type of lesion is not associated with a period of spinal shock and the neurological disturbances on the two sides are different. On the side of the lesion the following are found below the level of the lesion: (1) an upper motor neuron syndrome, (2) greatly impaired discriminatory tactile sense, (3) loss of kinesthetic sense, and (4) reduced muscle tone. At the level of the lesion, there usually is bilateral impairment of pain and thermal sense and variable degrees of lower motor neuron involvement on the lesion side. Contralateral to the lesion there is: (1) loss of pain sensibility from one segment below the level of the lesion and (2) loss of thermal sense from about two segments below the level of the lesion. Sensory disturbances contralateral to the lesion are due to interruption of crossed ascending fibers in the spinothalamic tracts. The spinal degeneration seen in the Brown-Séquard syndrome is almost entirely on the side of the lesion, and conforms to the same principle as described for complete spinal cord transection (5, in Fig. 4-17).

Spinal Cord Syndromes. There are many varieties of spinal cord lesions and syndromes. *Amyotrophic lateral sclerosis* is a progressive degenerative disease involving both upper and lower motor neurons bilaterally. *Combined system disease*, representing the neurological manifestations of pernicious anemia, is associated with degenerative changes in peripheral nerves and in the central nervous system. Degeneration in the spinal cord is evident in the posterior white columns and in the corticospinal tracts, but is not confined to these systems. *Syringomyelia* is a chronic disease characterized by cavities that develop in relationship to the central canal of the spinal cord. The hallmark of the disease is an early impairment, or loss, of pain and thermal sense with preservation of tactile sense. The central cavities which develop in this disease interrupt the decussating fibers of the spinothalamic tracts in several consecutive segments. *Tabes dorsalis* is a central nervous system form of syphilis which produces degeneration in the central processes of spinal ganglion cells. Sensory loss, impairment of position and vibratory sense, radicular (i.e., root) pains and paresthesias all are related to dorsal root pathology. Ataxia and difficulty in walking are related to loss of position and kinesthetic sense. Muscle tone and myotatic reflexes are greatly reduced in the lower extremities. Vascular lesions of the spinal cord are not common, but sometimes occur in relationship to surgical procedures. The blood supply of the spinal cord is discussed in Chapter 14 (Figs. 14-1 and 14-2).

CHAPTER 5

The Medulla

The medulla (myelencephalon), the most caudal brain stem segment, begins rostral to the highest rootlets of the first cervical spinal nerve. The external transition from upper cervical spinal cord to medulla is gradual and appears as a cylindrical expansion. Above the level of transition, the medulla increases in size and develops distinctive external features (Figs. 5-1 and 5-2). The development of the fourth ventricle causes structures located posteriorly to shift posterolaterally. The appearance of the pyramids rostral to the corticospinal decussation obliterates the anterior median fissure, and the development of the inferior olivary complex above the transitional zone produces an oval eminence posterolateral to the pyramids. The principal structural changes in the transition from spinal cord to medulla are: (1) the development of the fourth ventricle (Fig. 1-4); (2) the decussation of the medullary pyramids (Figs. 4-7, 4-8, 4-9, 5-3, and 5-4); (3) the termination of the fasciculi gracilis and cuneatus upon their respective nuclei and formation of the medial lemniscus (Figs. 4-1 and 5-5); (4) the replacement fibers in the zone of Lissauer by descending fibers of the spinal trigeminal tract (Fig. 5-5); (5) replacement of the spinal gray by cellular aggregations of the reticular formation; (6) the development of cranial nerve nuclei; and (7) the appearance of relay nuclei, most of which project fibers to the cerebellum (Fig. 5-7).

SPINOMEDULLARY TRANSITION

Transverse sections at the junction of spinal cord and medulla resemble those of upper cervical spinal segments (Fig. 5-3). The substantia gelatinosa has increased in size, and coarse descending spinal trigeminal fibers are found posterolateral to it. These fibers arise from cells of the trigeminal ganglion, enter the brain stem at pontine levels, and some of them descend caudally as far as the second cervical segment (Fig. 6-21). The substantia gelatinosa gradually becomes the spinal trigeminal nucleus at high cervical levels and this nucleus retains its position and size throughout the medulla. There is an increase in the central gray matter surrounding the central canal. The lateral corticospinal tract presents a somewhat reticulated appearance as its fibers project dorsally, laterally and caudally

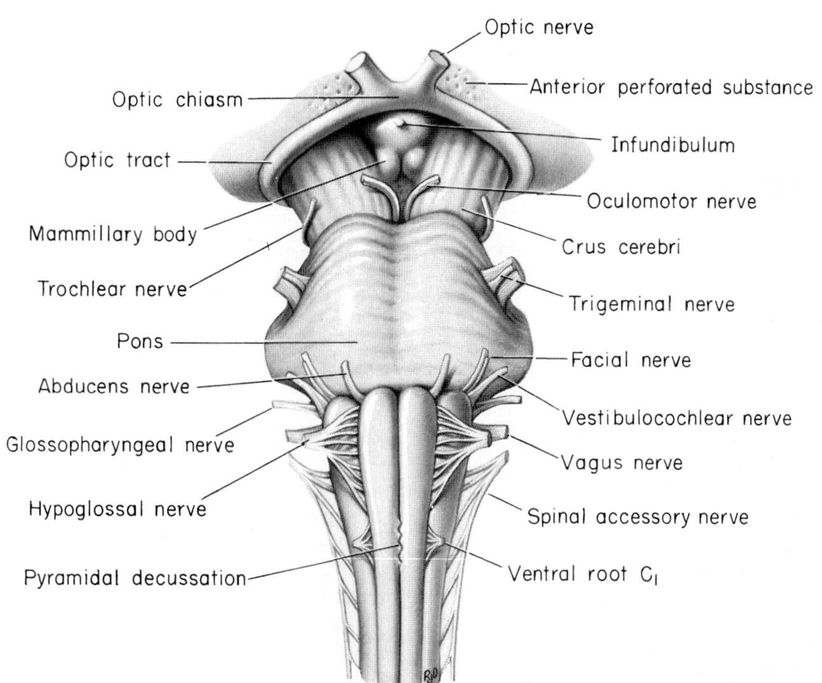

Figure 5-1. Drawing of the anterior aspect of the medulla, pons and midbrain. (From Carpenter and Sutin, *Human Neuroanatomy*, 1983; courtesy of Williams & Wilkins.)

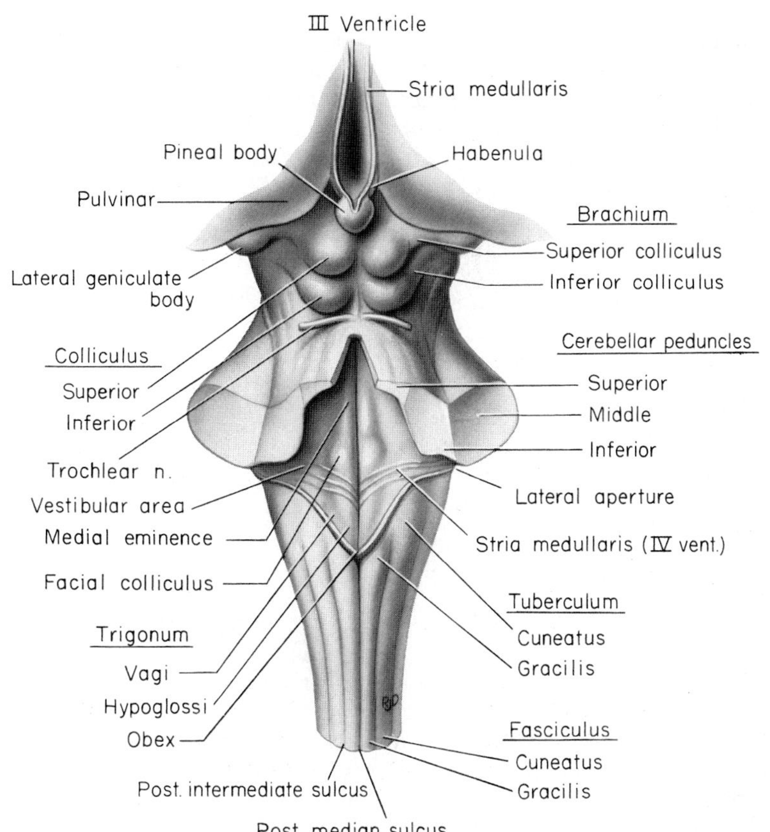

Figure 5-2. Drawing of the posterior aspect of the brain stem with the cerebellum removed. (From Carpenter and Sutin, *Human Neuroanatomy*, 1983; courtesy of Williams & Wilkins.)

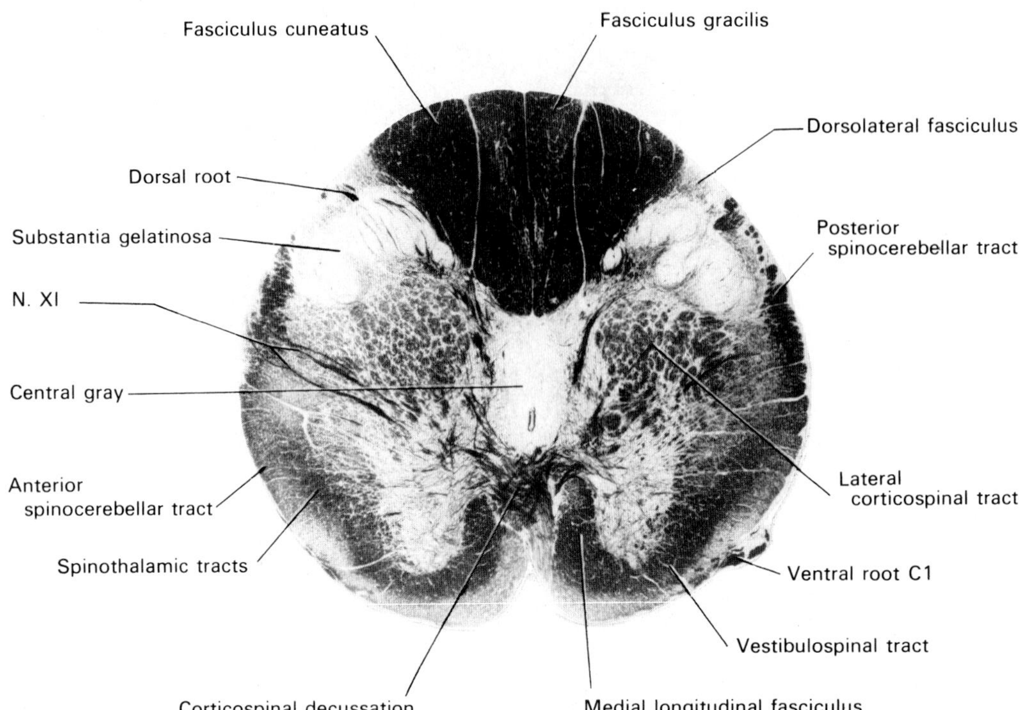

Figure 5-3. Transverse section through the junction of spinal cord and medulla. The most caudal decussating fibers of the corticospinal tract can be seen passing into the posterior part of the lateral funiculus. The structure labeled substantia gelatinosa also contains cell groups of the spinal trigeminal nucleus. (Weigert's myelin stain; photograph.) (From Carpenter and Sutin, *Human Neuroanatomy*, 1983; courtesy of Williams & Wilkins.)

into the lateral funiculus of the spinal cord. The anterior horn is relatively small and is covered anteromedially by fibers of the medial longitudinal fasciculus (MLF) and anterolaterally by fibers of the vestibulospinal tract. A few fibers of the spinal part of the spinal accessory nerve arch posterolaterally to emerge from the lateral aspect of the spinal cord. Anterior horn cells which extend into the lower medulla constitute the *supraspinal nucleus.*

Corticospinal Decussation. The most conspicuous feature of the spinomedullary transition is the corticospinal decussation (Figs. 4-8 and 5-4). These fibers, all contained in the medullary pyramid, cross the midline in large fascicles anterior to the central gray, and project posterolaterally across the base of the anterior horn. Interdigitating fiber bundles project downward and posteriorly so that in transverse sections most of the bundles are cut obliquely. The crossed fibers of the lateral corticospinal tract descend in the dorsal part of the lateral funiculus, while uncrossed fibers of the anterior corticospinal tract descend in the anterior funiculus (Figs. 4-9 and 4-10). In a graded series of ascending sections the corticospinal decussation is seen in reverse sequence. The corticospinal decussation forms the anatomical basis for voluntary motor control of one half of the body by impulses from the contralateral cerebral cortex.

Decussation of the Medial Lemniscus. At levels through the corticospinal decussation, relatively large nuclear masses begin to appear in the posterior white columns. These are the nuclei gracilis and cuneatus (Figs. 5-4 and 5-5). The long ascending branches of cells in the spinal ganglia, contained in the fasciculi gracilis and cuneatus, terminate respectively upon these nuclei (Figs. 4-1 and 5-5). The nuclei gracilis appear first as slender collections of cells posterior to the central gray and anterior to the fibers of the fasciculi gracilis (Fig. 5-4). The nuclei cuneatus develop at more rostral levels as triangular-shaped cell aggregations in the most anterior part of

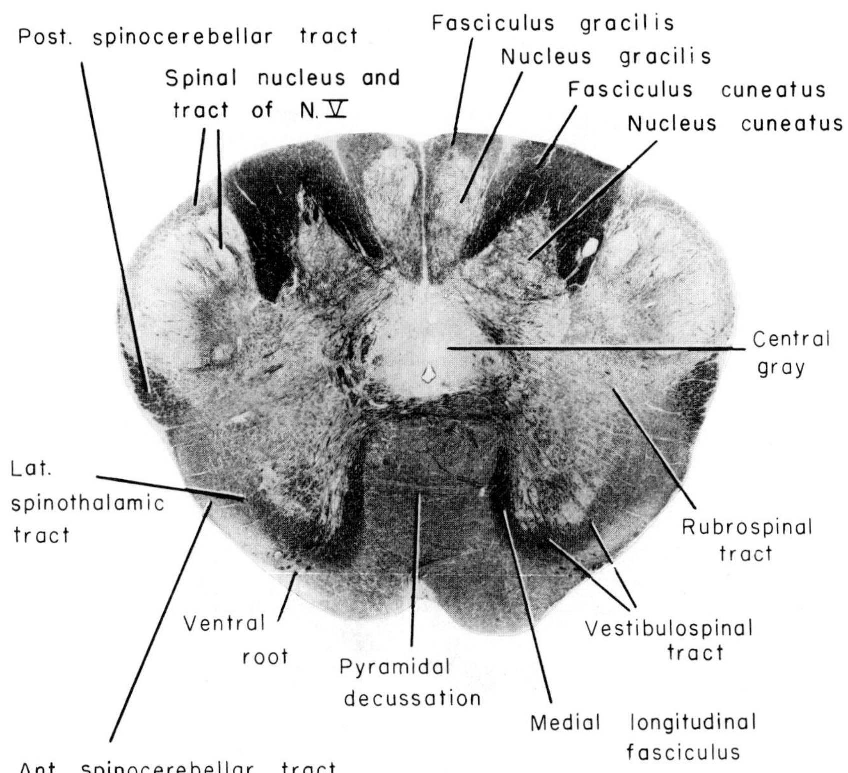

Figure 5-4. Transverse section of the medulla through the upper part of the corticospinal decussation. (Weigert's myelin stain; photograph.) (From Carpenter and Sutin, *Human Neuroanatomy*, 1983; courtesy of Williams & Wilkins.)

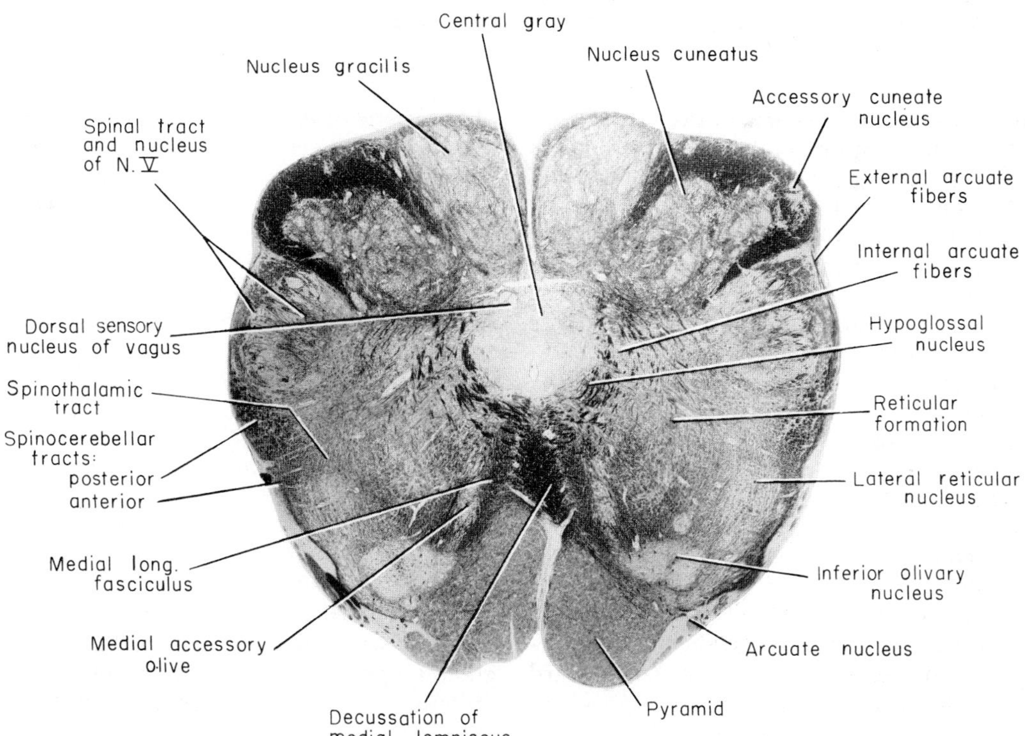

Figure 5-5. Transverse section of medulla through the decussation of the medial lemniscus. (Weigert's myelin stain; photograph.) (From Carpenter and Sutin, *Human Neuroanatomy*, 1983; courtesy of Williams & Wilkins.)

the fasciculi cuneatus. At higher levels these posterior column nuclei progressively enlarge and the posterior white columns show a corresponding reduction (Fig. 5-5). Fibers in the posterior white column terminate somatotopically throughout most of the rostrocaudal extent of the nuclei gracilis and cuneatus.

Three cytological regions of the nucleus gracilis have been recognized: (1) a reticular region rostral to the obex characterized by a loose cellular organization, (2) a "cell nest" region caudal to the obex made up of cell clusters, and (3) a caudal region of scattered cells (Taber, '61; Kuypers and Tuerk, '64). Ascending branches of dorsal root fibers projects somatotopically upon the nucleus gracilis and exhibit a somatotopic lamination chiefly in the "cell nest" region; terminals in the reticular region are diffuse (Hand, '66; Carpenter et al., '68a). The nucleus cuneatus also exhibits regional differences in cytoarchitecture (Olszewski and Baxter, '54). Dorsal regions of the cuneate nucleus contain clusters of round cells with bushy dendrites, while basal areas contain triangular, multipolar, and fusiform cells (Kuypers and Tuerk, '64). Clusters of round cells are considered to receive the principal afferents from distal parts of the body and to be related to small cutaneous receptive fields, while triangular cells receive afferents from proximal parts of limb related to larger cutaneous receptive fields. Dorsal root fibers terminate somatotopically in the nucleus cuneatus in exclusive and overlapping zones (Shriver et al., '68).

Comparisons of the patterns of dorsal root terminations in the nuclei gracilis and cuneatus in the monkey indicate: (1) overlapping terminations are more extensive and irregular in the nucleus gracilis, and (2) there is less autonomous terminal representation of individual dorsal root fibers in the nucleus gracilis.

Physiological studies in the cat suggest that neurons in different parts of the nucleus gracilis are related to: (1) peripheral receptive fields of different sizes, and (2) different sensory modalities. Other studies indicate that the somatotopic organization of the posterior columns and the medial lemniscus is maintained at the level of the posterior column nuclei and neural elements related to kinesthesis and tactile sense are intermingled in a single and mutual somatotopic pattern (Poggio and Mountcastle, '60).

Myelinated fibers arising from the nuclei gracilis and cuneatus sweep anteromedially around the central gray, as *internal arcuate fibers* (Figs. 4-1 and 5-5). These fibers decussate completely and form a well-defined ascending bundle, the *medial lemniscus*, which terminates in the ventral posterolateral (VPL) nucleus of the thalamus. The decussation of the medial lemniscus provides part of the anatomical basis for the sensory representation of half of the body in the contralateral cerebral cortex.

Cells in rostral parts of the nuclei gracilis and cuneatus, classified as multipolar and triangular neurons, give rise to fibers which cross the midline with the internal arcuate fibers, but terminate in the dorsal accessory olivary nucleus (Ebbesson, '68). These fibers from the posterior column nuclei are a link in the dorsal spino-olivocerebellar pathways. This pathway to the cerebellar vermis is activated exclusively by flexor reflex afferents (i.e., myelinated afferents which evoke the flexon reflex in spinal preparations (Oscarsson, '73)).

The *accessory cuneate nucleus*, lateral to the cuneate nucleus at slightly more rostral levels, is composed of large cells similar to those of the dorsal nucleus of Clarke (nucleus thoracicus) (Figs. 5-5, 5-6, and 5-7). These nuclei share the following features: (1) cells are morphologically similar, (2) afferents are derived from dorsal roots, (3) both nuclei give rise to uncrossed cerebellar afferent fibers (Fig. 4-5), and (4) both nuclei relay impulses from muscle spindles, Golgi tendon organs, type II muscle afferents, and cutaneous afferents. Fibers terminating in the accessory cuneate nucleus are derived from the same dorsal root ganglia as those projecting to the cuneate nucleus, namely cervical and upper thoracic. Ascending fibers in the fasciculus cuneatus terminate somatotopically in the accessory cuneate nucleus, with fibers from C5 through C8 terminating in the central core region. Cells of the accessory cuneate nucleus give rise to uncrossed *cuneocerebellar fibers* which enter the cerebellum via the inferior cerebellar peduncle (Fig. 4-5). Axonal transport studies indicate that the

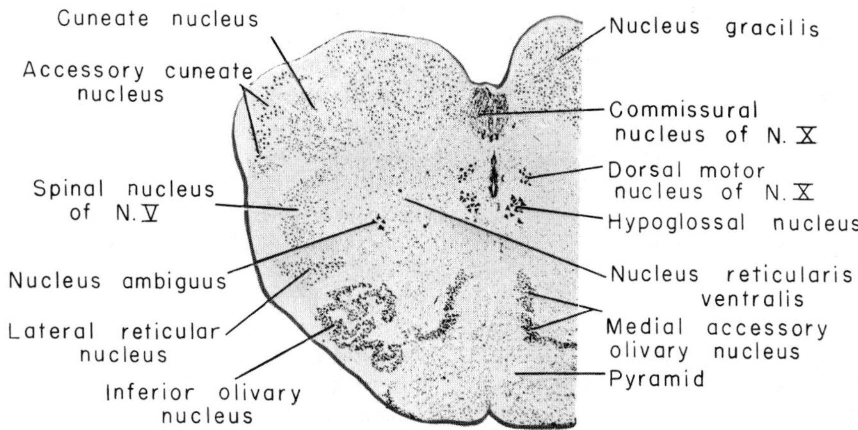

Figure 5-6. Section through medulla of 1-month infant at about the same level as in Figure 5-5. (Cresyl violet; photograph, with cell groups blocked in schematically.) (From Carpenter and Sutin, *Human Neuroanatomy*, 1983; courtesy of Williams & Wilkins.)

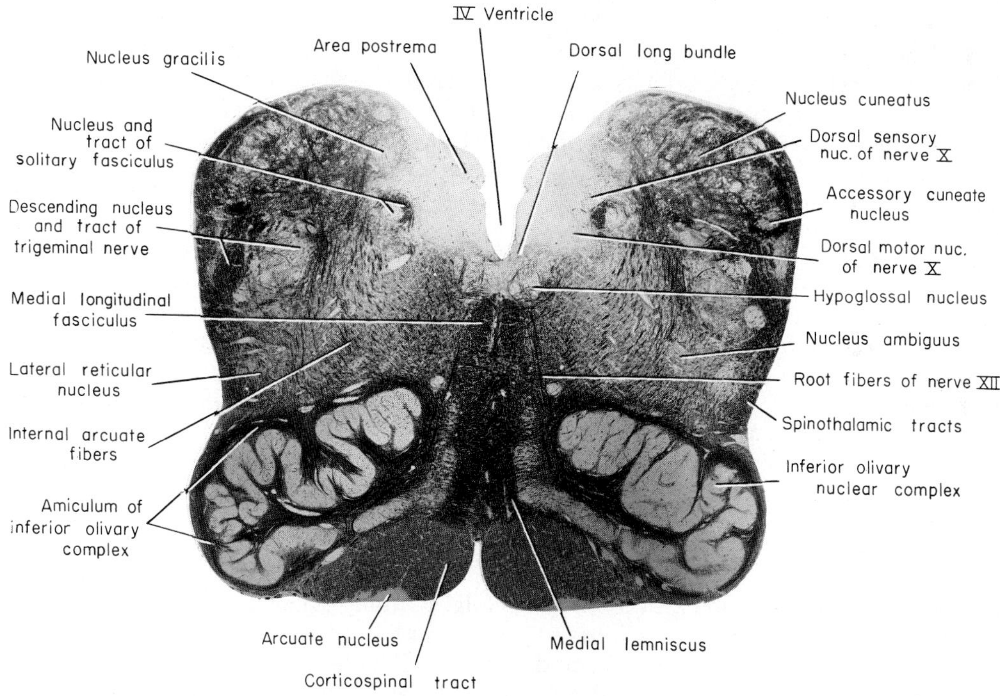

Figure 5-7. Transverse section of the medulla through the caudal part of the fourth ventricle, the area postrema and the lower part of the inferior olivary nucleus. (Weigert's myelin stain; photograph.) (From Carpenter and Sutin, *Human Neuroanatomy*, 1983; courtesy of Williams & Wilkins.)

main cerebellar projection of the accessory cuneate nucleus is ipsilateral to parts of lobule V and to the paramedian lobule (Rinvik and Walberg, '75). The cuneocerebellar tract is regarded as the upper limb equivalent of the posterior spinocerebellar tract.

Spinal Trigeminal Tract. Afferent trigeminal root fibers, which enter at upper pons levels, descend in the dorsolateral part of the brain stem, and project as far caudally as the C2 spinal level, constitute the spinal trigeminal tract (Figs. 5-4, 5-5, and 5-7). These descending fibers, originating from cells of the trigeminal ganglion, have a definite topographic organization, so that: (1) fibers of the mandibular division are most dorsal, (2) fibers of the ophthalmic division are most ventral, and (3) fibers of the maxillary division are intermediate (Fig. 6-21). Although previously fibers of the different divisions were regarded as extending caudally for different distances, experimental studies indicate that some fibers from all divisions extend into upper cervical spinal segments (Kerr, '63; Rhoton et al., '66). As this tract descends, it becomes progressively smaller as fibers of the tract terminate in the adjacent spinal trigeminal nucleus (Fig. 5-6). The tract contains general somatic afferent fibers from the trigeminal nerve, as well as fibers of the same functional category from the vagus, glossopharyngeal, and facial nerves which descend (Torvik, '56). Some visceral afferent fibers descending in the dorsal part of the spinal trigeminal tract project medially and terminate in ventrolateral parts of the nucleus solitarius (Kerr, '61; Rhoton et al., '66).

Spinal Trigeminal Nucleus. This nucleus lies along the medial border of the tract from the level of the trigeminal root in the pons to the second cervical spinal segment (Figs. 5-5, 5-6, 5-7, and 5-8). Fibers of the spinal trigeminal tract terminate upon cells of the nucleus throughout its extent. Cytoarchitecturally, the spinal trigeminal nucleus is subdivided into three parts (Olszewski, '50): (1) *pars oralis*, which extends caudally to the rostral pole of the hypoglossal nucleus, (2) *pars interpolaris*, which extends caudally to the level of the obex, and (3) *pars caudalis*, which begins near the level of the obex and extends into the upper cervical spinal cord. Cells in the caudal part of this nuclear complex resemble those of the posterior horn, and an inner part composed of large cells is referred to as the magnocellular subnucleus. Detailed studies reveal a cytoarchitectural lamination in the caudal part of the spinal trigeminal nucleus, similar to that described for the spinal cord (Gobel, '78, '78a). Four laminae are recognized: (1) lamina I (marginal zone) containing cells responding to nociceptive or thermal stimulation, (2) lamina II which corresponds to the substantia gelatinosa, and (3) laminae III and IV which constitute magnocellular layers (Olszewski, '50) (Fig. 5-8). Fibers in different parts of the spinal trigeminal tract terminate in corresponding circumscribed parts of the spinal trigeminal nucleus (e.g., mandibular fibers terminate in dorsal parts of the nucleus). Some neurons in the spinal trigeminal nucleus give rise to an axonal plexus of small fibers which emit collaterals that link together different levels of the spinal trigeminal nucleus (Gobel and Purvis, '72).

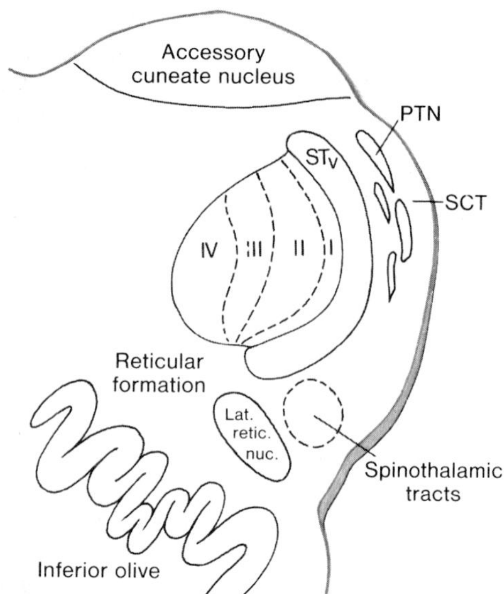

Figure 5-8. Schematic diagram of the laminar organization of the spinal trigeminal nucleus. Lamina I adjacent to the spinal trigeminal tract (ST_v) is called the marginal layer. Lamina II corresponds to the substantia gelatinosa and laminae III and IV form the magnocellular layers. *PTN*, indicates the paratrigeminal nucleus and *SCT* the spinocerebellar tracts. (From Carpenter and Sutin, *Human Neuroanatomy*, 1983; courtesy of Williams & Wilkins.)

Fibers in the spinal trigeminal tract convey impulses concerned with pain, thermal sense and tactile sense from the face, forehead, and mucous membranes of the nose and mouth. The spinal trigeminal tract and nucleus appear to be the only part of the trigeminal complex uniquely concerned with the preception of pain and thermal sense. Medullary trigeminal tractotomy (i.e., section of the spinal trigeminal tract) markedly reduces pain and thermal sense ipsilaterally without impairing tactile sense. Lesions in the dorsolateral region of the medulla involving the spinal trigeminal tract and the adjacent spinothalamic tracts produce a curious alternating hemianalgesia and hemithermo-anesthesia of the face and body (Figs. 4-4 and 6-21). This condition, known as the lateral medullary syndrome, is characterized by diminished pain and thermal sense in the face ipsilaterally (spinal trigeminal tract) and over the opposite side of the body (spinothalamic tracts).

Secondary trigeminal fibers arise from cells of the spinal trigeminal tract at multiple levels, cross through the reticular formation to the opposite side, and ascend to thalamic levels in association with the contralateral medial lemniscus (Fig. 6-23). These trigeminothalamic fibers constitute the second neuron in a sensory pathway from the face to the cortex. Other trigeminal fibers: (1) terminate upon reticular neurons, (2) project to the cerebellum via the inferior cerebellar peduncle, or (3) establish reflex connections with motor cranial nerve nuclei.

Reticular Formation. The reticular formation at the level of the decussation of the medial lemniscus occupies the region anterior to the posterior column nuclei and the spinal trigeminal complex and posterolateral to the pyramid (Figs. 5-5 and 5-6). It contains numerous cells of various sizes arranged in more or less definite groups which are traversed by both longitudinal and transverse fiber bundles. The internal arcuate fibers and many smaller bundles, including secondary trigeminal fibers, course through the reticular formation. Cells in the above described region constitute the *ventral reticular nucleus* (Fig. 5-6).

One of the more discrete and distinct nuclei at this level is the *lateral reticular nucleus of the medulla*, located anterolaterally (Figs. 5-5, 5-6, and 5-7). This nucleus begins caudal to the inferior olivary complex and extends to midolivary regions. Three cytoarchitectonic regions of the nucleus are recognized: magnocellular, parvicellular, and subtrigeminal. Large cells are located ventromedially dorsal to the inferior olive, while small cell groups are situated dorsolaterally within the nucleus. The lateral reticular nucleus of the medulla is a cerebellar relay nucleus. It receives afferent fibers from the spinal cord (i.e., spinoreticular and collaterals from the spinothalamic tracts) and descending fibers from the red nucleus (rubrobulbar). Spinal afferents to the lateral reticular nucleus are topographically organized with the magnocellular part of the nucleus receiving fibers from cervical and upper thoracic spinal segments (i.e., C1 to T3) and the parvicellular part and a transitional zone receiving fibers from more caudal spinal segments (Künzle, '73). Fibers from all subdivisions of the lateral reticular nucleus enter the cerebellum via the inferior cerebellar peduncle. These fibers terminate as mossy fibers in the anterior lobe, in both vermal and intermediate parts, in the paramedian lobule, and in lobule VII of the vermis (Künzle, '75; Matsushita and Ikeda, '76). The cerebellar projection is bilateral with ipsilateral dominance. Fibers ending in the anterior lobe and paramedian lobule are topographically organized (Brodal, '75; Dietrichs and Walberg, '79).

On the anterior aspect of the pyramid is a small collection of cells which varies in size, position and level. These cells, constituting the *arcuate nucleus* (Figs. 5-5 and 5-7), frequently become continuous with the pontine nuclei at higher levels. Afferent fibers are derived from the cerebral cortex and efferents project to the cerebellum as *external arcuate fibers* (Fig. 5-5).

Area Postrema. Immediately rostral to the obex on each side of the fourth ventricle is a small rounded eminence, the *area postrema* (Fig. 5-7), containing astroblast-like cells, arterioles, sinusoids and some apolar or unipolar neurons. The area postrema is one of several specialized ependyma regions which lie outside the blood-brain barrier collectively referred to as circumventricular organs (Fig. 1-19). All of the circumventricular organs, except the area postrema, are unpaired and related to portions of the diencephalon. Fibers from the solitary nucleus and spinal cord project to the area postrema (Morest, '60, '67). Fields of terminals surrounding this area contain neurophysin, oxytocin, and vasopressin, although these peptides cannot be demonstrated within the area postrema. Physiological studies have demonstrated that the area postrema is an emetic chemoreceptor, sensitive to apomorphine and intravenous digitalis glycosides (Borison and Wang, '49, '53).

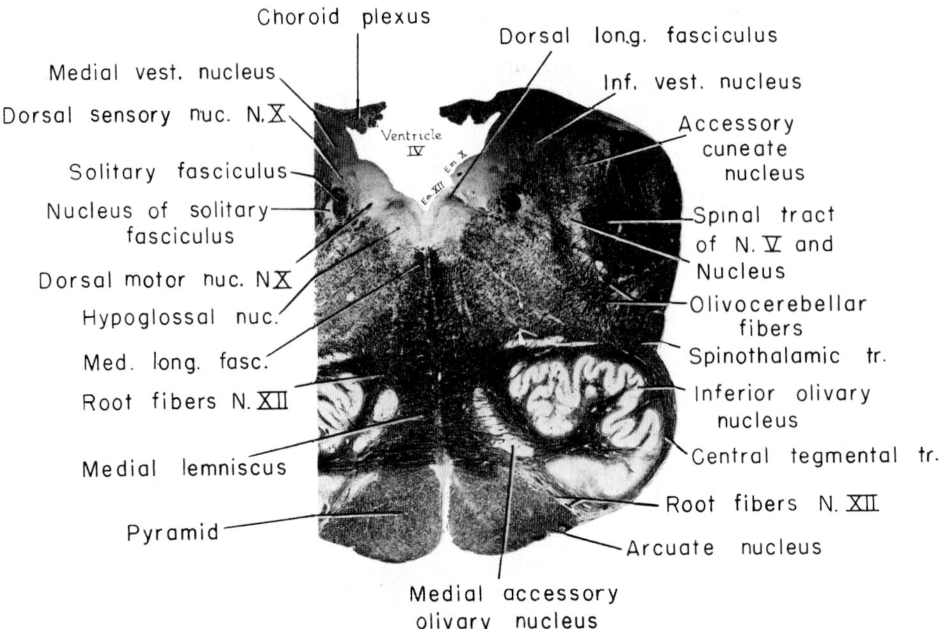

Figure 5-9. Transverse section of the medulla through the inferior olive complex rostral to that shown in Figure 5-7. *Em. X*, eminentia vagi; *Em. XII*, eminentia hypoglossi. (Weigert's myelin stain; photograph.) (From Carpenter and Sutin, *Human Neuroanatomy*, 1983; courtesy of Williams & Wilkins.)

Cranial Nerve Nuclei. At these levels, the cranial nerve nuclei, other than the spinal trigeminal nucleus, include the hypoglossal (N.XII) and those of the vagus (N.X) nerve (Figs. 5-6 and 5-7). The latter nuclei are in the gray surrounding the central canal. Anterolateral to the central canal are small collections of typical large motor neurons which constitute the caudal portions of the hypoglossal nucleus. Lateral to the central canal collections of smaller spindle-shaped cells form the dorsal motor nucleus of the vagus nerve. These cells give rise to preganglionic parasympathetic fibers. Dorsal to the central canal on each side of the median raphe is the commissural nucleus of the vagus nerve (Fig. 5-6). These cells, the most caudal extension of the medial portion of the nucleus solitarius, receive general visceral afferent fibers. The nucleus ambiguus lies in the reticular formation dorsal to the inferior olivary complex and medial to the lateral reticular nucleus (Figs. 5-6 and 5-7).

OLIVARY LEVELS OF THE MEDULLA

The most characteristic features of the medulla are present in transverse sections through the inferior olivary complex (Figs. 5-9 and 5-10). The cental canal has opened into the fourth ventricle; its roof is formed by the tela choroidea and the choroid plexus in the inferior medullary velum. The floor of the fourth ventricle contains three eminences which overlie cranial nerve nuclei. The most medial is the *hypoglossal eminence* overlying the nucleus of N.XII (Fig. 5-2 and 5-15); an *intermediate eminence* overlies the vagal nuclei. The most medial of these nuclei is the dorsal motor nucleus of the vagus; the lateral part of the intermediate eminence overlies the nuclei of the solitary fasciculus. The sulcus limitans, often an indistinct sulcus, passes through the intermediate or vagal eminence; cranial nerve cell columns medial to the sulcus are efferent while those lateral to it are afferent (Fig. 5-15). The most *lateral eminence* overlies the vestibular nuclei and is referred to as the *area vestibularis* (Fig. 5-2). In the reticular formation, internal arcuate fibers sweep ventromedially to enter the contralateral medial lemniscus (Fig. 5-7). The medial lemnisci occupy triangular-shaped areas on each side of the raphe, bounded ventrally by the pyr-

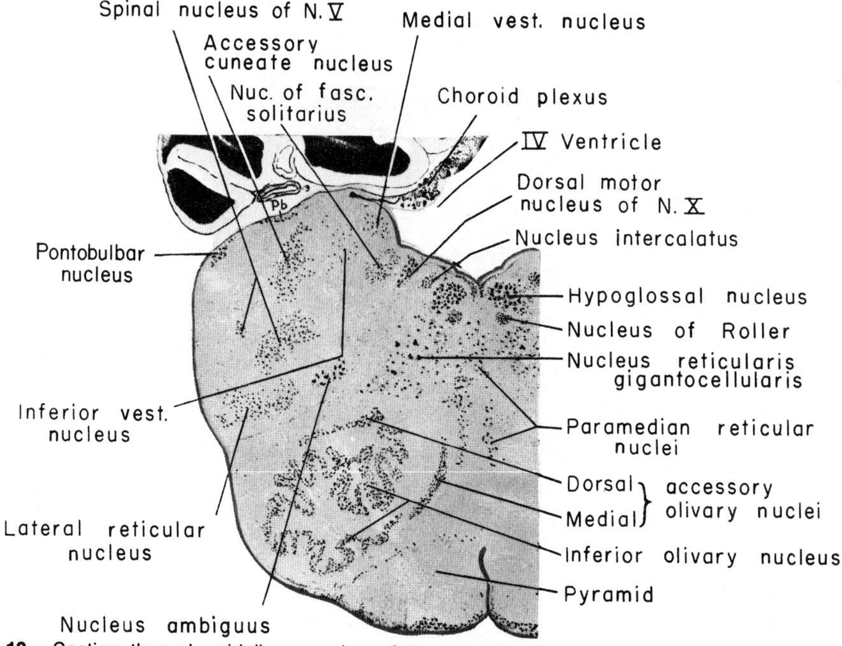

Figure 5-10. Section through midolivary region of the medulla. Cresyl violet. Photograph, with schematic representation of main cell groups. (From Carpenter and Sutin, *Human Neuroanatomy*, 1983; courtesy of Williams & Wilkins.)

amids and laterally by the inferior olivary nuclei. The accessory cuneate nucleus lies dorsolaterally, posterior to the spinal trigeminal tract and nucleus.

Inferior Olivary Nuclear Complex. The most characteristic and striking nuclear structure in the medulla is the inferior olivary complex (Figs. 5-6, 5-7, 5-9, and 5-10). This complex consists of three parts: (1) the *principal inferior olivary nucleus* appearing as a folded bag with the opening or hilus directed medially, (2) a *medial accessory olivary nucleus* located along the lateral border of the medial lemniscus, and (3) a *dorsal accessory olivary nucleus* located dorsal to the principal nucleus. These nuclei are composed of small round cells with numerous short dendrites. Axons of cells of the complex cross the median raphe, sweep posterolaterally, and enter the opposite side of the cerebellum via the inferior cerebellar peduncle. Crossed *olivocerebellar fibers*, constituting the largest single component of the inferior cerebellar peduncle (Figs. 5-9 and 5-14), project to all parts of the cerebellar cortex and to the deep cerebellar nuclei (Brodal, '40). Fibers of this massive projection end as climbing fibers which have a powerful excitatory action upon individual Purkinje cells. Olivocerebellar fibers terminate in a series of strips perpendicular to the long axes of the folia (Courville, '75).

The accessory olivary nuclei and the most medial part of the principal olivary nucleus project fibers mainly to the cerebellar vermis. The larger lateral part of the principal olivary nucleus projects fibers to the contralateral cerebellar hemisphere. The principal olivary nucleus is surrounded by a band of myelinated fibers, most of which terminate in the nucleus. These myelinated fibers form the *amiculum olivae* (Fig. 5-7).

Descending fibers terminating upon cells of the inferior olivary complex arise from the cerebral cortex, the red nucleus and the periaqueductal gray of the midbrain. *Cortico-olivary fibers* arise from frontal, parietal, temporal and occipital cortex, descend with corticospinal fibers and terminate bilaterally, primarily in the ventral lamella of the principal olive. Uncrossed olivary afferent fibers from the midbrain descend in the *central tegmental tract.* Rubro-olivary fibers end in the dorsal lamella of the principal olive while fibers from the periaqueductal gray terminate in rostral parts of the principal and medial accessory olivary nuclei. Afferent fibers to parts of the inferior olive also originate from the inferior vestibular nucleus (Saint-Cyr and Courville, '79), parts of the spinal trigeminal nucleus, and the contralateral deep cerebellar nuclei (Tolbert, et al., '76; Berkley and Hand, '78; Berkley and Worden, '78).

Spino-olivary fibers are among the most important afferents to the inferior olivary complex. Fibers ascending in the anterior funiculus of the spinal cord form the anterior spino-olivary tract which terminates in parts of the dorsal and medial accessory olivary nuclei; more than half of these fibers cross in the medulla. Spino-olivary fibers ascending in the posterior white columns, end upon cells in rostral parts of the nuclei gracilis and cuneatus; these cells give rise to fibers that terminate in the contralateral accessory olivary nuclei (Ebbesson, '68; Kalil, '79). Collectively these fibers form a dorsal spino-olivary pathway. Spinal afferents to parts of the inferior olivary complex constitute a link in spinocerebellar circuitry which resembles that of other spinocerebellar tracts.

Medullary Reticular Formation. Phylogenetically, this constitutes the oldest part of the brain stem and is the structure which forms its core. It is composed of diverse types of cells, organized in both compact and diffuse aggregations, and enmeshed in a complex fiber network (Figs. 5-5, 5-6, 5-7, 5-9, and 5-10). Detailed anatomical studies indicate that the brain stem reticular formation can be subdivided into regions having distinctive cytoarchitecture, fiber connections and intrinsic organization (Brodal, '57). In spite of these features, various subdivisions cannot be regarded as entirely independent entities, because complex fiber connections provide innumerable possibilities for interaction between subdivisions. Golgi studies of the reticular core indicate that reticular neurons project axons in both rostral and caudal directions (Scheibel and Scheibel, '58). Although primary bifurcating axons are oriented longitudinally, collateral axons pass in all directions and terminate in a variety of different endings. Many collaterals arborize about cells in both motor and sensory cranial nerve nuclei. These studies have failed to demonstrate Golgi type II cells (i.e., short axons), a finding which suggests that polysynaptic transmission of impulses probably is due to dispersion of impulses along collateral fibers. Thus the organization of the reticular formation suggests that a single reticular neuron can convey impulses both rostrally and caudally, may exert its influences both locally and at a distance, and impulses can be conducted both rapidly (primary axon) and slowly (via synapsing collateral axons).

The brain stem reticular formation begins in the caudal medulla rostral to the corticospinal decussation. Reticular nuclei present at this level are: the *lateral reticular nucleus* of the medulla and the *ventral reticular nucleus*, which have been described (Fig. 5-6). At midolivary levels the *gigantocellular reticular nucleus* occupies the area dorsal and medial to the inferior olivary complex (Figs. 4-6, 4-14, and 5-10). As its name implies, it has characteristic large cells, but it also contains many medium-sized and small cells. This nucleus, the rostral expansion of the ventral reticular nucleus, occupies the medial two-thirds of the reticular formation and extends to the medullary-pontine junction.

The *parvicellular reticular nucleus* is a small-celled collection of cells located posterolaterally in the reticular formation, medial to the spinal trigeminal nucleus and anterior to the vestibular nuclei. This nucleus, occupying roughly the lateral third of the medullary reticular formation has been referred to as the "sensory" part because it receives collaterals from secondary sensory pathways.

The *paramedian reticular nuclei* consist of several small nuclear groups which lie close to, and sometimes among, fibers of the medial longitudinal fasciculus and the medial lemniscus (Fig. 5-10). These reticular neurons project most of their fibers to the cerebellar vermis.

In essence the medullary reticular formation consists of three principal nuclear masses: (1) a *paramedian reticular nuclear group*; (2) a *central group* (i.e., the ventral reticular and gigantocellular reticular nuclei); and (3) a *lateral nuclear group* consisting of the lateral reticular and parvicellular reticular nuclei. The raphe nuclei, consisting of several distinct groups of neurons, also belong to the reticular formation, but will be described separately.

Afferent fibers projecting into the medullary reticular formation arise in the spinal cord, from secondary sensory cranial nerve nuclei, and from the cerebral cortex and cerebellum. *Spinoreticular fibers* ascend in the anterolateral funiculus and terminate in the caudal and lateral portions of the medullary reticular formation. A considerable number of these fibers end in the gigantocellular reticular nucleus, though some project to more rostral parts of the reticular formation. Collaterals of spinothalamic fibers terminate somatotopically upon cells of the lateral reticular nucleus, a cerebellar relay nucleus. *Collateral fibers* from second order sensory neurons in cranial nerve nuclei (i.e., auditory, vestibular, trigeminal, and visceral (solitary fasciculus)), project to the parvicellular reticular nucleus. No collaterals of the medial lemniscus terminate in any part of the brain stem reticular formation.

Cerebelloreticular fibers terminate mainly in the paramedian reticular nuclei. These reticular projections originate from the fastigial (Carpenter and Batton, '82) and dentate nuclei (Carpenter and Nova, '60; Brodal and Szikla, '72). The paramedian reticular nuclei are involved in a feedback system in that they project and receive fibers from the cerebellum.

Corticoreticular fibers arise from widespread areas of cortex, but the largest number of these fibers are derived from sensorimotor areas. Most of these fibers terminate in portions of the reticular formation in the pons and medulla. These fibers are both crossed and uncrossed. Regions of the brain stem reticular formation receiving corticoreticular fibers give rise to reticulospinal fibers. Impulses from a wide variety of sources converge upon the reticular nuclei. The maximal overlap of afferent fibers from different sources occurs in the medullary reticular formation which gives rise to a large number of long ascending and descending axons.

Efferent fibers arise from the medial two-thirds of the medullary reticular formation, which corresponds to the gigantocellular reticular nucleus; this nuclear mass gives rise to both long ascending and descending fibers. Ascending fibers from this nuclear mass ascend in the *central tegmental tract*, are uncrossed and terminate mainly upon portions of the intralaminar thalamic nuclei (Fig. 2-25). This system plays an important role in the mechanism of arousal from sleep. Descending fibers from this medial region of the reticular formation give rise to the medullary reticulospinal tracts which are bilateral but predominantly uncrossed (Fig. 4-14). Axons of medullary reticular neurons form long descending reticulospinal projections that provide collaterals to all spinal levels and shorter projections only to cervical spinal segments (Peterson, '79). Stimulation of the rostral and dorsal part of the nucleus reticularis gigantocellularis and regions of the caudal pontine reticular formation produce monosynaptic excitatory postsynaptic potentials in motor neurons supplying the axial muscles of the neck and back (Peterson, '80). Stimulation of the caudal and medial medullary reticular formation produces disynaptic and multisynaptic inhibitory postsynaptic potentials in motor neurons at all levels. Thus the medullary reticular formation can be divided into a dorsorostral facilitatory region and a caudal inhibitory zone. Cells in this "effector" area of the medullary reticular formation receive axons of cells of the parvicellular reticular nucleus. The latter reticular region is considered to serve "receptive" or "associative" functions, while the larger, more medial reticular region is organized to exert "effector" influences at both spinal and higher brain stem levels.

Raphe Nuclei. Cell groups lying in the midline of the medulla, pons, and midbrain collectively are called the raphe nuclei. The major raphe nuclei of the brain stem are shown in a schematized midsagittal section in Figure 5-11. Many, but not all, of the raphe nuclei have neurons that synthesize serotonin (5-hydroxytryptamine, 5-HT). Fibers originating from cells in the raphe nuclei are distributed widely in the neuraxis and release serotonin at their terminals. While serotonin is a neurotransmitter of major importance, over 95% of it is in blood platelets and the gastrointestinal tract (Angevine and Cotman, '81). In the medulla serotonergic neurons lie in the nuclei raphe magnus, raphe obscurus, and raphe pallidus

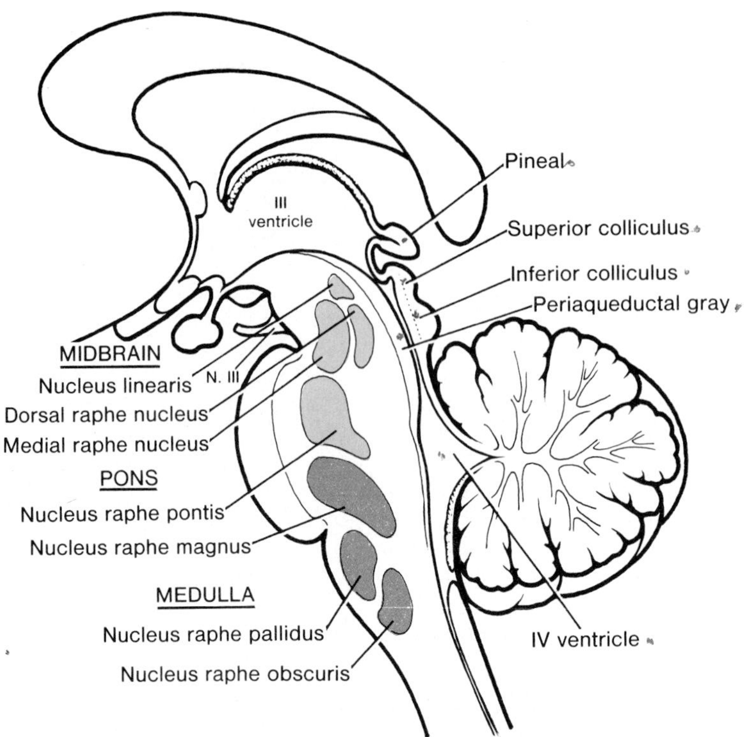

Figure 5-11. Schematic drawing of a midsagittal section of the brain stem indicating the positions of the raphe nuclei. Nuclei in *red* project to spinal levels, while nuclei in *blue* have projections to brain stem nuclei and to parts of the telencephalon. Projections to diencephalic structures are most numerous from the dorsal and medial raphe nuclei and from the nucleus raphe pontis. The dorsal and medial raphe nuclei also project widely to telencephalic structures (Bobillier et al.,'76; Basbaum and Fields, '79). (From Carpenter and Sutin, *Human Neuroanatomy*, 1983; courtesy of Williams & Wilkins.)

(*red* in Fig. 5-11) which give rise to descending spinal projections. Cells in the nucleus raphe magnus (Fig. 5-12) give rise to bilateral spinal projections that descend in the dorsolateral funiculus and terminate mostly in laminae I and II (Basbaum et al., '78). Stimulation of the nucleus raphe magnus produces an analgesic effect by an inhibitory action upon sensory neurons (Basbaum et al., '76). Other serotonergic fibers descending in anterior and lateral funiculi appear to end in the anterior and lateral gray horns. Sympathetic preganglionic neurons can be inhibited by stimulation of the raphe nuclei. The medulla also contains serotonergic nerve terminals in the caudal part of spinal trigeminal nucleus and in the nucleus of the solitary tract (Steinbusch, '81).

Ascending and Descending Tracts. Ascending fibers of the medial lemniscus occupy an "L"-shaped area on each side of the median raphe posterior to the pyramid and medial to the inferior olivary complex (Figs. 4-1, 5-9 and 5-14). The spinothalamic tracts, which can no longer be designated as anterior and lateral, have merged and form essentially a single entity in the retro-olivary area. These tracts are considerably smaller than at spinal levels, because an appreciable number of fibers terminate in the lateral reticular nucleus and a number of spinoreticular fibers, which at spinal levels ascend in close association with these tracts, have passed medially into the gigantocellular reticular nucleus. The posterior spinocerebellar tract moves posteriorly at medullary levels and becomes incorporated in the inferior cerebellar peduncle (Fig. 5-14). The anterior spinocerebellar tract maintains a retro-olivary position and ultimately enters the cerebellum by coursing along the superior surface of the superior cerebellar peduncle (Fig. 4-5). About one third of the fibers of the rostral spinocerebellar tract enter the cerebellum via the inferior cerebellar peduncle; all other fibers of this uncrossed tract enter the cerebellum in association with the anterior spinocerebellar tract.

The medial longitudinal fasciculus (MLF) lies anterior to the hypoglossal nucleus adjacent to the median raphe (Figs. 5-7, 5-9 and 5-14). Descending fibers in this complex bundle are derived from various brain stem nuclei. Vestibular fibers in this bundle arise from the medial and inferior vestibular nuclei. The pontine reticular formation contributes the largest number of descending fibers in the MLF; smaller groups of fibers arise from the interstitial nucleus of Cajal (interstitiospinal tract) and the superior colliculus (tectospinal tract). Rubrospinal fibers descend in retro-olivary position close to the lateral reticular nucleus; some crossed descending rubral efferent fibers, terminating in this cerebellar relay nucleus, are called *rubrobulbar fibers*. Uncrossed rubrobulbar fibers, arising from rostral parts of the red nucleus, descend in the central tegmental tract and end upon cells in the dorsal lamella of the principal inferior olivary nucleus. At mid-medullary levels fibers of the vestibulospinal tract, which arise only from the lateral vestibular nucleus, are scattered obliquely in an area posterior to the inferior olivary complex (Fig. 4-12). At more caudal levels, these fibers form a more compact bundle in the retro-olivary region. The medullary reticulospinal tract is not evident at these levels, but its cells of origin, the gigantocellular reticular nucleus, are present posteromedial to the inferior olivary complex (Figs. 4-6, 4-14 and 5-10). The spinal trigeminal tract and nucleus occupy the same location as at more caudal levels.

Inferior Cerebellar Peduncle. This peduncle is a composite bundle of tracts and fibers which assembles along the posterolateral border of the medulla. This bundle rapidly increases in size in the upper medulla by the addition of more fibers, and enters the cerebellum (Fig. 5-14 and 5-24). Fibers forming this peduncle arise from cell groups in the spinal cord and medulla. Crossed olivocerebellar fibers constitute the largest component of the inferior cerebellar peduncle (Fig. 5-14). Other medullary nuclei relaying impulses to the cerebellum via this peduncle are: (1) the lateral reticular nucleus of the medulla, (2) the accessory cuneate nucleus, (3) the paramedian reticular nuclei, (4) the arcuate nucleus, and (5) the perihypoglossal nuclei (see p. 120). Projections of the lateral reticular and accessory cuneate nuclei are uncrossed; those from other medullary relay nuclei are both crossed and uncrossed. The posterior spinocerebellar tract and approximately one third of fibers of the rostral spinocerebellar tract project to the cerebellum via this peduncle.

CHEMICALLY IDENTIFIED NEURONS AND CIRCUITS

The functional organization of the central nervous system is dependent upon neurotransmitters to carry impulses across synapses. Chemical coding of neural circuits only recently has been perceived as being as essential to understanding of neuroanatomy as the cell groups and their connections. There are a large number of neurotransmitters recognized as having unique properties in certain neural circuits and probably a great many more that remain to be identified. Neurotransmitters not only turn the signals on or off as impulses arrive at the synapses, but different neurotransmitters can modify the signal, act over a different time course, influence neuronal metabolism, or prepare cells for later neural events. Knowledge of neurotransmitters is essential to understanding the organization of the central nervous system, a variety of neurological diseases and the nature of many drug actions. Recently developed immunohistochemical methods have revealed information concerning the sites of synthesis and storage of known or suspected neurotransmitters and neuromodulators. Autoradiographic technics provide information concerning the distribution of transmitter binding sites. The functional significance of many putative neurotransmitters remains obscure.

Acetylcholine (ACh), the first neurotransmitter identified, is the major transmitter of the peripheral nervous system, but is less prominent in the central nervous system. Neurons containing ACh can be identified only indirectly by labeling its synthesizing enzyme choline acetyltransferase or visualizing the hydrolytic enzyme acetylcholinesterase (AChE). While there

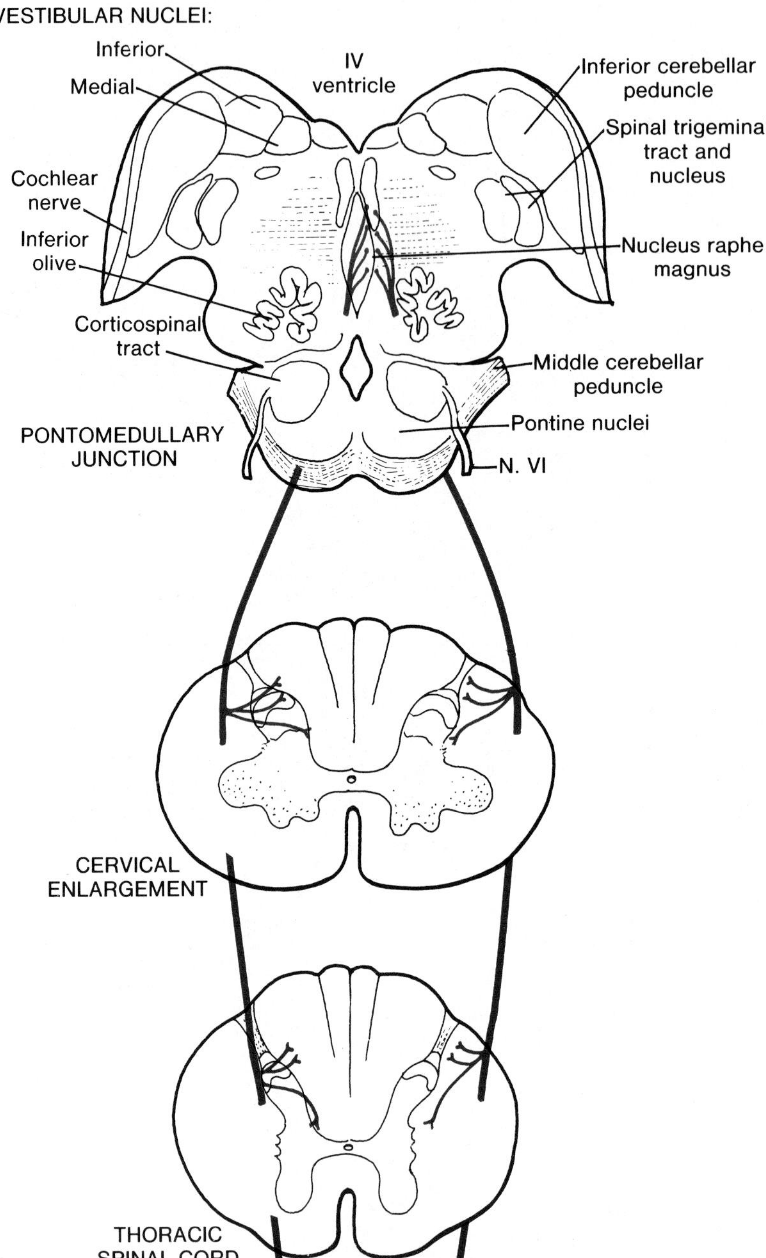

Figure 5-12. Schematic diagram of spinal serotonergic projections from the nucleus raphe magnus. These projections are bilateral, descend in the dorsal part of the lateral funiculus and terminate upon cells in laminae I, II and V, considered to receive nociceptive inputs. Adjacent large reticular neurons have similar spinal projections, but are not serotonergic. Both of these pathways are considered links in an endogenous analgesia-producing system. Fibers from the nuclei raphe pallidus and obscurus (not shown) descend in the ventral quadrant of the spinal cord (Basbaum et al., '78; Basbaum and Fields, '79). (From Carpenter and Sutin, *Human Neuroanatomy*, 1983; courtesy of Williams & Wilkins.)

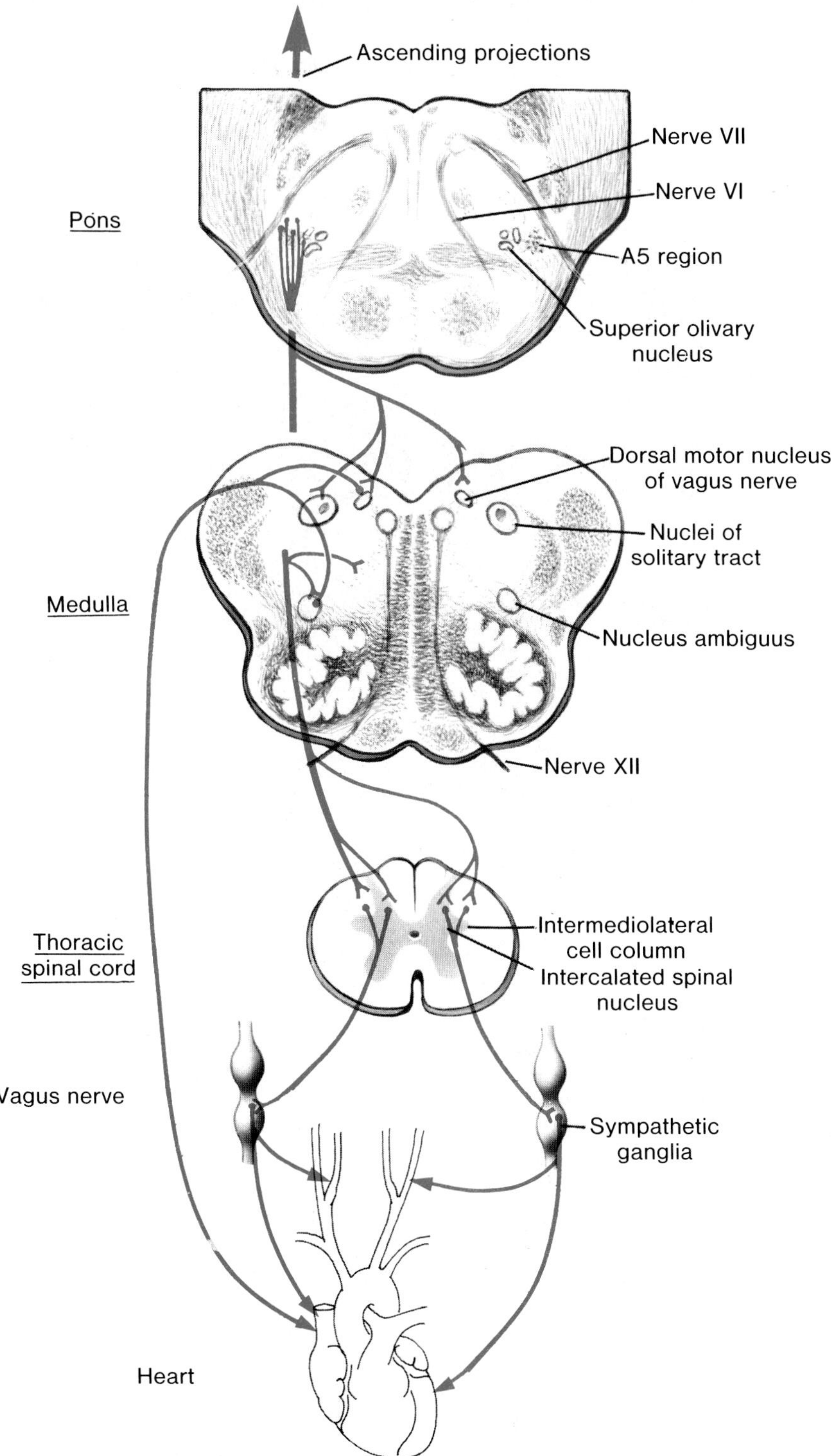

Figure 5-13. Schematic diagram of descending projections from the catecholamine cell group (A5) which lies lateral to the superior olviary nucleus and projects to: (1) medullary vasomotor areas, (2) preganglionic sympathetic neurons, and (3) intercalated spinal neurons. Medullary nuclei receiving fibers from the A5 cell group include: (1) the dorsal motor nucleus of the vagus nerve, (2) the nucleus ambiguus, (3) the nuclei of the solitary tract, and (4) paramedian (not shown) and medial medullary reticular neurons. Inputs to cells of the intermediolateral cell column and intercalated spinal neurons from this cell group are relayed via preganglionic and postganglionic sympathetic neurons to the cardiovascular system. Stimulation of the A5 cell group produces an increase in systemic blood and pulse pressure. Ascending projections from this catecholamine cell group have been described but not fully characterized (Lewy and McKellar, '80). (From Carpenter and Sutin, *Human Neuroanatomy*, 1983; courtesy of Williams & Wilkins.)

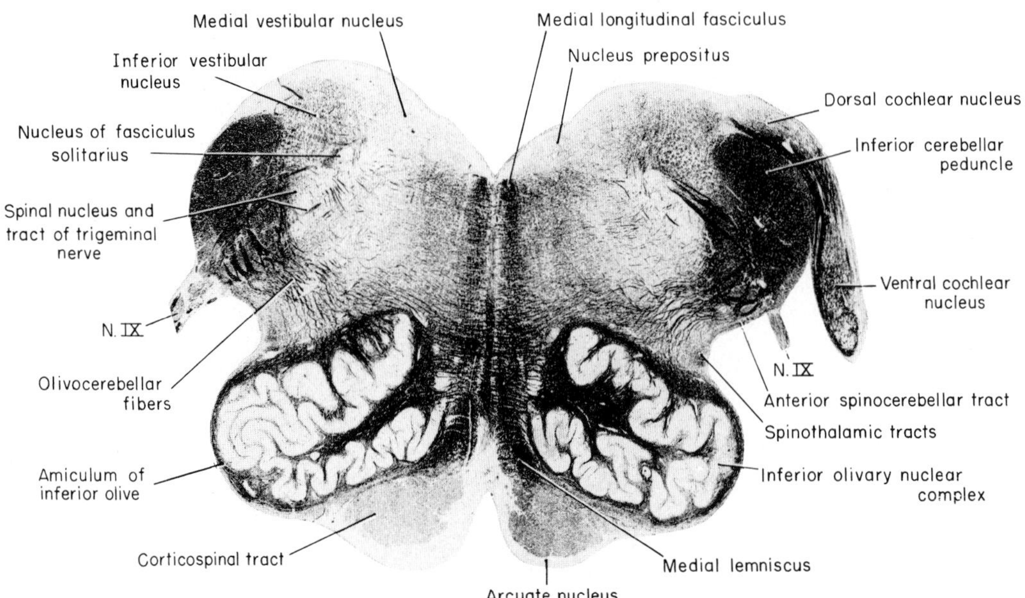

Figure 5-14. Transverse section of medulla of 1-month infant through the cochlear nuclei and ninth nerve. (Weigert's myelin stain; photograph.) (From Carpenter and Sutin, *Human Neuroanatomy*, 1983; courtesy of Williams & Wilkins.)

is a general correspondence between AChE and ACh, AChE is present in noncholinergic neurons and is by itself not a definitive marker. ACh is the chemical messenger that brings about contractions of striated muscle and is released at the terminals of all preganglionic neurons. Cell bodies containing AChE are found in all motor cranial nerve nuclei, including the dorsal motor nucleus of the vagus (Palkovits and Jacobwitz, '74).

Biogenic amines present in the medulla are norepinephrine, epinephrine, and serotonin. The locus ceruleus represents the largest concentration of norepinephrine-containing cell bodies in the brain stem (Figs. 4-15, 6-27 and 6-26). Fibers of this pigmented nucleus located at isthmus levels are widely distributed throughout the central nervous system (Ungerstedt, '71). Most of the noradrenergic cell bodies in the medulla and pons are scattered throughout the region of the lateral reticular formation, but others are present near the commissural and dorsal motor nuclei of the vagus (Dahlström and Fuxe, '64; Ungerstedt, '71). Noradrenergic neurons in the caudal brain stem have been collectively referred to as the lateral tegmental group (Fig. 5-13). Studies of the distribution of noradrenergic fibers from these two sources indicate that the locus ceruleus innervates primary sensory and association nuclei while the lateral tegmental norepinephrine-containing neurons innervate primary motor and visceral nuclei (Levitt and Moore, '79). The highest norepinephrine content is present in the trigeminal motor nucleus, the nucleus of the solitary tract, the dorsal motor nucleus of the vagus and the dorsal nucleus of the raphe. Bilateral lesions of the locus ceruleus do not diminish norepinephrine content in these nuclei (Levitt and Moore, '79).

The indoleamine serotonin occurs largely in neurons of the raphe nuclei, although some serotonergic cells are in the reticular formation (Figs. 5-11 and 5-12). The serotonin system resembles the norepinephrine system in that both are components of the brain stem reticular formation and have widespread and partially overlapping projections. The ascending projections of the serotonin-containing neurons in the midbrain are more selective in their targets than the noradrenergic fibers, and they innervate the ependyma and circumventricular organs. The raphe nuclei and the serotonergic neurons in the medulla have been described in a previous section.

Two pentapeptides, methionine-enkephalin (met-enkephalin) and leucine-enkephalin (leu-enkephalin), isolated from both central and peripheral nervous tissue appear to be endogenous ligands for opiate receptors (Hughes et al., '75). Both enkephalins are widely distributed in the central nervous system where their ratios differ; leu-enkephalin generally is present in higher concentrations. The distribution of opiate receptor binding sites parallels that of the opiate peptides. Enkephalin immunoreactive cell bodies in the medulla occur in laminae I and II in caudal portions of the spinal trigeminal nucleus (Fig. 5-8), in the solitary nucleus (Fig. 5-19), in the hypoglossal nucleus, and in parts of reticular formation adjacent to the nucleus raphe magnus. These opiate-like peptides appear to act as neurotransmitters or neuromodulators to suppress pain (Fields, '81).

Substance P is a peptide of 10 amino acids found in several neural subsystems. It is found in about 20% of the cell bodies in spinal ganglia and in the terminals of dorsal root fibers in laminae I and II (Fig. 3-21). In sensory neurons this peptide is associated with small, poorly myelinated fibers that encode nociceptive information. In the medulla substance P terminals are found in the superficial laminae of the caudal part of the spinal trigeminal nucleus, in the solitary nucleus, and in certain cells in the raphe nuclei (Cuello and Kanazawa, '78). In some neurons substance P may coexist with other neurotransmitters. Dale's principle which states that one neuron produces and releases only one transmitter no longer holds. Substance P produces a prolonged excitation of central sensory neurons (Jessell, '81).

CRANIAL NERVES OF THE MEDULLA

The schematic arrangement of the functional components of the cranial nerves of the medulla and the cell columns to which they are related are shown in Figure 5-15. The functional components of a typical spinal nerve are four: (1) *general somatic afferent* (GSA), (2) *general visceral afferent* (GVA), (3) *general somatic efferent* (GSE), and (4) *general visceral efferent* (GVE). Functional components of the cranial nerves include the four types found in spinal nerves, plus three additional special categories: (1) *special somatic afferent* (SSA), (2) *special visceral afferent* (SVA), and (3) *special visceral efferent* (SVE). Somatic efferent fibers in both spinal and cranial nerves are regarded as a general component.

In the medulla, as in the spinal cord the sulcus limitans divides afferent and efferent cell columns. Within the medulla special somatic afferent (SSA) cranial nerves are represented by the auditory and vestibular components of the vestibulocochlear nerve (N.VIII). General somatic afferent (GSA) fiber components of cranial nerves V, VII, IX, and X descend in the spinal trigeminal tract. Fibers conveying taste (special visceral afferent, SVA) and general visceral afferent (GVA) impulses from components of cranial nerves VII, IX and X form a well defined tract, the solitary fasciculus, which is embedded in the solitary nucleus (Figs. 5-7, 5-9, 5-10, and 5-20). The above cell columns lie posterolateral to a hypothetical extension of the sulcus limitans (Fig. 5-15). Ventromedial to this hypothetically projected line are the efferent cell columns. The dorsal motor nucleus of the vagus nerve and the inferior salivatory nucleus of the glossopharyngeal nerve give rise to general visceral efferent (GVE) fibers. Cells of the nucleus ambiguus located in the ventrolateral reticular formation posterior to the inferior olivary nuclear complex, give rise to special visceral efferent (SVE) fibers that pass peripherally as components of the XI, X and IX cranial nerves (Fig. 5-10). These fibers innervate muscles of the pharynx and larynx derived from the third and fourth branchial arches (i.e., branchiomeric muscles). The hypoglossal nucleus located in the floor of the fourth ventricle near the median raphe gives rise to general somatic efferent (GSE) fibers which innervate the muscles of the tongue (Fig. 5-10). The general somatic efferent cranial nerve nuclei all lie near the median raphe and in the floor of the fourth ventricle or cerebral aqueduct. Other nuclei, at more rostral levels, belonging to this group are: the abducens, trochlear and oc-

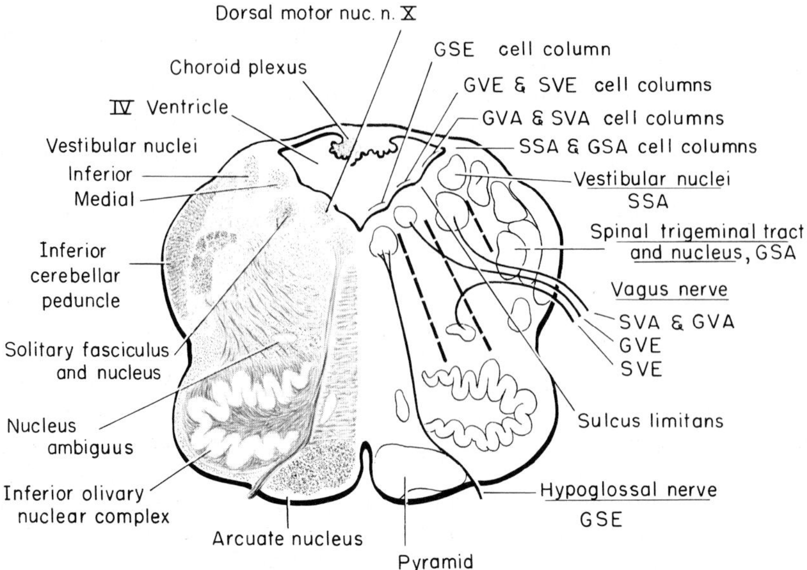

Figure 5-15. Schematic transverse section of the medulla showing its basic features. Cell columns related to functional components of the cranial nerve are indicated on the *right*. Functional components of cranial nerves are both general and special. The vestibular nuclei shown at this level (and auditory nuclei at higher levels) form the special somatic afferent (*SSA*) cell columns. The spinal trigeminal nucleus forms the general somatic afferent (*GSA*) cell column and receives fibers from cranial nerves with this functional component (i.e., N. V, N. VII, N. IX, N. X). Functional components of the vague nerve (except *GSA*) are shown in relation to particular nuclei. The hypoglossal nucleus (and the nuclei of N. VI, N. IV and N. III at higher brain stem levels) gives rise to general somatic efferent (*GSE*) fibers. Heavy dashes separate the nuclei of the various cell columns on the right side. (From Carpenter and Sutin, *Human Neuroanatomy*, 1983; courtesy of Williams & Wilkins.)

ulomotor. Schematic diagrams showing these nuclei and their intramedullary course (Figs. 5-16 and 5-17) should help to understand the organization of the cranial nerves and their various components.

Hypoglossal Nerve. This is a *general somatic efferent* (GSE) cranial nerve which supplies the somatic skeletal muscles of the tongue. The hypoglossal nucleus forms a column of typical motor cells about 18 mm long (Fig. 5-16 and 5-17). Root fibers of the nerve emerge ventrally, pass along the lateral margin of the MLF and the medial lemniscus, traverse medial parts of the inferior olivary complex and exit from the medulla in the pre-olivary sulcus, between the pyramid and the inferior olive (Figs. 5-1, 5-7, and 5-9). In the gray matter surrounding the hypoglossal nuclei are several discrete nuclear groups, collectively known as the *perihypoglossal nuclei.* These are the *nucleus intercalatus*, the *nucleus prepositus*, and the *nucleus of Roller* (Figs. 5-10 and 5-14). The nucleus intercalatus lies between the hypoglossal and dorsal motor vagal nuclei. The nucleus prepositus extends from the rostral pole of the hypoglossal nucleus almost to the level of the abducens nucleus (Figs. 5-14 and 5-24). The nucleus of Roller lies ventral to the rostral part of the hypoglossal nucleus adjacent to nerve rootlets (Fig. 5-10). Immediately posterior to the hypoglossal nucleus is a small bundle of descending fibers in the periventricular gray known as the *dorsal longitudinal fasciculus* (Schütz). This bundle consists of both ascending and descending components which are thought to be visceral in nature (Fig. 5-9).

Lesions of the hypoglossal nerve produce a lower motor neuron paralysis of the ipsilateral tongue muscles with loss of muscle tone and ultimately, atrophy of the muscles. Due to paralysis of the genioglossus muscle, a muscle which effects protrusion of the tongue to the opposite side, the tongue will deviate to the side of the lesion when protruded. The intrinsic muscles alter the shape of the tongue, while the extrinsic muscles alter its shape and position.

Intramedullary lesions involving the medullary pyramid and the hypoglossal nerve (due to vascular lesions of the anterior spinal artery) produce a combined upper and lower motor neuron syndrome referred to as *inferior alternating hemiplegia.* This syndrome is characterized by: (1) a contralateral hemiplegia (upper motor neuron) and (2) an ipsilateral paralysis of the tongue (lower motor neuron).

Spinal Accessory Nerve. This nerve consists of two distinct parts referred to as the cranial and spinal portions (Figs. 1-4 and 5-18). The *cranial part* of the nerve arises from cells in the most caudal part of the nucleus ambiguus. Axons of these cells emerge from the lateral surface of the medulla caudal to the filaments of the vagus nerve. Fibers of the cranial part of the accessory nerve join the vagus nerve, form the inferior (recurrent) laryngeal nerve, and innervate the intrinsic muscles of the larynx (Figs. 5-16 and 5-17). This component of the accessory nerve innervates branchiomeric musculature and is regarded as a *special visceral efferent* (SVE) component.

The *spinal portion* of the accessory nerve originates from a column of cells in the anterior horn of the upper five (or six) cervical segments (Figs. 1-4, 5-3, and 5-18). Root fibers from these cells arch posterolaterally and emerge from the lateral aspect of the spinal cord between the dorsal and ventral roots. Rootlets of the spinal portion of the nerve unite to form a common trunk which ascends posterior to the denticulate ligaments, enters the skull through the foramen magnum and ultimately makes its exit from the skull in association with the vagus and glossopharyngeal nerve via the jugular foramen (Fig. 1-4). The spinal part of the accessory nerve innervates the ipsilateral sternocleidomastoid and the upper parts of the trapezius muscles. Although contraction of one sternocleidomastoid muscle turns the head to the opposite side, a unilateral lesion of the spinal accessory nerve usually does not produce any abnormality in the position of the head. Weakness in turning the head to the opposite side against resistance, however, is obvious. Paralysis of the upper part of the trapezius muscle is evidenced by: (1) downward and outward rotation of the scapula, and (2) moderate sagging of the shoulder on the affected side.

Vagus Nerve. This is a complex mixed branchiomeric nerve containing: (1) *general somatic afferent* (GSA) fibers distributed to cutaneous areas back of the ear and in the external auditory meatus, (2) *general visceral afferent* (GVA) fibers from the pharynx, larynx, trachea, esophagus and thoracic and abdominal viscera, (3) *special visceral afferent* (SVA) fibers from taste buds in the region of the epiglottis, (4) *general visceral efferent* (GVE) fibers distributed to parasympathetic ganglia located near to thoracic and abdominal viscera, and (5) *special visceral efferent* (SVE) fibers which innervate the striated (branchiomeric) muscles of the larynx and pharynx (Figs. 5-15 and 5-16).

General somatic afferent fibers of the vagus nerve arise from cells of the superior ganglion of the vagus nerve, located in, or immediately beneath, the jugular foramen (Fig. 5-18). Both general and special visceral afferent fibers of the vagus nerve arise from the larger inferior vagal ganglion (nodosal ganglion). Afferent vagal fibers enter the lateral surface of the medulla ventral to the inferior cerebellar peduncle and usually traverse the spinal trigeminal tract and nucleus (Fig. 5-15). Cutaneous afferent fibers enter the dorsal part of the spinal trigeminal tract along with similar general somatic afferents from other branchiomeric cranial nerves. More numerous visceral afferent fibers of the vagus nerve pass dorsomedially into the nucleus and tractus solitarius (Fig. 5-16, 5-19, and 5-20). Fibers entering the solitary fasciculus bifurcate into short ascending and longer descending components. Descending vagal components in the solitary fasciculus gradually diminish in number as collaterals and terminals are given off to the solitary nucleus. Some vagal visceral fibers descend caudal to the obex, where the solitary nuclei of the two sides merge to form the *commissural nucleus* of the vagus nerve (Fig. 5-6).

The *fasciculus solitarius* is formed by visceral afferent fibers contributed by the vagus, glossopharyngeal and facial (intermediate) nerves (Figs. 5-16 and 5-17). Fibers conveying taste from the anterior two-thirds of the tongue (chorda tympani) and from the posterior third of the tongue (glos-

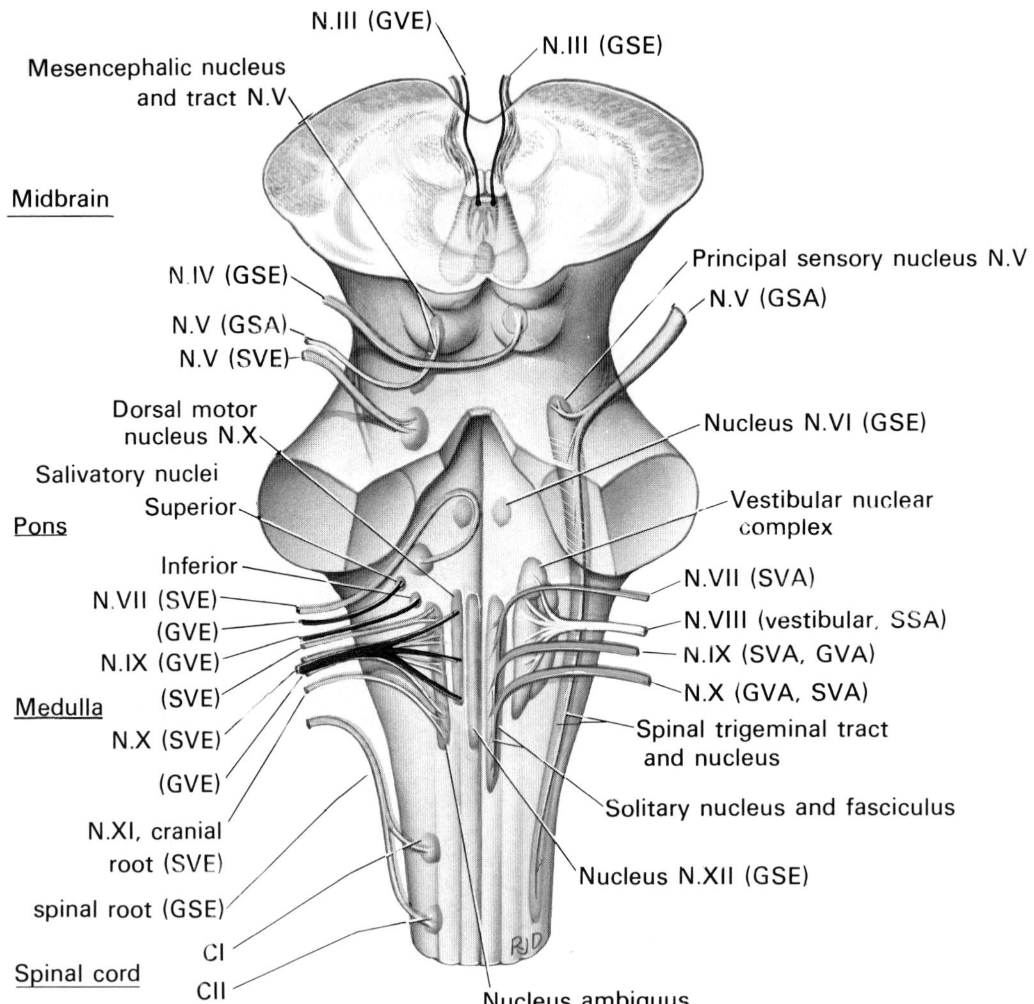

Figure 5-16. Schematic representation of the infratentorial cranial nerves showing their nuclei of origin and termination, their intramedullary course and their functional components. The cochlear nerve and nuclei are not shown (see Fig. 6-10). General somatic afferent (*GSA*) components of the trigeminal nerve (N. V) are shown in *light blue*. General and special visceral afferent (*GVA*, *SVA*) components of the facial (N. VII), glossopharyngeal (N. IX) and vagus (N. X) nerves are shown in *dark blue*. The vestibular nerve which distributes special somatic afferent (*SSA*) fibers to the vestibular nuclear complex is *white*. Similarities in the intramedullary course of fibers in the spinal trigeminal tract, the vestibular nerve root and the solitary fasciculus are evident on the *right*. General somatic efferent (*GSE*) fibers from the oculomotor (N. III) and trochlear (N. IV) nuclei and those of the spinal root of the accessory nerve (N. XI) are *light red*. Only contributions from the first and second cervical segments to the spinal root of the accessory nerve are shown. Root fibers of the abducens (N. VI) and hypoglossal (N. XII) nuclei which exit ventrally and contain *GSE* fibers are not shown. Special visceral efferent (*SVE*) fibers from the branchiomeric cranial nerves (N. V, N. VII, N. IX, N. S and N. XI) are shown in *light red*. General visceral efferent (*GVE*) fibers, representing preganglionic parasympathetic components, of the oculomotor (N. III), facial (N. VII), glossopharyngeal (N. IX) and vagus (N. X) nerves are in *dark red*. (From Carpenter and Sutin, *Human Neuroanatomy*, 1983; courtesy of Williams & Wilkins.)

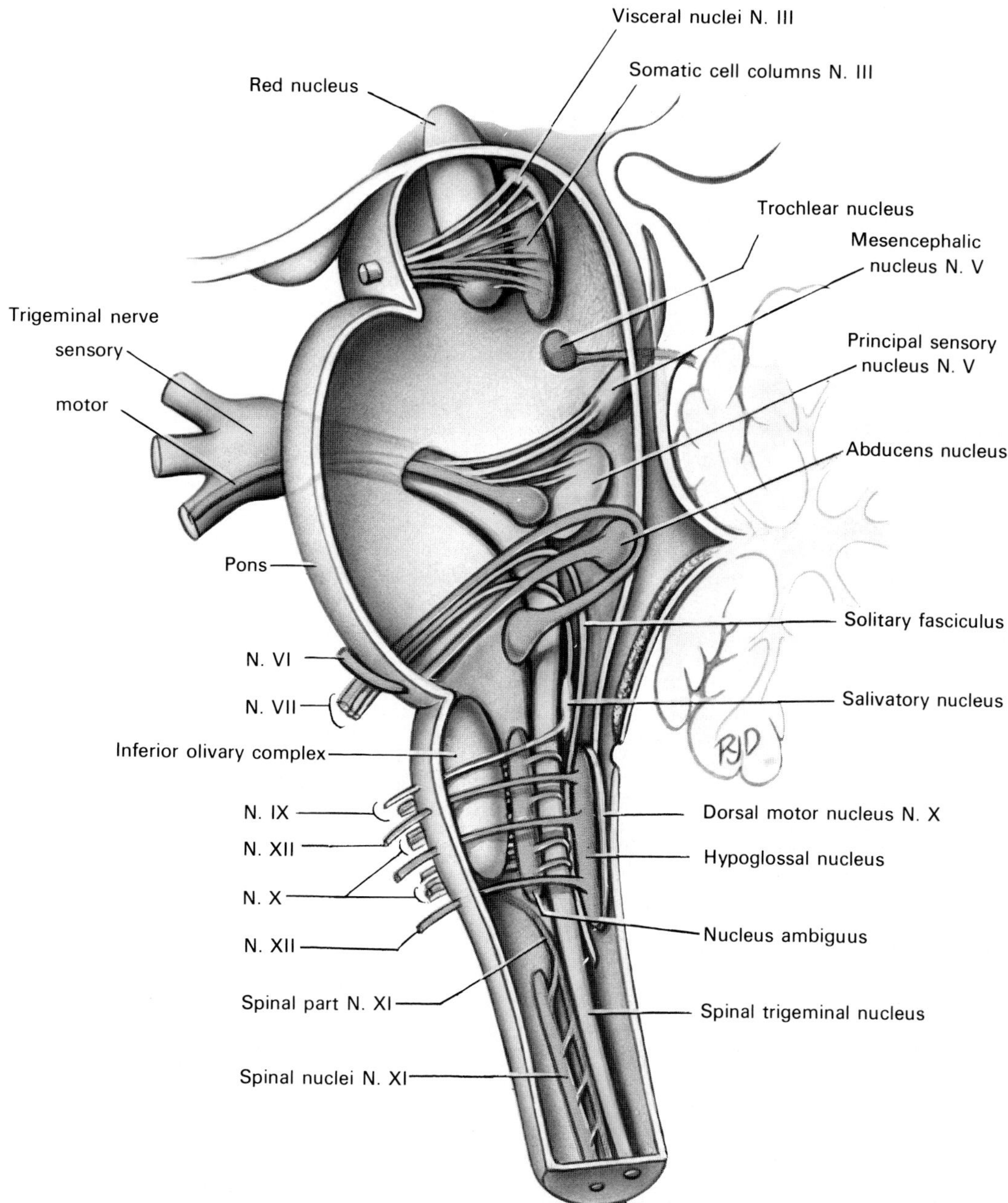

Figure 5-17. Schematic diagram of the intramedullary course of the cranial nerves in a midsagittal view. The brain stem is represented as a hollow shell except for cranial nerve components. General somatic (*GSE*) and special visceral (*SVE*) efferent components of cranial nerves innervating striated muscles are shown in *red*. General visceral efferent (*GVE*) components of cranial nerves III, VII, IX, and X, representing preganglionic parasympathetic fibers, are shown in *yellow*. General somatic (*GSA*), general visceral (*GVA*) and special visceral (*SVA*) afferent components of the cranial nerves are in *blue*. (Modified from Elze, '32.) (From Carpenter and Sutin, *Human Neuroanatomy*, 1983; courtesy of Williams & Wilkins.)

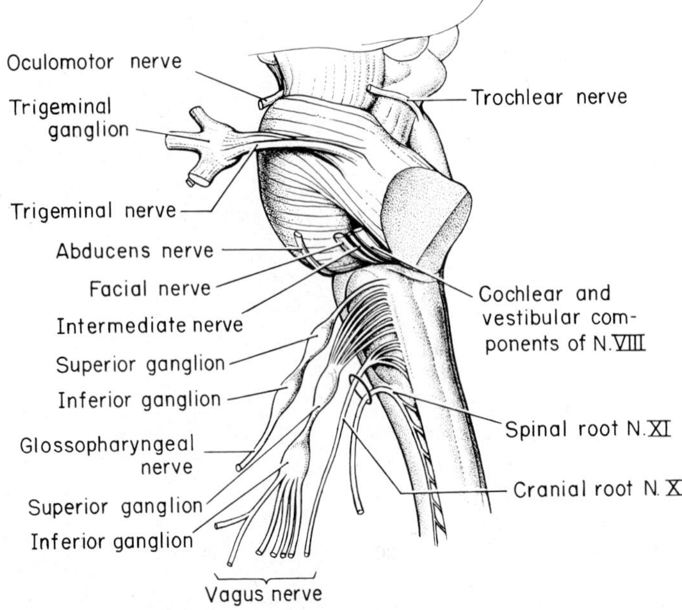

Figure 5-18. Semidiagrammatic sketch of brain stem and cranial nerves showing the peripheral ganglia. (From Carpenter and Sutin, *Human Neuroanatomy*, 1983; courtesy of Williams & Wilkins.)

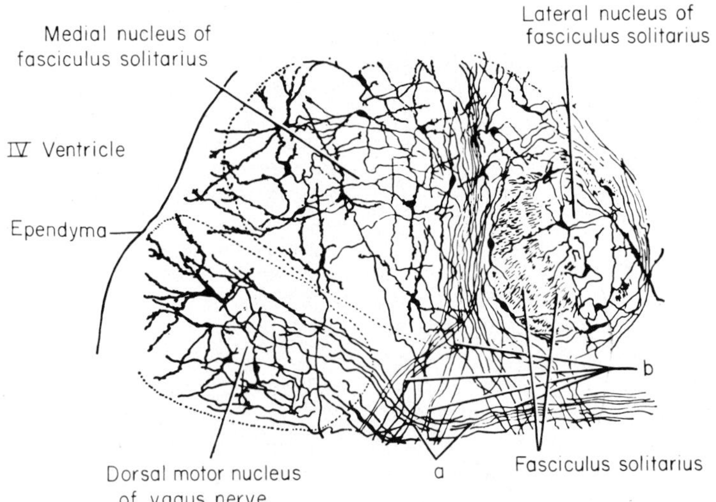

Figure 5-19. The vagal nuclei in the floor of the fourth ventricle based upon a drawing of a Golgi preparation of newborn cat (Cajal, '09). Efferent (preganglionic) fibers from the dorsal motor nucleus of the vagus nerve are indicated by *a*, while *b* indicates fibers from the medial and lateral (sensory) nuclei of the fasciculus solitarius forming secondary vagoglossopharyngeal pathways. The medial nucleus of the fasciculus solitarius extends caudal to the fourth ventricle and merges with the corresponding cell group on the opposite side, forming the commissural nucleus of the vagus nerve (Fig. 5-6). The lateral nucleus of the fasciculus solitarius extends rostrally, increases in size and parallels the fasciculus solitarius throughout most of its length. (From Carpenter and Sutin, *Human Neuroanatomy*, 1983; courtesy of Williams & Wilkins.)

sopharyngeal nerve) enter rostral parts of the solitary fasciculus and mainly terminate in rostral parts of the solitary nucleus. Portions of the solitary fasciculus at the level of entry of the vagus nerve, and caudal to it, contain mainly general visceral afferent fibers, largely from the vagus nerve.

The *nucleus solitarius* can be divided into several parts: (1) a medial part, dorsolateral to the dorsal motor nucleus of the vagus, (2) dorsomedial, dorsolateral and ventrolateral subnuclei which surround the *tractus solitarius*, and (3) a parvicellular subnucleus beneath the area postrema (Fig. 5-19). Cells of the medial part extend rostrally slightly beyond the dorsal motor nucleus of the valgus; this part of the nucleus also extends caudal to the fourth ventricle and merges with the corresponding cell column on the opposite side to form the commissural nucleus of the vagus nerve (Fig. 5-6).

The lateral nuclei form columns of larger cells which partially or completely surrounds the solitary fasciculus (Figs. 5-7, 5-9, and 5-19). This part of the nucleus parallels the fasciculus throughout most of its length; rostrally it extends into the lower part of the pons, while caudally its cells diminish in number and are difficult to distinguish from reticular neurons. The enlarged rostral part of the solitary nucleus (i.e., the lateral part) receives mainly special visceral afferent (taste) fibers from the facial (intermediate) and glossopharyngeal nerves and is referred to as the gustatory nucleus. The caudal and medial solitary nucleus receives mainly general visceral afferent fibers from the vagus nerve, along with some facial and glossopharyngeal fibers. Although visceral afferents terminate over the rostrocaudal extent of the solitary nuclear complex (Fig. 5-20), there is a viscerotopic pattern in that: (1) gastrointestinal afferents end in the parvicellular subnucleus (Gwyn et al., '79); (2) pulmonary afferents end in the ventrolateral subnuclei (Kalia and Mesulam, '80); and (3) carotid sinus afferents end in medial and dorsomedial subnuclei (Panneton and Loewy, '80).

Secondary fiber systems arising from the solitary nucleus project ipsilaterally to: (1) the nucleus ambiguus and surrounding reticular formation, (2) the parabrachial nuclei in the rostral pons (Fig. 5-21), and (3) the thalamic nucleus concerned with gustatory sensation, namely the ventral posteromedial nucleus (pars parvicellularis) (Fig. 9-14) (Beckstead et al., '80). Other secondary fibers from the solitary nucleus projecting to the hypoglossal and salivatory nuclei mediate lingual and secretory reflexes. Projections from this nucleus to the dorsal motor nucleus of N. X, the phrenic nerve nucleus and anterior horn cells of thoracic spinal segments are involved in coughing, vomiting, and respiration (Fig. 4-15). The nucleus of the solitary tract is

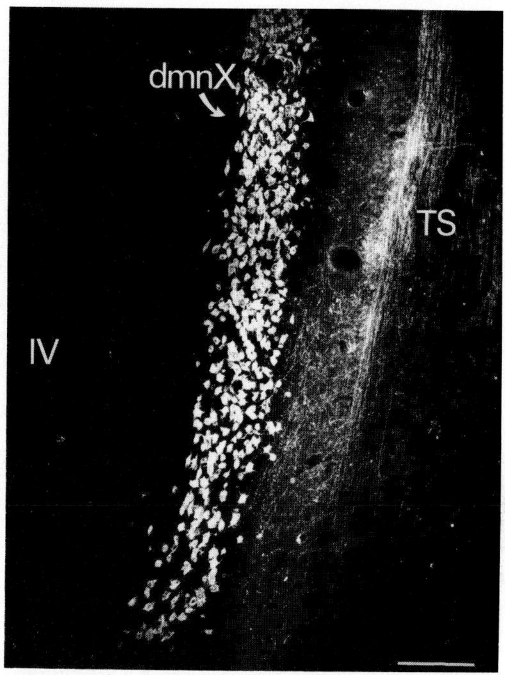

Figure 5-20. Dark-field photomicrograph of a horizontal section of the medulla of a cat in which horseradish peroxidase (HRP) was injected into the inferior ganglion (nodose) of the vagus nerve. Rostral is toward the top and lateral is to the right; *IV* indicates the fourth ventricle. Cells of the dorsal motor nucleus of the vagus nerve (*dmnX*) are retrogradely labeled and form a long column. Fibers of the tractus solitarius (*TS*) are anterogradely labeled with HRP. Note the region of finely labeled terminals from the tractus solitarius situated in the solitary nucleus between TS and dmnX. These terminals parallel the TS for an appreciable distance. (Calibration bar equals 500 μm.) (From Carpenter and Sutin, *Human Neuroanatomy*, 1983; courtesy of Williams & Wilkins.)

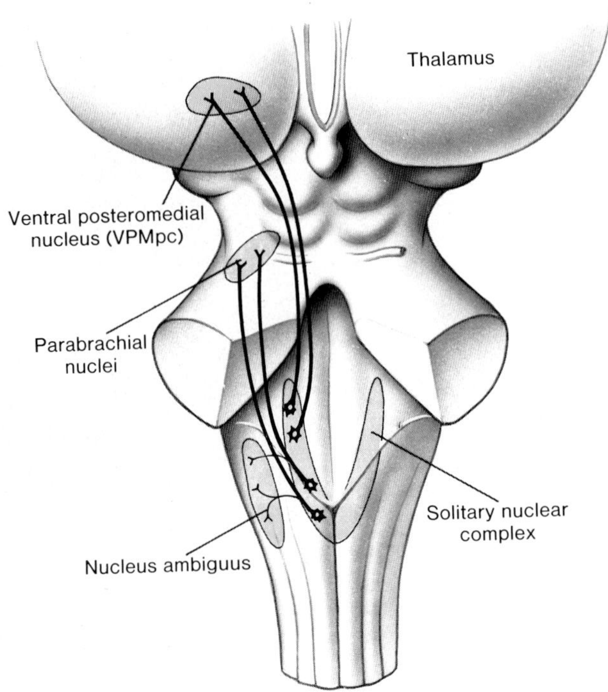

Figure 5-21. Schematic diagram of ascending projections of the solitary nuclear complex. Special visceral afferent (SVA) neurons in the geniculate ganglion (intermediate nerve) and both special (SVA) and general (GVA) visceral neurons in the inferior ganglia of the glossopharyngeal and vagus nerves project to portions of the solitary nuclear complex (*blue*). Cells in rostral portions of the nucleus solitarius project ipsilaterally via the central tegmental tract to the small-celled part of the ventral posteromedial (VPMpc) nucleus of the thalamus (Fig. 9-14). Cells of VPMpc project thalamocortical fibers to the cortex of the parietal operculum. Caudal parts of the solitary nucleus which receive afferents from the vagus and glossopharyngeal nerves project rostrally to the ipsilateral medial and lateral parabrachial nuclei. Caudal parts of solitary nucleus also project fibers to the ipsilateral nucleus ambiguus. The solitary nuclear complex, the nucleus ambiguus, the parabrachial nuclei and VPMpc are shown in *blue*. (Based upon Beckstead et al., '80.) (From Carpenter and Sutin, *Human Neuroanatomy*, 1983; courtesy of Williams & Wilkins.)

coextensive with the physiologically defined medullary respiratory "center" which includes the nucleus ambiguus and surrounding portions of the reticular formation (Kalia, '77). Cells of the medullary "respiratory center" are activated by vagal impulses and directly by changes in their chemical environment (CO_2 accumulation). A medullary vasomotor "center" consisting of separate pressor and depressor zones has been poorly defined. Recent emphasis has been on neural networks concerned with cardiovascular control. A group of noradrenergic neurons (designated as group A5) (Fig. 5-13), located in the caudal pons between the superior olive and root fibers of the facial nerve and projecting axons to the nucleus solitarius, the nucleus ambiguus, the dorsal motor nucleus of N. X, and preganglionic sympathetic neurons in the thoracic spinal cord, appears to be part of this neural network (Loewy and McKellar, '80).

The *dorsal motor nucleus* of the vagus nerve is situated in the floor of the fourth ventricle posterolateral to the hypoglossal nucleus (Figs. 5-9, 5-10, 5-16, and 5-17). This column of relatively small spindle-shaped cells extends both rostrally and caudally slightly beyond the hypoglossal nucleus. Some larger cells in the nucleus contain coarse chromophilic bodies and scattered melanin pigment. Cells of this nucleus give rise to preganglionic parasympathetic fibers (GVE). Axons of these cells emerge from the lateral surface of the medulla by traversing the spinal trigeminal tract and nucleus (Fig. 5-15). The dorsal motor nucleus of the vagus is the vagal secretomotor center (Kerr and Preshaw, '69). Destruction of this nucleus greatly reduces insulin-induced secretion of gastric acid.

The *nucleus ambiguus* is a column of cells in the reticular formation about half way between the spinal trigeminal nucleus and the inferior olivary complex (Figs. 5-6 and 5-10). This nucleus, extending from the level of the decussation of the medial lemniscus to levels through the rostral third of the inferior olivary complex, is composed of typical multipolar lower motor neurons. Fibers from the nucleus arch dorsally, join efferent fibers from the dorsal motor nucleus of the vagus nerve and emerge from the lateral surface of the medulla dorsal to the inferior olivary complex (Fig. 5-15). Caudal parts of the nucleus ambiguus give rise to the cranial part of the spinal accessory nerve, while rostral parts of this cell column give rise to glossopharyngeal special visceral efferent fibers (which innervate the stylopharyngeus muscle). Special visceral efferent fibers of the vagus nerve (and those from the cranial part of the accessory nerve which rejoin the vagus nerve) innervate the muscles of the pharynx and larynx (Figs. 5-16 and 5-17).

A unilateral lesion of the vagus nerve produces ipsilateral paralysis of the soft palate, pharynx and larynx which results in hoarseness of the voice, dyspnea and dysphagia. During phonation the soft palate is elevated on the normal side and the uvula deviates to the normal side. The palatal reflex is lost on the side of the lesion. Anesthesia of the pharynx and larynx results in an ipsilateral loss of the cough reflex, while destruction of visceral motor fibers of the vagus nerve abolishes the carotid sinus reflex ipsilaterally.

Bilateral lesions of the vagus nerve cause complete paralysis of the pharynx and larynx and will result in death due to asphyxia unless a tracheostomy is performed immediately. With complete paralysis of the larynx, the vocal cords lie close to the midline and cannot be abducted on attempted inspiration. Paralysis and atonia of the esophagus and stomach produce pain and vomiting. The heart rate becomes rapid and irregular due to removal of vagal inhibitory influences. This condition is associated with marked dysphagia and dysarthria.

Glossopharyngeal Nerve. This nerve is closely related to the vagus nerve, having certain common intermedullary nuclei, and similar functional components. Fibers of this nerve enter and emerge at levels rostral to the vagus nerve, but like the vagus nerve, they traverse the spinal trigeminal tract and nucleus (Figs. 5-14, 5-16, 5-17, and 5-18). The glossopharyngeal is a mixed branchiomeric cranial nerve with the following functional components: (1) *general visceral afferent* (GVA) fibers, (2) *special visceral afferent* (SVA) fibers (taste), (3) a few *general somatic afferent* (GSA) fibers, (4) *general visceral efferent* (GVE) fibers, and (5) a small number of *special visceral efferent* (SVE) fibers. Like the vagus nerve it has two peripheral ganglia, a small *superior ganglion* in the jugular foramen and a larger extracranial *inferior (petrosal) ganglion* (Fig. 5-18).

Primary sensory neurons mediating general somatic sense (GSA) from cutaneous areas back of the ear lie in the superior ganglion; central processes of these cells enter the spinal trigeminal tract and nucleus. Cell bodies of visceral afferent fibers lie in the inferior ganglion. General visceral afferent fibers convey impulses concerned with tactile sense, thermal sense and pain from the mucous membranes of the posterior third of the tongue, the tonsil, the posterior wall of the upper pharynx and the Eustachian tube. Special visceral afferent fibers convey taste sensation from the posterior third of the tongue. Visceral afferent fibers enter the posterolateral part of the medulla and are distributed to rostral portions of the solitary fasciculus and its nucleus (Figs. 5-16 and 5-17). Rostral and lateral parts of the nucleus solitarius which receive fibers from the facial (intermediate) and glossopharyngeal nerves constitute what is called the "gustatory nucleus." The carotid sinus nerve conveys impulses from the carotid sinus, a baroreceptor, located at the bifurcation of the common carotid. Increases in carotid arterial pressure excite carotid sinus baroreceptors and impulses are conveyed centrally by the glossopharyngeal nerve to the nucleus of the solitary tract (Panneton and Loewy, '80). Second order neurons in the solitary nucleus project to the dorsal motor nucleus of the vagus nerve and bring about reductions in heart rate and arterial pressure via pre- and postganglionic vagal fibers that convey impulses to the sinoatrial and atrioventricular nodes, as well as to atrial heart muscle. The *carotid sinus reflex* involving glossopharyngeal visceral afferents and vagal general visceral efferents constitutes a mechanism for the regulation of arterial blood pressure.

General visceral efferent fibers, arising from the *inferior salivatory nucleus*, pass via the lesser petrosal nerve to the otic ganglion, situated below the foramen ovale and medial to the mandibular division of the trigeminal nerve. Postganglionic fibers originating from cells of the otic ganglion convey parasympathetic secretory impulses to the parotid gland. Cells of the inferior salivatory nucleus are virtually impossible to distinguish from reticular neurons, but they are considered as a separate rostral cell group equivalent to the dorsal motor nucleus of the vagus.

Special visceral efferent fibers, as already described, arise from rostral portions of the nucleus ambiguus (Figs. 5-10 and 5-16). These fibers, small in number, innervate the stylopharyngeus muscle and perhaps portions of the superior pharyngeal constrictor muscle.

As the above description indicates, the glossopharyngeal nerve is predominately a sensory nerve, and a nerve contributing preganglionic parasympathetic fibers to the otic ganglion. Isolated lesions of the glossopharyngeal nerve are rare. Disturbances associated with lesions of the nerve include: (1) loss of the pharyngeal (gag) reflex, (2) loss of the carotid sinus reflex, and (3) loss of taste and general sensation in the posterior third of the tongue. *Glossopharyngeal neuralgia* resembles trigeminal neuralgia in that the excruciating pain is paroxysmal and may be triggered by seemingly trivial stimuli such as coughing or swallowing. The pain associated with this syndrome radiates to regions behind the ear.

CORTICOBULBAR FIBERS

Corticofugal fibers projecting to, and terminating in, portions of the lower brain stem are referred to as *corticobulbar fibers.* These fibers arise mainly from cortex on both sides of the central sulcus and project to: (1) sensory relay nuclei, (2) parts of the reticular formation, and (3) certain motor cranial nerve nuclei (Fig. 5-22).

Sensory relay nuclei receiving corticobulbar fibers include: (1) the nuclei gracilis and cuneatus, (2) sensory trigeminal nuclei, and (3) the nucleus of the solitary fasciculus. Corticobulbar fibers to the posterior column nuclei leave the pyramid and enter these nuclei by either traversing the medial lemniscus or the reticular formation. There are suggestions of somatotopic relationships between cortical areas and the nuclei gracilis and cuneatus, but details are incomplete and considerable overlap is evident. Corticofugal fibers do not appear to terminate upon cells receiving ascending fibers from spinal dorsal roots via the posterior columns.

Corticobulbar fibers projecting to all trigeminal sensory nuclei and the nucleus solitarius are derived predominantly, but not exclusively, from frontoparietal cortical areas. Fibers passing to the solitary nucleus terminate chiefly in its rostral part.

Corticobulbar fibers, projecting to the above described sensory relay nuclei, underlie the physiological mechanism by which descending cortical impulses can influence the transmission of sensory impulses at the second neuronal level. Both excitatory and inhibitory influences upon these relay nuclei can be produced following stimulation of certain cortical regions.

Corticoreticular fibers projecting to the lower brain stem arise predominantly from the motor, premotor and somesthetic cortex. Fibers descend in association with the corticospinal tract, leave the tract at various levels, and enter the reticular formation. The bulk of these fibers terminate in two fairly circumscribed areas, one in the medulla and one in the pons. In the medulla these fibers terminate in the area of the gigantocellular reticular nucleus; in the pons most of the fibers end in the oral pontine reticular nucleus (Figs. 4-6 and 4-14). Corticoreticular fibers are distributed bilaterally but with slight contralateral preponderance. Some corticoreticular fibers project to other nuclei, such as: (1) the reticulotegmental nucleus (pons), (2) the lateral reticular nucleus of the medulla, and

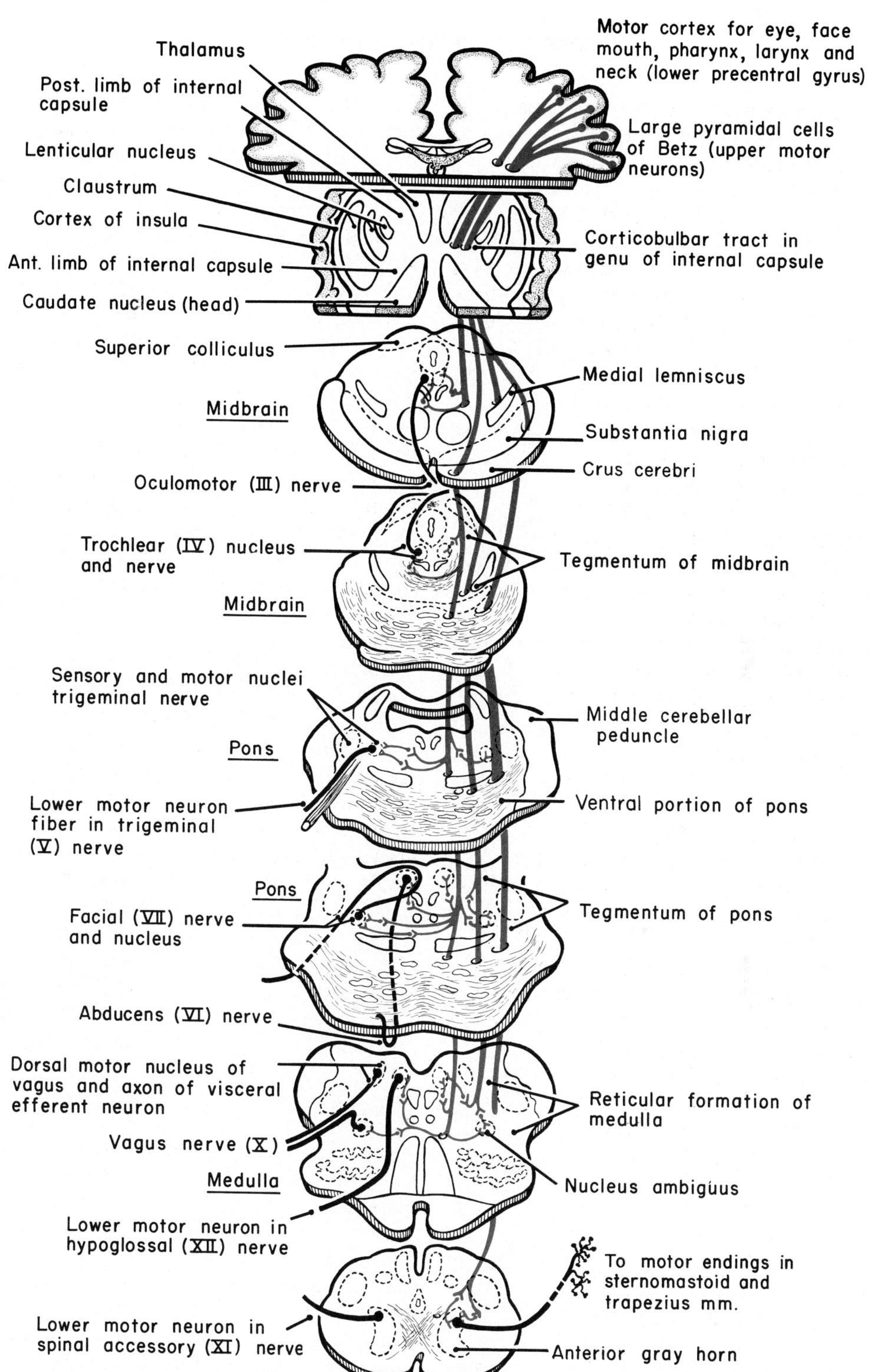

Figure 5-22. Schematic diagram of "corticobulbar" pathways in the brain stem. Fibers of this upper motor neuron pathway to the motor cranial nerve nuclei arise in the cerebral cortex; pass caudally in the internal capsule, the crus cerebri and the ventral portion of the pons; and are distributed largely to neurons in the reticular formation bilaterally. Reticular neurons conveying the impulses to the motor cranial nerve nuclei correspond to the intercalated or internuncial neurons found at spinal levels. In man and primates this indirect system is paralleled by more recently developed direct corticobulbar fibers distributed to the motor nuclei of the trigeminal, facial and hypoglossal nerves (Kuypers, '58). (From Carpenter and Sutin, *Human Neuroanatomy*, 1983; courtesy of Williams & Wilkins.)

(3) the paramedian reticular nuclei (medulla). Regions of the reticular formation, receiving corticofugal fibers, give rise to: (1) long ascending and descending projections, (2) projections to the cerebellum, and (3) collateral fibers projecting to cranial nerve nuclei (Scheibel and Scheibel, '58).

The *motor cranial nerve nuclei* innervating striated muscle receive impulses via corticobulbar pathways. These fibers arise mainly from portions of the precentral gyrus and constitute the upper motor neurons for motor cranial nerve nuclei. Most of the so-called "corticobulbar" fibers conveying impulses to motor cranial nerve nuclei are actually corticoreticular fibers; neurons in the reticular formation serve to relay impulses to the motor cranial nerve nuclei (Fig. 5-22). In the rat and cat it has not been possible to trace corticofugal fibers to direct terminations in any motor cranial nerve nucleus. This indirect system is supplemented in man and primates by direct corticobulbar fibers that project to particular motor cranial nerve nuclei. Nuclei receiving these direct cortical projections are the trigeminal, facial, hypoglossal and supraspinal (Kuypers, '58). These fibers are bilateral and nearly equal in number, except for those passing to parts of the facial nucleus. The more numerous corticoreticular fibers represent a phylogenetically older indirect corticobulbar pathway in which neurons in the reticular core serve as internuncials. Direct corticobulbar fibers found in man and primates represent a more recently developed parallel system.

The *supranuclear innervation of motor cranial nerve nuclei* is largely bilateral and more complex than that present at spinal levels. Corticobulbar projections are bilateral to those cranial nerve nuclei that innervate muscle groups which, as a rule, cannot be contracted voluntarily on one side. These include laryngeal, pharyngeal, palatal, and upper facial muscles. The same principle applies to the muscles of mastication and the extraocular muscles. Because unilateral stimulation of the motor cortex produces isolated contraction of the contralateral lower facial muscles, and certain lesions involving corticobulbar fibers produce paralysis only of contralateral lower facial muscles, certain cell groups of the facial nucleus are regarded as receiving predominantly crossed corticobulbar fibers.

Because the supranuclear innervation of the motor cranial nerve nuclei is bilateral, unilateral lesions interrupting corticobulbar fibers produce comparatively mild forms of paresis. Slight weakness of tongue and jaw movements contralateral to the lesions usually can be detected, and is expressed by modest deviation of the tongue or jaw to the side opposite the lesion. However, marked weakness in the contralateral lower facial muscles is evident with such lesions.

Pseudobulbar palsy results from bilateral lesions involving corticobulbar fibers. This syndrome is characterized by weakness or paralysis of the muscles involved in swallowing, chewing, breathing and speaking, and may occur with relatively little paralysis in the extremities. Loss of emotional control, characterized by inappropriate laughing and crying, forms an important part of this syndrome.

MEDULLARY-PONTINE JUNCTION

The fourth ventricle reaches its greatest width at the level of the lateral recess (Figs. 2-18) and 2-20). At this level the *nodulus* of the cerebellum lies in the roof of the fourth ventricle and the *peduncle of the flocculus* forms the dorsal surface of the lateral recess (Fig. 5-23). The cochlear nerve and the *dorsal* and *ventral cochlear nuclei* lie on the medial and ventral surfaces of the lateral recess. The *inferior cerebellar peduncle* has achieved its maximum size, and fibers of the cochlear nerve curve around its lateral and superior surfaces. At slightly more rostral levels, above the lateral recess, the inferior cerebellar peduncle enters the cerebellum by passing posterolaterally. The fibers of this peduncle lie medial to the middle cerebellar peduncle (Fig. 5-24).

In the floor of the fourth ventricle the nucleus prepositus lies medially in the position previously occupied by the hypoglossal nucleus. Lateral to this nucleus are the vestibular nuclei (Fig. 5-24). At this level portions of the *medial* and *inferior vestibular nuclei* are seen. The inferior vestibular

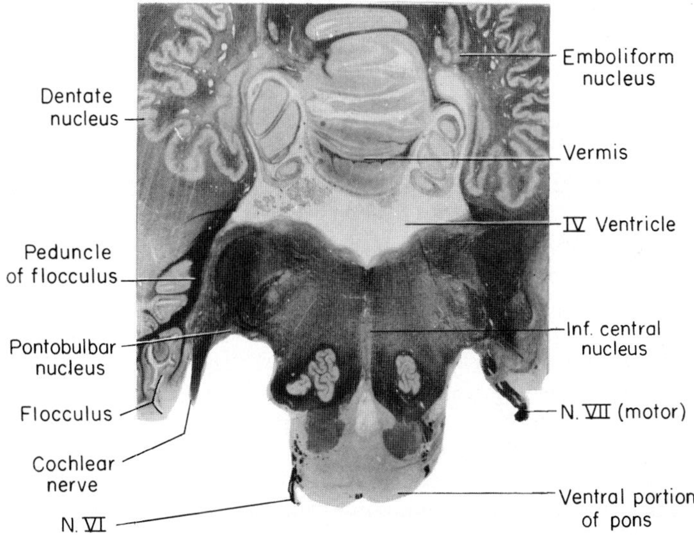

Figure 5-23. Asymmetrical transverse section through the junction of the medulla and pons in a 1-month infant. Attached portions of the cerebellum contain large portions of the deep cerebellar nuclei and the peduncle of the flocculus is seen on the left near the lateral recess of the fourth ventricle. Structures in the tegmentum are identified in Figure 5-24. (Weigert's myelin stain; photograph.) (From Carpenter and Sutin, *Human Neuroanatomy*, 1983; courtesy of Williams & Wilkins.)

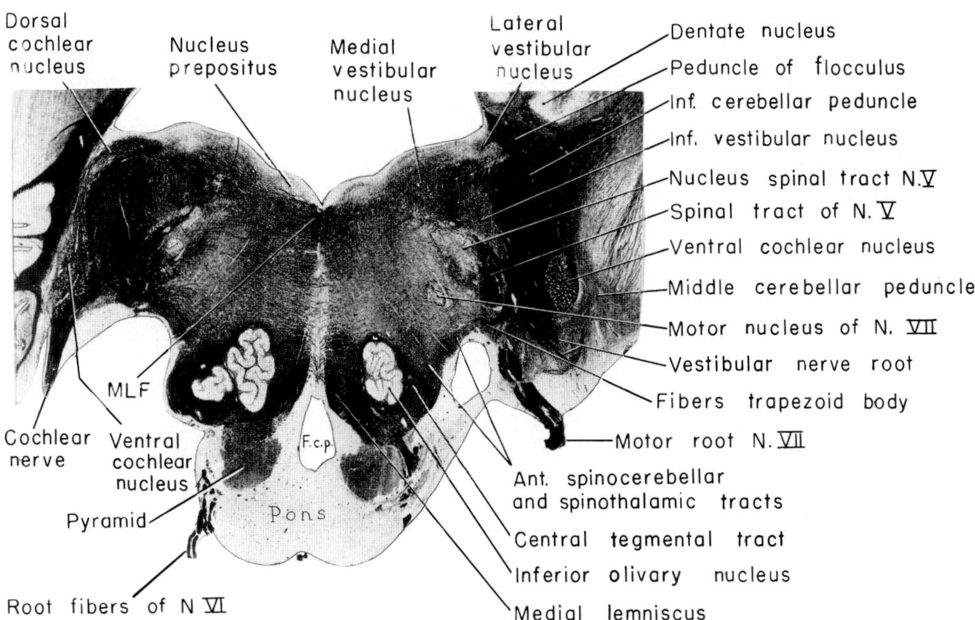

Figure 5-24. Transverse section of medulla of 1-month infant through caudal border of pons. Fibers of the inferior cerebellar peduncle are seen entering the cerebellum on the right. *F.c.p.*, Foramen cecum posterior; *MLF*, medial longitudinal fasciculus. (Weigert's myelin stain; photograph.) (From Carpenter and Sutin, *Human Neuroanatomy*, 1983; courtesy of Williams & Wilkins.)

nucleus, adjacent to the medial surface of the inferior cerebellar peduncle, is characterized by numerous coarse myelinated fiber bundles which course through it (Fig. 5-24). These fibers coursing longitudinally in the axis of the nucleus are primary vestibular fibers and cerebellar efferent fibers which descend. The medial vestibular nucleus is highly cellular and contains finer fibers most of which are not myelinated. In some preparations myelinated fibers of the *striae medullares* of the medulla can be seen in the floor of the fourth ventricle dorsal to the nucleus prepositus and the vestibular nuclei (Fig. 5-2). These fibers probably arise from the arcuate nucleus, pass dorsally in the raphe, and then project laterally in the floor of the fourth ventricle to the cerebellum.

The inferior olivary complex is reduced in size, and the accessory olivary nuclei have disappeared. Anterior to the olivary complex the fibers of the pyramid are surrounded by pontine nuclei and some transverse fibers. The medial lemniscus and medial longitudinal fasciculus occupy the same positions as at more caudal levels, although they are slightly separated from the corresponding tract on the opposite side by more fully developed nuclei in the median raphe (i.e., nucleus raphe magnus). Other ascending and descending tracts maintain the same relative positions as at lower medullary levels.

The junction of medulla and pons (Fig. 5-24) is characterized by: (1) passage of the inferior cerebellar peduncle into the cerebellum; (2) reduction in size and, ultimately, disappearance of the inferior olivary complex; (3) gradual incorporation of the corticospinal tracts within the ventral part of the pons; (4) enlargement of the reticular formation; and (5) appearance of cranial nerve nuclei and root fibers typical of this higher level.

Cranial nerves present at the junction of medulla and pons are the abducens, cochlear, vestibular and facial (Fig. 5-24). The abducens nerve emerges at the lower border of the pons lateral to the pyramids. All other cranial nerves at this level are grouped together at the *cerebellopontine angle*, formed by the junction of medulla, pons and cerebellum. All of these nerves emerge from, or enter, the internal auditory meatus. The cochlear nerve is the most caudal and lateral, while the facial nerve is the most rostral and medial. The vestibular nerve lies between the cochlear and facial nerves (Fig. 6-2). These cranial nerves will be described and discussed in the next chapter.

Lesions of the medulla or structures within it can be produced by a variety of causes, but those due to demyelinating diseases, neoplasms and vascular pathology are the most common. Demyelinating diseases usually are disseminated and involve multiple systems at different sites. Neoplasms tend to extend in the axis of the brain stem. Vascular lesions show great variation but often give rise to characteristic syndromes. The vascular syndrome most commonly seen in the medulla is attributed to occlusion of the posterior inferior cerebellar artery, a vessel which supplies structures in the posterolateral region (Fig. 14-14). While it seems likely that this syndrome may more frequently result from involvement of the vertebral artery and its smaller branches, the symptoms and signs are similar and unmistakable. The *lateral medullary syndrome* is characterized by: (1) loss of pain and thermal sense over the ipsilateral half of the face and the contralateral half of the body, (2) nausea, (3) vertigo, (4) disturbances of equilibrium, (5) persistent hiccup, and (6) dysphonia (hoarse voice). Disturbances forming parts of this syndrome frequently can be correlated with the extent and precise location of the medullary lesion. The blood supply of the medulla is discussed and illustrated in Chapter 14.

CHAPTER 6

The Pons

The pons (metencephalon) represents the rostral part of the hindbrain. It consists of two distinctive parts: (1) a *dorsal portion*, the pontine tegmentum, and (2) a *ventral portion*, referred to as the pons proper (Fig. 6-1).

CAUDAL PONS

Dorsal Portion of the Pons. This part of the pons, known as the pontine tegmentum, is the rostral continuation of the medullary reticular formation. It contains cranial nerve nuclei, ascending and descending tracts, and reticular nuclei (Fig. 6-1). Cranial nerve nuclei found in the pons are those of nerves V, VI, VII, and VIII (Figs. 6-2, 6-5, 6-6, and 6-20). The ascending tracts in the part of the brain stem are the same as those found in the medulla. The medial lemniscus occupies a different position and its configuration is changed. This large bundle, present on each side of the median raphe, lies anteriorly, just above the ventral portion of the pons (Fig. 6-1 and 6-2). Crossing fibers of the trapezoid body traverse ventral parts of the bundle on each side. The medial longitudinal fasciculi (MLF) are situated dorsally on each side of the median raphe. The spinothalamic and anterior spinocerebellar tracts are difficult to distinguish but occupy positions in the anterolateral tegmentum. The spinal trigeminal tract and nucleus lie medial and ventral to the inferior cerebellar peduncle. The vestibular nuclei (i.e., medial and lateral) are present in the floor of the fourth ventricle, dorsal to the reticular formation (Fig. 6-2).

The pontine reticular formation, more extensive than the medullary reticular formation, occupies a similar region. The major part of the pontine reticular formation is represented by the *pontine reticular nuclei* (pars caudalis and pars oralis; Figs. 6-1 and 6-22). The *pars caudalis* replaces the gigantocellular reticular nucleus of the me-

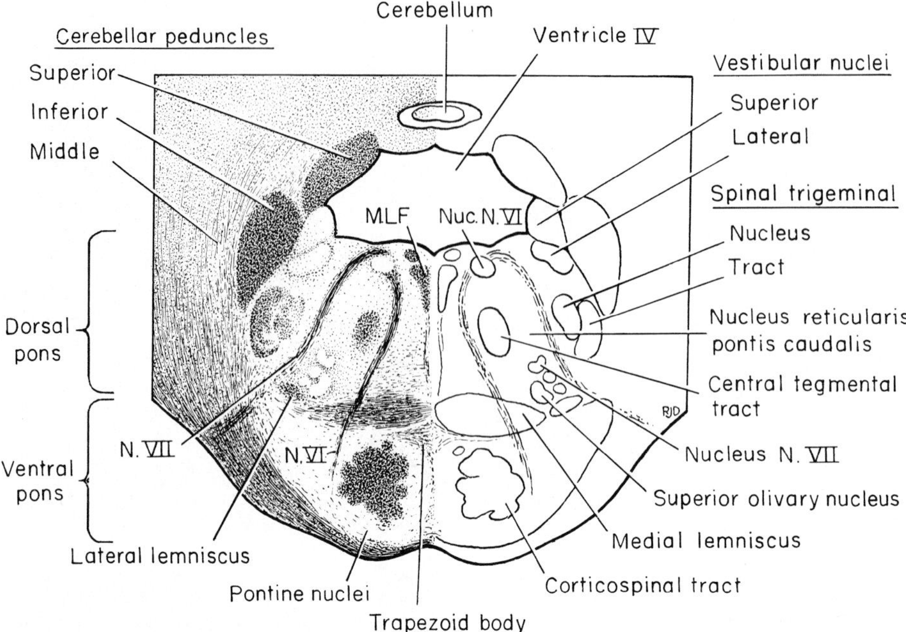

Figure 6-1. Semidiagrammatic drawing of a transverse section of the pons at the level of the abducens nucleus. The dorsal portion of the pons, constituting the tegmentum, contains the reticular formation, cranial nerve nuclei, and ascending and descending tracts. The ventral portion of the pons contains the pontine nuclei, massive bundles of corticofugal fibers and the transverse fibers of the pons which form the middle cerebellar peduncle. (From Carpenter and Sutin, *Human Neuroanatomy*, 1983; courtesy of Williams & Wilkins.)

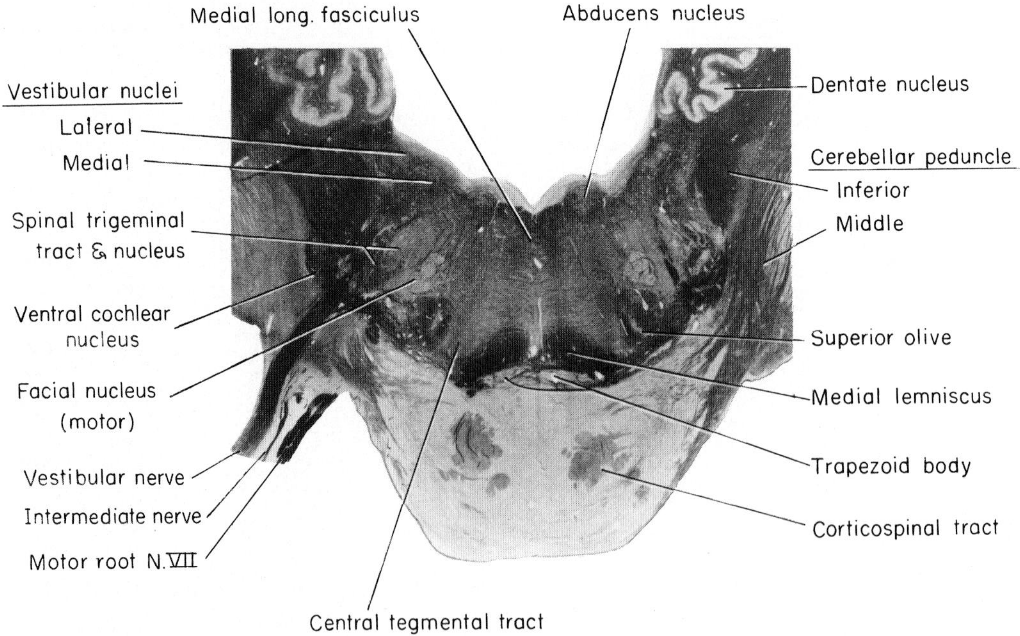

Figure 6-2. Slightly asymmetrical section of the pons of a 1-month infant. Root fibers of the vestibular, intermediate, and facial nerves are present on the left at the cerebellopontine angle. (Weigert's myelin stain; photograph.) (From Carpenter and Sutin, *Human Neuroanatomy*, 1983; courtesy of Williams & Wilkins.)

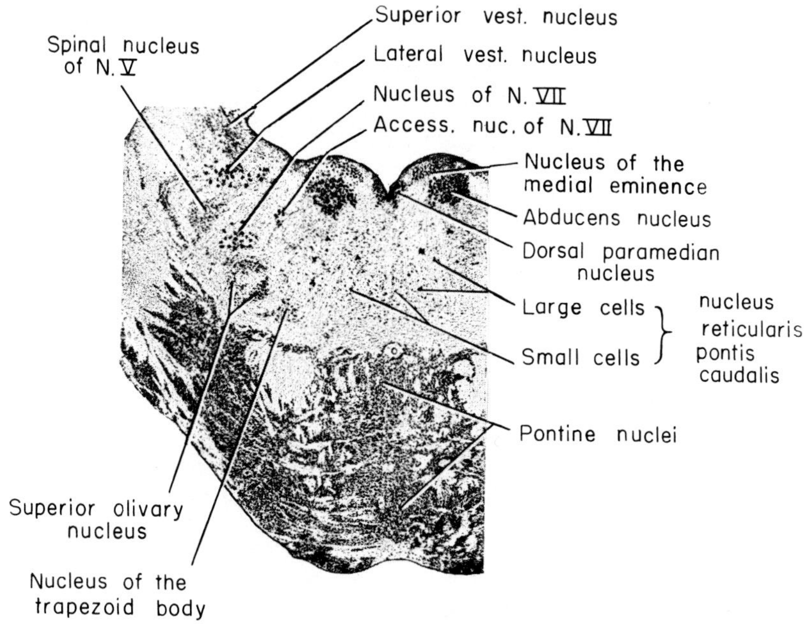

Figure 6-3. Section through pons and pontine tegmentum of 3-month infant at about same level as Figure 6-2. (Cresyl violet; photograph, with schematic representation of cell groups.) (From Carpenter and Sutin, *Human Neuroanatomy*, 1983; courtesy of Williams & Wilkins.)

dulla and extends rostrally to the level of the trigeminal motor nucleus (Fig. 6-22). The *pars oralis*, present in more rostral pontine levels, extends into the caudal mesencephalon. The pontine reticular nuclei give rise to the pontine reticulospinal tract (Figs. 4-6 and 4-14). Lateral to the pars caudalis is a small-celled reticular nucleus (parvicellularis) similar to that described in the medulla. The median raphe contains the inferior central nucleus (nucleus raphe magnus) (Figs. 5-11 and 6-4).

The reticular formation posterolateral to the medial lemniscus contains a relatively large discrete bundle, the *central tegmental tract* (Figs. 6-1 and 6-4). This is a composite tract consisting of descending fibers from midbrain nuclei that project to the inferior olivary complex, and ascending fibers from the reticular formation that project to certain thalamic nuclei.

Ventral Portion of the Pons. The massive ventral part of the pons consists of orderly arranged transverse and longitudinal fiber bundles, and large collections of pontine nuclei (Figs. 6-1, 6-3, and 6-4). Longitudinal fiber bundles coursing through central regions of the ventral pons are: (1) corticospinal fibers, (2) corticobulbar fibers, and (3) corticopontine fibers. Corticospinal fibers traverse the ventral part of the pons and in sagittal sections can be traced into the medullary pyramid. Corticopontine fibers, arising from the frontal, parietal, temporal, and occipital cortex, descend without crossing and terminate upon the pontine nuclei. The pontine nuclei surround the fibers of the corticospinal and corticopontine tracts. These nuclei give rise to the transverse fiber bundles of the pons, which cross the midline and enter the cerebellum as the middle cerebellar peduncle (Figs. 6-1 and 6-3). These fibers cross above and below the fascicles of descending fibers. The ventral portion of the pons may be considered as a massive relay station in a two-neuronal pathway by which impulses from the cerebral cortex are transmitted to the contralateral cerebellar hemisphere. Corticobulbar fibers descending in the ventral part of the pons project into the pontine tegmentum (Fig. 5-22).

VESTIBULOCOCHLEAR NERVE

The eighth cranial nerve (N VIII) consists of two distinctive parts: (1) the coch-

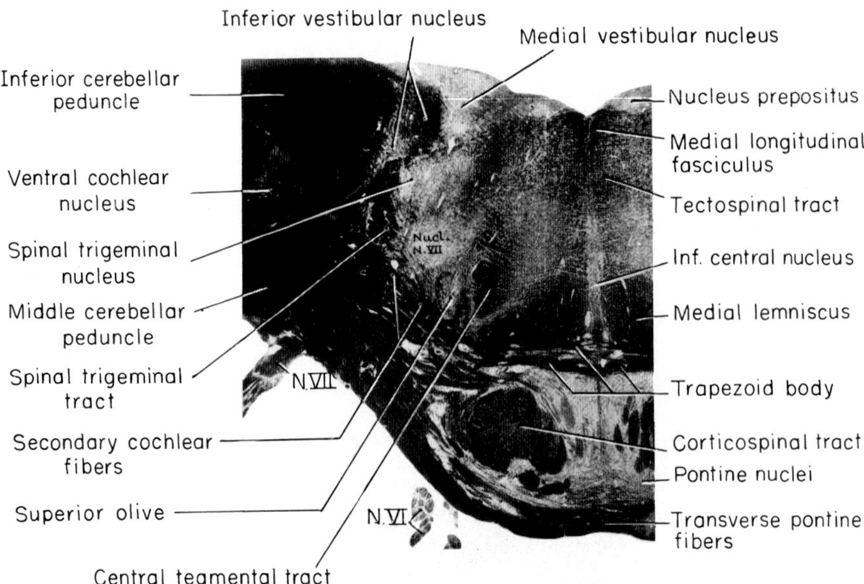

Figure 6-4. Transverse section of the adult pons at the level of emergence of the facial nerve root. (Weigert's myelin stain; photograph.) (From Carpenter and Sutin, *Human Neuroanatomy*, 1983; courtesy of Williams & Wilkins.)

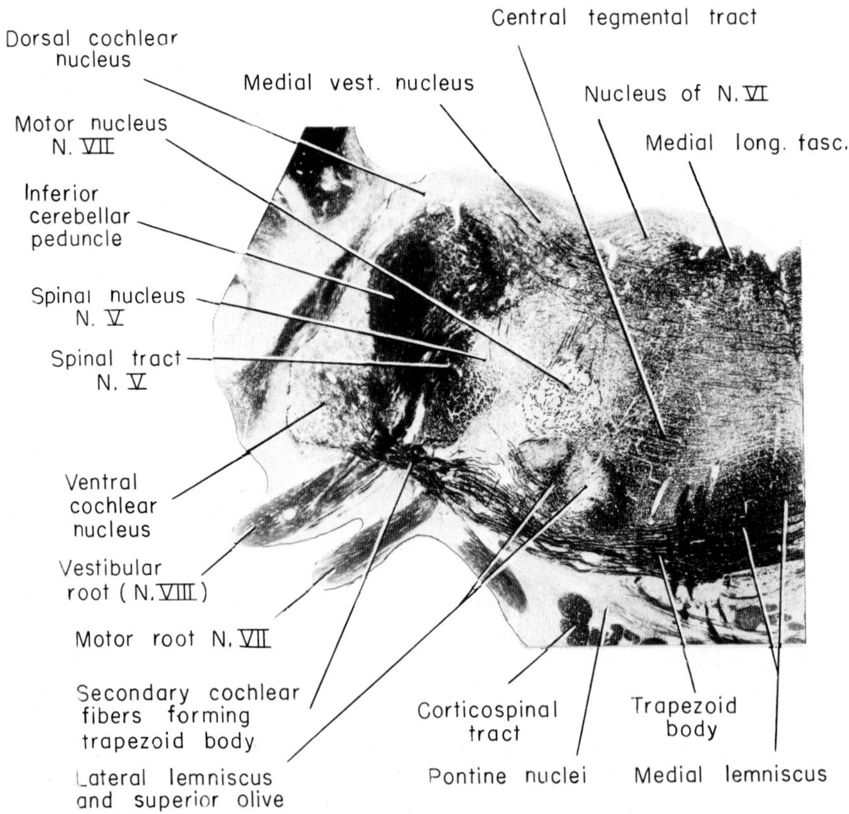

Figure 6-5. Section of left half of the pontine tegmentum of 3-year-old child whose brain showed a complete absence of the left cerebellar hemisphere and middle cerebellar peduncle. Fibers of the trapezoid body arising from the ventral cochlear nucleus are clearly shown. Smaller numbers of fibers in the dorsal acoustic stria are seen passing into the tegmentum from the dorsal cochlear nucleus (Strong, '15). (Weigert's myelin stain; photograph.) (From Carpenter and Sutin, *Human Neuroanatomy*, 1983; courtesy of Williams & Wilkins.)

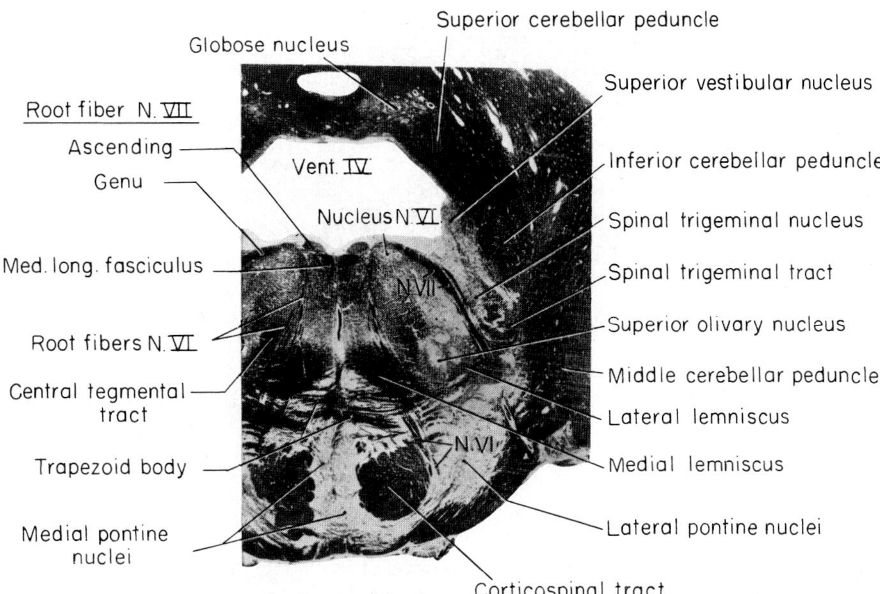

Figure 6-6. Transverse section of the adult pons through the abducens nucleus showing the root fibers of the abducens and facial nerves. (Weigert's myelin stain; photograph.) (From Carpenter and Sutin, *Human Neuroanatomy*, 1983; courtesy of Williams & Wilkins.)

lear part concerned with audition and (2) the vestibular part conveying impulses concerned with equilibrium and orientation in three dimensional space. These two components of the vestibulocochlear nerve run together from the internal auditory meatus to the cerebellopontine angle, where they enter they enter the brain stem (Figs. 1-4, 2-21, 5-1, and 6-5). Each of these nerves has distinctive central nuclei and connections.

Cochlea. The cochlea consists of a fluid-filled coil tube of two and a half turns (Fig. 6-7) that contains the auditory transducer (Fig. 6-8). The basilar and vestibular (Reissner's) membranes partition the cochlea to form the scala vestibuli, the scala tympani, and cochlear duct (scala media). Energy from sound waves reaching the tympanic membrane is transmitted via the ear ossicles to the scala vestibuli (ovale window) by the foot plate of the stapes. The membrane covering the round window at the base of the scala tympani accommodates to changes in hydrostatic pressure. The *organ of Corti*, the auditory transductor, lies in the cochlear duct and consists of one row of inner hair cells and three rows of outer hair cells (Fig. 6-8). The tectorial membrane, attached to the spiral limbus, overlies the hair cells. The piston-like action of the stapes transmits the energy of sound waves to the perilymph in the scala vestibuli. Energy transmitted to the perilymph produces traveling waves in the basilar membrane that move from the base of the cochlear to its apex (Békésy, '60). Displacement of the basilar membrane in response to acoustic stimuli causes bending of hair cells in contact with the tectorial membrane. Maximum displacement of the basal membrane at different distances from the stapes can be correlated with specific sound frequencies. High frequencies are perceived at the base of the cochlear and low frequencies at its apex.

Cochlear Nerve and Nuclei. The cochlear nerve originates from cells of the *spiral ganglion* situated about the modiolus of the cochlea (Figs. 6-8 and 6-9). Peripheral processes of the bipolar cells of the ganglion end in relation to the hair cells of the organ of Corti. The central processes of ganglion cells form the cochlear nerve, which enters the brain stem lateral, dorsal, and slightly caudal to the vestibular nerve. Fibers of the cochlear nerve terminate in two cell masses on the lateral surface of the

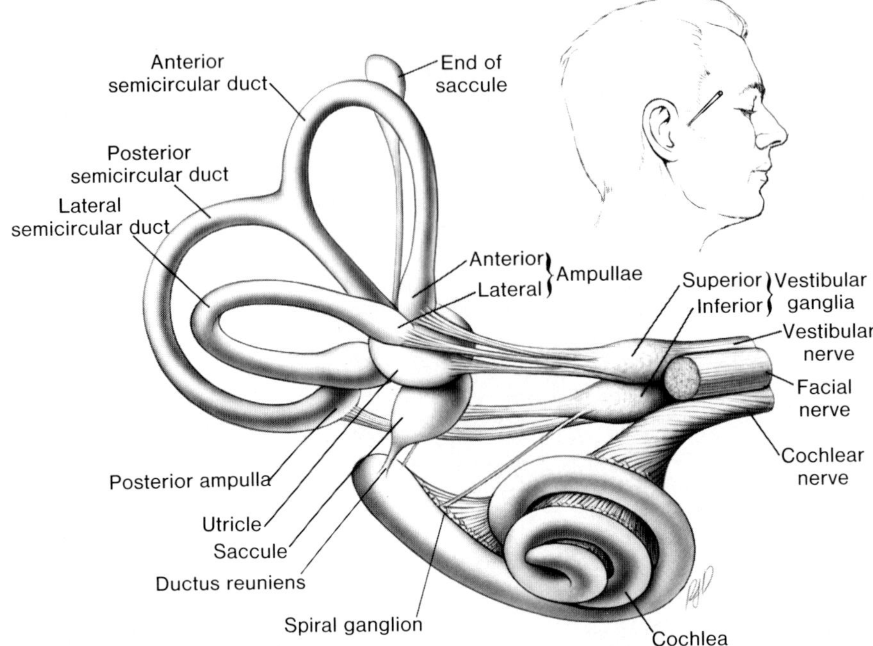

Figure 6-7. Drawing of the labyrinthine and cochlear apparatus, their ganglia and nerves with anatomical orientation. The cochlea has been rotated downward and laterally to expose the vestibular ganglia. (From Carpenter and Sutin, *Human Neuroanatomy*, 1983; courtesy of Williams & Wilkins.)

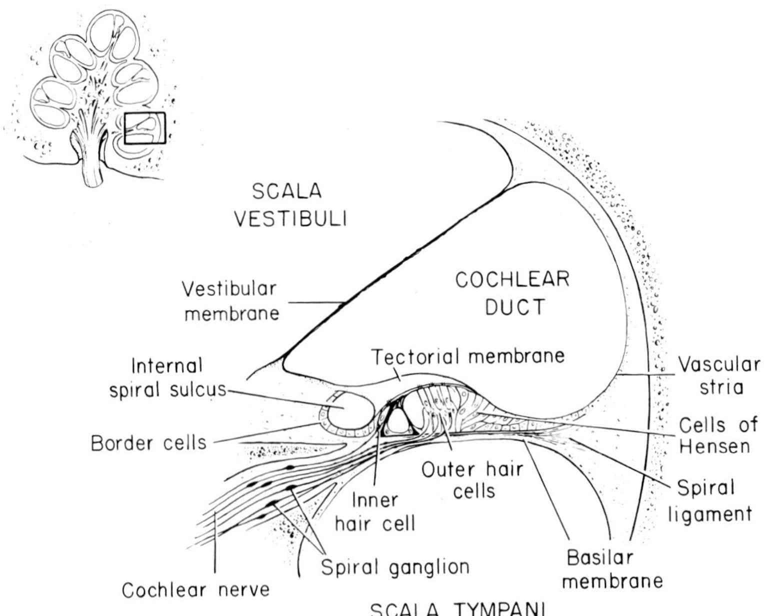

Figure 6-8. Drawing of a radial section through the cochlea showing the cochlear duct, the basilar membrane, the organ of Corti, and the tectorial membrane. The small *diagram in the upper left* is an axial section of the cochlea. The *area enclosed in the rectangle* is reproduced in detail in the large drawing. (From Carpenter and Sutin, *Human Neuroanatomy*, 1983; courtesy of Williams & Wilkins.)

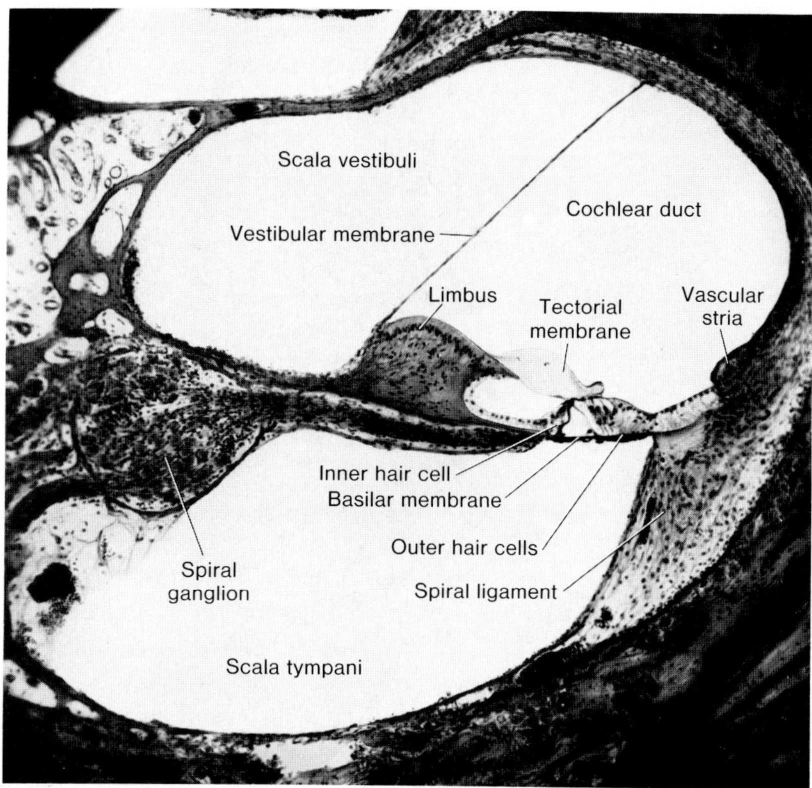

Figure 6-9. Photomicrograph of a radial section through the cochlea in man similar to the schematic drawing in Figure 6-8. (From Carpenter and Sutin, *Human Neuroanatomy*, 1983; courtesy of Williams & Wilkins.)

inferior cerebellar peduncle, the ventral and dorsal cochlear nuclei (Figs. 5-24 and 6-10). These nuclei represent a more or less continuous cell mass, but they have distinctive cells and cytoarchitecture. The *dorsal cochlear nucleus* forms an eminence on the most lateral part of the floor of the fourth ventricle, known as the *acoustic tubercle* (Fig. 6-5). Cells of this nucleus, in most mammals, are distinctly laminated; three layers are recognized: (1) molecular, (2) fusiform, and (3) polymorphic. In man these layers are indistinct.

The *ventral cochlear nucleus* is subdivided into anteroventral and posteroventral nuclei on a topographical and cytological basis. Cells of the *anteroventral cochlear nucleus* in the rostral region contain densely packed ovoid cells. The *posteroventral cochlear nucleus*, located near the entrance of the cochlear nerve root, contains several types of neurons with a predominance of multipolar cells (Osen, '69; Brawer, et al., '74). Each of the subdivisions of the cochlear nuclei is tonotopically organized and has a sequential representation of the auditory spectrum (Rose et al., '59; Rose, '60).

On entering the brain stem, fibers of the cochlear nerve bifurcate in orderly sequence and are distibuted to both dorsal and ventral cochlear nuclei (Powell and Cowan, '62; Fig. 6-10). Anatomical studies suggest that apical cochlear fibers terminate in ventral parts of the dorsal cochlear nucleus and in the ventral cochlear nucleus, while fibers from the basal coils end in dorsal parts of the dorsal cochlear nucleus. Physiological studies indicate a multiple tonotopic representation in the cochlear nuclear complex, due to the orderly bifurcation and distribution of fibers throughout the complex. In all divisions of the cochlear nuclear complex neurons responding to

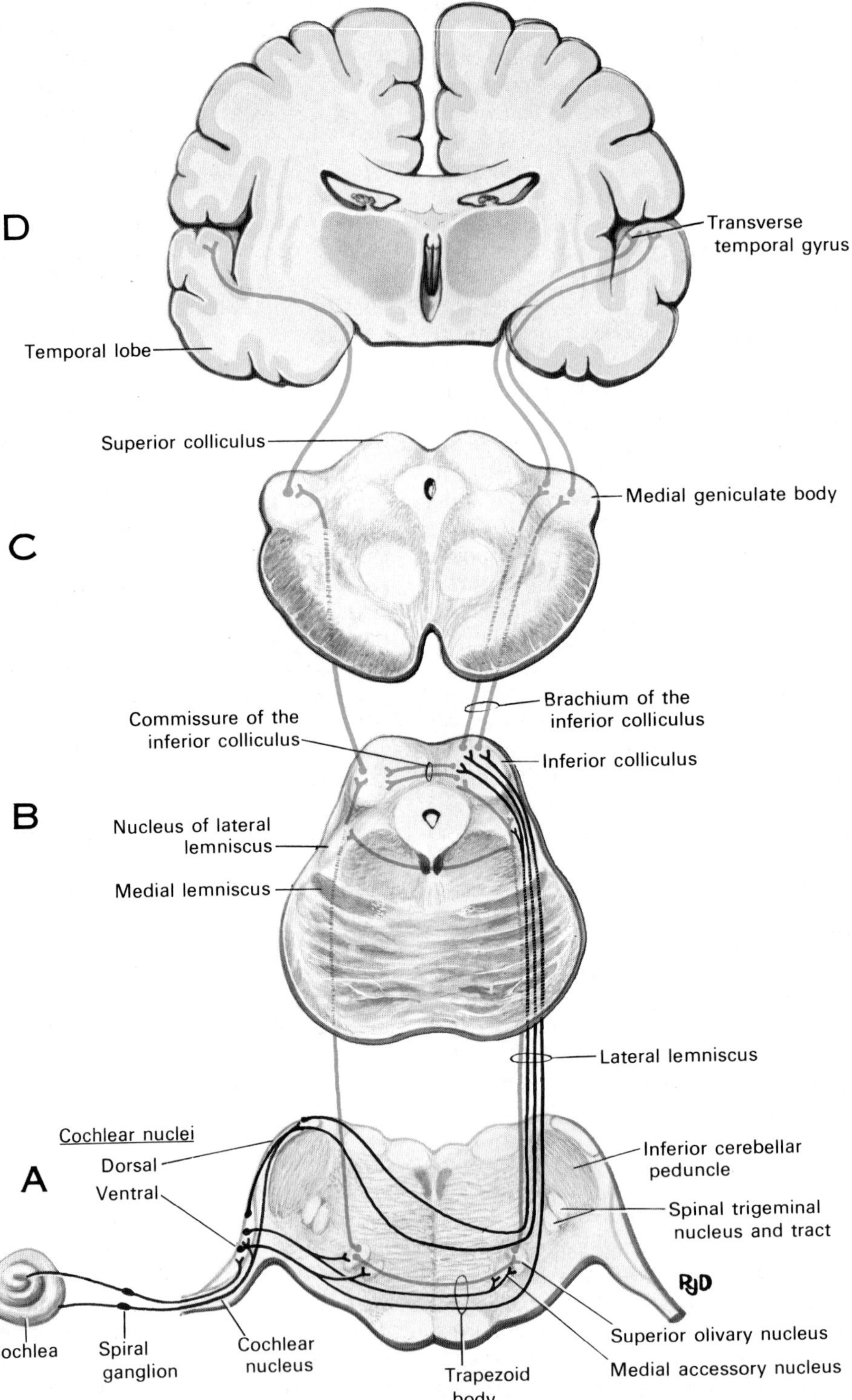

Figure 6-10. Schematic diagram of the auditory pathways. Primary auditory fibers arising from the spiral ganglion are in *black*. Secondary auditory fibers arising from the cochlear nuclei and forming the acoustic striae are in *red*. Auditory fibers arising from relay nuclei are in *blue*. (*A*) Medulla, (*B*) level of inferior colliculus, (*C*) level of superior colliculus, and (*D*) transverse section through the cerebral hemisphere.

higher frequencies are located dorsally (Rose, '60).

Auditory Pathways. Secondary auditory pathways in the brain stem are exceedingly complex and many details concerning their composition are uncertain (Fig. 6-10). These fibers are grouped into three acoustic striae: (1) a *ventral acoustic stria* which arises from the ventral cochlear nucleus and courses medially along the ventral border of the pontine tegmentum (Fig. 6-5), (2) a *dorsal acoustic stria* which arises from the dorsal cochlear nucleus, and (3) an *intermediate acoustic stria* which arises from the dorsal part of the ventral cochlear nucleus. Fibers of the dorsal and intermediate acoustic striae pass medially dorsal to the inferior cerebellar peduncle (Fig. 6-10). The dorsal acoustic stria crosses the median raphe ventral to the MLF, and its fibers join the lateral lemniscus of the opposite side. The intermediate stria courses through the reticular formation in an intermediate position, crosses the midline, and enters the contralateral lateral lemniscus. The ventral acoustic stria is larger than the combined dorsal and intermediate striae. In their passage through the tegmentum fibers terminate in the reticular formation, the superior olivary nuclei, and the nuclei of the trapezoid body (Fig. 6-5). The superior olivary and trapezoid nuclei give rise to tertiary auditory fibers which ascend mainly in the contralateral lateral lemniscus (Fig. 6-10). No fibers from the cochlear nuclei ascend in the ipsilateral lateral lemniscus. Many fibers of the ventral acoustic stria pass through ventral parts of the medial lemniscus to reach the superior olivary nucleus of the opposite side. These ventrally crossing fibers form part of the trapezoid body. Intercalated cell aggregations among these fibers constitute the *nuclei of the trapezoid body* (Figs. 6-3, 6-4, and 6-10). Laterally most of the fibers of the trapezoid body enter the lateral lemniscus. Close to the place where fibers enter the lateral lemniscus there is a large collection of cells called the superior olivary nuclear complex. This complex consists of an "S"-shaped principal nucleus and a wedge-shaped accessory nucleus (Figs. 6-3, 6-4, and 6-10). The superior olivary nuclei receive secondary auditory fibers and project fibers into the lateral lemniscus. The lateral lemniscus, the principal ascending auditory pathway in the brain stem, ascends in the lateral part of the tegmentum (Fig. 6-10).

The *lateral lemniscus* ascends in the lateral tegmentum to midbrain levels, where most of the fibers terminate in the inferior colliculus (Figs. 6-10, 7-2, and 7-3). Interposed in the lateral lemniscus at isthmus levels are the *nuclei of the lateral leminiscus* which receive and contribute fibers to the main bundle (Fig. 6-25). The inferior colliculus gives rise to fibers that project to the medial geniculate body via the brachium of the inferior colliculus (Fig. 5-2).

Destruction of the cochlea, the cochlear nerve, or of the cochlear nuclei (both dorsal and ventral), results in complete ipsilateral deafness, Lesions of the lateral lemniscus cause bilateral partial deafness, greatest in the contralateral ear, because fibers in this pathway are both crossed and uncrossed.

Efferent Cochlear Bundle. Crossed and uncrossed components of the *olivocochlear bundle* or the *efferent cochlear bundle* project peripherally from the brain stem to the cochlea and form a pathway by which the central nervous system may influence its own sensory input (Rasmussen, '46, '60; Gacek, '61). Electrical stimulation of the crossed fibers of this bundle in the cat reduce auditory nerve fiber responses to acoustic stimuli (Galambos, '56). The crossed component of this bundle originates from the region dorsal to the medial accessory superior olive, passes dorsomedially toward the facial genu, crosses the midline and exits from the brain stem in association with the vestibular nerve (Fig. 6-11). A smaller uncrossed component arises from the region dorsal to the principal superior olivary nucleus and joins the crossed fibers from the opposite side. Peripherally crossed and uncrossed fibers of the efferent cochlear bundle are associated initially with the vestibular nerve, but in the inner ear they enter the cochlear nerve via the vestibulocochlear anastomosis. These fine fibers pass to the organ of Corti and make synaptic contact with hair cells (Smith and Rasmussen, '63) and cells of the spiral ganglion (Smith, '67). The finding that stimulation of the efferent cochlear bundle suppresses auditory nerve activity,

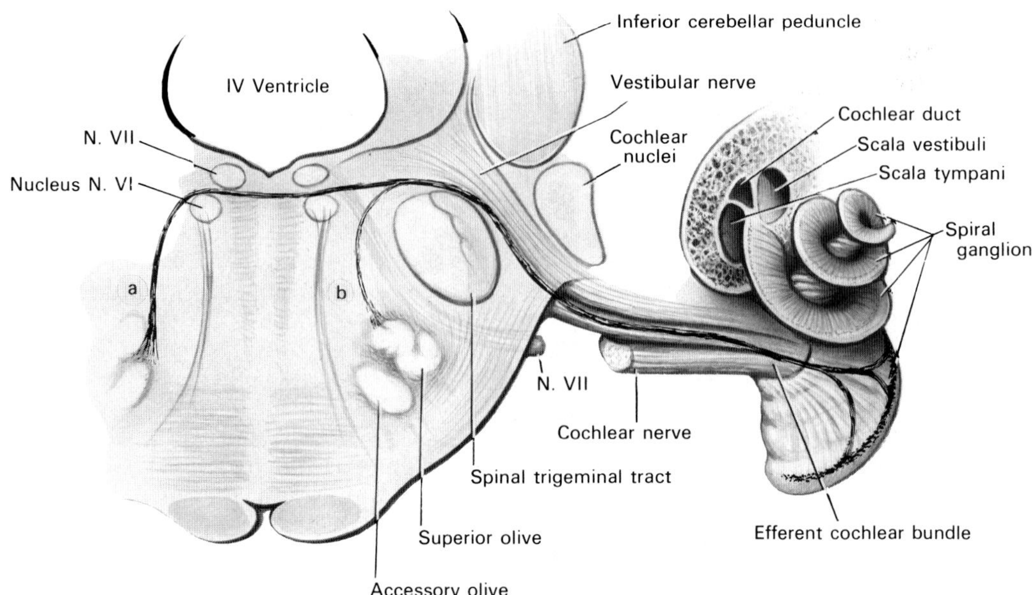

Figure 6-11. Schematic drawing of efferent cochlear fibers in the cat. Crossed fibers of the *olivocochlear bundle* (*red*, *a*) arise from cells dorsal to the accessory superior olivary nucleus, pass dorsomedially toward the floor of the fourth ventricle and cross to the opposite side. Uncrossed fibers of the olivocochlear bundle (*red*, *b*) arise from the region dorsal to the superior olivary nucleus, join the crossed fibers and pass peripherally in association with the vestibular nerve. Peripherally efferent cochlear fibers pass via the vestibulocochlear anastomosis to the cochlear nerve and are distributed to the hair cells of the cochlea and to ganglion cells. (Modified from Rasmussen, '60.) (From Carpenter and Sutin, *Human Neuroanatomy*, 1983; courtesy of Williams & Wilkins.)

indicates this bundle serves as a feedback that inhibits the receptivity of the end organ.

Other feedback mechanisms in the auditory system involve relay nuclei in the auditory pathway. Fibers from the inferior colliculus, the nuclei of the lateral lemniscus and the superior olivary nuclei descend, or pass distally, to relay nuclei. These pathways inhibit impulses concerned with certain frequencies of the auditory spectrum and in this way enhance frequencies not subject to central inhibition. This phenomenon is known as auditory sharpening. Acoustic reflex mechanisms also involve middle ear muscles such as the stapedius and tensor tympani. In the reflex involving the stapedius muscle, fibers from the medial accessory superior olive project bilaterally to facial motor neurons (Borg. '73). Contractions of the stapedius muscle dampen the oscillations of the ear ossicles.

Labyrinth. The vestibular part of the inner ear consists of the *semicircular* ducts, the *utricle*, and the *saccule* (Fig. 6-7). These parts of the labyrinth are concerned with orientation in three-dimensional space, equilibrium, and modification of muscle tone. The semicircular ducts, concerned with kinetic equilibrium, are arranged at right angles to each other and represent the three planes of space. One end of each duct has a dilatation, the ampulla, containing a transversely oriented ridge, known as the *crista ampullaris.* Columnar epithelium of the crista ampullaris is composed of neuroepithelial hair cells which constitute the vestibular receptor (Fig. 6-15). Each crista has opposite it a gelatinous *cupula* whch moves across the hair cells in response to movement of the endolymphatic fluid. Angular acceleration causes displacement of endolymphatic fluid and movement of the cupula which stimulates the hair cells. Endolymphatic flow is greatest in the pair of semicircular ducts most nearly perpendicular to the axis of rotation.

The utricle and saccule (the otolithic organs) each have a similar patch of sensory epithelium known as the macula. The mac-

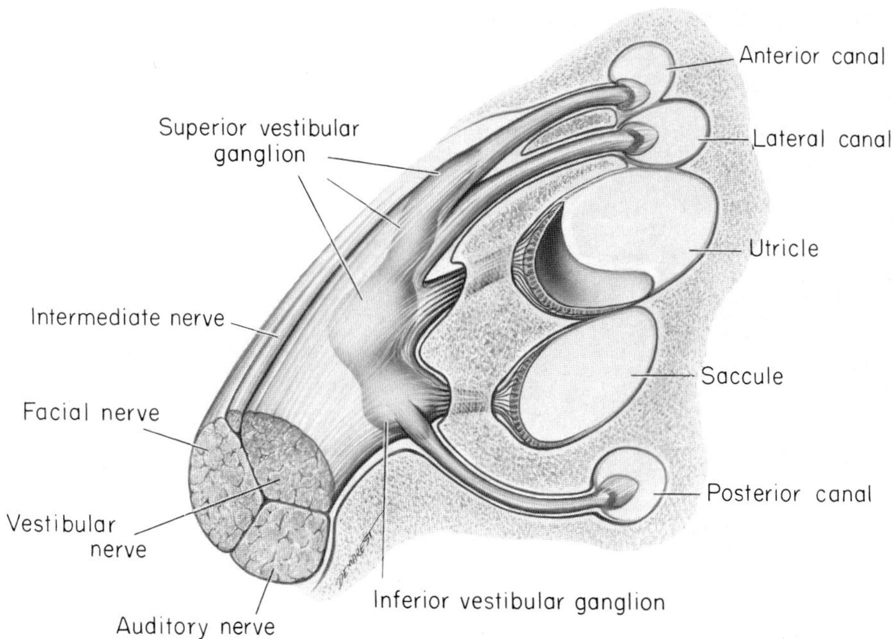

Figure 6-12. Semischematic drawing of the vestibular ganglia and peripheral branches innervating distinctive portions of the labyrinth. Cells in the superior vestibular ganglion are arranged in a spiral fashion and cells in the distal portion of the ganglion innervate the cristae of the anterior and lateral semicircular ducts. Cells in the broader proximal part of the superior vestibular ganglion innervate the macula of the utricle. Cells of the inferior vestibular ganglion innervate the macula of the saccule and the crista of the posterior semicircular duct. The superior and inferior vestibular ganglia are joined by an isthmus of cells. Relationships between the facial, intermediate, vestibular and auditory nerves are shown (Stein and Carpenter, '67). (From Carpenter and Sutin, *Human Neuroanatomy*, 1983; courtesy of Williams & Wilkins.)

ulae contain hair cells in contact with a gelatinous covering containing small calcareous particles, the otoliths. The utricular macula responds to changes in gravitational forces and to linear acceleration in the long axis of the body, and conveys impulses concerning the position of the head in space (i.e., static equilibrium). The macula of the saccule is less sensitive, but responds to linear acceleration in the ventrodorsal axis of the body (Fernández et al., '72).

Vestibular Ganglion and Nerve. The maculae and cristae are innervated by cells in the vestibular ganglion (Fig. 6-12). This ganglion can be divided into superior and inferior vestibular ganglia which are connected by a narrow isthmus. Peripheral processes of bipolar cells located in the ganglia pass to the maculae and cristae, while the central processes form the vestibular nerve. The vestibular root enters the cerebellopontine angle where the root fibers pass dorsally between the inferior cerebellar peduncle and the spinal trigeminal tract (Fig. 6-2). On entering the vestibular nuclear complex, the fibers bifurcate into short ascending and long descending fibers; a small number of fibers pass directly to parts of the cerebellum.

Vestibular Nuclei. The vestibular nuclei lie in the floor of the fourth ventricle and extend from levels rostral to the hypoglossal nucleus to slightly beyond the level of the abducens nucleus. The nuclei of this complex are arranged in two longitudinal columns (Figs. 6-13 and 14). The lateral column consists of three distinctive nuclei, the inferior, lateral and superior vestibular nuclei. The medial vestibular nucleus constitutes the medial cell column.

The *inferior vestibular nucleus* begins in the medulla, medial to the accessory cuneate nucleus, and extends rostrally to the

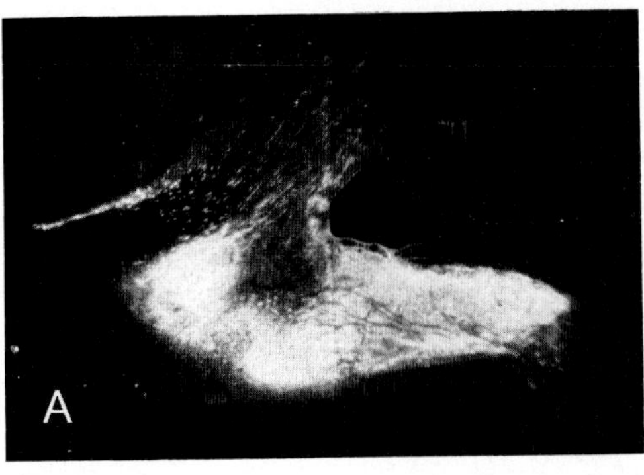

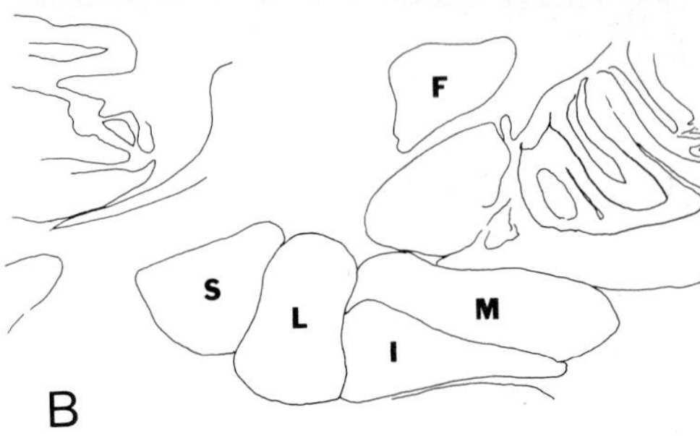

Figure 6-13. (*A*) Sagittal section through the brain stem in a rhesus monkey demonstrating the transport of [^{3}H] amino acids from the labyrinth to the vestibular nuclei in an autoradiograph. (Cresyl violet, dark-field, ×20.) (*B*) Outline drawings of the fastigial (*F*) and vestibular nuclei: *S*, superior vestibular nucleus; *L*, lateral vestibular nucleus; *I*, inferior vestibular nucleus; *M*, medial vestibular nucleus. Although primary vestibular afferents project to all ipsilateral vestibular nuclei, only the ventral half of the lateral vestibular receives terminals from this source. (From Carpenter and Sutin, *Human Neuroanatomy*, 1983; courtesy of Williams & Wilkins.)

level of entrance of the vestibular nerve (Figs. 5-14, 5-24, and 6-4). This nucleus is composed mostly of small and medium-sized cells, except in its most rostral part where large cells resemble those of the lateral vestibular nucleus. In ventrolateral and caudal parts of the nucleus the cells of group "f" form a large cluster (Brodal and Pompeiano. '57). In fiber-stained sections the nucleus is characterized by bundles of longitudinally oriented fibers.

The *lateral vestibular nucleus*, located at the level of entrance of the vestibular nerve, is composed of giant cells, but some regional differences are evident in the number and size of cells (Fig. 6-3). Fibers of the vestibular root traverse ventral parts of the nucleus. The *superior vestibular nucleus* lies dorsal and rostral to the lateral vestibular nucleus in the lateral angle of the fourth ventricle (Fig. 6-6). Cells of this nucleus are small and medium-sized, and round or spindle-shaped.

The *medial vestibular nucleus*, composed of small and medium-sized cells, contains relatively few fibers. This is the largest vestibular nucleus; it extends from the oral pole of the hypoglossal nucleus to the abducens nucleus and rostrally fuses with the superior vestibular nucleus.

Primary Vestibular Fibers. These fibers project to all four vestibular nuclei and to the interstitial nucleus of the vestibular nerve, a collection of relatively large cells between vestibular fibers near the root entry zone (Fig. 6-13 and 6-14). Upon entering the vestibular complex virtually all fibers bifurcate into ascending and descending branches. Ascending branches project mainly to the superior, lateral, and rostral parts of the medial vestibular nuclei. Descending branches provide fibers to the inferior vestibular nucleus and collaterals to caudal parts of the medial vestibular nucleus. Primary vestibular fibers are distributed within all vestibular nuclei but some regions of each nucleus contain fewer endings. (Brodal et al., '62; Carleton and Carpenter, '84). In the superior vestibular nucleus primary fibers terminate most profusely about large central cells but extend into all peripheral regions. In the lateral vestibular nucleus primary fibers terminate only in ventral regions (Fig. 6-13); the dorsal part of the lateral vestibular nucleus is the largest regional area devoid of terminal vestibular fibers. The medial vestibular nucleus receives vestibular fibers throughout its length, but caudally terminations are mainly in lateral regions. Primary vestibular fibers in the inferior vestibular nucleus end most profusely in dorsal regions. The cristae of the semicircular ducts give rise to fibers that project primarily to the superior vestibular nucleus and to rostral parts of the medial vestibular nucleus (Stein and Carpenter, '67). Cells of the superior vestibular ganglion, which innervate the macula of the utricle, give rise to fibers which descend in the dorsomedial part of the inferior vestibular nucleus and project collaterals into adjacent portions of the medial vestibular nucleus. Cells of the inferior vestibular

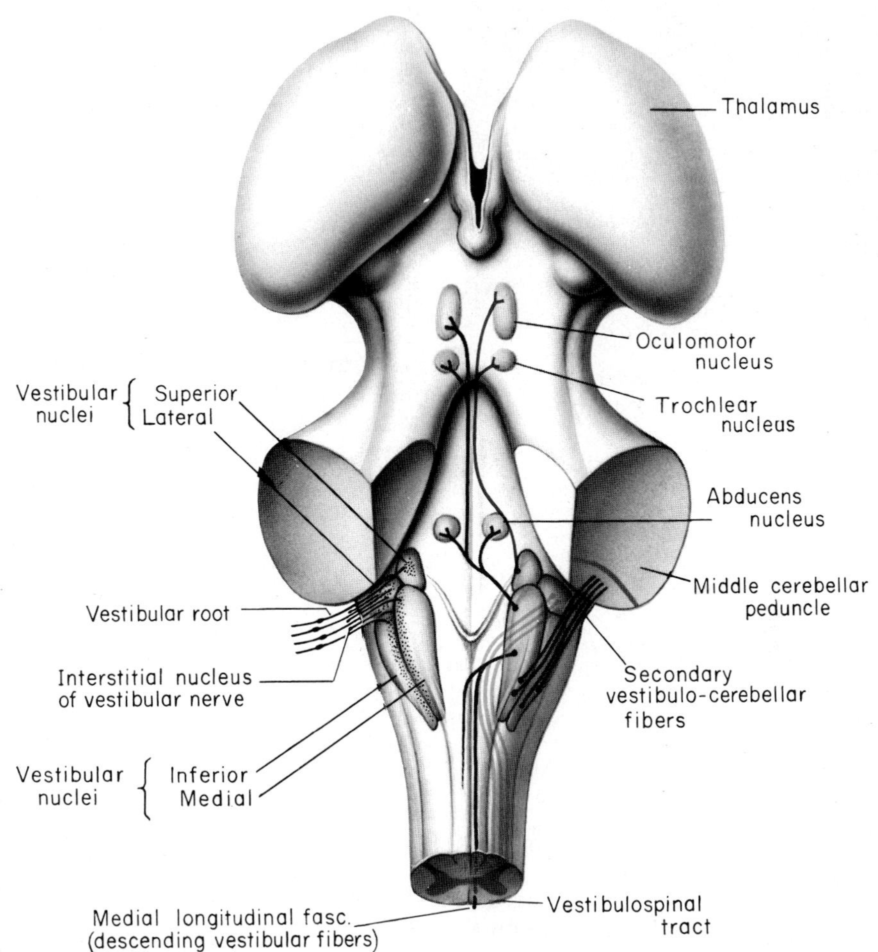

Figure 6-14. Schematic diagram of some of the principal projections of the vestibular system. Relationships and spatial disposition of the four main vestibular nuclei are indicated on the *left*. Among the afferent root fibers are the cells of the interstitial nucleus of the vestibular nerve. *Dotted areas* (*black*) in the vestibular nuclei represent the regions of the nuclear complex which receive the largest number of *primary vestibular fibers*. These areas are: (1) the ventral half of the lateral vestibular nucleus, (2) the lateral part of the medial vestibular nucleus, (3) the dorsomedial part of the inferior vestibular nucleus, and (4) the central part of the superior vestibular nucleus. *Secondary vestibular fibers* originating from individual vestibular nuclei are shown on the right. Fibers from the superior vestibular nucleus (*red*) ascend largely uncrossed in the medial longitudinal fasciculus (MLF) and terminate in the trochlear and parts of the oculomotor nuclei. Ascending projections from the medial vestibular nucleus (*black*) to the nuclei of the extraocular muscles are predominantly crossed. Descending fibers from the medial vestibular nucleus in the MLF are shown in *black*. The somatotopically organized vestibulospinal tract (*blue*) arises only from cells of the lateral vestibular nucleus. Secondary vestibulocerebellar fibers (*black*) arise from caudal parts of the inferior and medial vestibular nuclei. (From Carpenter and Sutin, *Human Neuroanatomy*, 1983; courtesy of Williams & Wilkins.)

ganglion, which innervate the macula of the saccule, give rise to central fibers that descend and terminate mainly in dorsolateral portions of the inferior vestibular nucleus and in an accessory nucleus known as cell group "y" (Gacek, '71). Cell groups within the vestibular ganglion, which innervate particular receptor components of the labyrinth, have major central projections within the ipsilateral vestibular nuclei and some overlapping projections in other parts of the complex (Figs. 6-12 and 6-13).

A small number of primary vestibular fibers enter the cerebellum via the juxtarestiform body (Fig. 6-20). In the monkey, cells in all parts of the vestibular ganglion project to the ipsilateral nodulus, uvula, and flocculus where these projections end as mossy fibers in the granular layer of the cerebellar cortex (Carpenter et al. '72; Carleton and Carpenter, '84).

Afferent Projections to the Vestibular Nuclei. Afferents to the vestibular nuclei, from sources other than the vestibular ganglion, include fibers from: (1) the vestibulocerebellum (i.e., the flocculus, nodulus, and uvula) to the superior, medial, and inferior vestibular nuclei (Carleton and Carpenter, '83); (2) the anterior lobe vermis of the cerebellum to the dorsal half of the lateral vestibular nucleus; (3) the fastigial nucleus bilaterally to symmetrical ventral portions of the inferior and lateral vestibular nuclei (Batton et al., '77; Carpenter and Batton, '82); (4) the interstitial nucleus of Cajal to the ipsilateral medial vestibular nucleus (Pompeiano and Walberg, '57); and (5) the contralateral vestibular nuclei, (largely from the medial and superior vestibular nuclei) which are commissural in nature (Gacek, '78; Carleton and Carpenter, '83). Projections from the cerebellar cortex, representing Purkinje cell axons, have inhibitory influences upon vestibular neurons mediated by γ-aminobutyric acid (GABA) (Chan-Palay, '78). Fastigial efferent projections are excitatory in nature. Commissural vestibular projections have inhibitory influences upon the contralateral vestibular nuclei mediated by GABA (Precht, '78).

Secondary Vestibular Fibers. The vestibular nuclei give rise to secondary fibers that project to specific portions of the cerebellum, certain motor cranial nerve nuclei, and to all spinal levels. These fibers are more widely dispersed within the neuraxis than those of any special sensory system, probably because the vestibular system is concerned with the maintenance of equilibrium and orientation in three-dimensional space.

Secondary vestibulocerebellar fibers arise mainly from caudal portions of the medial and inferior vestibular nuclei and project ipsilaterally to the cortex of the nodulus, uvula and flocculus. Vestibulocerebellar fibers, both primary and secondary, enter the cerebellum via the juxtarestiform body (Fig. 6-20). None of these fibers ends in the fastigial nucleus.

Cells of the lateral vestibular nucleus give rise to the somatotopically organized, uncrossed vestibulospinal tract which descends the length of the cord in the anterior part of the lateral funiculus (Fig. 4-12). In the medulla the vestibulospinal tract is a loosely organized bundle extending obliquely from the region of the medial longitudinal fasciculus (MLF) to the retro-olivary area. The dorsal half of the lateral vestibular nucleus receives inhibitory influences from Purkinje cells in the anterior lobe vermis, while ventral regions of the nucleus receive crossed and uncrossed excitatory inputs from the fastigial nuclei. Impulses relayed to spinal levels via the vestibulospinal tract have facilitating influences upon extensor muscle tone.

Fibers of the MLF arise from parts of the superior, medial, and inferior vestibular nuclei and many of these fibers bifurcate into ascending and descending branches (Fig. 6-14). Descending fibers projecting to spinal levels arise from portions of the medial and inferior vestibular nuclei. In the medulla the inferior vestibular nucleus projects fibers ipsilaterally to parts of the medial accessory olive (nucleus β) and the medial vestibular nucleus projects bilaterally to the perihypoglossal and paramedian reticular nuclei (Carleton and Carpenter, '83). Although descending fibers in the MLF from these nuclei are bilateral in the medulla, at spinal levels almost all fibers are ipsilateral. Most of these descending vestibular fibers extend only to cervical spinal segments. Some vestibular fibers in the MLF terminate monosynaptically upon anterior horn cells and exert inhibitory influences (Wilson and Yoshida, '69). The MLF also contains nonvestibular descending fibers from: (1) the interstitial nucleus of Cajal, (2) the superior colliculus, and (3) the pontine reticular formation. The largest group of descending fibers in the MLF is the pontine reticulospinal tract that descends the length of the spinal cord.

Medial Longitudinal Fasciculus (MLF). Ascending fibers of the MLF arise from parts of all vestibular nuclei, are crossed and uncrossed, and project primarily to the nuclei of the extraocular muscles (i.e., the abducens, trochlear, and oculomotor). Ascending fibers from the medial vestibular nucleus are predominantly crossed and project bilaterally upon the abducens nuclei and asymmetrically upon portions of the oculomotor nuclei; projections to the trochlear nucleus are crossed (Carleton and Carpenter, '83). Projections of the rostral part of the inferior vestibular nucleus are entirely crossed and end upon the trochlear and parts of the oculomotor nuclei. The superior vestibular nucleus gives rise to mainly uncrossed projections, while the lateral vestibular nucleus in the cat projects a small number of fibers ipsilaterally to a particular part of the oculomotor nucleus. Retrograde transport studies in the cat and monkey indicate that vestibular projections to the oculomotor nuclear complex arise mainly from the superior and medial vestibular nuclei (Graybiel and Hartwieg, '74; Steiger and Büttner-Ennever, '79). Projections from the superior vestibular nucleus are mainly ipsilateral while those from the medial vestibular nucleus and cell group "y" are largely crossed.

In addition the MLF contains an impressive crossed ascending projection originating from abducens internuclear neurons that terminates upon cells of the medial rectus subdivision of the oculomotor nuclear complex (Fig. 6-19) (Baker and Highstein, '75); Carpenter and Batton, '80; Spencer and Sterling, '77; Steiger and Büttner-Ennever, '78). This projection interrelates activities of the abducens nucleus of one side with neurons of the oculomotor nucleus which innervates the medial rectus muscle on the opposite side. This pathway provides a neural mechanism for simultaneous contractions of the lateral rectus muscle on one side and the medial rectus muscle on the opposite side, as required for lateral gaze.

A small number of ascending fibers in the MLF bypass the oculomotor nucleus and terminate in the interstitial nucleus of Cajal, a small group of neurons partially embedded in the MLF (Figs. 7-11 and 7-14). The medial vestibular nucleus projects to the opposite interstitial nucleus, while the superior vestibular nucleus provides terminals to the ipsilateral interstitial nucleus. Secondary vestibular projections to thalamic relay nuclei are bilateral and end about clusters of cells in the ventral posterior inferior (VPI) and ventral posterolateral (VPL) nuclei (Lang et al., '79). Thalamic neurons receiving vestibular inputs, part of which ascend outside of the MLF, are intermingled with cells responding to somatosensory signals, suggesting there is no specific vestibular relay nucleus in the thalamus (Büttner and Henn, '76; Deecke et al., '77).

Efferent Vestibular Projections. Like the cochlea, the vestibular end organ receives an efferent innervation which arises bilaterally from brain stem neurons. These efferent neurons lie along the lateral border of the abducens nucleus and give rise to fibers that pass peripherally with the vestibular nerve on each side to innervate hair cells in the cristae of the semicircular ducts and the maculae of the utricle and saccule (Fig. 6-15) (Gacek and Lyon, '74; Goldberg and Fernández, '80). Efferent vestibular fibers appear to exert excitatory effects bilaterally upon each of the five end organs of the labyrinth. It has been postulated that the efferent vestibular projection may modulate the dynamic range of afferents to match expected accelerations.

FUNCTIONAL CONSIDERATIONS

Secondary vestibular fibers contained in the MLF play an important role in conjugate eye movements. Selective stimulation of the nerve from the ampulla of individual semicircular ducts produces specific deviations of both eyes which are regarded as primary responses.

Stimulation of the ampullary nerve from the horizontal duct produces conjugate deviation of the eyes to the opposite side. Bilateral stimulation of the ampullary nerves of the anterior ducts produces upward movement of both eyes; similar bilateral stimulation of the ampullary nerves of the posterior ducts causes downward movements of the eyes. Section of the MLF rostral to the abducens nuclei abolishes these primary oculomotor responses, but nystagmus still results from labyrinthine stimulation, suggesting that impulses essential for nystagmus probably pass via the reticular formation.

Labyrinthine stimulation, irritation, or disease cause vertigo, postural deviations, unsteadiness in standing and walking, deviations of the eyes, and nystagmus. *Vertigo*

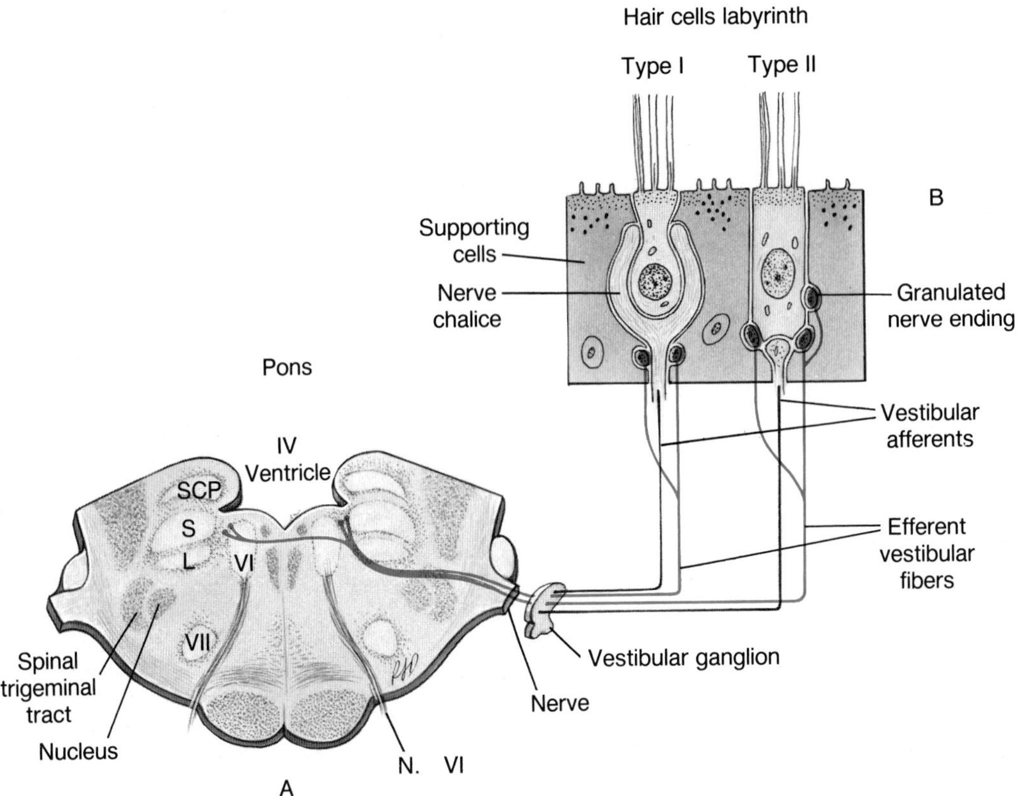

Figure 6-15. Schematic diagram of efferent vestibular fibers (*red*) and their relationship to hair cells of the labyrinth. Efferent vestibular fibers arise bilaterally from small groups of neurons along the lateral border of the abducens nuclei (VI), emerge via the vestibular nerve and terminate in granulated nerve endings at the base of type I and type II hair cells. (*A*) schematic transverse drawing of the pons at level of abducens nuclei and (*B*) hair cells of the labyrinth. Efferent vestibular fibers exert excitatory influences upon the hair cells which may modulate their dynamic range. (Based upon Wersäll, '60; and Goldberg and Fernández, '80.) Abbreviations used: *L*, lateral vestibular nucleus; *S*, superior vestibular nucleus; *SCP*, superior cerebellar peduncle.

implies a subjective sense of rotation, either of the individual or his environment. The most prominent objective sign of vestibular involvement is *nystagmus*, a rhythmic, involuntary oscillation of the eyes characterized by alternate slow and rapid ocular excursions. By convention the direction of the nystagmus is named for the rapid phase, even though the slow ocular excursion is the primary movement (the rapid phase is the automatic reflex correction). Tests of vestibular function are based upon stimulation of the semicircular canals or vestibular nerve endings by: (1) the rotating-chair test (Bárány chair) or (2) the caloric test (irrigation of the external auditory canal with water of temperatures appropriate to induce convection currents in the endolymphatic fluid). Following a period of rotation in the Bárány chair, the chair is abruptly stopped, but the endolymphatic fluid continues to circulate for a time. In this postrotational phase, the slow phase of the nystagmus, the deviations of the eyes, postural deviation (standing) and past-pointing are all in the direction of the previous rotation and can be correlated with the direction of persistent endolymphatic flow. The patient experiences a sense of vertigo opposite to that of the prior rotation.

Lesions of the MLF rostral to the abducens nuclei produce a disturbance of conjugate horizontal eye movements known as *anterior internuclear ophthalmoplegia* (Carpenter and Strominger, '65). A unilateral lesion in the MLF rostral to the abducens nuclear levels results in: (1) paresis of ipsilateral ocular adduction on attempted lateral gaze to the opposite side, (2) monocular horizontal nystagmus in the contralateral abducted eye, and (3) no impairment of ocular convergence. The paresis of ocular adduction on attempted lateral gaze to the opposite side occurs ipsilateral to a unilateral lesion of the MLF (Fig. 6-16). Bilateral lesions of the MLF rostral to the abducens nuclei result in dissociated horizontal eye movements on attempted lateral gaze to both the right and left. In the bilateral syndrome no ocular adduction is seen on attempted lateral gaze to either side. An adequate explanation for the monocular horizontal nystagmus seen in the abducting eye has eluded clinicians and investigators. This syndrome has been produced in the monkey, and occurs in man, mainly as a consequence of brain stem vascular lesions or in association with demyelinating disease (i.e., multiple sclerosis). The paresis of ocular adduction on attempted lateral gaze to the opposite side results from interruption of ascending fibers from abducens internuclear neurons after they have crossed from the opposite side (Fig. 6-16).

Mechanisms governing equilibrium (i.e., maintenance of appropriate body position) and orientation in three-dimensional space are largely reflex in character and depend upon afferent inputs from several sources. The most important of these are: (1) kinesthetic sense conveyed by the posterior column-medial lemniscal system from receptors in joints and joint capsules, (2) impulses conveyed centrally by spinocerebellar systems from stretch receptors in muscles and tendons, (3) the suprasegmental kinesthetic sense provided by the vestibular end organ, and (4) visual input from the retina. The labyrinth is a highly specialized receptor stimulated by the change of position, or changes in the position of the head. When the head is moved the cristae are stimulated and effect compensatory reflexes of the eyes and limbs. Sustaining or static reflexes are initiated by gravitational forces acting upon the macular hair cells.

The vestibulospinal tracts and descending fibers from the pontine reticular formation exert strong excitatory influences upon muscle tone, particularly extensor muscle tone. Normally, muscle tone is maintained by a balance of inhibitory and facilitatory influences, a large part of which are mediated by the brain stem reticular formation. If the influences of higher centers acting upon brain stem structures are removed by transection of the brain stem at the intercollicular level (i.e., between the superior and inferior colliculi) a condition known as *decerebrate rigidity* develops. This condition is characterized by tremendously increased tone in the antigravity muscles, due to an increased rate of firing of muscle spindles by gamma (γ) motor neurons. The increased firing rate of the muscle spindle afferents activates alpha (α) motor neurons which maintain the tonic state (Fig. 3.23). In this experimental preparation facilitatory pathways from the reticular formation of the pons and from the lateral vestibular nucleus (vestibulospinal tract) remain active, while inhibitory elements of the medullary reticular formation no longer function. Inhibitory regions of the reticular formation are considered to be dependent upon descending inpulses from higher levels, while facilitating regions of the reticular formation remain active. Midbrain transection removes the input to the reticular inhibitory system, but has little effect upon brain stem facilitating mechanisms. Decerebrate rigidity can be abolished, or diminished, by a variety of different lesions, including section of the vestibular nerve, destruction of the vestibular nuclei, or section of the vestibulospinal tract. Surgical section of several successive dorsal or ventral spinal roots will abolish the phenomenon segmentally because either will interrupt the γ loop.

FACIAL NERVE

The facial nerve, and the intermediate nerve, usually are discussed together although they subserve separate functions (Figs. 6-1, 6-2, 6-6, and 6-17). Functional components of these nerves include: (1) *special visceral efferent* (SVE, branchiomotor) fibers, (2) *general visceral efferent* (GVE, parasympathetic) fibers, (3) *special visceral afferent* (SVA, taste), and (4) a few

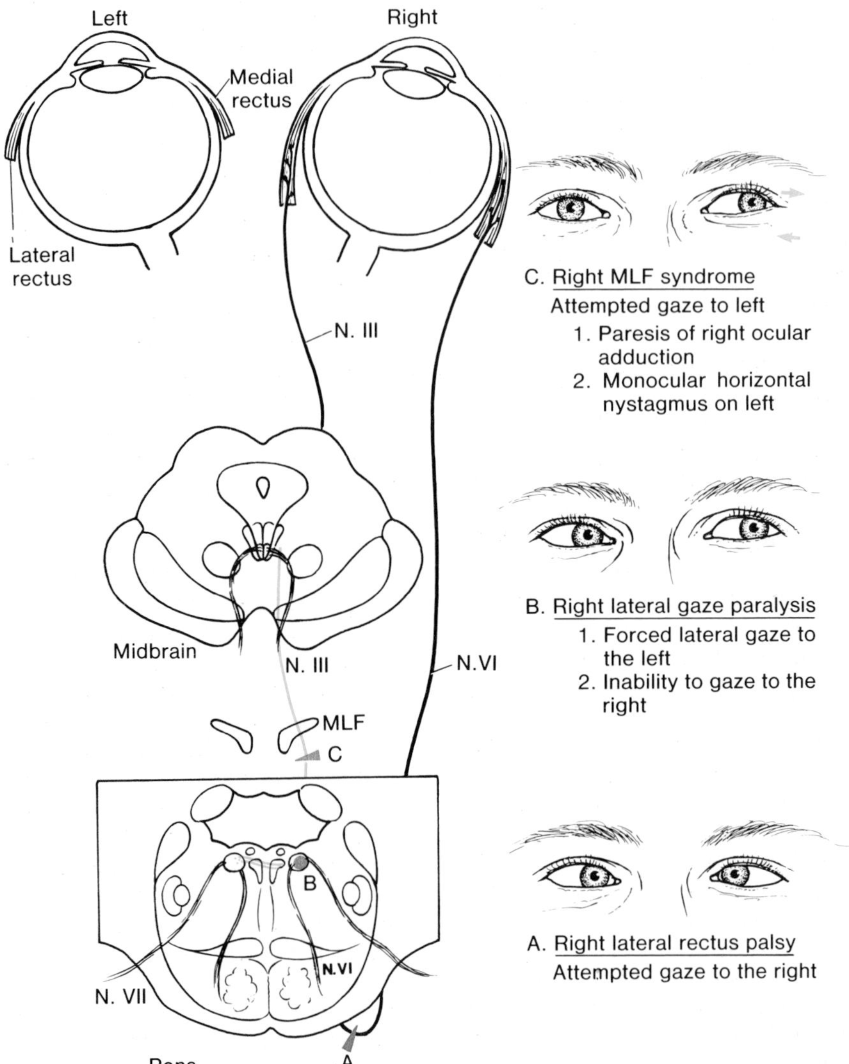

Figure 6-16. Diagrammatic drawing of lesions affecting conjugate horizontal gaze. The lesion (*red*) at *A*, involving the right abducens nerve as it leaves the brain stem, produces a paralysis of the right lateral rectus muscle. In sketch of the eyes at *A* the patient is attempting to gaze to the right: the right eye is somewhat adducted and the left eye is fully adducted. This patient would experience horizontal diplopia on attempted right lateral gaze. The lesion (*red*) in the abducens nucleus (*B*) would destroy lower motor neurons and abducens internuclear neurons whose axons enter the opposite MLF and ascend to the medial rectus subdivision of the oculomotor complex. A patient with such a lesion would have a right lateral gaze paralysis and both eyes would be forcefully directed to the left field of gaze. A unilateral lesion (*red*) in the MLF (*blue*) at *C* would interrupt axons of abducens internuclear neurons arising from the left abducens nucleus. This lesion would produce dissociated horizontal eye movements. On attempted gaze to the left there would be a paresis of right ocular adduction (*C*) and monocular horizontal nystagmus in the left abducting eye, indicated by arrows. (From Carpenter and Sutin, *Human Neuroanatomy*, 1983; courtesy of Williams & Wilkins.)

general somatic afferent (GSA, sensory) fibers.

Special visceral efferent (SVE) *fibers* of the motor component innervate the muscles of facial expression, the platysma, the buccinator and the stapedius muscles. The motor nucleus of N. VII forms a column of multipolar neurons in the ventrolateral tegmentum dorsal to the superior olivary nucleus and ventromedial to the spinal trigeminal nucleus (Figs. 6-1, 6-2, 6-3, and 6-5). At least four distinct cell groups which innervate specific muscles have been recognized: (1) dorsomedial (auricular and occipital muscles), (2) ventromedial (platysma), (3) intermediate (orbicularis oculi and upper mimetic facial muscles), and (4) lateral (buccinator and buccolabial muscles). Efferent fibers, emerging from the dorsal surface of the nucleus, project dorsomedially into the floor of the fourth ventricle. These fibers ascend longitudinally medial to the abducens nucleus and dorsal to the MLF (Figs. 6-6 and 6-17), but near the rostral pole of the abducens nucleus they make a sharp lateral bend and project ventrolaterally. In their emerging course these fibers pass medial to the spinal trigeminal complex and exit from the brain stem near to caudal border of the pons, at the cerebellopontine angle (Figs. 6-2, 6-6, and 6-17).

The *intermediate nerve*, which emerges between the facial motor root and the vestibular nerve (Fig. 6-2), contains afferent and general visceral efferent fibers. Afferent fibers (SVA and GSA) arise from cells of the geniculate ganglion, located at the external genu of the facial nerve (Fig. 6-18). *Special visceral afferent* (SVA) *fibers* convey gustatory sense (taste) from the anterior two-thirds of the tongue. Centrally these fibers enter the solitary fasciculus and terminate upon cells in the rostral part of the solitary nucleus, referred to as the gustatory nucleus. *General somatic afferent* (GSA) *fibers* convey cutaneous sensation from the external auditory meatus and the region back of the ear; centrally these fibers enter the dorsal part of the spinal trigeminal tract.

General visceral efferent (GVE) *fibers* in the intermediate nerve arise from the superior salivatory nucleus, which probably consists of scattered neurons in the dorsolateral reticular formation (Fig. 6-18). Preganglionic parasympathetic fibers from these cells pass peripherally as a component of the intermediate nerve, but near the external genu of the facial nerve they divide so that: (1) one group passes to the pterygopalatine ganglion via the major superficial petrosal nerve, and (2) another group projects via the chorda tympani and branches of the lingual nerves to the submandibular ganglion. Synapses with postganglionic neurons occur in the pterygopalatine and submandibular ganglia. Postganglionic fibers from the pterygopalatine ganglion give rise to secretory and vasomotor fibers that innervate the lacrimal gland and the mucous membrane of the nose and mouth. Postganglionic parasympathetic fibers from the submandibular ganglion pass to the submandibular and sublingual salivary glands.

Lesions of the Facial Nerve. (Bell's palsy) produce paralysis of facial muscles and other sensory and autonomic disturbances which depend upon the location and extent of the peripheral lesion. A complete lesion of the motor part of the facial nerve as it emerges from the stylomastoid foramen (*A*, Fig. 6-18) results in a complete paralysis of the ipsilateral facial muscles. On the side of the lesion, the patient is unable to wrinkle the forehead, close the eye, show his teeth, or purse his lips. The palpebral fissure is widened, the nasolabial fold is flattened and the corner of the mouth droops. The corneal reflex is abolished on the side of the lesion, but corneal sensation remains. A lesion distal to the geniculate ganglion (*B*, Fig. 6-18) produces the deficits associated with a lesion at *A*, but in addition produces impairment of sublingual and submandibular salivary secretions, hyperacusis and frequently loss of taste in the anterior two-thirds of the tongue ipsilaterally. Salivary secretions are impaired due to interruption of preganglionic parasympathetic fibers, and loss of taste is due to interruption of SVA fibers. Hyperacusis results from paralysis of the stapedius muscle which serves to dampen the oscillations of the ear ossicles, and causes sounds to be abnormally loud on the affected side. Lesions of the facial nerve proximal to the geniculate ganglion (*C*, Fig. 6-18) produce all of the disturbances described for lesions at *A* and *B*, and in addition result invariably in loss of taste over the anterior two-thirds of the tongue and impairment of ipsilateral lacrimation. This lesion interrupts all SVA fibers as they course centrally and all preganglionic parasympathetic fibers en route to both the pterygopalatine and submandibular ganglia. Following complete lesions proximal to the geniculate ganglion, taste is perma-

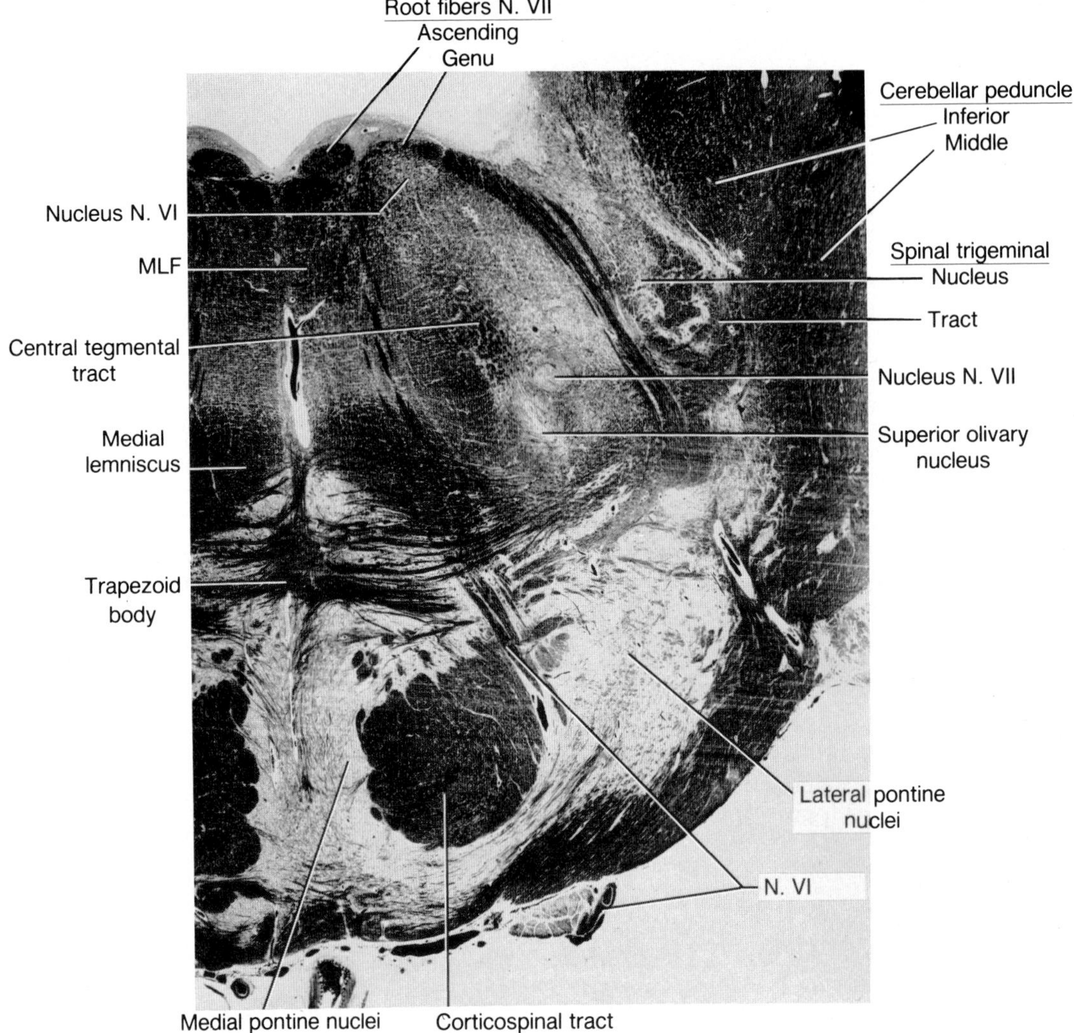

Figure 6-17. Photomicrograph of the right half of the pons showing the intramedullary course of the abducens and facial nerves. (Weigert's myelin stain.)

nently lost and no regeneration of sensory fibers takes place. Preganglionic parasympathetic fibers may regenerate, but this frequently occurs in an aberrant manner. Fibers that previously projected to the submandibular ganglion may regrow and enter the major superficial petrosal nerve. As a consequence of this aberrant regeneration a salivary stimulus may produce lacrimation (syndrome of "*crocodile tears*").

Central type facial palsies involve corticobulbar and corticoreticular fibers which directly and indirectly convey impulses to cells of the facial nucleus. Two types of central facial paralysis are recognized: (1) voluntary and (2) mimetic. Voluntary central type facial palsy occurs contralateral to a lesion involving corticobulbar fibers and affects only the muscles of the lower half of the face, especially those in the perioral region. The accepted explanation is that corticobulbar fibers projecting to cell groups of the facial nucleus innervating muscles in the upper part of the face and forehead are distributed bilaterally; those projecting to cell groups which innervate the lower part of the face are predominantly crossed. Thus a lesion interrupting corticobulbar pathways results in paralysis only of the lower facial muscles contralaterally.

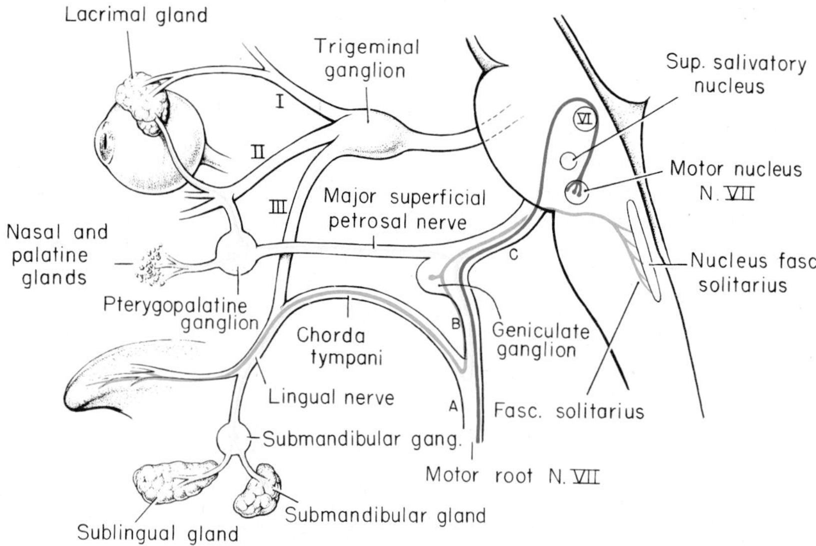

Figure 6-18. Diagram showing the functional components, organization, and peripheral distribution of the facial and intermediate nerves. *Special visceral efferent* (SVE) fibers (motor) are shown in *red. General visceral efferent* (GVE) fibers (parasympathetic) are in *yellow*, and *special visceral afferent* (SVA) fibers (taste) are in *blue. A*, *B*, and *C* denote lesions of the facial nerve at the stylomastoid foramen, distal to the geniculate ganglion, and proximal to the geniculate ganglion. Disturbances resulting from lesions at these locations are described in the text (p. 151). (From Carpenter and Sutin, *Human Neuroanatomy*, 1983; courtesy of Williams & Wilkins.)

A lesions involving corticobulbar and corticospinal fibers in the internal capsule produces a contralateral voluntary central type facial paralysis an a contralateral hemiplegia. Such a lesion never impairs taste, salivary or lacrimal secretions, or the corneal reflex.

Mimetic or emotional innervation of the muscles of facial expression may be preserved even in the presence of a voluntary central type facial palsy. In response to a genuine emotional stimulus, the muscles of the lower part of the face will contract symmetrically. Mimetic facial innervation is involuntary and presumably is mediated by pathways which are independent of those arising from the cerebral cortex. While is is recognized that these pathways are separate from those mediating voluntary facial expression, their origin and course are unknown. Thus certain neural lesions can produce a mimetic facial paralysis without impairing voluntary facial contractions. More extensive lesions can produce combined voluntary and mimetic facial palsies.

ABDUCENS NERVE

The abducens nerve arises from a collection of typical motor cells in the floor of the fourth ventricle which are within the complicated loop formed by fibers of the facial nerve (Figs. 6-1, 6-2, 6-3, 6-6, and 6-17). This motor nerve (GSE) innervates the lateral rectus muscle. Root fibers emerge from the medial aspect of the nucleus, pass ventrally through the pontine tegmentum and emerge from the brain stem at the caudal border of the pons (Figs. 5-1, 5-23, and 6-17). This slender nerve has a long intracranial course and traverses the cavernous sinus and superior orbital fissure en route to the lateral rectus muscle. The abducens nucleus contains two populations of neurons: (1) typical motor neurons which project fibers via the nerve root to innervate the ipsilateral lateral rectus muscle and (2) internuclear neurons whose axons cross the midline, ascend in the contralateral MLF, and terminate upon cells of the oculomotor complex that innervate the medial rectus muscle of the opposite side

(Baker, '77; Highstein, '77; Spencer and Sterling, '77; Steiger and Büttner-Ennever, '79; Carpenter and Batton, '80; Carpenter and Carleton, '83). Abducens internuclear neurons are uniformly distributed throughout the nucleus and are virtually impossible to distinguish from motor neurons.

The abducens nucleus receives inputs from the medial vestibular nucleus, the reticular formation, and the nucleus prepositus. Afferents from the medial vestibular nucleus are predominantly ipsilateral and both populations of abducens neurons receive the same profile of disynaptic excitation and inhibition from the labyrinth (Baker and Highstein, '75; Carleton and Carpenter, '83). Afferents to the abducens nucleus from the paramedian pontine reticular formation (PPRF) and the nucleus prepositus hypoglossi are uncrossed (Büttner-Ennever, '77; Baker and Berthoz, '75). Corticobulbar fibers convey impulses bilaterally to the abducens nuclei via intercalated neurons in the reticular formation.

Lesions of the abducens nerve produce a paralysis of the ipsilateral lateral rectus muscle that results in horizontal diplopia (double vision), which is maximal on attempted lateral gaze to the side of the lesion. Because of the unopposed action of the medial rectus muscle, the affected eye maintains a strongly adducted position. Diplopia is a phenomenon which results when light reflected by an object in the visual field does not fall upon corresponding points of the two retinae.

Discrete unilateral lesions of the abducens nucleus produce a paralysis of lateral gaze to the side of the lesion. (Fig. 6-16). The syndrome of "*lateral gaze paralysis*" differs from paralysis of the lateral rectus muscle in that neither eye can be directed laterally towards the side of the lesion and both eyes tend to be forcefully and conjugately deviated to the opposite side. Ocular convergence usually is not affected. Thus the abducens nerve appears unique in that it is the only cranial nerve in which lesions of the root fibers and nucleus do not produce the same effects (Carpenter et al., '63).

While the general somatic efferent (GSE) cranial nerves innervating the extraocular muscles are regarded the simplest of all the cranial nerves, this simplicity applies only to their peripheral activities. Because the extraocular muscles of the two sides must function synergistically and precisely to produce a full range of conjugate eye movements, a central neural mechanism must control activities of the abducens, trochlear and oculomotor nuclei. The central neural mechanism underlying conjugate lateral eye movements is just beginning to be understood. The observation that paralysis of vertical or horizontal eye movements can occur independently implies separate anatomical sites at some distance from each other that generate vertical and horizontal eye movements. However, conjugate eye movement have both vertical and horizontal components so precisely synchronized that centers controlling vertical and horizontal eye movements must be functionally connected and coordinated. Considerable evidence suggests that the pontine "center for lateral gaze" and the abducens nucleus probably constitute a single entity (Carpenter et al., '63; Carpenter, '71; Graybiel and Hartwieg, '74; Spencer and Sterling, '77; Steiger and Büttner-Ennever, '78).

The localized region most concerned with vertical eye movements lies in the tegmental area rostral to the oculomotor complex in the zone of transition between diencephalon and mesencephalon (Büttner et al., '77). Large cells in this area lie in the medial part of Forel's field H, rostral to the fasciculus retroflexus, and have been referred to as the *rostral interstitial nucleus of the MLF*. They form an entity distinct from interstitial of Cajal which lies lateral to the oculomotor complex. The important question as to how horizontal and vertical components of conjugate eye movements are coordinated suggests that the *paramedian pontine reticular formation* (PPRF) which projects directly to the abducens nucleus and to the rostral interstitial nucleus of the MLF may be the encoding site (Büttner et al., '77). Bilateral lesions of the PPRF may cause paralysis of both horizontal and vertical gaze (Bender and Shanzer, '64). Projections from the PPRF to the abducens nucleus are uncrossed; those to the rostral interstitial nucleus of the MLF are uncrossed and ascend outside of the MLF. The rostral interstitial nucleus of the MLF projects ipsilaterally to the oculomotor nuclear complex (Fig. 6-19) (Steiger and Büttner-Ennever, '79).

Lateral gaze paralysis, due to discrete lesions in the abducens nucleus, is caused by: (1) destruction of motor neurons in the abducens nucleus which results in paralysis of the ipsilateral lateral rectus muscle, and (2) destruction of internuclear neurons within the abducens nucleus which give rise to ascending fibers that project via the opposite MLF to the medial rectus subdivision (see p. 149) of the contralateral oculomotor complex. The paresis of ocular adduction in the contralateral eye, which forms part of the syndrome of lateral gaze paralysis, appears to be due to destruction of abducens internuclear neurons that are intermingled with cells whose axons form the abducens nerve root.

Root fibers of the abducens nerve may be concomitantly destroyed along with fibers of the corticospinal tract in the caudal pons as a consequence of a vascular lesion. Such a lesion results in the so-called *middle alternating hemiplegia*, characterized by an ipsilateral lateral rectus paralysis and a contralateral hemiplegia.

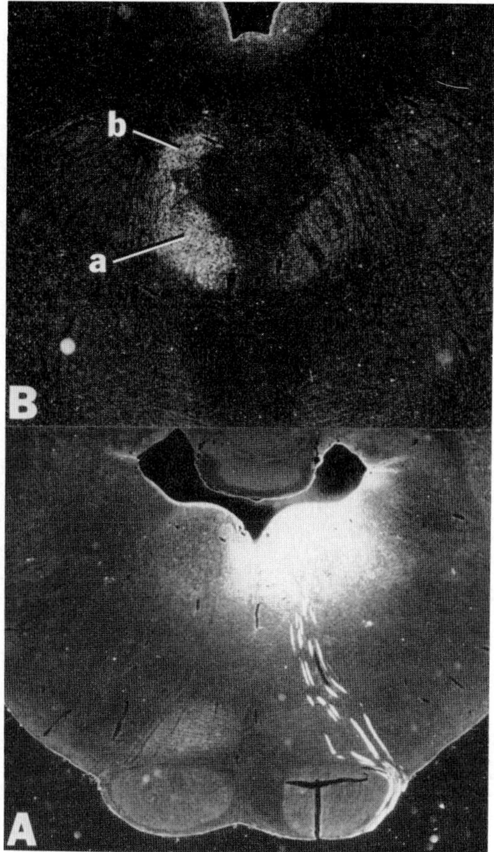

Figure 6-19. Dark-field photomicrographs of [^{3}H] amino acids injected into the right abducens nucleus in a monkey showing transport via abducens root fibers and the contralateral medial longitudinal fasciculus (MLF) (*A*). Ascending isotope transported from abducens internuclear neurons via the MLF terminates in the medial rectus subdivision of the opposite oculomotor complex (*B*). The medial rectus subdivisions in the caudal oculomotor complex are represented by cell groups designated *a* and *b*. (From Carpenter and Carleton, '83.)

TRIGEMINAL NERVE

The trigeminal, the largest cranial nerve, contains both sensory (GSA) and motor (SVE) components. The *general somatic afferent* component conveys both exteroceptive and proprioceptive impulses. Exteroceptive impulses (i.e., pain, thermal and tactile sense) are transmitted from: (1) the face and forehead, (2) mucous membranes of the nose and mouth, (3) the teeth, and (4) large portions of the cranial dura. Deep pressure and kinesthesis are conveyed from the teeth, periodontium, hard palate, and temporomandibular joint. In addition impulses are transmitted centrally from stretch receptors in the muscles of mastication. *Special visceral efferent* fibers (branchiomotor) innervate the muscles of mastication, the tensor tympani and the tensor veli palatini.

Trigeminal Ganglion. Afferent fibers, except for those associated with proprioceptive and stretch receptors, have their cell bodies in the trigeminal ganglion. This ganglion, composed of typical unipolar cells, lies on the petrous bone in the middle cranial fossa (Fig. 1-3). Peripheral processes of these cells form the ophthalmic, maxillary and mandibular divisions of the trigeminal nerve which innervate distinctive regions of the face, head and intraoral structures. All three divisions of the trigeminal nerve contribute sensory fibers to the dura.

Central processes of trigeminal ganglion

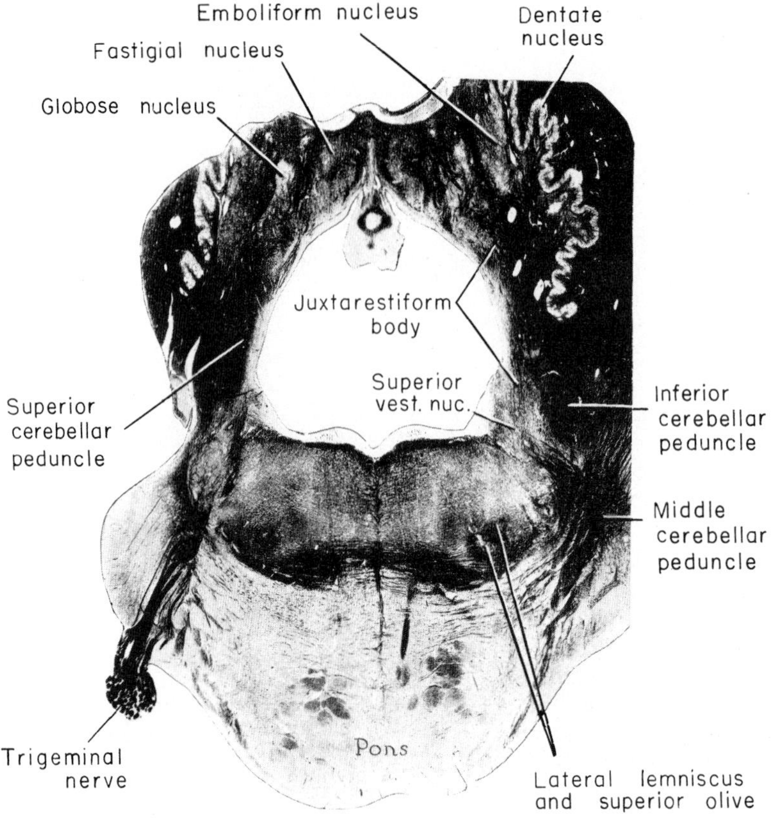

Figure 6-20. Section of pons, pontine tegmentum, and part of cerebellum through the trigeminal nerve root. One-month infant. (Weigert's myelin stain; photograph.) (From Carpenter and Sutin, *Human Neuroanatomy*, 1983; courtesy of Williams & Wilkins.)

cells form the sensory root of this nerve, which traverses the lateral part of the pons, to enter the pontine tegmentum and terminate upon sensory relay nuclei distributed in the pons and medulla (Figs. 2-21, 6-20, and 6-21). Many sensory root fibers bifurcate into short ascending and long descending branches; other fibers ascend or descend without branching. Ascending fibers terminate upon cells of the principal sensory nucleus, while descending fibers form the spinal trigeminal tract (Fig. 6-24).

Spinal Trigeminal Tract and Nucleus. Root fibers entering the spinal trigeminal tract have a definite topographical organization. Fibers of the ophthalmic division are most ventral, fibers of the mandibular division are most dorsal and those of the maxillary division are intermediate (Fig. 6-21). This inverted laminar arrangement of fibers results from medial rotation of the trigeminal sensory root as it enters the brain stem and persists throughout the length of the tract. The tract extends from the level of the trigeminal root in the pons to the uppermost cervical spinal segments. Fibers of the spinal trigeminal tract terminate upon cells of the spinal trigeminal nucleus, which form a long laminated cell column medial to the tract. Rostrally the nucleus merges with the principal sensory nucleus, while caudally it blends into the substantia gelatinosa of the first two cervical spinal segments. Fibers of the spinal trigeminal tract project into that part of the spinal trigeminal nucleus immediately adjacent to it. There is a sharp segregation of terminal fibers within parts of the nucleus and virtually no overlap of fibers from the different divisions of the nerve. The spinal trigeminal tract also contains small groups of GSA fibers from the facial, glossopharyngeal and vagus nerves which occupy dorsomedial regions.

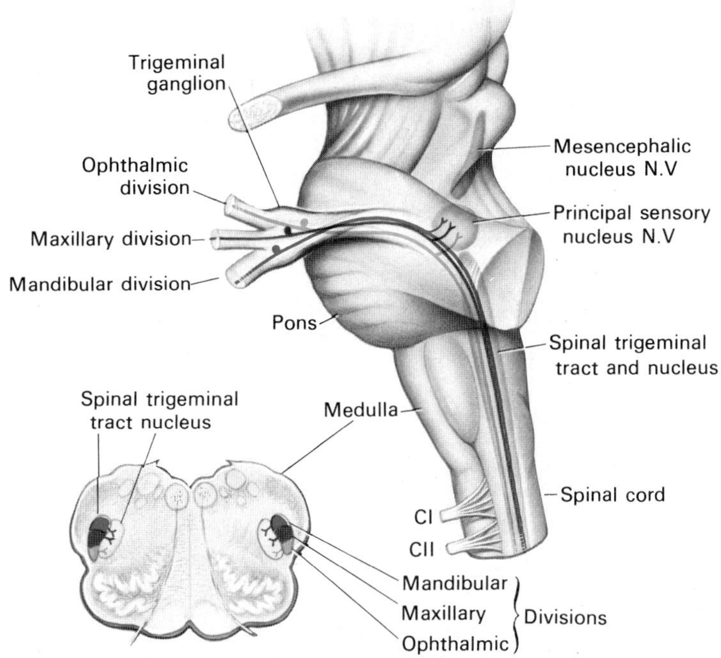

Figure 6-21. Diagram of the topographical arrangement of the fibers in the spinal trigeminal tract. The laminar arrangement of fibers from the different divisions of the trigeminal nerve persists throughout its length, although fibers leave the tract at all levels to terminate upon adjacent cells of the spinal trigeminal nucleus.

Cytoarchitecturally the spinal trigeminal nucleus consists of three parts: (1) a *pars oralis*, (2) a *pars interpolaris*, and (3) a *pars caudalis*. The laminar configurations within caudal parts of the spinal trigeminal nucleus consist of four layers (Fig. 5-8) and resemble those of the posterior gray horn at spinal levels (Gobel, '75, '78, '78a; Kruger, '79). Cells in lamina I respond to nociceptive and thermal stimuli; lamina II corresponds to the substantia gelatinosa and laminae III and IV (magnocellular layers) correspond to the proper sensory nucleus. Throughout the nucleus the face is represented in an upside down fashion, with the jaw dorsal and the forehead ventral (Fig. 6.21). The pars oralis receives impulses predominantly from internal structures of the nose and mouth. The pars interpolaris is related mainly to cutaneous facial regions, while the pars caudalis has large receptive fields over the forehead, cheek and jaw (Wall and Taub, '62).

Lesions of the spinal trigeminal tract result chiefly in loss or diminution of pain and thermal sense in areas innervated by the trigeminal nerve. Such lesions have little effect upon tactile sense, although neurons at all levels of the nucleus respond to tactile stimuli. Tactile sense may be mediated by fibers that bifurcate and send branches to both the spinal trigeminal nucleus and the principal sensory nucleus (Fig. 6-24). Virtually no overlap exists between cutaneous areas supplied by the three peripheral divisions of the trigeminal nerve, in contrast to the extensive overlap seen for spinal nerves. Trigeminal tractotomy (i.e., sectioning of the spinal trigeminal tract) can relieve various forms of facial pain, including trigeminal neuralgia (tic douloureux). This procedure eliminates or greatly reduces pain and thermal sense without impairing tactile sense. Corneal sensation remains, as does the corneal reflex, though it may not be as brisk.

Principal Sensory Nucleus. This nucleus lies lateral to the entering trigeminal root fibers in the upper pons (Figs. 6-20, 6-21, 6-22, and 6-24). Root fibers conveying impulses for tactile and pressure sense enter the principal sensory nucleus and are

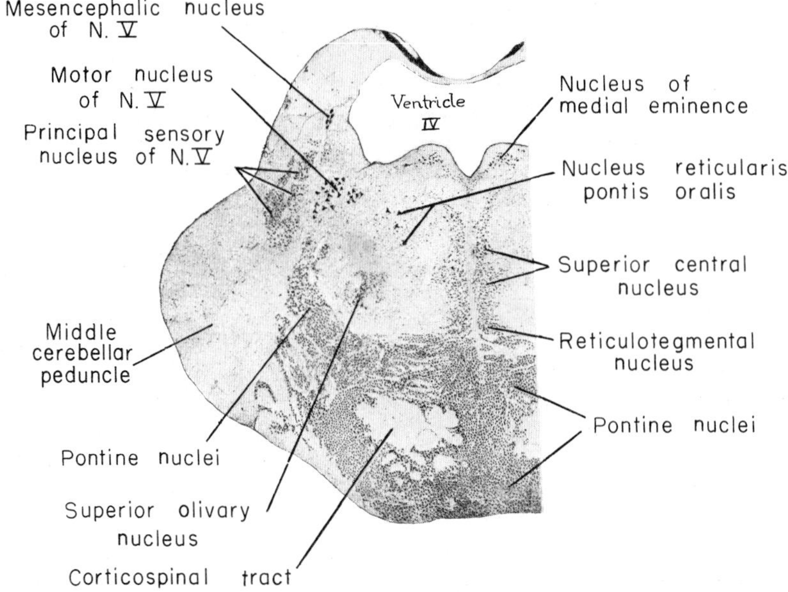

Figure 6-22. Section through the pons of a 1-month infant at about same level as shown in Figure 6-20. (Cresyl violet; photograph, with cell groups schematically blocked in.) (From Carpenter and Sutin, *Human Neuroanatomy*, 1983; courtesy at Williams & Wilkins.)

distributed in a manner similar to that described for the spinal trigeminal nucleus. Fibers of the ophthalmic division terminate ventrally, fibers of the maxillary division are intermediate, and fibers of the mandibular division are most dorsal. Cells of the principal sensory nucleus have large receptive fields, show high spontaneous activity, and respond to a wide range of pressure stimuli with little adaptation.

Mesencephalic Nucleus. This trigeminal nucleus forms a slender cell column near the lateral margin of the central gray of the upper fourth ventricle and cerebral aqueduct. The nucleus, composed of large unipolar neurons, extends from the level of the motor nucleus of N.V to the rostral midbrain (Figs. 6-22 and 6-24). Cells resemble those of the dorsal root ganglion but are not encapsulated and lie within the central nervous system. The principal processes of these cells form the sickle-shaped mesencephalic tract of the trigeminal nerve (Figs. 5-17, 6-22, and 6-24), which descends to the level of the motor nucleus of N.V. Collaterals of these processes enter the motor nucleus, while the main fibers emerge as part of the motor root. The cells of this nucleus are considered to be primary sensory neurons which have been "retained" within the central nervous system. Afferent fibers of the mesencephalic nucleus of the trigeminal nerve convey, pressure and kinesthesis sense from the teeth, periodontium, hard palate and joint capsules. This nucleus is concerned with mechanisms that control the force of the bite. It also receives impulses from stretch receptors in the muscles of mastication. While afferent fibers of the mesencephalic nucleus travel with fibers of the motor root, some fibers from this nucleus pass peripherally with all three divisions of the trigeminal nerve.

Motor Nucleus. The *motor nucleus of the trigeminal nerve* forms an oval column of typical large motor neurons medial to the motor root and the principal sensory nucleus (Figs. 6-20 and 6-22). Fibers from this nucleus exit from the brain stem medial to the entering sensory root, pass underneath the trigeminal ganglion, and become incorporated in the mandibular division. The motor nucleus receives collaterals from the mesencephalic root which form a two-neuron reflex arc. Secondary trigeminal fibers, both crossed and uncrossed, establish reflex connections between the muscles of mastication and cutaneous regions as well as with lingual and oral mucous membranes. Some corticobulbar fibers terminate directly upon trigeminal motor neurons, while others pass to reticular neurons which in turn project to the motor nucleus.

Secondary Trigeminal Pathways. These pathways originate from cells in the principal sensory and spinal trigeminal nuclei and project to higher levels of the brain stem, the cerebellum and the spinal cord (Ruggiero et al., '81; Matsushita et al., '82). Collaterals of these fibers provide numerous projections to motor nuclei of the brain stem involved in complex reflexes (Fig. 6-24).

Trigeminothalamic projections arise largely from cells in laminae I and IV of the pars caudalis and interpolaris of the spinal trigeminal nucleus. Axons from these cells in the spinal trigeminal nucleus project ventromedially into the reticular formation, cross the median raphe, and come into close association with the contralateral medial lemniscus (Fig. 6-23). These secondary trigeminal fibers terminate in a selective manner about cells of the ventral posteromedial (VPM) nucleus of the thalamus. Crossed axons from cells of the spinal trigeminal nucleus which ascend in the brain stem with the contralateral medial lemniscus form the ventral trigeminal tract (*ventral trigeminothalamic tract*).

Trigeminocerebellar fibers arise from cells in lamina IV in all parts of the spinal trigeminal nucleus with the largest number originating from rostral parts of the nucleus (Matsushita et al., '82). Additional trigeminocerebellar fibers come from cells in ventral portions of the principal sensory nucleus. These portions of the trigeminal nuclei project uncrossed fibers to the paramedian lobule, the simple lobule and posterior parts of crus II. A large number of these fibers enter the cerebellum via the inferior cerebellar peduncle.

Trigeminospinal projections arise from cells in laminae I and III in all subdivisions of the spinal trigeminal nucleus. Fibers from the pars caudalis and interpolaris are ipsilateral while those from pars oralis are bilateral in distribution. These descending projections may modulate incoming sensory information in the posterior horn, contribute to a variety of reflexes and link receptors in the trigeminal distribution with somatic and visceral effectors in the spinal cord (Ruggiero et al., '81).

Secondary trigeminal fibers from the principal sensory nucleus are both crossed and uncrossed. Cells in the dorsomedial part of the nucleus give rise to a small bundle of uncrossed fibers which ascend close to the central gray of the mesencephalon and enter the ipsilateral ventral posteromedial (VPM) nucleus of the thalamus. These fibers form the *dorsal trigeminal tract* and appear to be associated in a unique way with the mandibular division of the trigeminal nerve (Fig. 6-23).

Cells in the ventral part of the principal sensory nucleus of N. V give rise to a larger, entirely crossed bundle of trigeminothalamic fibers which ascends in association with the contralateral medial lemniscus, in a manner similar to that described for the ventral trigeminal tract. These crossed secondary trigeminal fibers terminate in the VPM nucleus of the thalamus.

The central connections of the mesencephalic nucleus of the trigeminal nerve are not established, although it has been suggested that they may project to the cerebellum. In the monkey, fibers from the mesencephalic nucleus of N. V are described as terminating in parts of the dentate nucleus and in the overlying cerebellar cortex (Chan-Palay, '77). Retrograde transport studies in the cat have failed to establish projections from this nucleus to the cerebellar cortex (Gould, '80; Matsushita et al., '82). Neurons of the mesencephalic nucleus of N. V are consistently labeled following horseradish peroxidase (HRP) injections of the upper cervical spinal cord (Matsushita et al., '79a).

Trigeminal Reflexes. Although secondary trigeminal fibers are involved in a large number of reflexes, the *corneal reflex* is one of the most important (Fig. 6-24). Normally stimulation of the cornea with a wisp of cotton produces bilateral blinking and closing of the eyes. The blinking and closing of the eyes is effected by impulses reaching the facial nuclei on both sides. Evidence suggests that secondary trigeminal fibers project bilaterally to the facial nuclei. Following an injury to the ophthalmic division of the trigeminal nerve, cor-

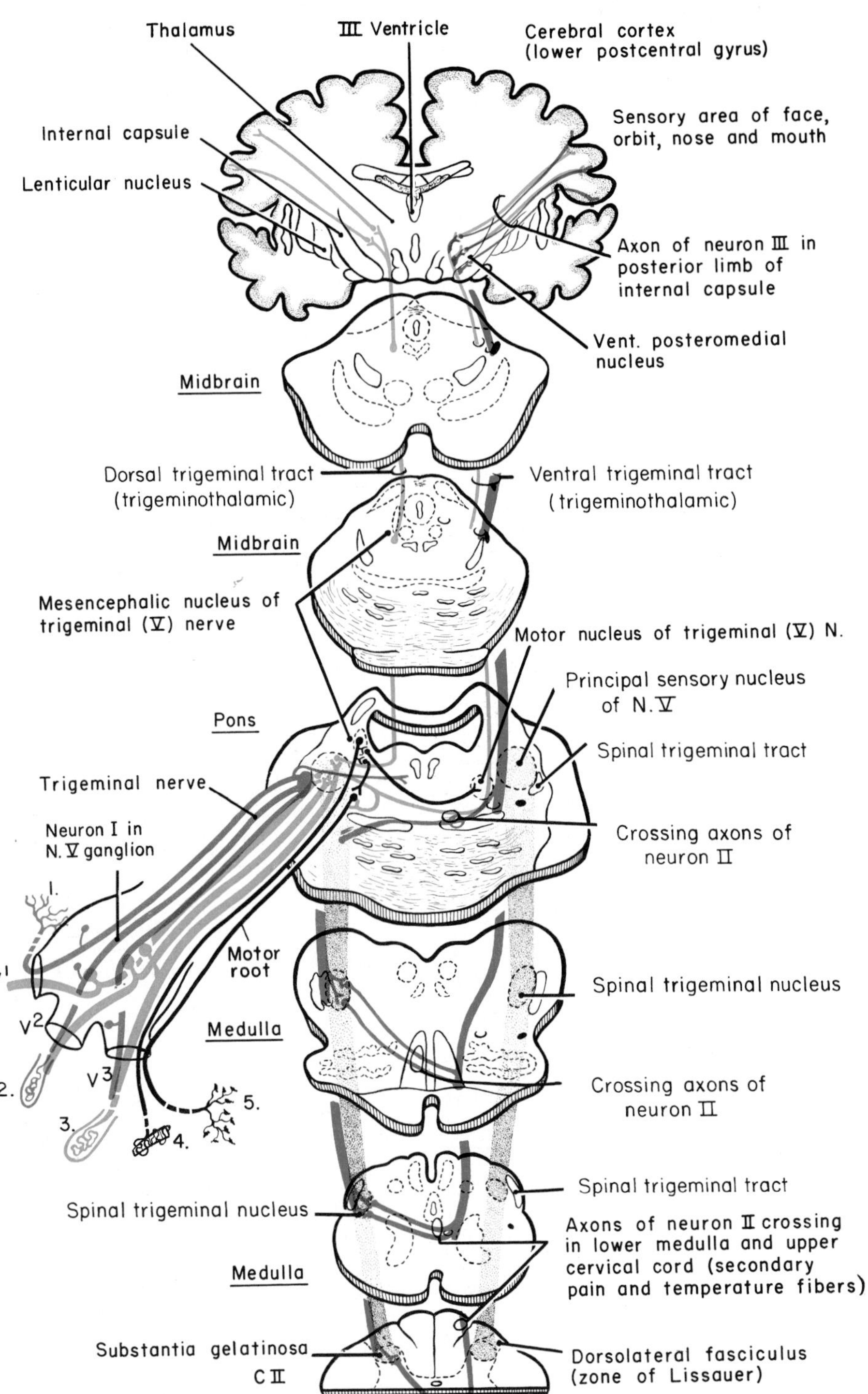

Figure 6-23. Diagram of the trigeminothalamic tracts. The *ventral trigeminal tract* (*red*) conveys tactile, pain and thermal sense. These fibers originate from the spinal trigeminal nucleus, cross in the lower brain stem at various locations and ascend in association with the contralateral medial lemniscus. Trigeminothalamic fibers from the principal sensory nucleus, conveying touch and pressure (*blue*) ascend by two separate pathways. Fibers from the ventral part of the principal sensory nucleus of N. V cross and ascend in association with the contralateral medial lemniscus. Fibers from the dorsomedial part of the same nucleus ascend uncrossed as the *dorsal trigeminal tract*. Both the ventral and dorsal trigeminal tracts project to the ventral posteromedial nucleus of the thalamus. The brain stem location of the ascending lateral spinothalamic tract is indicated in *black* on the *right side*. The ophthalmic (V^1), maxillary (V^2), and mandibular (V^3) divisions of the trigeminal nerve are identified. *1*, Free nerve ending; *2*, thermal receptor, *3*, Meissner's corpuscle; *4*, neuromuscular spindle; *5*, motor end plate in muscle of mastication. (From Carpenter and Sutin, *Human Neuroanatomy*, 1983; courtesy of Williams & Wilkins.)

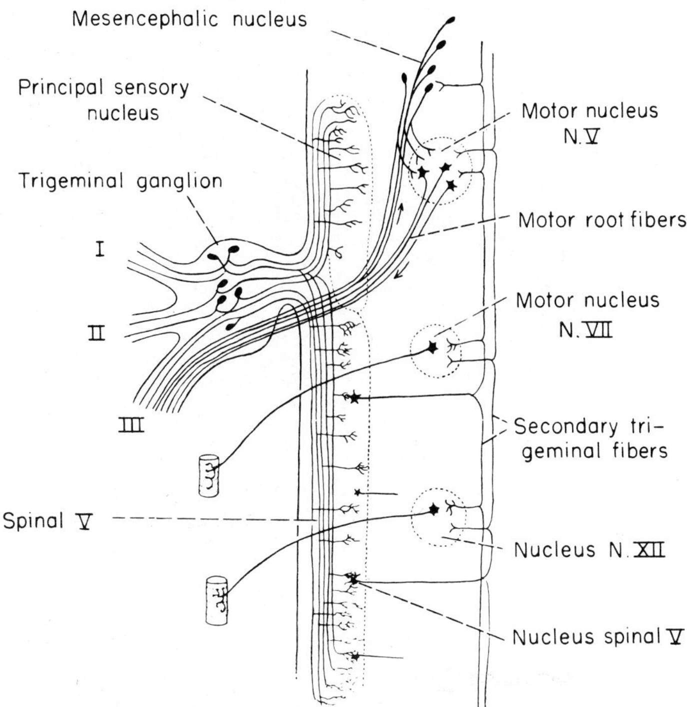

Figure 6-24. Diagram of the trigeminal nuclei and some of the pathways involved in trigeminal reflexes. *I*, Ophthalmic division; *II*, maxillary division; *III*, mandibular division. (Modified from Cajal, '09.) (From Carpenter and Sutin, *Human Neuroanatomy*, 1983; courtesy of Williams & Wilkins.)

neal sensation and the corneal reflex are lost on that side because the afferent limb of the reflex arc has been destroyed. However, corneal sensation remains on the opposite side and stimulation of that cornea will produce bilateral blinking and eye closure, indicating that the efferent limb (facial nucleus and nerve) of the reflex arc is intact. In patients with peripheral facial palsies, corneal sensation will be present on both sides, but no corneal reflex can be elicited on the side of the lesion because the efferent limb of the reflex arc has been destroyed. However, stimulation of the cornea on the side of the lesion will cause blinking and closure of the opposite eye (consensual response).

Secondary trigeminal fibers ascending and descending in dorsolateral regions of the brain stem reticular formation give off collaterals to various motor nuclei that mediate specific reflexes (Fig. 6-24). These reflexes include: (1) the *tearing reflex*, in which impulses pass to the superior salivatory nucleus of N. VII; (2) *sneezing*, in which trigeminal impulses pass to the nucleus ambiguus, respiratory centers in the reticular formation and to certain cell groups of the spinal cord (i.e., phrenic nerve nuclei and anterior horn cells innervating the intercostal muscles); (3) *vomiting*, in which impulses pass to vagal nuclei; and (4) *salivary reflexes* in which secondary trigeminal fibers project to the salivatory nuclei. Secondary trigeminal fibers probably also pass to the hypoglossal nuclei and mediate reflex movements of the tongue in response to stimulation of the tongue and the mucous membranes of the mouth.

The *jaw jerk*, or masseter reflex, a monosynaptic reflex, is elicited by gently tapping the patient's chin (with mouth open slightly). The response is bilateral contractions of the masseter and temporal muscles. This myotatic reflex involves stretch receptors in the muscles of mastication, the mesencephalic nucleus, and collaterals from that nucleus which terminate in the motor

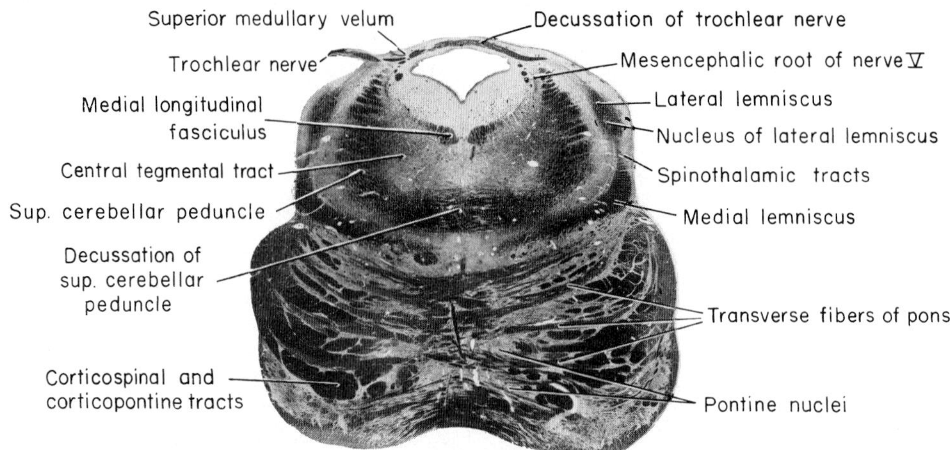

Figure 6-25. Section of the isthmus of an adult brain at the level of the decussation and exit of the trochlear nerves. (Weigert's myelin stain; photograph.) (From Carpenter and Sutin, *Human Neuroanatomy*, 1983; courtesy of Williams & Wilkins.)

trigeminal nucleus. The jaw reflex is absent in peripheral lesions of the trigeminal nerve.

PONTINE TEGMENTUM

Transverse sections through the pons at the level of the trigeminal nerve root (Figs. 5-1, 6-20 and 6-22) reveal significant changes when compared with lower pontine levels. These changes include the following: (1) the fourth ventricle is narrower, (2) fibers of the superior cerebellar peduncle form the dorsolateral wall of the fourth ventricle, (3) fibers of the inferior and middle cerebellar peduncles can be seen entering the cerebellum, and (4) portions of the cerebellum dorsal to the pons contain parts of all the deep cerebellar nuclei. The ventral portion of the pons is larger than at lower levels, the mass of pontine nuclei is greater, and longitudinally descending fiber bundles (i.e., corticospinal, corticopontine and corticobulbar tracts) are less compact.

In the dorsal part of the pons the medial lemniscus is located ventrally and is traversed in part by fibers of the trapezoid body. Portions of the superior olivary nuclei retain their same position. Dorsomedial to the superior olivary complex is the central tegmental tract. The spinothalamic and anterior spinocerebellar tracts are located lateral to the medial lemniscus, and the MLF is located dorsally on each side of the median raphe. The central part of the pontine tegmentum contains the pontine reticular formation.

Pontine Reticular Formation. Two relatively large nuclear masses, the *nucleus reticularis pontis caudalis* and *oralis*, compose the bulk of the pontine reticular formation. The pars caudalis which replaces the gigantocellular reticular nucleus of the medulla extends rostrally to levels of the trigeminal motor nucleus (Figs. 6-1 and 6-3). It contains some scattered giant cells similar to those seen in the medulla. The pars oralis extends rostrally into the caudal mesencephalon where its precise boundary is indistinct (Fig. 6-22). Cells of the pontine reticular formation give rise to uncrossed reticulospinal fibers which in the brain stem descend as a component of the MLF. Other cells give rise to fibers which ascend as part of the central tegmental tract (Figs. 6-4 and 6-25). Many cells have dichotomizing axons which project branches both rostrally and caudally. Ascending pontine reticular fibers project via the central tegmental fasciculus to the intralaminar thalamic nuclei. Impulses passing to these thalamic nuclei profoundly influence the electrical activity of broad areas of the cerebral cortex.

Other reticular nuclei present at pontine levels are the reticulotegmental and the superior central nuclei (Figs. 6-22 and 6-26). The reticulotegmental nucleus lies near the median raphe dorsal to the medial

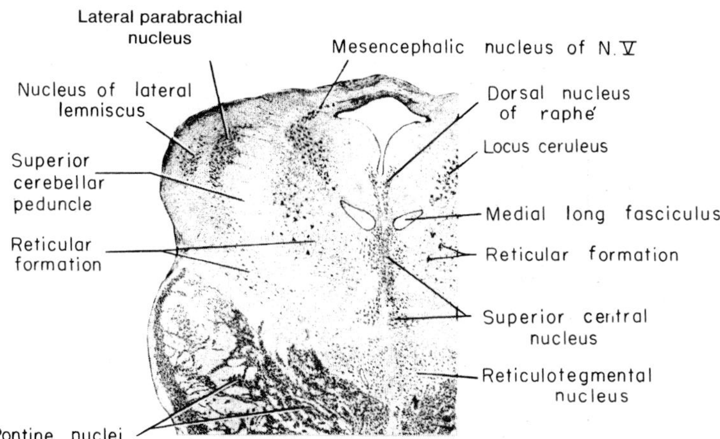

Figure 6-26. Section through isthmus of a 3-month infant. (Cresyl violet; photograph, with cell groups schematically blocked in.) (From Carpenter and Sutin, *Human Neuroanatomy*, 1983; courtesy of Williams & Wilkins.)

lemniscus and is regarded as a tegmentally displaced pontine nuclear group. The superior central nucleus develops in the median raphe and enlarges at isthmus levels.

ISTHMUS OF THE HINDBRAIN

The narrowest portion of the hindbrain, situated rostral to the cerebellum and immediately caudal to the midbrain, is known as the *isthmus rhombencephali* (Figs. 6-25 and 6-26). As in other parts of the brain stem three regions are recognized, namely, a roof plate, a tegmental region, and a ventral cortically dependent part. The roof is formed by a thin membrane, the *superior medullary velum.* This membrane contains the decussating fibers of the trochlear nerve and forms the roof of the most rostral part of the fourth ventricle (Fig. 6-25).

The tegmental region, ventral to the fourth ventricle, is smaller than at caudal levels. The more abundant central gray resembles that seen at mesencephalic levels. The lateral border of the central gray contains the mesencephalic nucleus and tract of the trigeminal nerve. Ventral to these structures is the relatively large collection of pigmented cells (melanin) which form the *locus ceruleus.* Lateral to the central gray are the fibers of the *superior cerebellar peduncle* which have passed into the tegmentum and are shifting ventromedially to undergo a complete discussion (Fig. 6-25). Fibers of the superior cerebellar peduncle arise from the dentate, emboliform and globose nuclei and constitute the largest and most important cerebellar efferent system.

The *lateral lemniscus* forms a well-defined bundle near the lateral surface of the tegmentum (Fig. 6-25). Groups of cells situated among the fibers of this tract constitute the *nuclei of the lateral lemniscus* (Fig. 6-26). Most of the fibers in the lateral lemniscus project rostrally and enter the inferior colliculus. The medial lemniscus is a flattened band of ascending fibers in the ventrolateral tegmentum; fibers of the spinothalamic tract are located laterally near the junction of the medial and lateral lemnisci. At this level the principal ascending sensory pathways form a peripheral shell of fibers which encloses most of the pontine tegmentum.

The ventral part of the pons at this level is larger than the tegmental part but it is not as massive as at midpontine levels. Corticospinal and corticopontine tracts are broken up into numerous bundles which are surrounded by pontine nuclei (Fig. 6-26).

Locus Ceruleus. Near the periventricular gray of the upper part of the fourth ventricle is an irregular collection of pigmented cells known as the locus ceruleus (Figs. 6-26, 6-27, and 6-28). Cells of this nucleus are partially intermingled with those of the mesencephalic nucleus of the

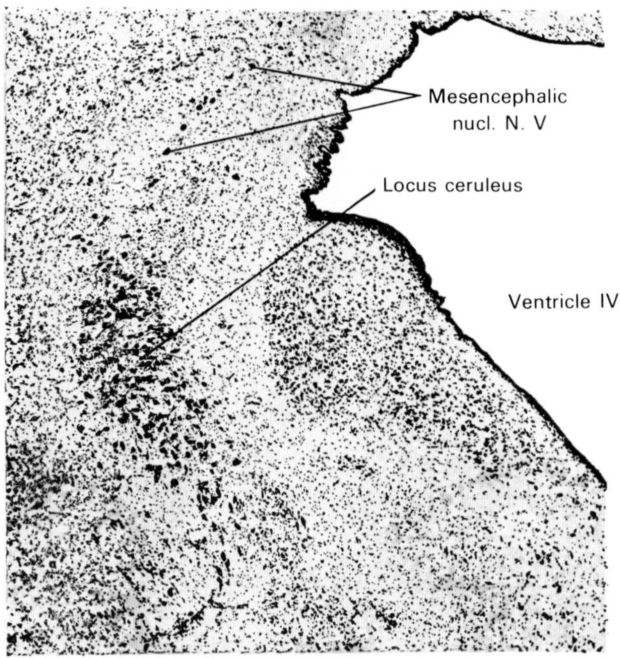

Figure 6-27. Photograph of the cell groups surrounding the periventricular gray at isthmus levels. Cells of the locus ceruleus contain melanin pigment granules and high concentrations of norepinephrine. Globular cells of the mesencephalic nucleus of N. V, present along the dorsal border of the locus ceruleus, extend dorsally and rostrally at the margin of the central gray. (From Carpenter and Sutin, *Human Neuroanatomy*, 1983; courtesy of Williams & Wilkins.)

trigeminal nerve, but the large globular neurons of the mesencephalic nucleus extend further dorsally and rostrally at the margin of the central gray (Fig. 6-27). Cells of the locus ceruleus are of two types: (1) medium-sized cells with eccentric nuclei containing clumps of melanin pigment granules and (2) small oval cells with scant cytoplasm and no pigment. Ventrolateral to the locus ceruleus is a diffuse collection of similar cells known as the nucleus subceruleus (Olszewski and Baxter, '54).

Although the locus ceruleus is a relatively small structure, it can be identified readily in gross sections of the brain stem. The significance of this small pigmented nucleus remained unknown until it was demonstrated by a sensitive fluorescence technic that its cells contain catecholamines, nearly all of which are norepinephrine (Fig. 6-28) (Dahlström and Fuxe, '64; Anden et al., '66; Olson and Fuxe, '71; Ungerstedt, '71; Kuhar et al., '72). Unlike other brain stem norepinephrine cells found as scattered neurons in the lateral tegmentum, the locus ceruleus is a compact nucleus that projects fibers to portions of the telencephalon, diencephalon, midbrain, cerebellum, pons, medulla, and spinal cord (Olson and Fuxe, '71; Ungerstedt, '71; Maeda and Shimizu, '72; Pickel et al., '74; McBride and Sutin, '76; Nygren and Olson, '77; Jones and Moore, '77; Levitt and Moore, '79). Information concerning the widespread projections of locus ceruleus and the nucleus subceruleus have been developed through a variety of different anatomical, histochemical, biochemical, and pharmacological methodologies.

Major ascending projections from the locus ceruleus pass rostrally in the medial forebrain bundle to and through the lateral hypothalamus (Fig. 10-9). Near the level of the anterior commissure the pathway divides into bundles which respectively innervate telencephalic and diencephalic structures. Noradrenergic fibers are distributed widely in the cerebral cortex and the

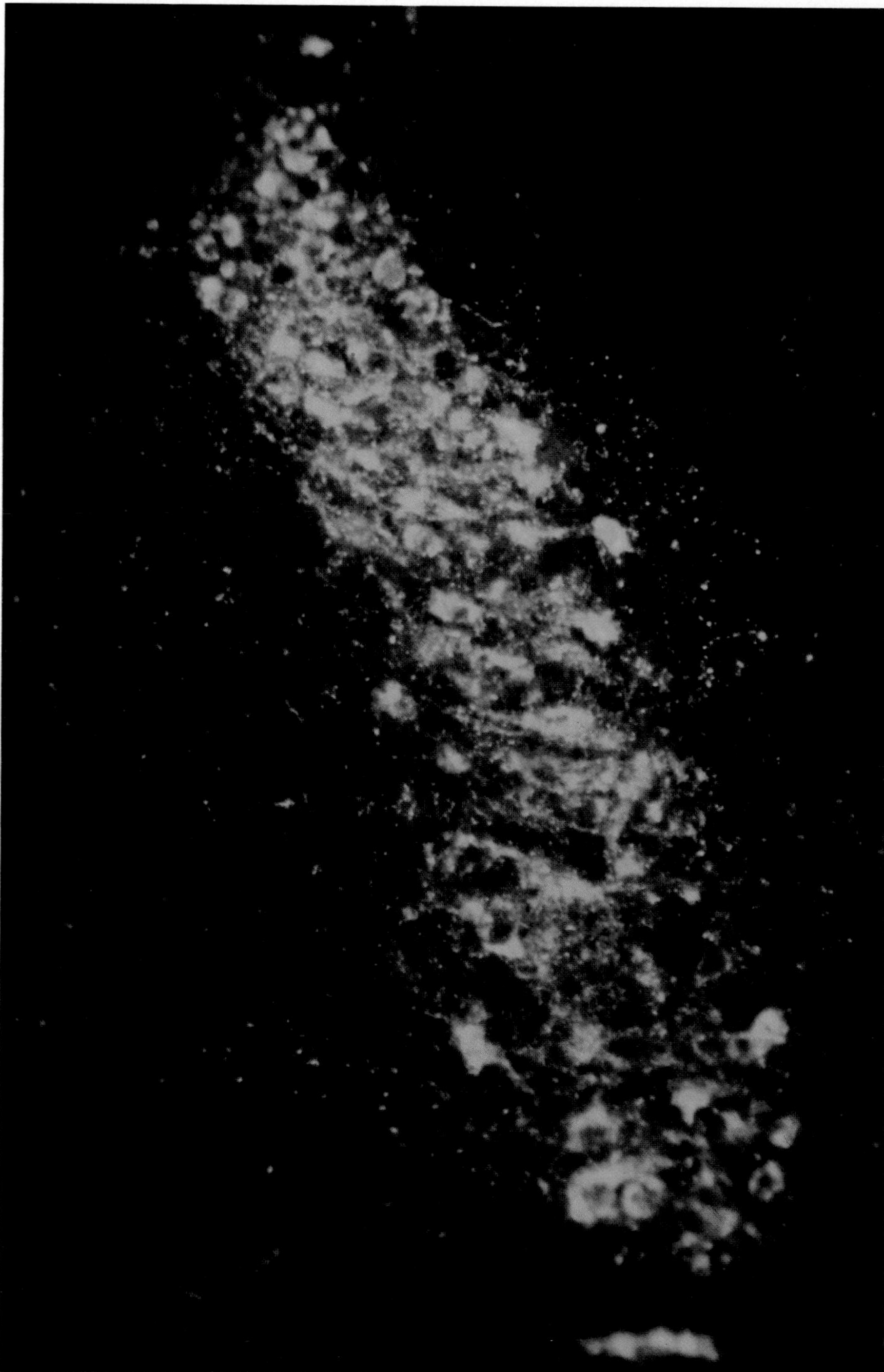

Figure 6-28. Photomicrograph of neurons containing norepinephrine in the locus ceruleus of the rat. The norepinephrine-containing cells were reacted with glyoxylic acid which converts norepinephrine into a fluorescent chemical derivative that can be viewed in the fluorescence microscope. (Courtesy of Drs. Jacqueline McGinty and Floyd Bloom, Salk Institute, La Jolla, Calif.) (From Carpenter and Sutin, *Human Neuroanatomy*, 1983; courtesy of Williams & Wilkins.)

hippocampal formation (Ungerstedt, '71; Maeda and Shimizu, '72). In the thalamus noradrenergic terminals are distributed to the intralaminar thalamic nuclei, the anterior nuclear group and the lateral geniculate body.

Noradrenergic fibers project to the cerebellar cortex via the superior cerebellar peduncle and terminate around Purkinje cell somata (Pickel et al., '74). Fluorescence histochemistry demonstrates the highest norepinephrine content in the trigeminal motor nucleus, the nucleus of the solitary tract, the dorsal motor nucleus of the vagus, and the dorsal raphe nucleus (Levitt and Moore, '79). Bilateral lesions of the locus ceruleus or subceruleus do not significantly alter the norepinephrine content of these nuclei, but such lesions decrease the norepinephrine content of the superior and inferior colliculi, the medial geniculate body, the interpeduncular nucleus, the pontine nuclei, and the principal sensory nucleus of the trigeminal nerve. These observations suggest that the locus ceruleus complex innervates mainly sensory and association nuclei, while norepinephrine-containing neurons scattered in the lateral tegmentum probably innervate primary motor and visceral nuclei. Both the locus ceruleus and the subceruleus project fibers to spinal levels via the anterior funiculus and ventral parts of the lateral funiculus (Kuypers and Maisky, '75; Nygren and Olson, '77).

The remarkable feature of the locus ceruleus projection is its wide distribution throughout the neuraxis. With the exception of the midbrain raphe-serotonin projection system, no other cell group of the reticular formation has been shown to have such an extensive projection. The projection of the locus ceruleus directly to the neocortex is unique in that it does not involve synaptic relays in the thalamus (Jones and Moore, '77). Retrograde HRP studies based upon transport of the enzyme from a large number of sites within the neuraxis suggest a regional topography within the locus ceruleus (Mason and Fibiger, '79). These data imply that the locus ceruleus is composed of several distinct subdivisions.

The locus ceruleus and its efferent projections have been considered to play a role in paradoxical sleep, facilitation and inhibition of sensory neurons, and control of cortical activation (Jouvet, '69; Chu and Bloom, '73; Sasa and Takaori, '73; Jones et al., '73; Lidbrink, '74; Nakai and Takaori, '74). In addition descending noradrenergic fibers from the locus ceruleus may supply preganglionic sympathetic neurons in the intermediolateral cell column at thoracic and upper lumbar levels (Nygren and Olson, '77).

Raphe Nuclei. Both the pons and medulla contain cell groups in the median raphe which properly belong to the reticular formation, but appear to serve distinctive functions (Taber et al., '60; Brodal et al., '60). Although the raphe nuclei of the human brain have not been studied extensively, these nuclei are similar to those found in animals. The raphe nuclei of the medulla are smaller and less conspicuous than those seen in the pons (Fig. 5-11). The *inferior central nucleus* appears in the median raphe at the junction of pons and medulla (Figs. 5-23 and 6-4) and represents the rostral part of the nucleus raphe magnus. The *nucleus raphe pontis* consists of several cell groups dorsal and rostral to the inferior central nucleus. The rostral extension of the pontine raphe nuclei is the *superior central nucleus*, also known as the *median nucleus of the raphe* (Fig. 6-26). Decussating fibers of the superior cerebellar peduncle pass through portions of the superior central nucleus (Fig. 6-25). The *dorsal nuclei of the raphe* are paired and lie on each side of the raphe within the anterior periaqueductal gray, dorsal to the medial longitudinal fasciculi (Fig. 6-26).

Histofluorescent technics demonstrate that the nuclei of the raphe region have a yellow fluorescence distinctive for serotonin (5-hydroxytryptamine, 5-HT) which can be demonstrated best with monoamine oxidase inhibitors (Dahlström and Fuxe, '64; Pin et al., '68). These cells present a sharp contrast with the norepinephrine containing neurons in the locus ceruleus which have a green fluorescence.

The principal ascending fibers arise from serotonin-containing cell bodies located in the dorsal nucleus of the raphe and in the superior central nucleus (Ungerstedt, '71; Bobillier et al., '75; Bobillier et al., '76).

The major ascending pathway from the rostral raphe nuclei passes through the ventral tegmental area (Tsai) and joins the medial forebrain bundle in the lateral hypothalamus (Fig. 10-9). Fibers leaving this main ascending bundle enter the substantia nigra, the intralaminar thalamic nuclei, the stria terminalis, the septum and the internal capsule. The most rostral projections terminate mainly in the frontal lobe, although some fibers are distributed throughout the neocortex. The dorsal nucleus of the raphe selectively innervates the substantia nigra, the lateral geniculate body, the neostriatum, the pyriform lobe, the olfactory bulb, and the amygdaloid nuclear complex. The superior central nucleus is particularly associated with serotonergic fibers projecting to the interpeduncular nucleus, the mammillary bodies, and the hippocampal formation. Ascending projections from the caudal raphe nuclei are less numerous and distributed to the superior colliculus, the pretectum, and the nuclei of the posterior commissure. Ascending serotonergic pathways from the superior central nucleus project mainly to mesolimbic structures, such as the hippocampus and the septal nuclei, while the dorsal nucleus of the raphe has a major projection to the meostriatum (neostriatum) (Geyer et al., '76).

Descending projections of the dorsal nucleus of the raphe are modest, but include the locus ceruleus. The superior central nucleus gives rise to descending projections to: (1) the cerebellum via the middle cerebellar peduncle, (2) the locus ceruleus, and (3) large regions of the pontine reticular formation. Autoradiographic studies of the nucleus raphe magnus suggest that descending fibers project primarily to structures concerned with nociceptive and/or visceral afferent input (Basbaum et al., '78). Structures receiving efferents from the nucleus raphe magnus include the dorsal motor nucleus of the vagus, the solitary nucleus, and the spinal trigeminal nucleus (pars caudalis). Spinal projections of this nucleus are bilateral and descend in the lateral funiculus. These fibers terminate in the marginal zone (lamina I), the substantia gelatinosa (lamina II), and in parts of laminae V, VI, and VII. Evidence suggests that this nucleus is linked to endogenous analgesic mechanisms (Basbaum, '76; Fields et al., '77; Willis et al., '77). Serotonin and the raphe nuclei have been implicated in the regulation of diverse physiological processes such as the regulation of sleep (Jouvet, '69), aggressive behavior (Sheard, '69), and a variety of neuroendocrine functions (Wurtman, '71; Conrad et al., '74).

Structurally, the serotonin molecule is similar to a portion of the larger D-lysergic acid diethylamide (LSD) molecule in that both contain an indole nucleus. LSD is a hallucinogenic drug considered to be the prototype of a psychotomimetic drug (i.e., a drug whose effects mimic psychosis (Gaddum and Hameed, '54; Wooley and Shaw, '54)). Microelectrode studies demonstrate that LSD produces a specific depression of activity in raphe neurons which contain serotonin (Aghajanian et al., '68; Haigler and Aghajanian, '74). These observations have led to the hypothesis that LSD acts to depress the activity of serotonin-containing neurons which, through disinhibition, cause a release of activity in neurons in the visual system, the limbic system, and in many other brain areas (Aghajanian et al., '75). Destruction of serotonin-containing neurons, inhibition of serotonin synthesis, or blockade of its receptors consistently produces an animal that is hypersensitive to virtually all environmental stimuli and hyperactive in virtually all situations. By a general inhibitory action in the central nervous system, serotonin may serve to modulate and maintain behavior within specific limits. Studies indicate that, as the overall level of motor activity or arousal increases, so does the activity of serotonin-containing cells. As an animal becomes quiescent and drowsy, the activity of these cells diminish. Neurons of the raphe fire slowly as an animal enters sleep and, during rapid eye movement (REM) sleep, the cells stop firing. These findings suggest that, under the influence of hallucinogenic drugs, the individual is fully awake but the brain-serotonin system is depressed and behaves as it does during sleep (Jacobs and Trulson, '79).

Both serotonin- and norepinephrine-containing neurons in the reticular formation have been considered to play active roles in the mechanisms that control sleep states (Jouvet, '69). Inhibition of serotonin synthesis, or total destruction of serotonin-containing neurons, in the raphe system leads to total insomnia. Serotonin appears to be involved in the neural mechanism related to so-called *slow sleep*, a state characterized by an electroencephalogram (EEG) with slow waves and spindles. In addition serotonin appears to have effects upon cells of the locus ceruleus which trigger what is called *paradoxical sleep* (Jouvet, '69; Chu and Bloom, '73). Paradoxical sleep is characterized by: (1) abolition of antigravity muscle tone; (2) reductions in blood pressure, bradycardia and irregular respirations; (3) bursts of REM; and (4) an EEG which resembles the waking state. Bilateral lesions of the locus ceruleus cause a selective suppression of paradoxical sleep for about 2 weeks, after which it returns to nearly the normal range (Jones et al., '77).

CHAPTER 7

The Mesencephalon

The midbrain, like other parts of the brain stem, can be divided into three parts: (1) the *tectum*, or quadrigeminal plate, (2) the *tegmentum*, representing the rostral continuation of the pontine tegmentum, and (3) the massive *crura cerebri* (Fig. 7-1).

Only two cranial nerves, the trochlear and oculomotor, arise in the midbrain, but relay nuclei in this part of the brain stem are of importance in the auditory and visual systems. The largest single nuclear mass in the midbrain, the *substantia nigra*, separates the tegmentum from the crus cerebri. The crus cerebri contains the massive bundles of corticofugal fibers in their passage to the lower brain stem and spinal cord. The nuclear masses and pathways in the midbrain are best presented at two typical levels, that of the inferior and superior colliculi.

INFERIOR COLLICULAR LEVEL

The transition from isthmus to midbrain is associated with changes mainly in the tectum and tegmentum (Figs. 6-25 and 7-2). Comparison of these levels reveals that: (1) the fourth ventricle has become the cerebral aqueduct, (2) the superior medullary velum is replaced by two rounded eminences, the inferior colliculi, and (3) fibers of the superior cerebellar peduncles have begun to decussate. The ventral part of the pons is reduced in size and, at slightly more rostral levels, undergoes a reorganization as the massive crura cerebri appear (Figs. 7-2 and 7-3).

Fibers of the lateral lemniscus, located near the lateral surface of the tegmentum, migrate dorsally and enter the inferior colliculus.

Inferior Colliculi. The distinctive paired ovoid cellular masses of the caudal tectum can be divided into three parts: (1) an ovoid cell mass called the central nucleus; (2) a thin dorsal cellular layer, the pericentral nucleus, referred to as the cortex; and (3) an external nucleus which surrounds the central nucleus laterally and ventrally (Geniec and Morest, '71; Rockel and Jones, '73; '73a).

The *central nucleus* of the inferior collic-

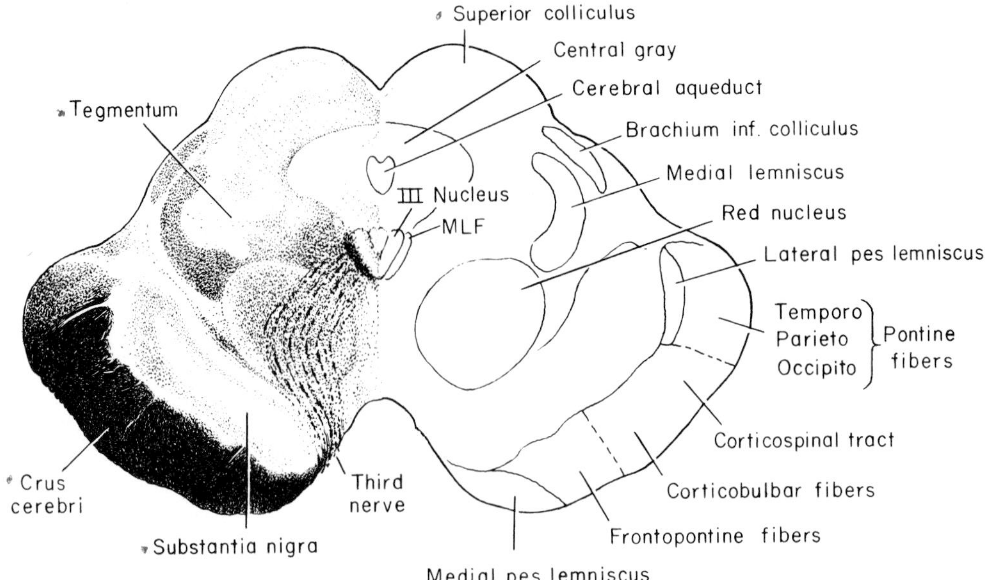

Figure 7-1. Schematic transverse section through the rostral midbrain. (From Carpenter and Sutin, *Human Neuroanatomy*, 1983; courtesy of Williams & Wilkins.)

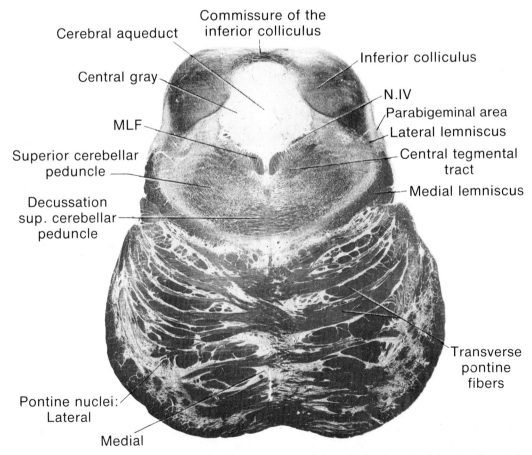

Figure 7-2. Transverse section of the adult midbrain through the inferior colliculus. Large fascicles of corticospinal and corticopontine fibers (unlabeled), cut in cross section, are located among the bundles of transverse pontine fibers. (Weigert's myelin stain; photograph.) (From Carpenter and Sutin, *Human Neuroanatomy*, 1983; courtesy of Williams & Wilkins.)

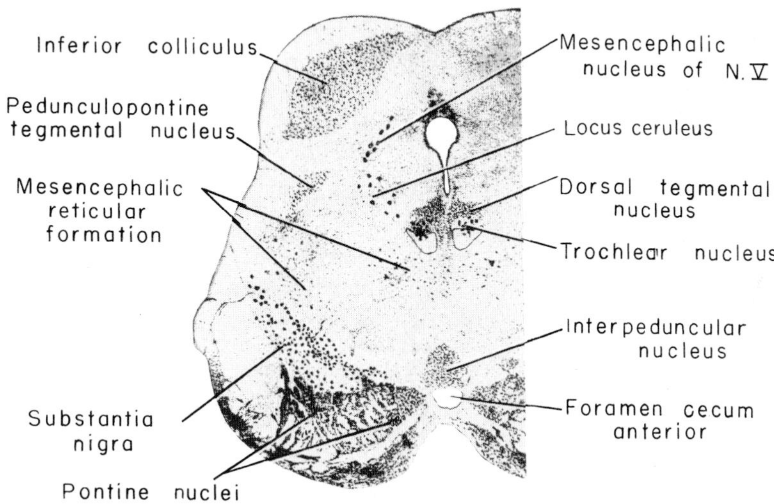

Figure 7-3. Section through inferior colliculi of midbrain. Three-month infant. (Cresyl violet; photograph, with schematic representation of main cell groups.) (From Carpenter and Sutin, *Human Neuroanatomy*, 1983; courtesy of Williams & Wilkins.)

ulus can be divided into a smaller dorsomedial division composed of large cells and a larger ventrolateral division composed of medium and small cells with a pronounced laminar arrangement (Fig. 7-4). Laminae in the ventrolateral division form an overlapping onion-like series of concentric shells, most of which are incomplete. The thickness of the laminae is determined by the dendritic ramifications of fusiform and bitufted cells which compose the layers. These laminae provide the basis for the tonotopic organization of neurons in the central nucleus. Each of these cellular laminae correspond to isofrequency contours (Merzenich and Reid, '74; Roth et al., '78).

The *pericentral nucleus* is a thin sheet of densely packed cells extending over the dorsal and posterior surfaces of the inferior colliculus which overlies both major divisions of the central nucleus (Fig. 7-4). The nucleus is composed of spiny and aspiny neurons. Small spiny neurons are found at all depths, while large spiny neurons overlie the large-celled division of the central nucleus and project axons into it. Large aspiny neurons project axons in the brachium of the inferior colliculus. The *external nucleus*, composed of cells of various sizes, appears continuous with the pericentral nucleus, but is traversed by fibers entering and leaving the inferior colliculus.

The inferior colliculus serves as a auditory relay nucleus transmitting signals received from the lateral lemniscus to the medial geniculate body, which in turn projects upon the auditory cortex. Both the dorsomedial and ventrolateral divisions of the central nucleus receive ascending fibers from the lateral lemniscus. Fibers entering the ventrolateral division of the inferior colliculus course along the length of each lamina following its curvature. As fibers traverse these laminae they establish synaptic contacts with collicular neurons (Rockel and Jones, '73). The dorsomedial division of the central nucleus receives commissural connections from the corresponding region of the opposite inferior colliculus (Fig. 7-2) and bilateral projections from the auditory cortex. The pericentral nucleus receives bilateral inputs from the auditory cortex and ascending projections from the dorsal nucleus of the lateral lemniscus (Rockel and Jones, '73a). Cells of the pericentral nucleus project fibers into the central nucleus which course parallel to its laminae.

Most cells of the inferior colliculus respond to binaural stimulation and many cells encode sound localization with spatiotemporal discharge patterns. Studies in the cat indicate a definite tonotopic localization within the central and pericentral nuclei of the inferior colliculus (Rose et al., '63; Merzenich and Reid, '74; Aitkin et al.,

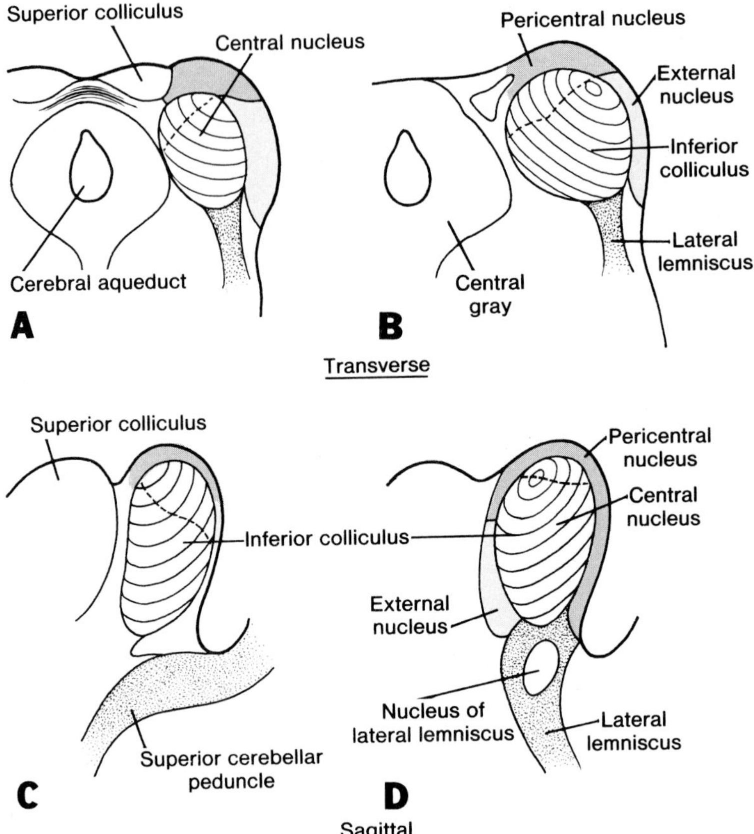

Figure 7-4. Drawing of transverse (*A*, *B*) and sagittal (*C*, *D*) sections through the inferior colliculus outlining the nuclear subdivisions. The pericentral nucleus is indicated in *red* and the external nucleus is *blue*. The central nucleus in *white* shows contours of the laminae in the ventrolateral division. *Black dots* indicate the division of the central nucleus into the large-celled dorsomedial part and the ventrolateral laminated part. Laminae in the central nucleus represent a given frequency band across the width of the nucleus and form the basis for the tonotopic organization of neurons. The disc-shaped laminae in dorsal regions are not as thick and represent the lower frequencies; high frequency octaves are represented ventrally (Rockel and Jones, '73, '73a; Merzenich and Reid, '74; Aitkin et al., '75). (From Carpenter and Sutin, *Human Neuroanatomy*, 1983; courtesy of Williams & Wilkins.)

'75). Neurons in the central nucleus of the inferior colliculus are arranged in a laminar pattern that represents a given frequency band of nearly constant thickness across the width of the nucleus. Isofrequency contours parallel the cellular laminae described in anatomical studies (Rockel and Jones, '73; Merzenich and Reid, '74) and are tilted down rostrally. Advancement of an electrode from dorsal to ventral in the inferior colliculus consistently gives a sequence of frequencies from low to high in the central nucleus. The disc-shaped laminae representing the lowest frequencies (i.e., dorsal regions) are not as thick or as extensive as those representing middle and high frequencies (i.e., ventral region). The frequency representation in the central nucleus reflects the proportional representation of frequencies along the cochlear partition, in which low frequencies are perceived at the apex of the cochlea and high frequencies at the base. The central nucleus of the inferior colliculus is a tightly organized structure bearing specific relationships to the cochlea with elements sharply tuned to different sound frequencies. These data suggest that small sections of the basilar membrane of approximately equal lengths are represented across individual anatomically defined cellular laminae within the nucleus (Merzenich and Reid, '74). This tonotopic organization applies only to the ventrolateral division of the central nucleus.

The pericentral nucleus demonstrates some evidence of a tonotopic organization in which high frequencies are located externally and low frequencies are found near the margins of the central nucleus (Aitkin et al., '75). This nucleus contains units with broad tuning characteristics. The majority of these units receive only a contralateral monaural input, and many units show habituation to repeated identical stimuli. The overall behavior of units in the pericentral nucleus and their monaural input suggests that cells in this nucleus may serve to direct auditory attention (Jane et al., '65). The external nucleus probably is not an auditory relay nucleus like the central nucleus of the inferior colliculus; this nucleus is related primarily to acousticomotor reflexes (Aitkin et al., '75).

Efferent fibers from the ventrolateral division of the central nucleus of the inferior colliculus project via the brachium of the inferior colliculus to the ventral laminated part of the medial geniculate body (Figs. 7-15 and 9-16) (Moore and Goldberg, '63; Powell and Hatton, '69; Rockel and Jones, '73; Kudo and Niimi, '78). Cells in the dorsal division of the central nucleus and in the pericentral nucleus send fibers to the dorsal part of the medial geniculate body. Thus, the dorsal division of the central nucleus and the pericentral nucleus of the inferior colliculus which receive fibers from the auditory cortex, ultimately send impulses back to the periauditory cortex (Kudo and Niimi, '78). Cells of the ventral part of the medial geniculate body project tonotopically upon the primary auditory cortex (Burton and Jones, '76).

Parabigeminal Area. Ventrolateral to the inferior colliculus and lateral to the lateral lemniscus is a cellular region known as the parabigeminal area (Fig. 7-2). This small oval-shaped nucleus in the lateral midbrain receives a substantial projection from the superficial layers of the superior colliculus and has a visuotopic organization (Graybiel, '72; Graham, '77; Sherk, '78). Cells of each parabigeminal nucleus project bilaterally upon superficial layers of the superior colliculi and show a regional organization; rostral parts of the nucleus project contralaterally and cells in caudal parts of the nucleus project to the ipsilateral superior colliculus (Graybiel, '78; Edwards et al., '79). Cells of the parabigeminal nucleus respond briskly and consistently to visual stimuli, can be activated by both moving and stationary light spots and have receptive fields similar in size to those of the superficial layers of the superior colliculus (Sherk, '78). The parabigeminal nucleus has a representation of the entire contralateral visual field and at least the central part of the ipsilateral field. Findings suggest that the parabigeminal nucleus functions with the superior colliculus in processing visual information.

Trochlear Nerve. The nucleus of the trochlear nerve appears as a small compact cell group at the ventral border of the central gray at levels through the inferior colliculus (Figs. 7-3 and 7-5). The nucleus (GSE) is a small caudal appendage to the oculomotor complex that indents the dorsal margin of the medial longitudinal fasciculus (MLF). Root fibers from the nucleus curve dorsolaterally and caudally near the margin of the central gray, decussate completely in the superior medullary velum (Fig. 6-25) and emerge from the dorsal surface of the brain stem caudal to the inferior colliculi (Figs. 2-20 and 2-21). The nerve root curves around the lateral surface of the midbrain, passes between the superior cerebellar and posterior cerebral arteries (Figs. 14-3 and 14-7), as do fibers of the oculomotor nerve, and enters the cavernous sinus. This nerve innervates the superior oblique muscle that serves to: (1) intort the eye when abducted, and (2) depress the eye when adducted. Although isolated lesions of the trochlear nerve are unusual, and detection of resulting disturbances by inspection is difficult, vertical diplopia results. Vertical diplopia is maximal on attempted downward gaze to the opposite side. Patients with trochlear nerve lesions complain of difficulty in walking downstairs.

Tegmental Nuclei. The periaqueductal gray surrounding the cerebral aqueduct contains several nuclear groups. The mesencephalic nucleus of the trigeminal nerve and the pigmented cells of the locus ceruleus occupy lateral regions at isthmus levels (Figs. 6-26 and 7-3). The raphe region con-

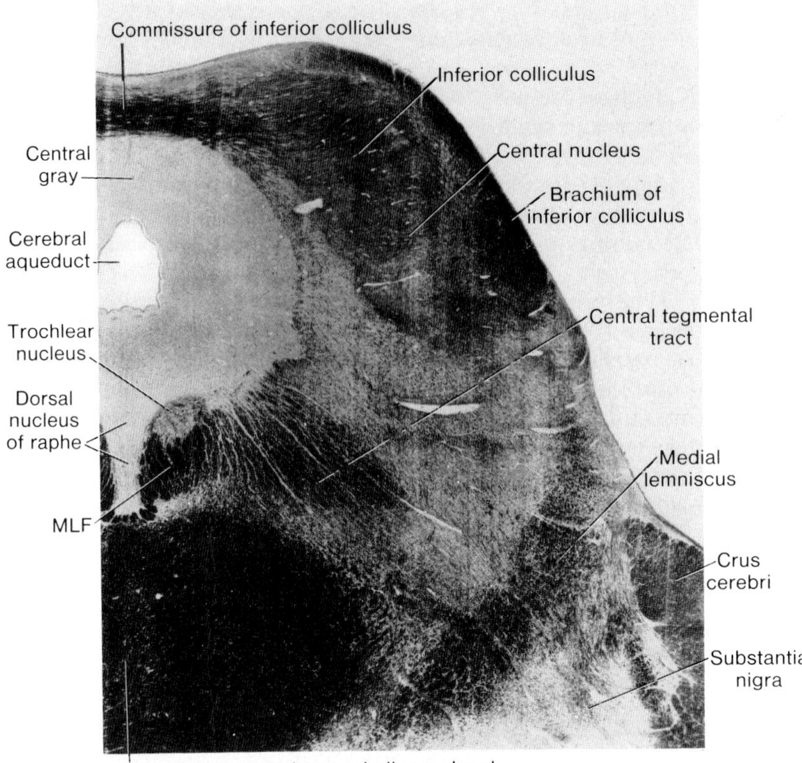

Figure 7-5. Photograph of the right dorsal quadrant of a section through the rostral part of the inferior colliculus. (Weigert's myelin stain.) (From Carpenter and Sutin, *Human Neuroanatomy*, 1983; courtesy of Williams & Wilkins.)

tains the *dorsal nucleus of the raphe* and is flanked laterally by the *dorsal tegmental nucleus* (Figs. 5-11 and 7-3). This dorsal nucleus of the raphe, composed mainly of small cells in the central gray dorsomedial to, and between, the trochlear nuclei, has been called the supratrochlear nucleus. Although the dorsal nucleus of the raphe and the dorsal tegmental nucleus are adjacent to each other, only cells in the dorsal nucleus of the raphe synthesize and transport serotonin. Ventral to the medial longitudinal fasciculus and lateral to the raphe are the cells of the *ventral tegmental nucleus*. These cells appear as a rostral continuation of the *superior central nucleus* (Fig. 6-26).

The dorsal nucleus of the raphe and the median nucleus of the raphe (i.e., the superior central nucleus) give rise to ascending serotonergic pathways which have both overlapping and distinctive features. Ascending projections from the dorsal nucleus of the raphe projecting to the substantia nigra and the putamen have been referred to as the mesostriatal system (Geyer et al., '76), while projections from the median raphe nucleus form the mesolimbic system. The median raphe nucleus projects to the midbrain reticular formation, the hypothalamus, the septal area, the entorhinal cortex, and the hippocampal formation. The median raphe nucleus also gives rise to descending fibers projecting to the cerebellum, the locus ceruleus, the reticular formation of the lower brain stem, and the raphe nuclei of the pons and the medulla (Bobillier et al., '76). Serotonin conveyed by these systems is believed to act as an inhibitory neurotransmitter (Haigler and Aghajanian, '74; Olpe and Koella, '77).

The *interpeduncular nucleus* lies dorsal to the interpeduncular fossa (Fig. 7-3). This nucleus receives fibers from the habenular nucleus via the fasciculus retroflexus (Figs. 9-4 and 10-8); some fibers of this bundle bypassing the interpeduncular nucleus are distributed to the superior central nucleus, the dorsal tegmental nucleus, and caudal

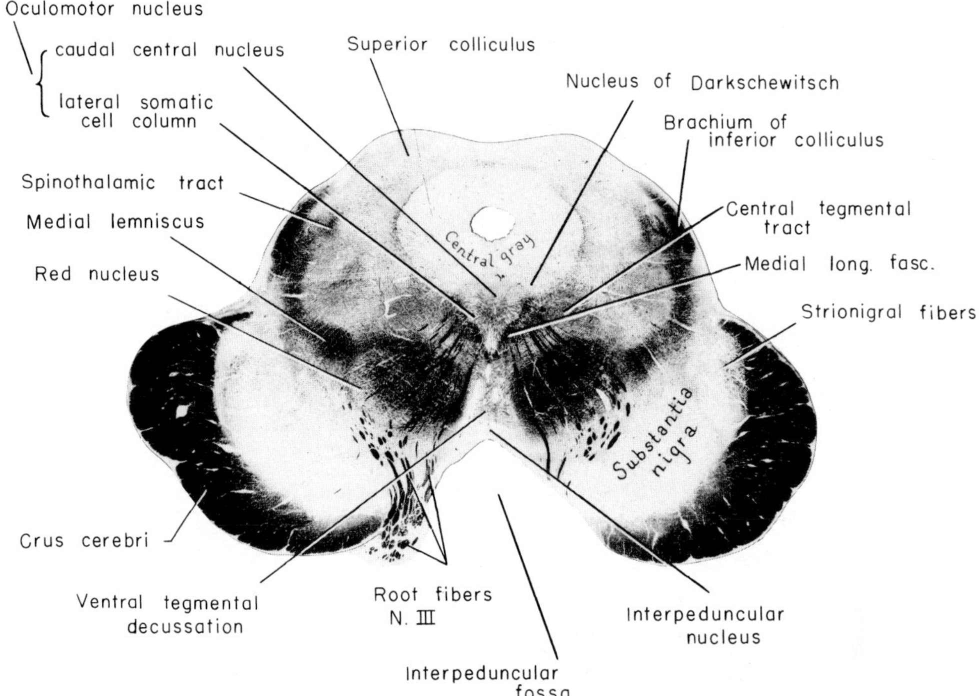

Figure 7-6. Transverse section of adult midbrain through the level of the oculomotor nerve. (Weigert's myelin stain; photograph.) (From Carpenter and Sutin, *Human Neuroanatomy*, 1983; courtesy of Williams & Wilkins.)

regions of the central gray (Nauta, '58). The dorsal tegmental nucleus also receives fibers from the interpeduncular nucleus and from the mammillary bodies via the mammillotegmental tract. The dorsal tegmental nucleus is closely related to the dorsal longitudinal fasciculus (of Schütz), a small pathway in ventromedial periaqueductal gray. These pathways constitute part of a complex system by which impulses related to the limbic system are projected to nuclei at midbrain levels. These pathways are concerned with visceral and behavioral functions.

SUPERIOR COLLICULAR LEVEL

Transverse sections of the rostral midbrain appear strikingly different from those through the inferior colliculus in that: (1) the flattened superior colliculi form the tectum; (2) the oculomotor nuclei form a V-shaped complex ventral to the central gray and root fibers of the nerve emerge from the interpeduncular fossa; (3) the red nuclei, surrounded by fibers of the superior cerebellar peduncle, occupy the central tegmental region; and (4) the substantia nigrae achieve their maximum size ventral to the tegmentum and dorsal to the crura cerebri (Fig. 7-6). Fibers of the brachium of the inferior colliculus lie on the lateral surface of the tegmentum. The medial lemniscus appears as a curved bundle dorsal to the substantia nigra and lateral to the red nucleus. The spinothalamic and spinotectal tracts lie together medial to the most dorsal part of the medial lemniscus.

Superior Colliculi. The superior colliculi are flattened, laminated eminences which form the rostral half of the tectum. In organization these structures resemble the cerebral cortex. Each colliculus has a laminated structure consisting of alternate gray and white layers. From the surface inward these layers are: (1) the *stratum zonale* (mainly fibrous), (2) the *stratum cinereum* (outer gray layer), (3) the *stratum opticum* (superficial white layer), and (4) the *stratum lemnisci* consisting of middle and deep gray and white layers (Fig. 7-7). The superior colliculus receives fibers from: (1) the retina via the optic tract, (2) the

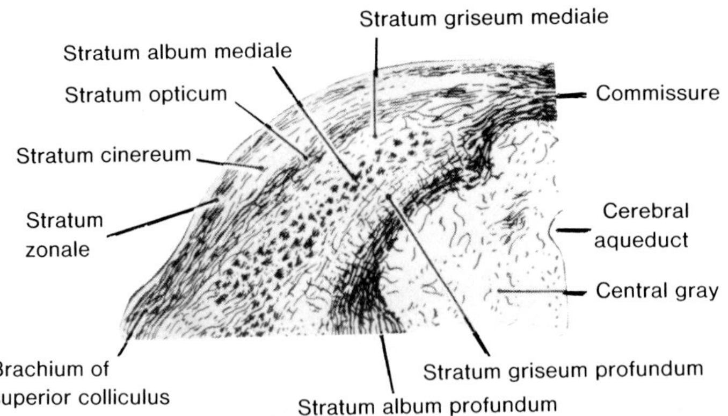

Figure 7-7. Drawing of the myelinated fiber structure of the superior colliculus based upon Weigert-stained sections. (From Carpenter and Sutin, *Human Neuroanatomy*, 1983; courtesy of Williams & Wilkins.)

cerebral cortex, (3) the inferior colliculus, and (4) the spinal cord. The superficial layers of the superior colliculus which receive most of their input from the retina and visual cortex are concerned with the detection of movement of objects in the visual field. The deep layers of the superior colliculus, which receive inputs from multiple sources (i.e., somesthetic and auditory systems, catecholamine-containing neurons, and various regions of the reticular formation), have many anatomical and physiological characteristics of the brain stem reticular formation (Edwards et al., '79). Efferent fibers arising from the superficial layers of the superior colliculus projecting to regions of the pulvinar form important links in the extrageniculate visual pathway which parallels the geniculostriate system (Altman and Carpenter, '61; Graybiel, '72; Harting et al., '73).

Retinotectal fibers leave the optic tract rostral to its principal termination in the lateral geniculate body and project to the superior colliculus via its brachium. Fibers come from homonymous portions of the retina of each eye, but crossed fibers are most numerous. Thus, the contralateral homonymous halves of the visual field are represented in each superior colliculus (Fig. 7-8). Optic tract fibers project to all parts of the superior colliculus, including the oral third where the fovea is represented (Cynader and Berman, '72; Hubel et al., '75). The upper quadrants of the contralateral visual field are represented in medial parts of the superior colliculus; the lower quadrants are related to lateral regions of this structure. The contralateral peripheral visual field is represented in the caudal two-thirds of the superior colliculus while central regions of the visual field are represented in the oral third. The region of the retina corresponding to the optic disc (the blind spot) has been identified near the center of the superior colliculus (Hubel et al., '75). In the superior colliculus representation of the contralateral eye is dominant, a finding that contrasts with the equal representation of the two eyes in the lateral geniculate body and the striate cortex.

Corticotectal fibers arise from portions of the frontal, temporal, parietal and occipital lobes. The most substantial and highly organized projection arises from the visual cortex and reaches the superior colliculus via the brachium of the superior colliculus (Fig. 7-8). These fibers enter the stratum opticum and pass into the superficial and middle gray layers. Fibers from the retina enter via the same route and appear to terminate in the same layers. Although retinal and visual cortical projections to the superior colliculus are similar, there are certain important differences: (1) retinal projections are bilateral and greatest contralaterally, while (2) striate cortical projections are unilateral. Anatomical data suggest that portions of the visual cortex and superior colliculus related to particular regions of the retina are interconnected (Garey et al., '68). Thus, essentially the same cells of the superior colliculus receive distinct, but related inputs, from the gan-

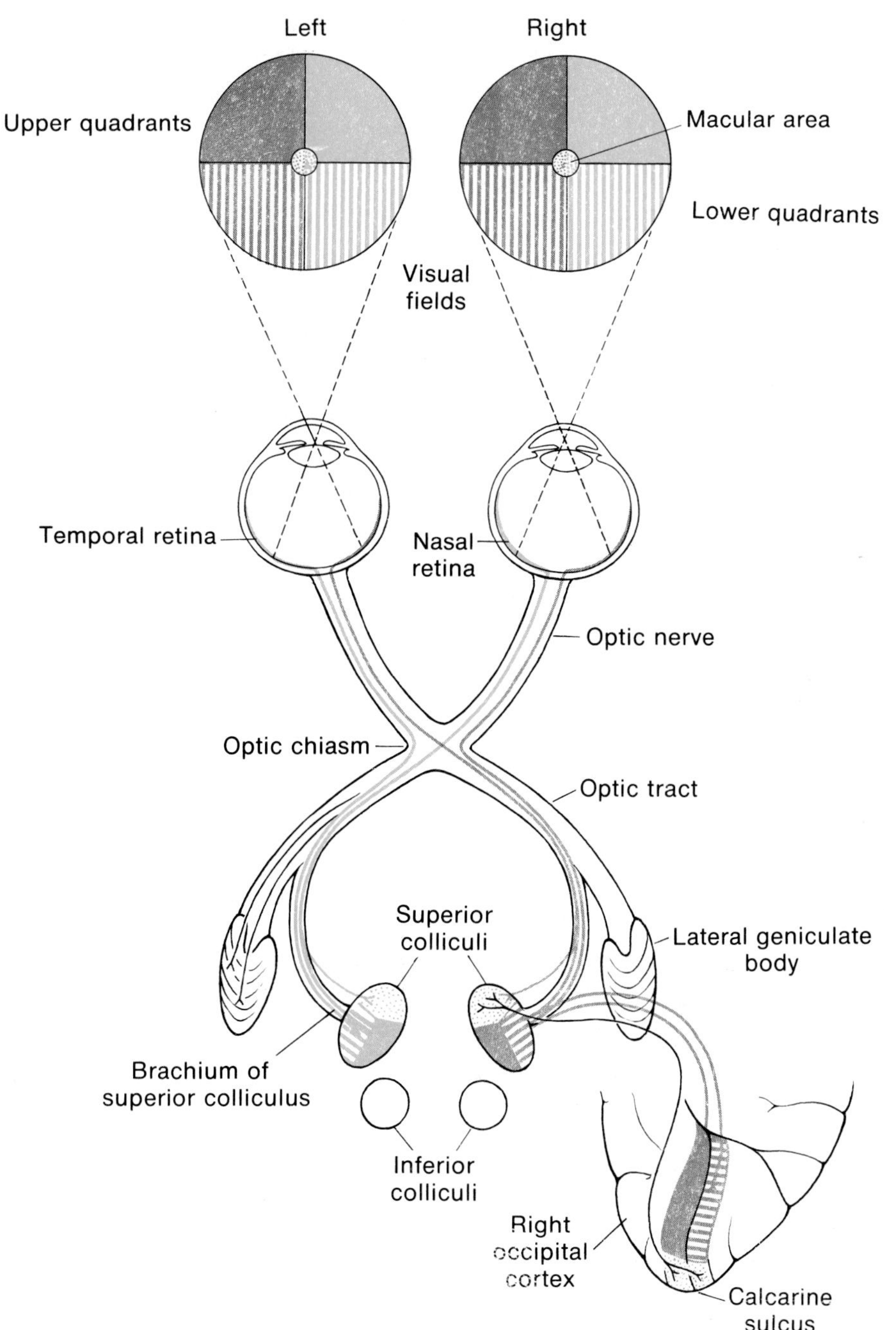

Figure 7-8. Diagrammatic representation of the projections of the retinae and striate cortex upon the superior colliculi in the monkey. Retinotectal fibers from the ipsilateral temporal and contralateral nasal halves of the retinae, which subserve the contralateral homonymous visual field, project to the superior colliculus. Cells in portions of the retinae concerned with the contralateral peripheral visual field project to the posterior two-thirds of the superior colliculus. Upper quadrants of the contralateral peripheral visual field (*solid blue* and *red*) are represented in medial region of caudal parts of the superior colliculus, while lower quadrants of the contralateral peripheral visual field (*blue* and *red stripes*) are represented in lateral regions. Portions of the retinae concerned with central vision (i.e., within 10° of the fovae centralis; *blue* and *red dots*) are represented in the rostral third of the superior colliculus. Although retinotectal fibers arise from all portions of the retina of each eye, crossed fibers are most numerous. Corticotectal fibers from the striate cortex, shown on the right, project to all superficial parts of the superior colliculus via its brachium. There is a correspondence in the superior colliculus of retinotectal and corticotectal terminations that represent both central and peripheral parts of the visual field. (From Carpenter and Sutin, *Human Neuroanatomy*, 1983; courtesy of Williams & Wilkins.)

glion cells of the retina and cells of the striate cortex. At this brain stem level there is the possibility of a potent interaction and integration of peripheral visual impulses with the more complex output of the visual cortex.

Corticotectal fibers from the frontal lobe (Brodmann's area 8) terminate in the middle gray layer, the stratum opticum and the stratum zonale (Künzle et al., '76). These fibers reach the superior colliculus via a transtegmental approach, and are thought to participate in motor mechanisms related to conjugate eye movements. Cells in the superficial layers respond to visual stimuli while cells in the middle gray layer discharge prior to saccadic eye movements. The auditory cortex projects to deeper layers of the superior colliculus that receive no visual input (Diamond et al., '69).

Brain stem afferents to the superior colliculus arise from the inferior colliculus and a number of auditory relay nuclei (Edwards et al., '79). Most of these fibers project to deep layers of caudal parts of the superior colliculus. Commissural connections (Figs. 7-7 and 7-12) primarily relate deep and intermediate gray layers in the rostral halves of the superior colliculi. These reciprocal connections may be related to motor functions, since all brain stem and spinal afferents arise from deep layers. Such fibers also may mediate mutually suppressive effects and contribute to visual tracking.

Spinotectal fibers projecting to the deep layers of the superior colliculus are not numerous. Although some somatosensory input to the superior colliculus arises from cells in lamina IV, the major inputs are from the nucleus cuneatus, the lateral cervical nucleus, and all parts of the spinal trigeminal nucleus (Edwards et al., '79). These inputs are topographically organized with the head represented rostrally.

As the preceding discussion indicates, the superior colliculus can be partitioned into two zones: (1) the superficial layers which receive primarily visual afferents, and (2) deep layers which receive heterogeneous multimodal inputs. Although the superficial layers of the superior colliculus, the stratum zonale, the stratum cinereum, and the stratum opticum, have projections distinct from that of all deeper layers, they also project to the deep layers (Harting, '77). In general the superficial layers give rise to ascending fibers and the deep layers project descending fibers to nuclei in the brain stem and spinal cord.

Tectothalamic fibers arising from superficial layers of the superior colliculus project ipsilaterally to the pulvinar, the dorsal and ventral lateral geniculate nuclei and the pretectum (Altman and Carpenter, '61; Casagrande et al., '72; Harting et al., '73; Benevento and Fallon, '75). The pulvinar receives the most extensive projection from the superficial layers of the colliculus and in turn projects upon extrastriate cortical areas (areas 18 and 19) (Benevento and Rezak, '76; Glendenning et al., '75). Thus the superficial layers of the superior colliculus give rise to tectothalamic fibers, part of which convey visual information to the extrastriate cortex via the pulvinar. Cells in the most superficial layers of the superior colliculus also project upon the dorsal lateral geniculate body (Harting et al., '78). These tectogeniculate fibers terminate in intralaminar geniculate regions adjacent to the magnocellular layers. Thus, visual pathways to the cortex via the superior colliculus and the lateral geniculate body are not entirely separate.

Descending tectofugal fibers arise from laminae of the superior colliculus ventral to the stratum opticum and can be grouped into uncrossed tectopontine and tectobulbar tracts, and crossed tectobulbar and tectospinal projections.

Uncrossed tectopontine and *tectobulbar fibers* project to the ipsilateral dorsolateral pontine nuclei, the lateral part of the reticulotegmental nucleus, and to the nucleus reticularis pontis oralis (Altman and Carpenter, '61; Harting et al., '73; Harting, '77). Superficial layers of superior colliculus give rise to a substantial ipsilateral projection to the parabigeminal nucleus, a structure that has bilateral regionally organized projections back to the superior colliculus (Harting, '77; Graybiel, '78). The dorsolateral region of the pontine nuclei which receives fibers from the superior colliculus also receives inputs from the visual and auditory cortex (Garey et al., '68; Brodal, '72); this collection of pontine nuclei projects to lobules VI and VII of the cerebellar vermis (Brodal and Jansen, '46).

Tectoreticular fibers project profusely

and bilaterally to dorsal regions of the midbrain reticular formation. Some of these fibers enter the accessory oculomotor nuclei (i.e., the nucleus of Darkschewitsch and the interstitial nucleus of Cajal), but none to enter the oculomotor complex.

Tectospinal and *tectobulbar fibers* cross in the dorsal tegmental decussation at midbrain levels and descend near the median raphe; at medullary levels these fibers become incorporated within the medial longitudinal fasciculus. Tectospinal fibers continuing to cervical spinal segments descend in the medial part of the anterior funiculus (Figs. 4-11 and 4-16).

Functional Considerations. Each superior colliculus receives a visual input largely from the contralateral visual field. In addition it receives an ipsilateral projection from the visual cortex supplying information concerning only the contralateral visual field. These two systems are precisely and topographically organized at all levels. Unilateral lesions of the superior colliculus in a variety of animals produce: (1) relative neglect of visual stimuli in the contralateral visual field, (2) deficits in perception involving spatial discriminations and tracking of moving objects, (3) heightened responses to stimuli in the ipsilateral visual field, and (4) no impairment of eye movements (Sprague and Meikle, '65; Sprague, '72). These disturbances suggest that the superior colliculus contributes to head and eye movements used to localize and follow visual stimuli. Physiological studies indicate that collicular receptive fields are two to four times larger than receptive fields in the visual cortex. The receptive field in the visual system is defined as that region of the retina (or visual field) over which one can influence the firing of a particular ganglion cell (Kuffler, '53). The receptive field consists of a central circular region (excitatory) and a concentric surround (inhibitory), or the reverse. Most collicular cells respond only to moving stimuli and three-fourths of these cells show a directional selectivity (Sterling and Wickelgren, '69). These cells respond well to movement in one direction, poorly, or not at all, to movement in the opposite direction and are nonresponsive to stationary stimuli flashed on and off within the receptive field. In the superior colliculus the preferred directional selectivity is parallel to the horizontal meridian of the visual field and toward the periphery of the visual field. Thus, most units in the left superior colliculus have receptive fields in the right visual field and respond best to stimuli moving from left to right.

Stimulation of the superior colliculus results in contralateral conjugate deviations of the eyes, even though this structure has no projections to the nuclei of the extraocular muscles. These responses may be mediated by collicular projections to: (1) the interstitial nucleus of Cajal which projects to specific subdivisions of the contralateral oculomotor complex (Carpenter et al., '70), or (2) the pontine paramedian reticular formation (PPRF) which projects to the ipsilateral abducens nucleus. Electrical stimulation of the superior colliculus in alert monkeys also elicits short-latency saccadic eye movements. The amplitude and direction of these saccades are a function of the site stimulated within the superior colliculus. The superior colliculus is involved in coding the location of an object in the visual field relative to the fovea and in eliciting saccadic eye movements that produce foveal acquisition of the object (Sparks et al., '76).

OCULOMOTOR NERVE

Oculomotor Nuclear Complex. This complex is a collection of cell columns and discrete nuclei which: (1) innervate the inferior oblique and the superior, medial and inferior recti muscles, (2) supply the levator palpebrae muscle, and (3) provide preganglionic parasympathetic fibers to the ciliary ganglion (Fig. 7-6). Functional components of the nerve are categorized as *general somatic efferent* (GSE) and *general visceral efferent* (GVE). This complex lies ventral to the periaqueductal gray in the midline in a "V"-shaped trough formed by the diverging fibers of the MLF; it extends from the rostral pole of the trochlear nucleus to the upper limit of the midbrain (Figs. 7-1, 7-6 and 7-9). The complex consists of paired lateral somatic cell columns, midline and dorsal visceral nuclei, and a somatic midline dorsal cell group called the caudal central nucleus (Figs. 7-9 and 7-10).

The *lateral somatic cell columns*, com-

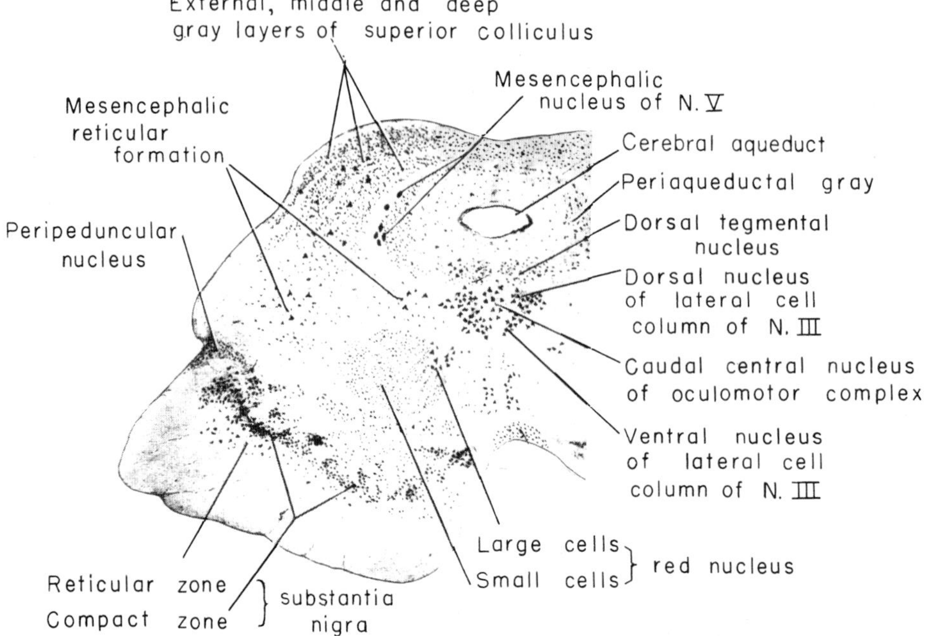

Figure 7-9. Section of the midbrain through the superior colliculi. Three-month infant. (Cresyl violet; photograph in which the main cell groups have been schematically blocked in.) (From Carpenter and Sutin, *Human Neuroanatomy*, 1983; courtesy of Williams & Wilkins.)

posed of large motor type neurons, innervate the extraocular muscles. The dorsal cell column (or nucleus) innervates the inferior rectus muscle, the intermediate cell column innervates the inferior oblique muscle, and the ventral cell column supplies fibers to the medial rectus muscle. Detailed studies of the medial rectus subdivision of the oculomotor complex in the monkey indicate that, although major representation is in the ventral cell column, discrete collections of cells in dorsal regions also innervate this muscle (Fig. 6-19) (Büttner-Ennever and Akert, '81). Root fibers arising from these cell columns are uncrossed. A cell column medial to both the dorsal and intermediate cell columns, referred to as the medial cell column, provides crossed fibers that innervate the superior rectus muscle (Fig. 7-10).

The *caudal central nucleus* is a midline somatic cell group found only in the caudal third of the complex. This nucleus gives rise to crossed and uncrossed fibers that innervate the levator palpebrae muscle (Figs. 7-9 and 7-10).

Visceral nuclei of the oculomotor nuclear complex consist of two distinct nuclear groups which are in continuity rostrally. The *Edinger-Westphal* nucleus consists of two slender columns of small cells dorsal to the rostral three-fifths of the somatic cell columns. In transverse sections through the middle third of the complex each of these paired columns divides into two smaller cell columns which taper and gradually disappear. Rostrally the cell columns of the Edinger-Westphal nucleus merge in the midline dorsally and become continuous with the visceral cells of the anterior median nucleus (Fig. 7-10). Cells of the anterior median nucleus lie in the raphe between rostral portions of the lateral somatic cell columns (principally the dorsal cell columns). Both the Edinger-Westphal and anterior median nuclei give rise to uncrossed preganglionic parasympathetic fibers that emerge with somatic root fibers and project to the ciliary ganglion. Although the visceral nuclei have been considered to supply preganglionic parasympathetic fibers only to the ciliary ganglion, retrograde transport studies demonstrate that these visceral neurons also project to the lower brain stem

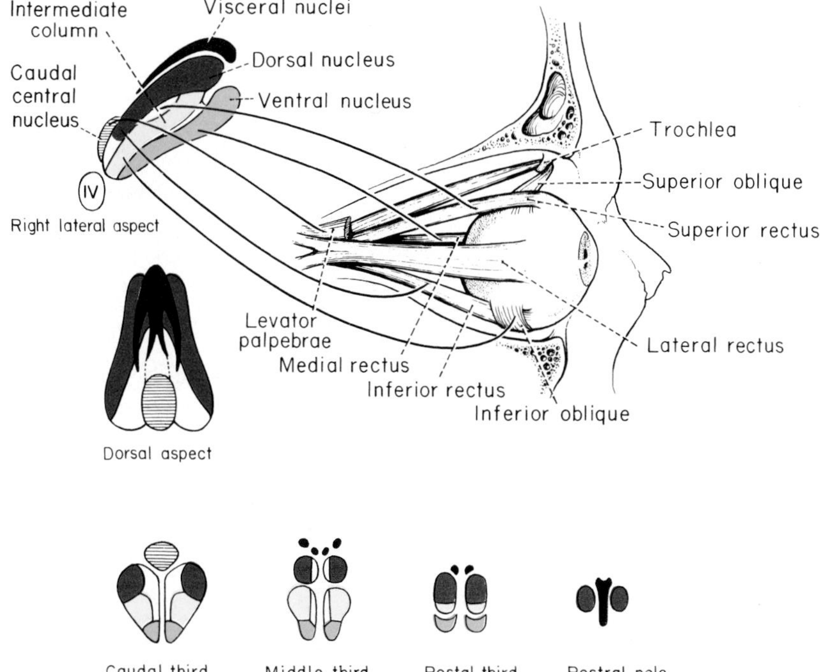

Figure 7-10. Schematic representation of the localization of the extraocular muscles within the oculomotor nuclear complex, based upon studies in the rhesus monkey (Warwick, '53). Cell columns composing the complex are shown in lateral, dorsal and in transverse views through various levels. The visceral motor (parasympathetic) cell columns are shown in *black*. The ventral nucleus (*blue*) innervates the medial rectus muscle. The dorsal nucleus (*red*) innervates the inferior rectus muscle. The intermediate cell column (*yellow*) innervates the inferior oblique muscle. The cell column (*white*) medial to the dorsal and intermediate cell columns innervates the superior rectus muscle. The caudal central nucleus (*lined*) supplies fibers to the levator palpebrae superioris. Fibers innervating the medial rectus, inferior rectus, and inferior oblique muscles are uncrossed; fibers supplying the levator palpebrae muscle are both crossed and uncrossed, while those to the superior rectus muscle are crossed. The *drawing in the upper right* shows the positions of the extraocular muscles in relation to the globe and the bony orbit. (From Carpenter and Sutin, *Human Neuroanatomy*, 1983; courtesy of Williams & Wilkins.)

and spinal cord (Loewy and Saper, '78; Loewy et al., '78).

The so-called *central nucleus of Perlia* has been regarded as a midline cell group particularly concerned with convergence. There has been great difficulty in identifying this nucleus in brains of man and monkey. Some cells of this nucleus may project to the ciliary ganglion (Burde and Loewy, '80), but its function remains in doubt.

Neuromuscular spindles in the extraocular muscles are thought to act as low threshold stretch receptors. Afferent impulses from eye muscle spindles are conveyed centrally by processes of cells in the trigeminal ganglion which form part of the ophthalmic branch (Manni et al., '66).

Root fibers of the oculomotor nerve pass ventrally in numerous small bundles, some of which traverse the red nucleus. The rootlets converge and emerge from the brain stem in the interpeduncular fossa (Figs. 5-1 and 7-6).

Accessory Oculomotor Nuclei. Grouped under this designation are three nuclei closely associated with the oculomotor complex. These nuclei are the interstitial nucleus of Cajal, the nucleus of Darkschewitsch, and the nuclei of the posterior commissure.

The *interstitial nucleus* is a small collection of multipolar neurons situated among, and lateral to, the fibers of the MLF in the rostral midbrain (Fig. 7-11). This nucleus receives projections from the superior colliculus (Altman and Carpenter, '61; Edwards and Henkel, '78) and from the vestibular nuclei (Carleton and Carpenter,

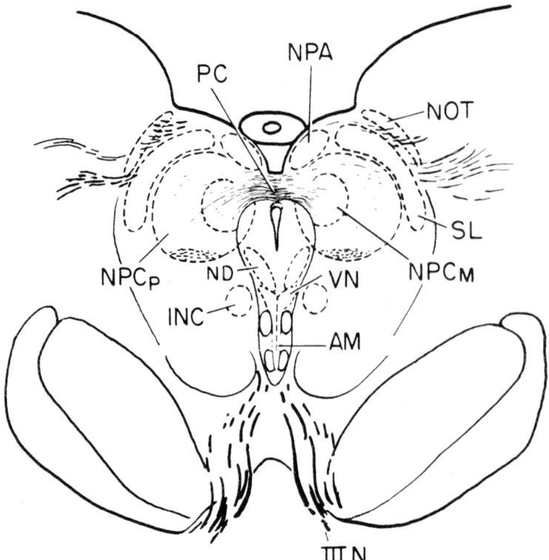

Figure 7-11. Outline drawing of a brain stem section through the most compact portion of the posterior commissure (*PC*). At this level, the nucleus of the optic tract (*NOT*), the sublentiform nucleus (*SL*), the nucleus of the pretectal area (*NPA*), and the nuclei of the posterior commissure (*NPC*) are well developed. The anterior median nucleus (*AM*) is present, but the dorsal visceral nuclei (*VN*) of the oculomotor complex have not separated into medial and lateral cell columns. Additional abbreviations: *INC*, interstitial nucleus of Cajal; *ND*, nucleus of Darkschewitsch; NPC_M, nucleus of posterior commissure, pars magnocellularis; NPC_P, nucleus of posterior commissure, pars principalis; III N. oculmotor nerve (Carpenter and Pierson, '73). (From Carpenter and Sutin, *Human Neuroanatomy*, 1983; courtesy of Williams & Wilkins.)

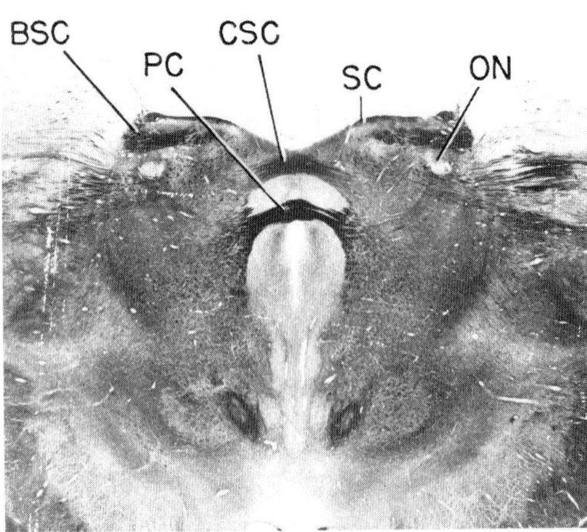

Figure 7-12. Photomicrograph of a myelin-stained section at the junction of pretectum and superior colliculus in the rhesus monkey. Abbreviations are as follows: *BSC*, brachium of the superior colliculus, *CSC*, commissure of the superior colliculus; *ON*, pretectal olivary nucleus; *PC*, posterior commissure; *SC*, superior colliculus. (Weil stain.) (From Carpenter and Sutin, *Human Neuroanatomy*, 1983; courtesy of Williams & Wilkins.)

'83). Efferent fibers from the interstitial nucleus crossing in the ventral part of the posterior commissure are distributed to all somatic cell columns of the oculomotor complex, except the ventral (Fig. 7-14) (Carpenter et al., '70). In addition the nucleus projects fibers bilaterally to the trochlear nuclei and ipsilaterally to the medial vestibular nucleus and spinal cord (i.e., interstitiospinal tract). This nucleus is considered to be concerned with rotatory and vertical eye movements and reflex movements involving head and eyes.

The *nucleus of Darkschewitsch* is formed by small cells which lie inside the ventrolateral border of the central gray, dorsal and lateral to the somatic cell columns of the oculomotor complex (Fig. 7-11). The nucleus projects fibers into the posterior commissure, but does not send fibers into the oculomotor complex or to lower brain stem levels.

The *nuclei of the posterior commissure* consists of collections of cells intimately associated with fibers of the posterior commissure (Figs. 7-11 and 7-13). Cells of these nuclei lie dorsolateral and dorsal to the central gray and have connections with the pretectal and posterior thalamic nuclei. In the monkey, interruption of fibers in the posterior commissure in the midline does not impair the pupillary light reflex, but lesions involving the nuclei of the posterior commissure and crossing fibers from the interstitial nuclei of Cajal produce bilateral eyelid retraction and impairment of vertical eye movements (Carpenter et al., '70; Carpenter and Pierson, '73).

Pretectal Region. This region lies immediately rostral to the superior colliculus at levels of the posterior commissure (Figs. 7-11 and 7-12). Several distinctive cell groups found in this region all appear related to the visual system. Some, but not all of these nuclei, receive fibers from the optic tract, the visual cortex and the lateral geniculate body (Scalia, '72; Pierson and Carpenter, '74). The nucleus of the optic tract consists of a plate of large cells along

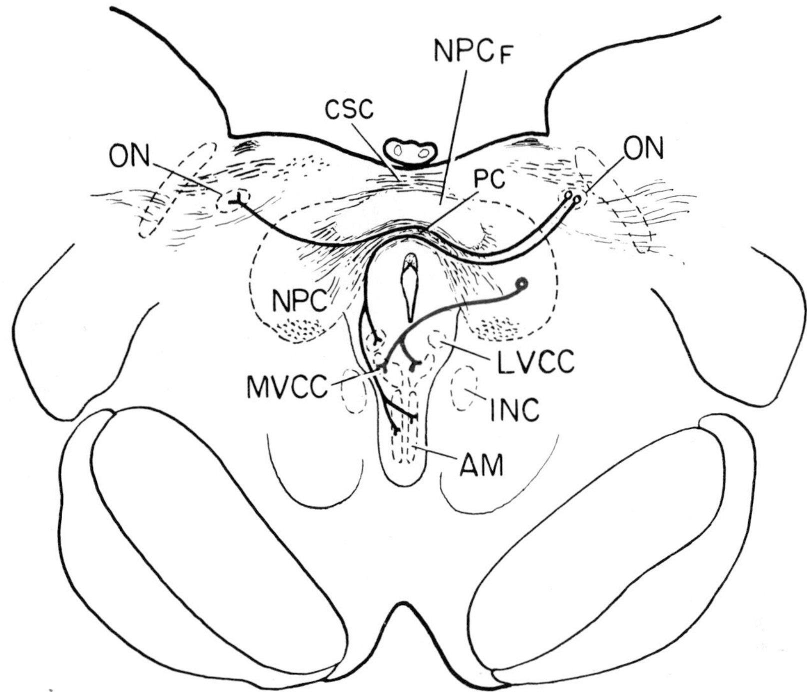

Figure 7-13. Schematic drawing of the brain stem through the caudal part of the posterior commissure, showing the course of fibers projecting to the visceral nuclei of the oculomotor complex. Fibers (*red*) from the nuclei of the posterior commissure (*NPC*) enter the ipsilateral central gray and project primarily to the medial visceral cell columns (*MVCC*); these fibers partially cross ventral to the cerebral aqueduct and some terminate in the anterior median nuclei. Fibers (*black*) from the pretectal olivary nucleus (*ON*) pass through the posterior commissure (*PC*), enter the central gray and project to the contralateral lateral visceral cell column (*LVCC*) and bilaterally to the anterior median nuclei (*AM*). There are some commissural projections from ON to the corresponding nucleus contralaterally. Additional abbreviations: *CSC*, commissure of superior colliculus; *INC*, interstitial nucleus of Cajal; NPC_F, nucleus of posterior commissure, pars infracommissuralis (Carpenter and Pierson, '73). (From Carpenter and Sutin, *Human Neuroanatomy*, 1983; courtesy of Williams & Wilkins.)

the dorsolateral border of the pretectum at its junction with the pulvinar (Fig. 7-11). The pretectal olivary nucleus, which forms a sharply delimited cell group at levels through caudal parts of the posterior commissure, receives crossed and uncrossed fibers of the optic tract and projects bilaterally to the visceral nuclei of the oculomotor complex (Carpenter and Pierson, '73; Steiger and Büttner-Ennever, '79) (Figs. 7-12 and 7-13). These fiber systems are involved in the direct and consensual pupillary light reflex.

Posterior Commissure. The transition from midbrain to diencephalon is marked dorsally by the posterior commissure (Figs. 2-22, 2-23, 7-11, and 7-12). This small commissure lies dorsal to the central gray and rostral to the superior colliculi at the point of transition between cerebral aqueduct and third ventricle. As fibers of this commissure fan out laterally they are surrounded by cells which collectively form the *nuclei of the posterior commissure.* The entire composition of this complex commissure is not known. Identified elements in the commissure include fibers from: (1) the pretectal nuclei, (2) the nuclei of the posterior commissure, (3) the interstitial nucleus, and (4) the nucleus of Darkschewitsch. Fibers involved in the pupillary light reflex partially cross in the posterior commissure.

The ependyma of the cerebral aqueduct beneath the posterior commissure consists of tall columnar cells with cilia. These modified ependyma cells form the *subcommissural organ* which is considered to have a

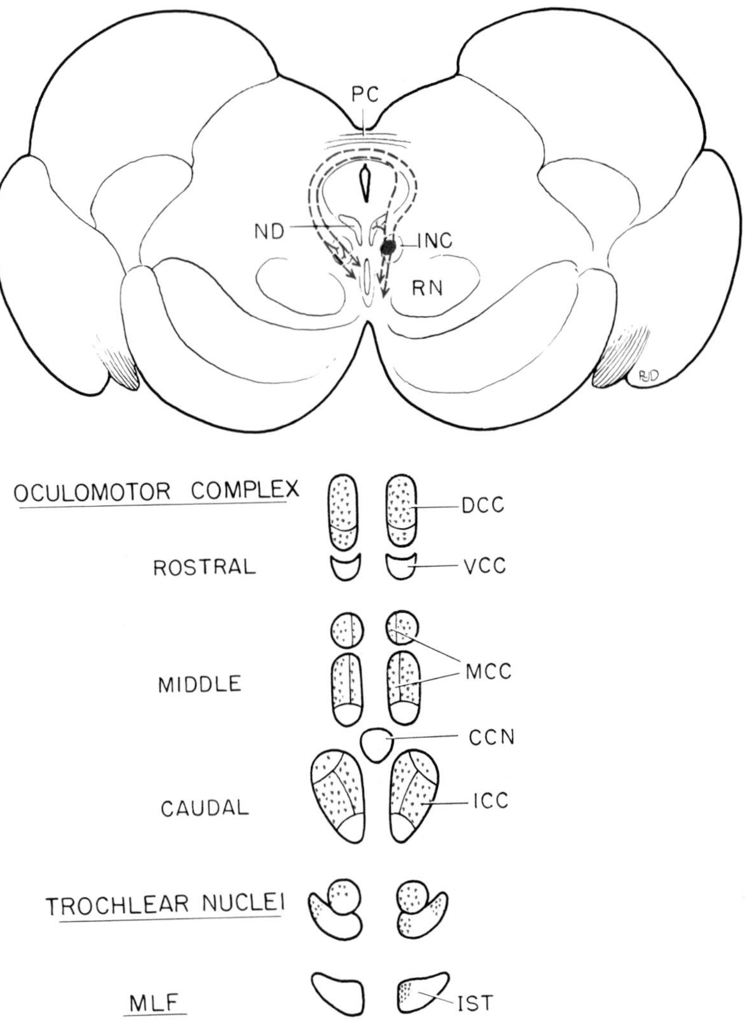

Figure 7-14 Schematic diagram of degeneration resulting from a lesion (*red*) in the right interstitial nucleus (*INC*). The lesion destroyed: (1) cells which give rise to fibers that cross in the ventral part of the posterior commissure and fibers which descend in the ipsilateral *MLF*, and (2) fibers from the opposite interstitial nucleus which have crossed in the posterior commissure and traverse the lesion *en route* to the oculomotor complex. Fairly symmetrical differential degeneration (*red stippling*) in the oculomotor complex was greatest in the intermediate (*ICC*) and medial cell columns (*MCC*), somewhat less profuse in the dorsal cell columns (*DCC*) and absent in the ventral cell columns (*VCC*) and in the caudal central nucleus (*CCN*). Degeneration in the trochlear nuclei was bilateral but greatest ipsilaterally. Fibers of the interstitiospinal tract (*IST*) were concentrated in the dorsomedial part of the MLF (Carpenter et al., '70). (From Carpenter and Sutin, *Human Neuroanatomy*, 1983; courtesy of Williams & Wilkins.)

secretory function and is recognized as a circumventricular organ (Fig. 1-16). The subcommissural organ is the only midbrain structure not included in the blood-brain barrier.

Afferent Connections of the Oculomotor Complex. The oculomotor complex receives impulses from the cerebral cortex, the vestibular nuclei, the superior colliculus, the reticular formation, and certain accessory oculomotor nuclei. Although no direct corticobulbar fibers reach the oculomotor complex, impulses from the cerebral cortex are conveyed by corticoreticular fibers and reticular neurons which relay these impulses. Direct projections to the oculomotor nuclear complex arise from parts of the vestibular nuclei, the interstitial nucleus of Cajal, the abducens nucleus, parts of the perihypoglossal nuclei, the rostral interstitial nucleus of the MLF, and the pretectal olivary nucleus. The superior colliculus does not give rise to direct projections to the oculomotor complex, but it projects to parts of the periaqueductal gray close to the oculomotor nuclei (Edwards and Henkel, '78). Secondary fibers from the medial and superior vestibular nuclei project to the oculomotor complex via the MLF (Steiger and Büttner-Ennever, '79; Carleton and Carpenter, '83). Projections from the medial vestibular nuclei via the MLF are bilateral while those from the superior vestibular nucleus via this bundle are mainly ipsilateral. Abducens internuclear neurons give rise to axons which ascend in the contralateral MLF and terminate selectively upon cells of the opposite medial rectus subdivision of the oculomotor complex (Steiger and Büttner-Ennever, '78; Carpenter and Batton, '80; Carpenter and Carleton, '83). The nucleus prepositus, which receives an input from the flocculus, projects ipsilaterally to the oculomotor complex and may be concerned with vertical eye movements (Fuchs, '77). The rostral interstitial nucleus of the MLF (RiMLF), situated among fibers of the MLF rostral to the oculomotor complex at the junction of mesencephalon and diencephalon, appears uniquely concerned with vertical eye movements (Büttner et al., '77). Cells in the RiMLF are activated in short bursts before vertical eye movements occur in response to vestibular or optokinetic stimuli. The RiMLF receives inputs from the superior vestibular nucleus via the MLF and uncrossed projections from the paramedian pontine reticular formation (PPRF) which ascend outside of the MLF (Büttner-Ennever and Büttner, '78). Cells of the RiMLF project ipsilateral to the oculomotor complex (Steiger and Büttner-Ennever, '79). Thus the PPRF projects fibers to both the principal center for conjugate horizontal eye movements, the abducens nucleus, and to an established center for vertical eye movements, the RiMLF. These data indicate that paralysis of conjugate horizontal or vertical eye movements can occur independently, yet a mechanism exists which integrates horizontal and vertical components of conjugate eye movements.

Pupillary Reflexes. Light shone on the retina of one eye causes both pupils to constrict. The response in the eye stimulated is called the *direct pupillary light reflex*, while that in the opposite eye is known as the *consensual pupillary light reflex*. Pathways involved in the pupillary light reflex are not entirely known, but involve: (1) axons of retinal ganglion cells which pass via the optic nerve, optic tract and brachium of the superior colliculus to the pretectal area, (2) axons of pretectal neurons which partially cross in the posterior commissure and presumably terminate bilaterally in visceral nuclei of the oculomotor complex, (3) preganglionic fibers from the visceral nuclei which course with fibers of the third nerve and synapse in the ciliary ganglion, and (4) postganglionic fibers from the ciliary ganglion which project to the sphincter of the iris. Cells of the pretectal olivary nucleus receive fibers of the optic tract and project bilaterally to the visceral nuclei of the oculomotor complex (Steiger and Büttner-Ennever, '79).

In man the direct and consensual pupillary light reflexes are normally equal. The term *anisocoria* is used to denote pupillary inequality. In man the principal central lesions producing anisocoria involve efferent pathways from the oculomotor complex.

The *accommodation-convergence* reaction occurs when gaze is shifted from a distant object to a near one. This reaction involves: (1) contractions of both medial recti muscles for convergence, (2) contraction of the ciliary muscle which relaxes the suspensory ligament of the lens and causes the lens to assume a more convex shape, and (3) pupillary constriction. In this reflex response retinal impulses must first reach the visual cortex and be relayed via corticofugal fibers to brain stem centers. It is presumed that the corticofugal fibers involved in this response reach the superior colliculus and pretectal region and are relayed to the oculomotor complex. Although under normal circumstances accommodation always is accompanied by pupillary constriction, certain central nervous system lesions can impair or abolish the pupillary light reflex without affecting accommodation. Such lesions occur with central nervous system syphilis (tabes dorsalis) in which the pupils are small (miosis) and do not react to light, but react to accommodation. This is the *Argyll-Robertson pupil.* The precise location of the responsible lesion is unknown.

The central pathways for pupillary dilatation are not entirely known, but dilatation occurs reflexly on shading the eyes, scratching the side of the neck, and in association with severe pain and extreme emotion. Impulses related to pain probably reach cells of the intermediolateral cell column in upper thoracic spinal segments which give rise to preganglionic sympathetic fibers that convey impulses to the superior cervical ganglion. Postganglionic fibers from the superior cervical ganglion pass via blood vessels to dilator muscle fibers in the iris. Interruption of descending autonomic pathways which course in the dorsolateral tegmentum of the brain stem at all levels caudal to the hypothalamus will produce a *Horner's syndrome.* This syndrome may also occur as a consequence of interrupting either preganglionic or postganglionic sympathetic fibers conveying impulses to, or from, the superior cervical ganglion. The syndrome is characterized by miosis, pseudoptosis, apparent enophthalmos, and dryness of the skin over the face. If Horner's syndrome is the result of a brain stem lesion, the pupil shows relatively little dilatation to adrenaline. If the provocative lesion involves postganglionic sympathetic fibers, adrenaline produces mydriasis and eyelid retraction on the affected side due to denervation sensitivity (Cogan, '56).

Lesions of the Oculomotor Nerve. Complete lesions of the third nerve produce an ipsilateral lower neuron paralysis of the muscles supplied by that nerve. There is a complete ptosis (drooping) of the eyelid, due to paralysis of the levator palpebrae muscle. The eye is deviated laterally (external strabismus) due to paralysis of the oculomotor-innervated muscles and the unopposed action of the lateral rectus muscle. The pupil is fully dilated (mydriasis), and there is a loss of the pupillary light reflex as well as a loss of lens accommodation. Loss of the pupillary light reflex and accommodation results from interruption of visceral efferent fibers. Lesions involving the oculomotor nerve and corticospinal fibers in the ventral part of the midbrain result in an ipsilateral oculomotor paralysis and a contralateral hemiplegia which clinically are known as *Weber's syndrome.*

MESENCEPHALIC TEGMENTUM

The midbrain tegmentum contains the reticular formation, the red nucleus and many smaller cell groups in addition to the oculomotor and trochlear nuclei.

Red Nucleus. The most conspicuous structure in the midbrain tegmentum is the red nucleus, a part of the reticular formation characterized by its pinkish-yellow color, its central position, and its "capsule" formed by fibers of the superior cerebellar peduncle (Figs. 7-6, 7-9 and 7-15). The nucleus is an oval column of cells extending from the caudal margin of the superior colliculus into the caudal diencephalon. In transverse sections the nucleus has a circular configuration. Cytologically the nucleus consists of a caudal magnocellular part and a rostral parvicellular part. Between the cells of the nucleus there are small bundles of myelinated fibers primarily from the superior cerebellar peduncle. Root fibers of the oculomotor nerve partially traverse the nucleus en route to the interpeduncular fossa (Fig. 7-6).

Afferent fibers projecting to the red nucleus are derived from two principal sources, the deep cerebellar nuclei and the cerebral cortex. Fibers from both sources terminate somatotopically within the red nucleus. Fibers of the superior cerebellar peduncle undergo a complete decussation in the caudal midbrain and enter and surround the contralateral red nucleus. Fibers and collaterals from the dentate nucleus terminate mainly in the rostral third of the opposite red nucleus, while those from the emboliform nucleus (anterior interposed nucleus) project somatotopically upon cells in the caudal two-thirds of the nucleus (Figs. 8-13 and 8-14). The latter connection links paravermal regions of the cerebellar cortex to cells of the red nucleus that in turn project somatotopically to spinal levels (Fig. 8-14). Two decussations are involved, that of the superior cerebellar peduncle and that of the rubrospinal tract. Terminals of fibers from the globose nucleus (posterior interposed nucleus) end in the medial mag-

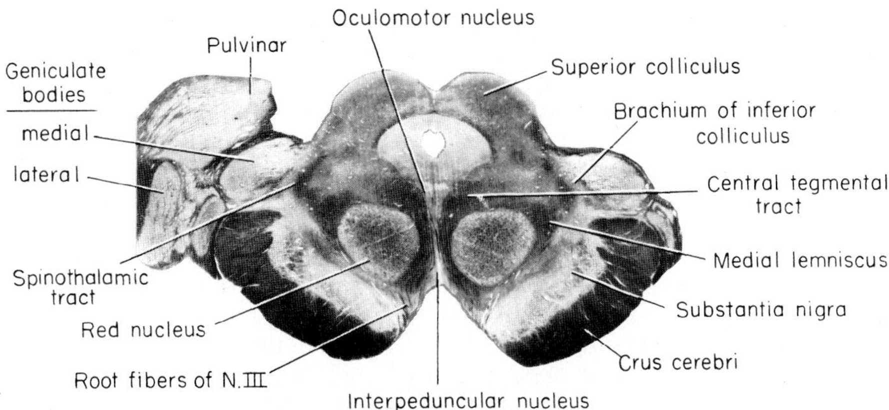

Figure 7-15. Traverse section through the rostral mesencephalon demonstrating the manner in which diencephalic nuclei surround dorsal and lateral portions of the mesencephalon. (Weigert's myelin stain; photograph.)

nocellular part of the red nucleus (Angaut, '70).

Corticorubral projections arise from precentral and premotor cortex; both of these areas project bilaterally and somatotopically upon cells in the parvicellular part of the red nucleus (Hartmann-von Monakow et al., '79). Projections from the medial part of area 6, coextensive with the supplementary motor area, are crossed and end in the magnocellular region of the nucleus. Projections from the precentral motor cortex to the magnocellular part of the red nucleus are ipsilateral and correspond to the somatotopic origins of rubrospinal fibers (Pompeiano and Brodal, '57). These fibers have a somatotopic linkage and, together with the rubrospinal tract (crossed), constitute a pathway by which impulses can be conveyed from the "motor" cortex to spinal levels.

Descending rubral efferent fibers cross in the *ventral tegmental decussation* and project to: (1) the anterior interposed nucleus of the cerebellum; (2) the principal sensory and spinal trigeminal nuclei (Edwards, '72; Miller and Strominger, '73); (3) parts of the facial nucleus; (4) the lateral reticular nucleus, the accessory cuneate nucleus, and the nuclei gracilis and cuneatus in the medulla; and (5) the spinal cord. Uncrossed descending rubral efferents from the parvicellular part of the nucleus enter the central tegmental tract and project to the dorsal lamella of the principal inferior olivary nucleus; these fibers are referred to a *rubro-olivary* and constitute part of a feedback system to the cerebellum. Although older studies suggested that cells of the red nucleus projected to thalamic nuclei in parallel with fibers of the superior cerebellar peduncle, the best evidence indicates no projection from this nucleus to the thalamus (Poirier and Bouvier, '66; Kuypers and Lawrence, '67; Edwards, '72).

Stimulation of the red nucleus in the decerebrate cat results in: (1) excitatory postsynaptic potentials in contralateral flexor alpha motor neurons, and (2) inhibitory postsynaptic potentials in contralateral extensor alpha motor neurons. These observations suggest that the rubrospinal tract transmits impulses which facilitate flexor muscle tone. Because somatotopic relationships exist between the anterior interposed nucleus of the cerebellum and the red nucleus, stimulation of the interposed nucleus in decerebrate animals produces flexion in the ipsilateral limb muscles (Fig. 8-14). These responses are ipsilateral because both fiber systems involved are crossed (i.e., the superior cerebellar peduncle and the rubrospinal tract).

Lesions involving the midbrain tegmentum and the red nucleus unilaterally produce a syndrome characterized by: (1) ipsilateral oculomotor disturbances, and (2) contralateral motor disturbances of an involuntary nature (i.e., tremor, ataxia or choreiform movements). This combination of disturbances is known as the *syndrome of Benedikt.* Experimental evidence suggests that the contralateral abnormal involuntary motor activity probably is due to involvement of crossed fibers of the superior cerebellar peduncle rather than cells of the red nucleus.

Mesencephalic Reticular Formation. The midbrain reticular formation is less extensive than that of the pons. Although the red nucleus is part of the reticular formation, this term usually is used to designate structures dorsal and lateral to the red nucleus. Three principal reticular nuclei are recognized: (1) cuneiformis, (2) subcuneiformis, and (3) tegmenti pedunculopontinus (pedunculopontine nucleus).

The *pedunculopontine nucleus* lies in the lateral tegmentum ventral to the inferior colliculus (Fig. 7-3). Fibers of the superior cerebellar peduncle traverse this nucleus as they course ventromedially toward their decussation. The pedunculopontine nucleus receives inputs from multiple sources that include: (1) the cerebral cortex (Hartmann-von Monakow et al., '79); (2) the medial pallidal segment (Kim et al., '76; Carpenter et al., '81); and (3) the pars reticulata of the substantia nigra (Beckstead et al., '79; Carpenter et al., '81). Projections of the pedunculopontine nucleus are ascending with the largest number of fibers projecting to the substantia nigra and the medial pallidal segment (Beckstead et al., '79; DeVito et al., '80). Connections of this small nucleus appear to form a mesencephalic loop that may function to modulate the activities of nigral and pallidal neurons which together constitute the major output systems of the corpus striatum (Fig. 11-24).

The *cuneiform* and *subcuneiform nuclei* lie ventral to the tectum and dorsal to the pedunculopontine nucleus, and extend rostrally. Fibers of the central tegmental tract lie medial to these reticular nuclei. The *interpeduncular nucleus*, composed of small cells, lies in the midline dorsal to the interpeduncular fossa (Figs. 7-6 and 7-9). This nucleus receives fibers from the habenular nuclei via the fasciculus retroflexus (Figs. 9-4 and 10-8).

The *dorsal tegmental nucleus* lies within the central gray caudal to the trochlear nuclei and lateral to the dorsal nucleus of the raphe. Fibers from this nucleus and the *ventral tegmental nucleus* ascend to lateral hypothalamic, preoptic and septal areas via the dorsal longitudinal fasciculus, the mammillary peduncle, and the medial forebrain bundle (Fig. 10-8).

FUNCTIONAL CONSIDERATIONS OF THE RETICULAR FORMATION

The anatomical organization of the brain stem reticular formation has been described regionally. In the medulla and pons four zones are recognized: (1) a median zone containing nuclei of the raphe, (2) the paramedian reticular nuclei, (3) a medial zone regarded as an "effector" area, and (4) a smaller lateral zone referred to as the "sensory" part, because it receives collaterals from secondary sensory pathways. In the medulla the paramedian reticular nuclei project mainly to the cerebellum. The effector zone, which is coextensive with the giant cell area of the reticular formation, gives rise to both ascending and descending fibers. The "sensory" zone, coextensive with the parvicellular area, projects its axons medially into the "effector" area. The pontine reticular formation has essentially the same zones, although the "sensory" part is much smaller and evident only caudally. Electrical stimulation of the caudal and medial "effector" zone of the medullary reticular formation inhibits most forms of motor activity (e.g., myotatic reflexes, flexion reflex, extensor muscle tone, and cortically induced movements). Regions of the medullary reticular formation from which inhibitory responses are obtained correspond roughly to the area of the gigantocellular part which gives rise to medullary reticulospinal fibers (Magoun and Rhines, '46). Stimulation of the rostral and dorsal part of the nucleus reticularis gigantocellularis produces monosynaptic excitatory postsynaptic potentials in motor neurons supplying axial muscles in the neck and back (Peterson, '80).

A far larger region of the brain stem reticular formation facilitates reflex activity and cortically induced movements. The facilitatory area extends rostrally from the upper medulla into the caudal diencephalon. Bilateral facilitatory effects can be evoked throughout this extensive region of the reticular formation. This region includes areas which do not give rise to direct reticulospinal fibers. Descending polysynaptic pathways must mediate effects from regions which have no direct reticulospinal projections.

Descending influences of the brain stem reticular formation are not limited to inhibition and facilitation of somatic motor functions. Inspiratory and vasodepressor effects can be obtained from the gigantocellular region in the medulla, while expiratory effects are obtained from the parvicellular region. Vasopressor effects are evoked from reticular regions which do not project fibers to spinal levels. Although nearly all parts of the central nervous system are capable of exerting detectable influences upon the heart and blood vessels, the primary vasomotor control center is located in the reticular formation of the medulla. Transections of the brain stem as far caudal as the lower third of the pons have no significant effect upon arterial pressure or on the tonic discharge of the inferior cardiac nerve. Successively more caudal transections produce: (1) an increasing drop in blood pressure and (2) a reduction in the discharge of cardiac accelerator impulses (Bard, '68). The bulbar pressor and depressor areas constitute a central cardiovascular mechanism which reflexly regulates blood pressure and the parameters of the heart rate. In the intact animal a normal arterial pressure is dependent upon the bulbar pressor area. A group of noradrenergic neurons located in the caudal pons and rostral medulla (Fig. 5-13) sends axons to the nucleus of the solitary tract, the nucleus ambiguus, and preganglionic sympathetic neurons in the intermediolateral cell column of the thoracic spinal cord. These noradrenergic neurons are part of a neural network related to the regulation of the cardiovascular system (Loewy and McKellar, '80).

The region surrounding the nucleus of the solitary tract is coextensive with the physiologically defined dorsal medullary respirator "center" (Kalia, '77). A ventral medullary respirator "center" includes the nucleus ambiguus and the surrounding reticular formation. Additional brain stem regions important in the control of respiration are the "pneumotaxic center" found in the pons near the medial parabrachial nucleus and an "apneustic center" which remains poorly defined. The parabrachial nuclei receive input from nucleus of the solitary tract and in turn project to both dorsal and ventral respiratory "centers" in the medulla (Bystrzycka, '80; Takeuchi et al., '80). The "pneumotaxic center" periodically releases the inhibition of the "apneustic center."

Stimulation of inhibitory and facilitatory regions of the reticular formation can decrease or increase the rates of discharge from the muscle spindles via gamma efferent fibers. A part of the effects exerted upon alpha motor neurons may result from the firing of gamma efferents which indirectly influence these neurons through the gamma loop (Fig. 3-23). The reticular formation also is thought to modify the transmission of other sensory impulses by facilitation and inhibition exerted at the second neuronal level.

Ascending influences of the reticular formation exert powerful influences upon the electrical activity of the cerebral cortex. Wakefulness, alertness and sleep are characterized by strikingly different electroencephalographic patterns (Berger, '29). Alertness is characterized by low voltage fast activity, while sleep is associated with high voltage slow activity. Fundamental insight into the underlying brain mechanisms was provided by Bremer ('37) who compared the electroencephalograms (EEG) of animals following high spinal transections (*encéphale isolé*) and decerebration (i.e., transection of the midbrain at the intercollicular level, *cerveau isolé*). In the encéphale isolé preparation the EEG displayed the waking pattern, while the cerveau isolé preparation exhibited an EEG pattern characteristic of the sleeping state. These experiments pointed to a potent electrotonic influence generated in the lower brain stem. While it was well known that a variety of different stimuli could change the EEG from a synchronized pattern (i.e., sleep state) to a desynchronized one (i.e., alert state), the puzzling feature was how impulses channeled in the classic pathways exerted such broad and diffuse electronic changes in the cerebral cortex. The observation that stimulation of the brain stem reticular formation could activate and desynchronize the EEG and produce behavioral arousal without discharging the classic lemniscal pathways, suggested the concept of a second ascending system (Moruzzi and Magoun, '49; Magoun, '63). This second ascending system with powerful influences upon broad regions of the cerebral cortex is known as the *ascending reticular activating system* (ARAS).

Interruption of the long ascending sensory pathways in the brain stem does not prevent impulses ascending in the reticular formation from provoking their characteristic EEG arousal response. Lesions in the rostromedial midbrain reticular formation abolish the EEG arousal response elicited by sensory stimulation, even though long ascending sensory pathways are intact. Thus two functionally distinct ascending sensory pathways must project to the diencephalon: (1) long ascending pathways, the *lemniscal systems,* concerned with specific sensory modalities (i.e., medial lemniscus, lateral lemniscus, spinothalamic tracts and secondary trigeminothalamic pathways) which end upon specific thalamic nuclei, and (2) the *ascending reticular activating system* which receives collaterals from surrounding specific systems and conveys impulses via the reticular core. Physiologically, the ascending reticular activating system is considered to be a multineuronal, polysynaptic system conveying impulses of a nonspecific nature related to wakefulness and arousal. Although physiologically the reticular formation behaves as if it consisted of chains of neurons that fire successively, the reticular formation does not contain short-axoned Golgi type II cells. The main ascending pathway in the reticular formation appears to be the *central tegmental tract* (Figs. 6-1, 6-4, 6-25 and 7-15). Ascending components of this bundle arise from effector regions of the reticular core and give rise to long axons with numerous collaterals that project laterally. Rapid conduction in the reticular core is via the long central axons, while slowly conducted impulses pass via collaterals and involve multiple synapses. The central tegmental tract projects into the subthalamic region and to the intralaminar nuclei of the thalamus. Ascending projections from medial regions of the midbrain reticular formation projecting to the hypothalamus are distinct from those contained in the central tegmental tract. Although there has been agreement that the intralaminar nuclei could influence electrical activity in broad cortical regions, it was impossible to demonstrate connections between these nuclei and the cerebral cortex by degeneration technics. Axonal transport studies have demonstrated that while the major projection of the intralaminar nuclei is to the striatum (i.e., caudate nucleus and putamen), these cells also give rise to a profuse collateral system distributed broadly in the cerebral cortex (Jones and Leavitt, '74).

In man lesions of the brain stem often produce disturbances of consciousness which range from fleeting unconsciousness to sustained coma. As Magoun ('54) has stated, "It is not easy for the physiologist to put his finger upon consciousness, though it is present abundantly and for long periods of time." In all forms of disturbed consciousness due to brain stem lesions there is a loss of crude awareness. With lesions of the lower brain stem unconsciousness is accompanied by respiratory and cardiovascular disturbances. The loss of consciousness frequently is sudden and depression of vital functions leads to extreme states. Lesions of the upper brain stem most commonly produce hypersomnia characterized by muscular relaxation, slow respiration and an EEG pattern showing large amplitude slow waves. The level of unconsciousness may not be deep and some patients can be aroused briefly. If the patient develops decerebrate rigidity, there is usually coma. A variant of hypersomnia seen with upper brain stem lesions is referred to as *akinetic mutism* (coma vigil). In this variant the EEG pattern mainly resembles that associated with slow sleep, but eye movements remain normal.

At all levels of the brain stem liability to unconsciousness is related to the rapidity with which the lesions develop. Lesions associated with hemorrhage usually produce sudden coma; slowly developing lesions, such as tumors, may not disturb consciousness for a considerable period of time. Although there is no center particularly concerned with consciousness, the functional integrity of the brain stem reticular formation is essential for its maintenance. A healthy cerebral cortex cannot by itself maintain the conscious state.

Major serotonergic neurons in the midbrain lie in the dorsal (supratrochlear) and median (superior central) raphe nuclei (Fig. 5-11). Ascending pathways from these nuclei pass through the ventral tegmental area and join the medial forebrain bundle (Fig. 10-8). Fibers of this bundle project medially into the hypothalamus and laterally into the striatum. Ascending fibers continuing in the medial forebrain bundle divide into several components that pass to: (1) the thalamus, (2) amygdala, (3) the hippocampus, (4) the cortex on the medial aspect of the hemisphere, and (5) the olfactory bulb (Moore et al., '78). The raphe nuclei of the midbrain have ascending fiber systems with functional relationships to the ascending reticular activating system and the limbic system. The general inhibitory action of serotonin in the central nervous system serves to modulate and maintain behavior within certain limits. Hallucinogenic drugs, such as LSD, depress the serotonergic system, and the release of inhibition results in a hypersensitivity to environmental stimuli and hyperactivity in a brain otherwise behaving as if it were asleep (Jacobs and Trulson, '79).

SUBSTANTIA NIGRA

The substantia nigra lies dorsal to the crus cerebri, ventral to the midbrain tegmentum and extends throughout the length of the mesencephalon (Figs. 7-1, 7-6, 7-9 and 7-15). Descriptively, the substantia nigra commonly is divided into two parts: (1) the *compact part,* a cell-rich region composed of large, pigmented cells, and (2) a *reticular part* which is a cell-poor region close to the crus cerebri. Three types of nigral neurons have been described: (1) large neurons distributed exclusively in the reticular part, (2) medium-sized and large neurons containing melanin pigment in the compact part, and (3) short-axoned (Golgi type II) cells found in both the compact and reticular parts (Gulley and Wood, '71). Some ultrastructural studies do not support the division of the substantia nigra into two parts, though cells vary in size and regional distribution (Rinvik and Grofová, '70).

Golgi studies demonstrate that nigral neurons give rise to long radiating dendrites with few branches. Relatively smooth dendrites are oriented in two main directions. Dendrites of cells in the pars reticulata and in the caudal pars compacta are oriented primarily in rostrocaudal directions. Dendrites of most cells in the pars compacta have a dorsoventral orientation. Thus the dendritic fields of cells in the pars compacta and pars reticulata overlap extensively in the pars reticulata (Rinvik and Grofová, '70). The surface of nigral dendrites is covered with boutons whose numbers increase with the distance from the soma and are separated from the neighboring neuropil by protoplasmic sheets of astroglia. Although axons of nigral neurons are difficult to impregnate by the Golgi technic, a prominent feature of the substantia nigra is the enormous number of thin, unmyelinated axons coursing in a rostrocaudal direction.

Dorsomedial to the substantia nigra is a region containing scattered cells of various sizes, some of which are pigmented. This tegmental region is regarded as a diffusely organized extension of the pars compacta and is referred to as the *ventral tegmental area* (Tsai). Lateral to the substantia nigra the small cells of the *peripeduncular nucleus* cap the dorsal margin of the crus cerebri (Fig. 7-9).

Neurotransmitters. Cells of the pars compacta contain high concentrations of dopamine (Fig. 7-16) and are recognized as the principal source of striatal (i.e., caudate nucleus and putamen) dopamine (Andén et al., '65; Andén et al., '66; Hökfelt and Ungerstedt, '69; Ungerstedt, '71). The enzyme glutamate decarboxylase (GAD) utilized in the synthesis of gamma (γ)-aminobutyric acid (GABA) is found in high concentrations in the pars reticulata (Fonnum et al., '74). About 85% of the GAD in the substantia nigra is present in synaptosomes. The substantia nigra also contains serotonin (5-HT) and its synthesizing enzyme tryptophan hydroxylase (Brownstein et al., '75; Hajdu et al., '73; Palkovitz et al., '74); serotonin is taken up by dense core vesicles in fiber terminals mainly within the pars reticulata. The dorsal nucleus of the raphe is

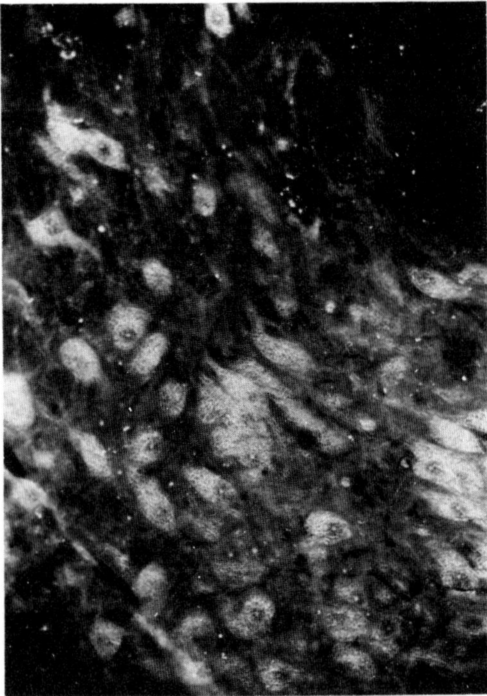

Figure 7-16. Dopamine-containing cell bodies in the pars compacta of the substantia nigra of the squirrel monkey. Green fluorescence in the cell bodies extends into some of the large processes which contribute to the background fluorescence. Fluorescence photomicrograph, X 400. (Courtesy of Dr. David L. Felton, School of Medicine, University of Rochester.) (From Carpenter and Sutin, *Human Neuroanatomy*, 1983; courtesy of Williams & Wilkins.)

the principal source of this serotonergic pathway (Bunney and Aghajanian, '76; Dray et al., '78; Carpenter et al., '81a). Stimulation of the dorsal nucleus of the raphe produces predominantly inhibition of spontaneous activity in single neurons of the substantia nigra.

The substantia nigra also contains a highly biologically active principal known as substance P characterized as an undecapeptide (von Euler and Gaddum, '31). Substance P (SP) has been synthesized and used to produce antibodies for radioimmunological determinations of the regional distribution of SP in the brain (Chang et al., '71; Tregear et al., '71). The highest concentration of SP in any brain region is found in the substantia nigra where the substance is concentrated in nerve ending particles (Powell et al., '73; Duffy et al., '75; Davies and Dray, '76). Neurons containing SP project from the striatum to the nigra and are presumed to synapse upon dendrites of dopaminergic neurons (Gale et al., '77; Hong et al., '77; Kanazawa et al., '77). SP has an excitatory action upon neurons in the central nervous system (Hökfelt et al., '77).

Sensitive radioimmunoassays indicate that some strionigral fibers have enkephalin as their neurotransmitter (Emson et al., '80; DiFiglia et al., '82). Evidence for neurotransmitter roles for the opioid pentapeptides leucine (leu) and methionine (met)-enkephalin has come from studies in laboratory mammals which show high content of these peptides in the caudate nucleus, putamen, parts of the globus pallidus and in the substantia nigra. Further opiate receptors are found in abundance in these same structures. Most of the striatal enkephalin terminals in the substantia nigra are found in the pars reticulata. The precise role of enkephalin in the substantia nigra is unknown, but it may have direct influences upon efferent systems. The substantia nigra is implicated in the metabolic disturbances which underlie parkinsonism (paralysis agitans) and may be involved along with other structures in Huntington's chorea (Hornykiewicz, '66, Bird and Iversen, '74). In Huntington's disease there is a substantial reduction of SP and met-enkephalin in the substantia nigra and in the globus pallidus (Emson et al., '80).

Nigral Afferent Fibers. Afferent fibers to the substantia nigra arise from the neostriatum (caudate nucleus and putamen), both segments of the globus pallidus, the subthalamic nucleus, the dorsal nucleus of the raphe, and the pedunculopontine nucleus. Although corticonigral fibers have been described by a number of investigators, electron microscopic studies (Rinvik and Walberg, '69) and axoplasmic transport technics (Bunney and Aghajanian, '76) indicate such fibers are very few in number. Quantitatively the largest number of nigral afferents arise from the caudate nucleus and the putamen and are known as strionigral fibers (Fig. 7-17).

Strionigral fibers are topographically organized in that fibers from the head of

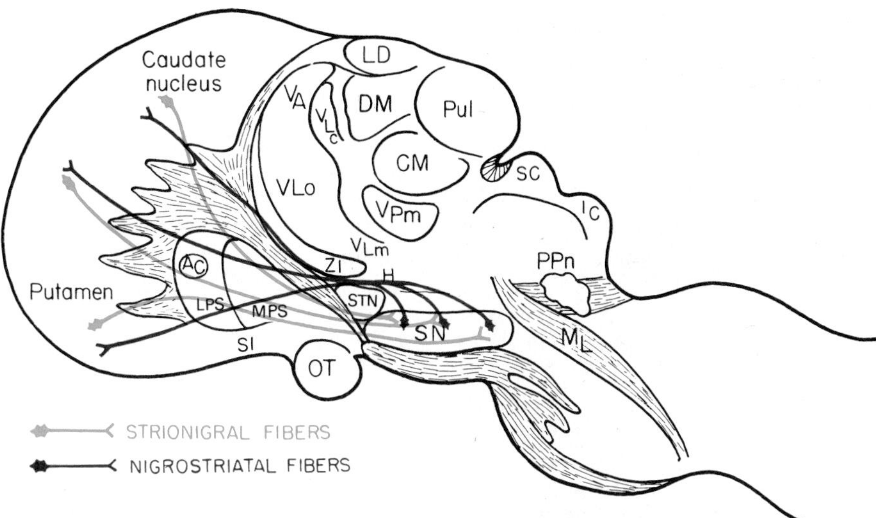

Figure 7-17. Schematic diagram of the strionigral and nigrostriatal feedback systems in a sagittal plane. Strionigral fibers (*blue*) project topographically upon cells of the pars reticulata of the nigra and have γ-aminobutyric acid (GABA) and substance P as their neurotransmitters; some fibers of a similar type convey the opioid peptide enkephalin to terminals in the pars reticulata. Enkephalin is considered to interact with known neurotransmitters. Cells of the pars compacta of the nigra give rise to reciprocally arranged nigrostriatal fibers (*red*) which convey dopamine to terminal varicosities within the striatum. Abbreviations: *AC*, anterior commissure; *CM*, centromedian nucleus; *IC*, inferior colliculus; *LD*, lateral dorsal nucleus; *LPS*, lateral segment of globus pallidus; *MD*, dorsomedial nucleus; *ML*, medial lemniscus; *MPS*, medial segment of globus pallidus; *OT*, optic tract; *PPn*, pedunculopontine nucleus; *Pul*, pulvinar; *SC*, superior colliculus; *SI*, substantia innominata; *SN*, substantia nigra; *STN*, subthalamic nucleus; *VA*, ventral anterior nucleus; *VLc, VLo* and *VLm*, ventral lateral nucleus, pars caudalis, pars oralis and pars medialis; *VPM*, ventral posterior medial nucleus; *ZI*, zona incerta. (From Carpenter and Sutin, *Human Neuroanatomy*, 1983; courtesy of Williams & Wilkins.)

the caudate nucleus project to the rostral third of the substantia nigra while the putamen projects to all other parts of the nigra (Szabo, '62, '67, '70). Virtually all of the strionigral fibers end upon dendrites of neurons in the pars reticulata (Grofová and Rinvik, '70). It has been suggested that strionigral fibers may be collaterals of stripallidal fibers (Fox and Rafols, '75; Fox et al., '75). Retrograde horseradish peroxidase (HRP) studies indicate that strionigral fibers arise from medium-sized, spiny striatal neurons (Grofová, '75; Bunney and Aghajanian, '76). Spiny striatal neurons projecting to the substantia nigra have at least three different neurotransmitters. Spiny neurons in all parts of the striatum appear to transport GABA to terminals in the substantia nigra (Okada et al., '71; Fonnum et al., '74). Rostral portions of the striatum give rise to an independent parallel projection that conveys substance P to particles in nerve endings in the pars reticulata (Davis and Dray, '76; Gale et al., '77). Spiny striatal neurons demonstrating enkephalin and projecting to the pars reticulata lie in medial regions of the caudate nucleus and ventromedial portions of the putamen (Emson et al., '80; DiFiglia et al., '82). In the cat a patch-like distribution of enkephalin-like immunoreactivity has been found in the caudate nucleus (Graybiel et al., '81a).

Pallidonigral projections have been identified by studies using horseradish peroxidase as a retrograde tracer; terminals in the pars reticulata have transported the enzyme to cells in the lateral pallidal segment (Grofová, '75; Bunney and Aghajanian, '76). Autoradiographic studies indicate that cells in both pallidal segments terminate preferentially upon dopaminergic neurons in the substantia nigra. These fibers are considered to have GABA as their neurotransmitter (Hattori et al., '75; Kanazawa et al., '77).

Subthalamonigral fibers have been demonstrated by both anterograde and retrograde transport studies (Kanazawa et al., '76; Nauta and Cole, '78; Carpenter et al., '81a). These fibers terminate in patchy areas in the pars reticulata. Fluorescent double-labeling studies suggest that in the rat virtually all cells in the subthalamic nucleus project axons to both the globus pallidus and the substantia nigra (Kooy and Hattori, '80).

Tegmentonigral fibers consist of projections from midbrain raphe nuclei that have serotonin (5-HT) as their neurotransmitter and projections from the pedunculopontine nucleus. The bulk of the serotonergic projections to the substantia nigra rise from the dorsal nucleus of the raphe; these neurons have an inhibitory action upon cells in the pars reticulata (Bunney and Aghajanian, '76; Dray et al., '76). Projections of the pedunculopontine nucleus appear to be mainly ascending (Fig. 11-24); the largest number of ascending fibers project to the substantia nigra, although smaller numbers of fibers project to the medial pallidal segment and the subthalamic nucleus (Moon Edley, '79; DeVito et al., '80; Nomura et al., '80; Carpenter et al., '81).

Nigral Efferent Projections. Efferent fibers arising from the pars compacta and pars reticulata of the substantia nigra are distinctive (Carpenter and Peter, '72) (Fig. 7-18). Nigrostriatal fibers originate from the pars compacta and project topographically upon all parts of the striatum (i.e., caudate nucleus and putamen) (Fig. 7-17). Nigrothalamic, nigrotectal and most of the nigrotegmental fibers arise from the pars reticulata.

Nigrostriatal fibers project dorsolaterally over the subthalamic nucleus and cross through the internal capsule (Figs. 7-17 and 7-18). These fibers traverse parts of the globus pallidus en route to the caudate nucleus and putamen. Retrograde transport studies of HRP in the cat and monkey provide data concerning the topographical organization of nigrostriatal projections (Szabo, '80, '80a). The projections of the pars compacta to the striatum are organized in all principal planes. The rostral two-thirds of the substantia nigra is related to the head of the caudate nucleus, while neurons projecting to the putamen are located posteriorly. An inverse relationship exists dorsoventrally between the substantia nigra and the caudate nucleus, so that ventral parts of the pars compacta project to dorsal regions of the caudate nucleus and dorsally situated neurons in the nigra pass to ventral regions of the caudate nucleus. Lateral and posterior regions of the nigra are related to dorsal and lateral parts of the putamen (Carpenter and Peter, '72). There is also a mediolateral correspondence between the cells of the substantia nigra and regions of fiber termination in the striatum. Biochemical and fluorescent histochemical studies not only provided convincing evidence that the large cells of the pars compacta project to striatum, but indicated that these fibers conveyed dopamine to their terminals (Andén et al., '64; Dahlström and Fuxe, '64; Fuxe and Andén, '66; Bedard et al., '69; Moore et al., '71). Histofluorescent studies indicated an extremely rich innervation of the striatum provided by neurons of the pars compacta. Data based upon this technic indicated that dopamine, stored in varicosities in nerve terminals, is mainly concentrated in three areas of the forebrain: (1) the striatum, (2) the nucleus accumbens septi, and (3) the olfactory bulb (Fuxe and Anden, '66). Varicosities, both terminal and nonterminal, in the striatum are fine, densely packed and exhibit a diffuse green fluorescence. Dopaminergic fibers form a matrix of fine varicose axons forming sworls around both small and large striatal neurons (Siggins et al., '76). In spite of difficulty in identifying "classic" terminations of dopamine fibers on caudate neurons, evidence indicates asymmetrical synapses on spiny processes with postsynaptic thickenings (Groves, '83). Nerve terminals containing dopamine have small granular vesicles about 50 nm in diameter (Hökfelt and Ungerstedt, '69). A consensus concerning the postsynaptic action of dopamine has not emerged (Groves, '83). Early evidence suggested an inhibitory influence upon striatal neurons, but intracellular recordings show that stimulation of the substantia nigra produces excitatory postsynaptic potentials (EPSPs) or excitatory-

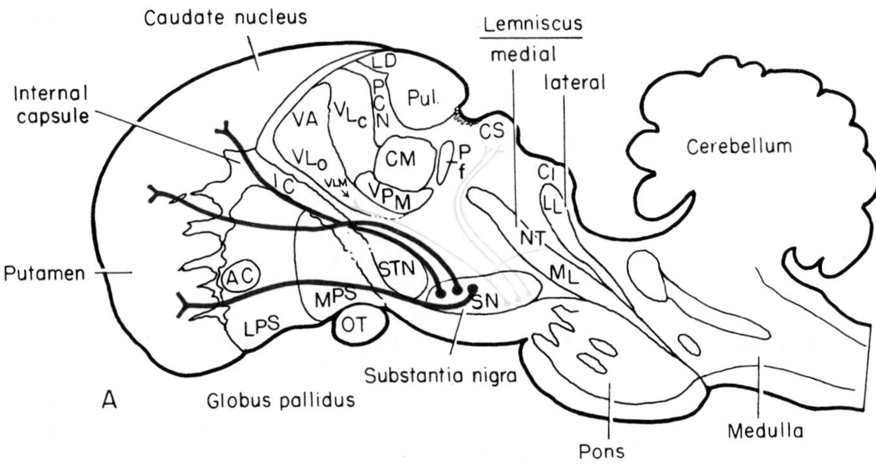

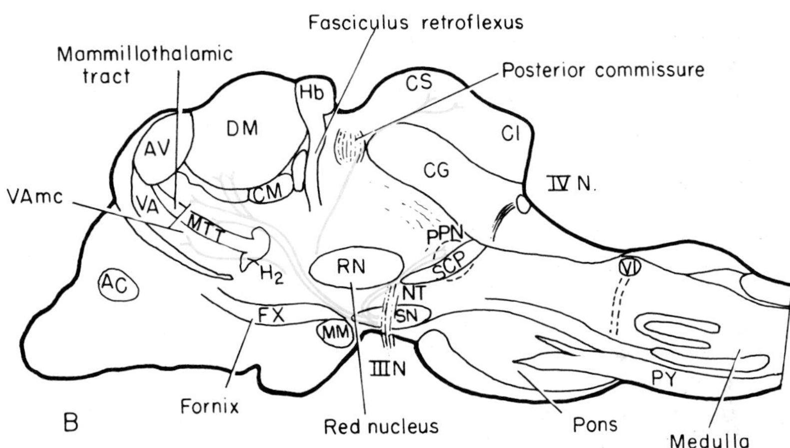

Figure 7-18. Schematic drawings of the efferent projections of the substantia nigra (*SN*) in sagittal sections. Ascending *nigrostriatal fibers* (*red*) arise from cells in the pars compacta and project through the internal capsule (*IC*) to terminations in the putamen and caudate nucleus (*A*). *Nigrothalamic*, *nigrotectal*, and *nigrotegmental* (*blue*) arise from cells in the pars reticulata (*A* and *B*). Nigrothalamic fibers (*blue*) project to medial parts of the ventral lateral nucleus (*VLM*), the magnocellular part of the ventral anterior nucleus (*VAmc*) and to the paralaminar part of the dorsomedial nucleus (*DM*). In part of their course these fibers parallel the mammillothalamic tract (*MTT*). Nigrotectal projections (*blue*) pass to middle gray layers in the caudal two-thirds of the superior colliculus (*A* and *B*). Nigrotegmental (*NT*) fibers (*blue*) project from the pars reticulata to the pedunculopontine nucleus (*PPN*) (see Fig. 11-24) or keep from the pars compacta to the raphe nuclei (not shown). Drawing *A* is lateral to drawing *B*. Abbreviations indicate the following: *AC*, anterior commissure; *AV*, anterior ventral thalamic nucleus; *CG*, central gray; *CI*, inferior colliculus; *CM*, centromedian thalamic nucleus; *CS*, superior colliculus; *DM*, dorsomedial thalamic nucleus; *FX*, fornix; H_2, lenticular fasciculus; *Hb*, habenular nucleus; *LD*, lateral dorsal thalamic nucleus; *LL*, lateral lemniscus; *LPS*, lateral pallidal segment; *ML*, medial lemniscus; *MM*, mammillary body; *MPS*, medial pallidal segment; *OT*, optic tract; *PCN*, paracentral thalamic nucleus; *Pf*, parafascicular nucleus; *PPN*, pedunculopontine nucleus; *Pul*, pulvinar; *PY*, medullary pyramid; *RN*, red nucleus; *SCP*, superior cerebellar peduncle; *STN*, subthalamic nucleus; *VA*, ventral anterior thalamic nucleus; *VLc* and *VLo*, ventral lateral thalamic nucleus (caudal and oral parts); *VPM*, ventral posteromedial thalamic nucleus; *VI*, abducens nucleus. (From Carpenter and Sutin, *Human Neuroanatomy*, 1983; courtesy of Williams & Wilkins.)

inhibitory (EPSP-IPSP) sequences in striatal neurons (Kitai et al., '76; Kitai, '81; Wilson et al., '82).

Strionigral and nigrostriatal fibers appear to form a closed feedback loop in which strionigral fibers form the afferent limb and nigrostriatal fibers constitute the efferent limb (Fig. 7-17). This reciprocal arrangement is evident in that HRP injected into the striatum is transported: (1) retrograde from axon terminals to cells of the pars compacta and (2) anterograde via striatal neurons to terminals in the pars reticulata of the substantia nigra (Nauta et al., '75). Spiny striatal neurons transport GABA, substance P and enkephalin to terminals in the pars reticulata of the substantia nigra. GABA appears to be inhibitory, while substance P is considered to be excitatory. The precise role of the opioid peptide, enkephalin, proposed to interact with known neurotransmitters, remains to be defined; it has been proposed that enkephalin may have a direct influence upon efferent systems originating from the substantia nigra (DiFiglia et al., '82).

Following lesions in the substantia nigra, dopamine in nigrostriatal nerve terminals disappears. In patients with paralysis agitans, there is a virtual absence of dopamine in the striatum and the substantia nigra (Hornykiewicz, '66). An effective treatment for this metabolic disorder is L-hydroxyphenylalanine (L-dopa), a precursor of dopamine, which passes the blood-brain barrier.

Nigrothalamic fibers arise from cells of the pars reticularis and project to: (1) the large-celled part of the ventral anterior nucleus (VAmc), (2) the medial part of the ventral lateral nucleus (VLm) and (3) parts of the dorsomedial nucleus (DMpl) (Carpenter and Peter, '72). These thalamic projections demonstrated by the retrograde transport of horseradish peroxidase (Rinvik, '75) and by autoradiographic tracing technics (Carpenter et al., '76), constitute a distinctive nigral efferent system (Fig 7-18).

Nigrotectal fibers have been described in almost all degeneration studies, but this finding originally was interpreted to be a consequence of interruption of corticotectal projections. Uncertainty concerning nigrotectal fibers has been resolved by axoplasmic transport studies which indicate that nigrotectal fibers: (1) arise only from cells of the pars reticulata (Graybiel and Sciascia, '75; Hopkins and Niessen, '76; Rinvik et al., '76); (2) project to the middle gray layers of the caudal two-thirds of the ipsilateral superior colliculus (Jayaraman et al., '77); and (3) may be topographically organized. Projections of nigrotectal fibers are to portions of the superior colliculus

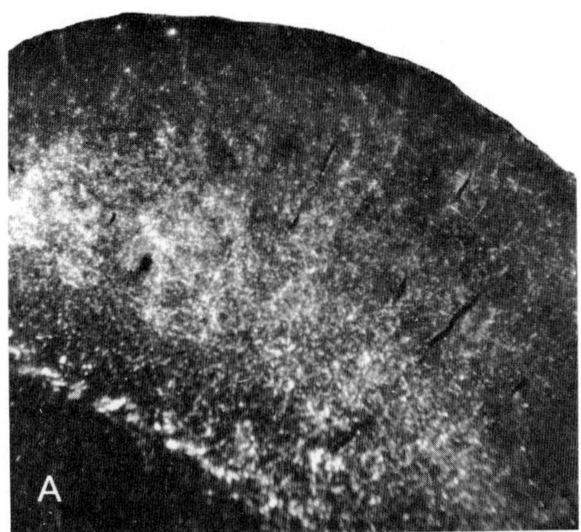

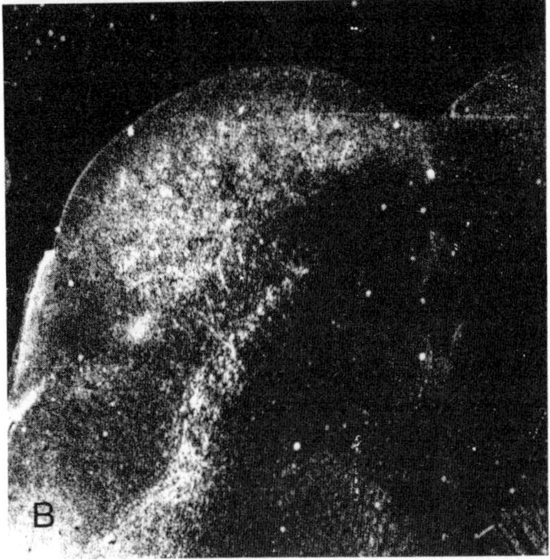

Figure 7-19. Dark-field photomicrograph of an autoradiograph demonstrating nigrotectal fibers in the monkey. Nigrotectal fibers arise from cells of the pars reticulata and project transtegmentally (*B*) to terminations mainly in the middle gray layers (*A*) of the superior colliculus (Jayaraman et al., '77). (From Carpenter and Sutin, *Human Neuroanatomy*, 1983; courtesy of Williams & Wilkins.)

which receive inputs not related to the visual system (Fig. 7-19).

The use of a fluorescent retrograde double labeling technic using Evans blue (fluoresces red) and mixture of DAPI-primuline (fluoresces a blue) has demonstrated that most cells in the pars reticulata of the substantia nigra project individudally to either the thalamus or the superior colliculus (Bentivoglio et al., '79). However, there are some cells in the pars reticulata with divergent axon collaterals that project to both the thalamus and the superior colliculus (double-labeled cells).

Nigrotegmental fibers arise from the pars reticulata and project nondopaminergic fibers to the pedunculopontine nucleus (Beckstead et al., '79; Moon Edley, '79; Carpenter et al., '81a). Cells of the pedunculopontine nucleus (Fig. 7-3) receive inputs from the cerebral cortex, the medial pallidal segment and the substantia nigra (Kuypers and Lawrence, '67; Beckstead et al., '79; Hartmann-von Monakow et al., '79; Carpenter et al., '81a). Subcortical inputs to the pedunculopontine nucleus are derived from structures that receive striatal afferents (i.e., the medial pallidal segment and the substantia nigra) and efferent projections of this nucleus are largely back to these same nuclei (Fig. 11-24). The pars compacta of the substantia nigra projects descending fibers into the tegmentum which terminate in the dorsal and median raphe nuclei (Beckstead et al., '79).

The substantia nigra is the brain stem nucleus most closely related to the largest part of the corpus striatum, the caudate nucleus, and the putamen and is the only brain nucleus that projects back to that massive structure in a reciprocal fashion. The pars reticulata receives its major input from the caudate nucleus and putamen. These strionigral fibers have GABA and substance P as their neurotransmitters, as well as the opioid peptide enkephalin, considered to interact with neurotransmitters. Cells in the pars compacta of the substantia nigra convey dopamine to terminals within the striatum. Cells of the pars reticulata constitute an important output component of the corpus striatum which is different from that arising from the medial pallidal segment. Projections of the pars reticulata of the substantia nigra are to different thalamic nuclei (VAmc, VLm, and DMpl) than the medial pallidal segment. Although both the pars reticulata and medial pallidal segment project to the pedunculopontine nucleus at midbrain levels, only the pars reticulata has projections to the superior colliculus. Nigrothalamic and pallidothalamic projections collectively constitute the major output system of the corpus striatum complex (Carpenter, '81). The substantia nigra is the principal site of the pathological process which underlies the metabolic disturbances associated with paralysis agitans (Hassler, '39; Hornykiewicz, '66). Discrete lesions of the substantia nigra nucleus do not produce tremor, alterations of muscle tone, or impairment of associated movements, although they interfere with a variety of neurotransmitters (Carpenter and McMasters, '64; Poirier and Sourkes, '65).

CRUS CEREBRI

The most ventral part of the midbrain contains a massive bundle of corticofugal fibers, the crus cerebri. Classically the medial two-thirds of the crus are thought to contain *corticospinal* and *corticobulbar fibers* (Fig. 7-1); the most lateral fibers in this part of the crus are related to the lower extremity, the most medial to the musculature of the face and larynx, and the intermediate fibers to the upper extremity. Extreme medial and lateral portions of the crus contain corticopontine fibers. Frontopontine fibers are medial while corticopontine fibers from the temporal, parietal and occipital areas are located laterally. More recent data indicate that corticospinal fibers in the internal capsule are largely confined to a compact region in the caudal part of the posterior limb of the internal capsule (Gillingham, '62; Bertrand et al., '65; Smith, '67; Englander et al., '75; Hanaway and Young, '77). Somatotopical organization of fibers destined for particular segmental levels appears relatively crude. These data suggest that the somatotopic arrangement of corticospinal fibers in the crus cerebri probably is much less precise than commonly depicted. In man, corticospinal fibers probably account for only 1 million of the 20 million fibers in the crus cerebri; the remaining fibers are largely corticopontine (Tomasch, '69).

CHAPTER 8

The Cerebellum

The cerebellum is derived from ectodermal thickenings about the cephalic borders of the fourth ventricle, known as the rhombic lip. Although the cerebellum is derived from portions of the embryonic neural tube dorsal to the sulcus limitans and receives sensory inputs from virtually all types of receptors, it is not concerned with conscious sensory perception. Sensory information transmitted to the cerebellum is used in the automatic coordination of somatic motor function, the regulation of muscle tone and the maintenance of equilibrium. This metencephalic derivative functions in a suprasegmental manner in that its integrative influences affect activities at all levels of the neuraxis. The major influences of the cerebellum upon segmental levels of the neuraxis are mediated indirectly by relay nuclei of the brain stem.

Structurally the cerebellum consists of: (1) a superficial gray mantle, the *cerebellar cortex*; (2) an internal white mass, the *medullary substance*; and (3) four pairs of *intrinsic nuclei* embedded in the white matter. The cerebellum is divided into a median portion, the *cerebellar vermis*, and two lateral lobes, referred to as the *cerebellar hemispheres*. The cerebellar cortex is composed of numerous narrow *laminae* or *folia*, most of which are oriented transversely. Five deep fissures divide the cerebellum into lobes and lobules (Fig. 8-1). All of these fissures can be identified in gross specimens as well as in midsagittal section (Figs. 2-26, 2-27, 2-28, and 2-29). The cerebellar fissures are: (1) the *primary*, (2) the *posterior superior*, (3) the *horizontal*, (4) the *prepyramidal*, and (5) the *posterolateral* (prenodular). These fissures form the basis for all subdivisions of the cerebellum (Fig. 8-1). Portions of the cerebellar vermis in Figure 8-1 are labeled by name and *Roman numerals*. The portion of the lateral lobe between the primary and the posterior superior fissures is known as the *simple lobule*. The *ansiform lobule* lies between the posterior superior fissure and the gracile lobule and is divided by the horizontal fissure into *crus I* (superior semilunar lobule) and *crus II* (inferior semilunar lobule). The *biventer lobule* and the *cerebellar tonsil* lie between

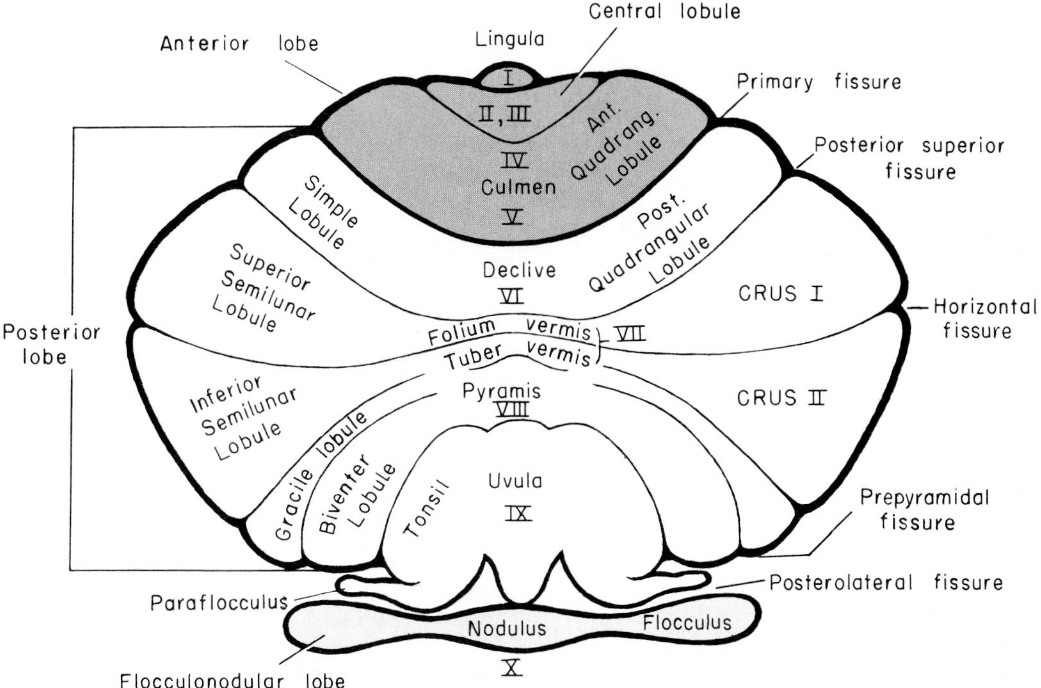

Figure 8-1. Schematic diagram of the fissures and lobules of the cerebellum (Larsell, '51; Jansen and Brodal, '58; Angevine et al., '61). Portions of the cerebellum caudal to the posterolateral fissure (*blue*) represent the flocculonodular lobule (archicerebellum), while portions of the cerebellum rostral to the primary fissure (*red*) constitute the anterior lobe (paleocerebellum). The neocerebellum lies between the primary and posterolateral fissure. *Roman numerals* refer to portions of the cerebellar vermis only. (From Carpenter and Sutin, *Human Neuroanatomy*, 1983; courtesy of Williams & Wilkins.)

the prepyramidal and posterolateral fissures in the cerebellar hemisphere (Fig. 2-28).

Embryologically and functionally the cerebellum can be divided into three parts. The *archicerebellum*, represented by the *nodulus*, the paired *flocculi* and their peduncular connections (i.e., the *flocculonodular lobule*), is phylogenetically the oldest part. This division of the cerebellum is most closely related to the vestibular system and is separated from the posterior lobe of the cerebellum by the posterolateral fissure (*blue* in Fig. 8-1). The *paleocerebellum* (i.e., the anterior lobe of the cerebellum) lies rostral to the primary fissure (*red* in Fig. 8-1). This division of the cerebellum receives impulses from stretch receptors via the spinocerebellar tracts and is the part most concerned with the regulation of muscle tone. The largest and phylogenetically newest portion of the cerebellum is the *neocerebellum*. This part of the cerebellum lies between the primary and posterolateral fissures (Fig. 8-1).

The gross anatomy of the cerebellum is described in Chapter 2, pages 47–50. The cerebellum is attached to the medulla, pons and midbrain by three paired cerebellar peduncles. These peduncles serve to connect the cerebellum with the spinal cord, brain stem and higher levels of the neuraxis.

CEREBELLAR CORTEX

The cerebellar cortex is uniformly structured in all parts and extends across the midline without evidence of a median raphe (Fig. 2-26). The cortex is composed of three well-defined layers containing five different types of neurons. These layers from the surface are: (1) the molecular layer, (2) the Purkinje cell layer, and (3) the granular layer (Fig. 8-2).

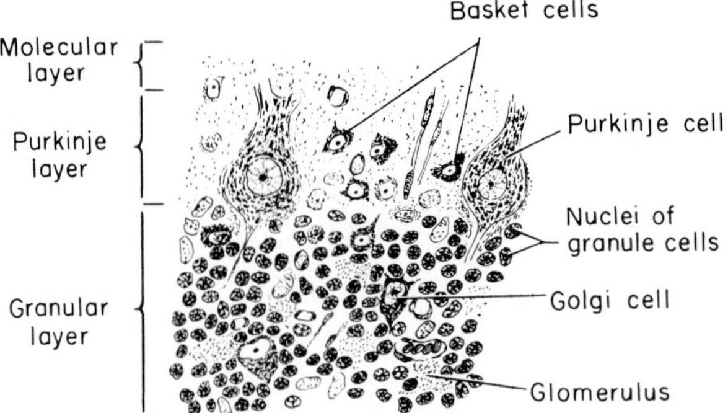

Figure 8-2. Drawing of portions of the three layers of the human cerebellar cortex (after Cajal, '11). (Nissl stain.) (From Carpenter and Sutin, *Human Neuroanatomy*, 1983; courtesy of Williams & Wilkins.)

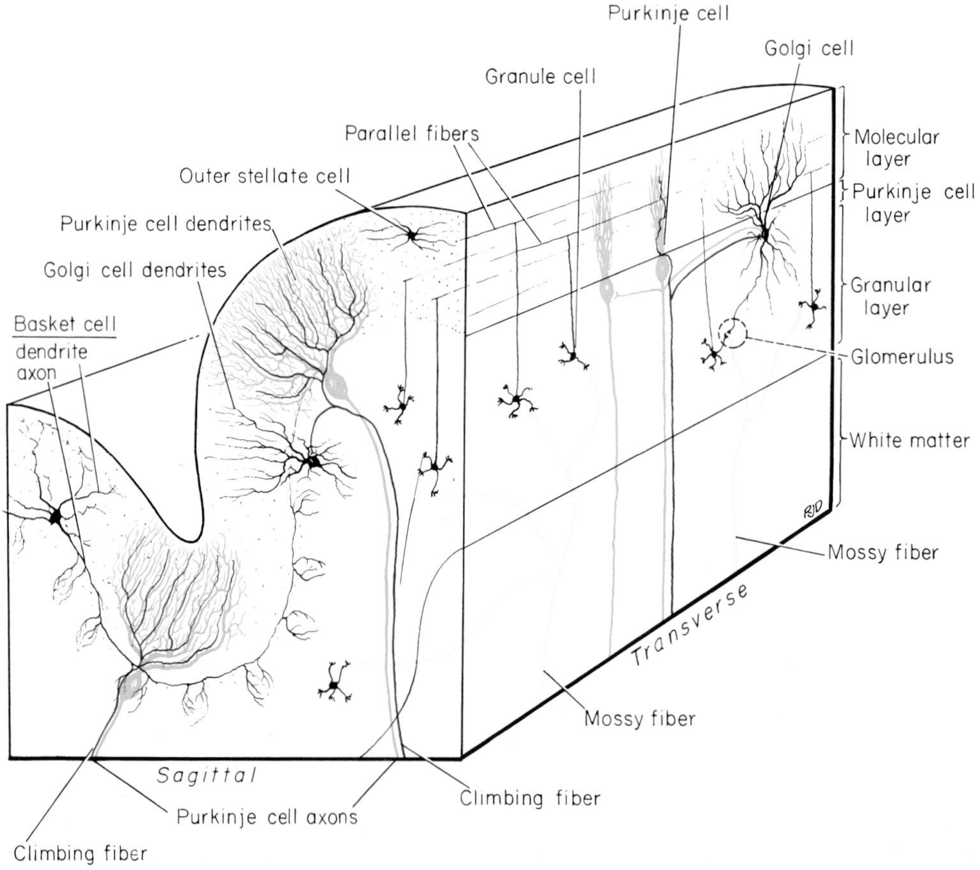

Figure 8-3. Schematic diagram of the cerebellar cortex in sagittal and transverse planes showing cell and fiber arrangements. Purkinje cells and cell processes (i.e., axons and dendrites) are shown in *blue*. Mossy fibers are in *yellow*; climbing fibers are shown in *red*. Golgi cells, basket cells, and outer stellate cells are in *black*. While the dendritic arborizations of Purkinje cells are oriented in a sagittal plane, dendrites of the Golgi cells show no similar arrangement. Layers of the cerebellar cortex are indicated. (From Carpenter and Sutin, *Human Neuroanatomy*, 1983; courtesy of Williams & Wilkins.)

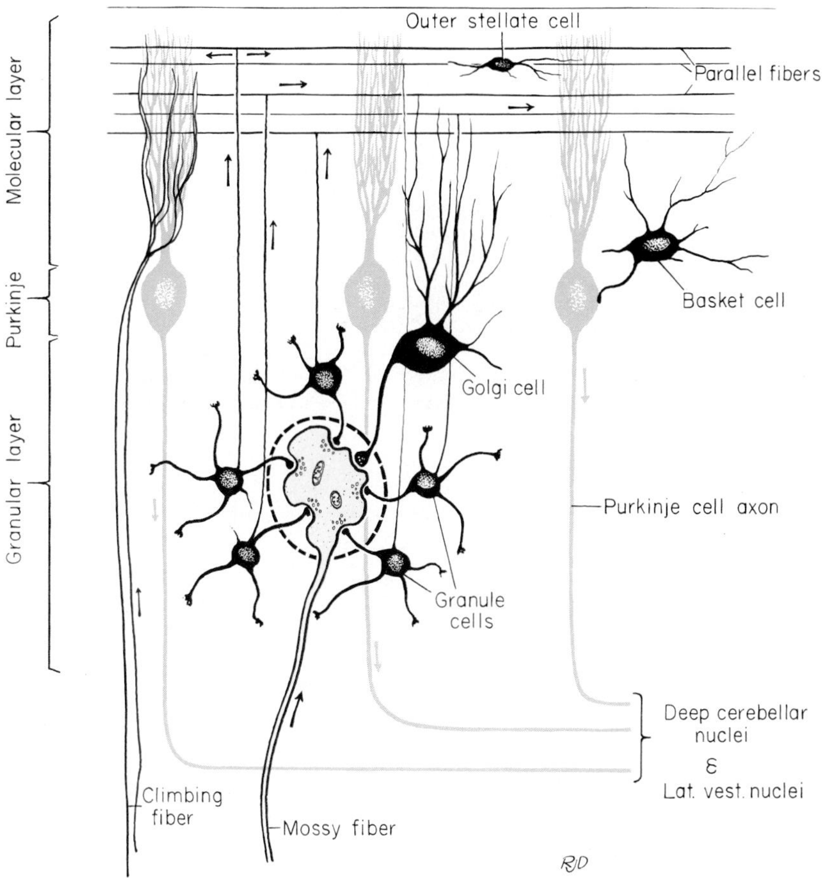

Figure 8-4. Schematic diagram of the cellular and fiber elements of the cerebellar cortex in the longitudinal axis of a folium. Excitatory inputs to the cerebellar cortex are conveyed by the mossy fibers (*yellow*) and the climbing fibers (*red*). The *broken line* represents a glia lamella ensheathing a glomerulus, containing: (a) a mossy fiber rosette, (b) several granule cell dendrites, and (c) one Golgi cell axon. Axons of granule cells ascend to the molecular layer, bifurcate, and form an extensive system of parallel fibers which synapse on the spiny processes of the Purkinje cells. Purkinje cells and their processes are shown in *blue*. Climbing fibers traverse the granular layer and ascend the dendrites of the Purkinje cells where they synapse on smooth branchlets. *Arrows* indicate the directions of impulse conduction. Outer stellate and basket cells are shown in the molecular layer, but the axons of the basket cells which ramify about Purkinje cell somata are not shown (based on Gray, '61; Eccles et al., '67.) (From Carpenter and Sutin, *Human Neuroanatomy*, 1983; courtesy of Williams & Wilkins.)

Molecular Layer. The molecular layer contains two types of neurons, dendritic arborizations, and numerous thin axons coursing parallel to the long axis of the folia. Cells found in the molecular layer are the basket cell and the outer stellate cell (Figs. 8-3 and 8-4). Dendrites of these cells are confined to the molecular layer, as are the axons of the outer stellate cells. Processes of both cells are oriented transversely to the long axis of the folia. Axons of *outer stellate cells* make synaptic contacts with Purkinje cell dendrites. *Basket cells*, located near Purkinje cell bodies, give rise to dendrites that ascend in the molecular layer and elaborate unmyelinated axons that form intricate terminal arborizations about the somata of many Purkinje cells. A single basket cell may establish synaptic relationships with 10 Purkinje cells in a plane transverse to the folia. In addition to the relatively few cells, the molecular layer contains the dendrites of Purkinje and Golgi type II cells and the transversely oriented axons of granule cells (i.e., parallel fibers).

Purkinje Cell Layer. This layer con-

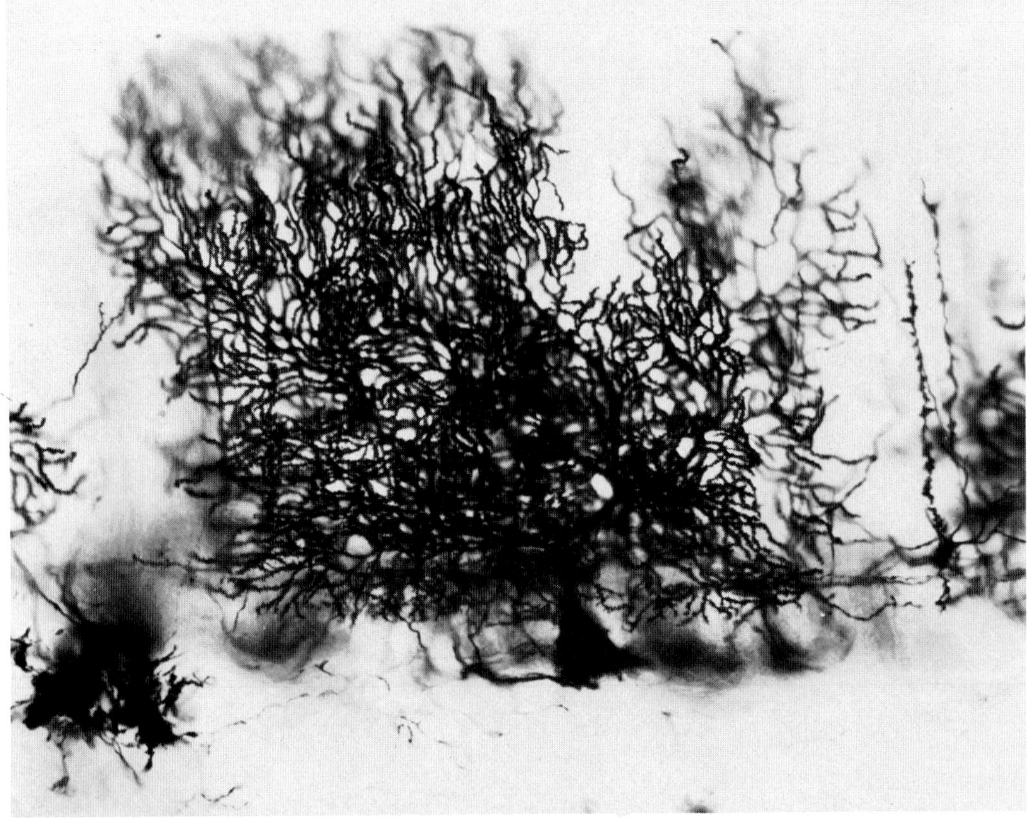

Figure 8-5. Photograph of a single Purkinje cell and its rich dendritic arborizations in the molecular layer (×300). (Courtesy of the late Dr. C. A. Fox, School of Medicine, Wayne State University.) (From Carpenter and Sutin, *Human Neuroanatomy*, 1983; courtesy of Williams & Wilkins.)

sists of great numbers of large flask shaped cells uniformly arranged along the upper margin of the granular layer (Figs. 8-2, 8-3, 8-4, 8-5, and 8-6). Purkinje cells have a clear vesicular nucleus with a deep staining nucleolus and irregular Nissl granules. Each cell gives rise to an elaborate flattened, fanlike dendritic tree oriented at right angles to the long axis of the folia. The full extent of the dendritic arborization can be appreciated only in sagittal sections (Figs. 8-3, 8-5 and 8-6). Primary and secondary dendritic branches are smooth, but tertiary dendritic branches have spines which are short, thick and rough. These thick dendritic spines are referred to as *spiny branchlets* or gemmules (Fig. 8-5). Larger dendritic processes bear stubbier spines known as *smooth branchlets.* Purkinje cell axons are myelinated, pass through the granular layer and white matter, and establish synaptic contacts with the deep cerebellar nuclei (Fig. 8-4). Some Purkinje cell axons from vermal cortex pass to the lateral vestibular nucleus. Axons of Purkinje cells represent the discharge pathway from the cerebellar cortex (Hámori and Szentágothai, '66). Purkinje cell collaterals make synaptic contact with Golgi type II cells in the granular layer (Fig. 8-3). Histochemical studies indicate that γ-aminobutyric acid (GABA) is the neurotransmitter released at the synapse (Fonnum et al., '70; Fonnum and Walberg, '73; Chan-Palay, '77). Intracellular iontophoresis of horseradish peroxidase (HRP) into a single Purkinje cell results in transport of the enzyme into the dendritic arborizations and into the axon (Fig. 8-6).

Granular Layer. This layer is composed of closely packed chromatic nuclei that in stained sections resemble lymphocytes (Fig. 8-2). Granule cells are so numerous (3 to 7 million cells per cubic mil-

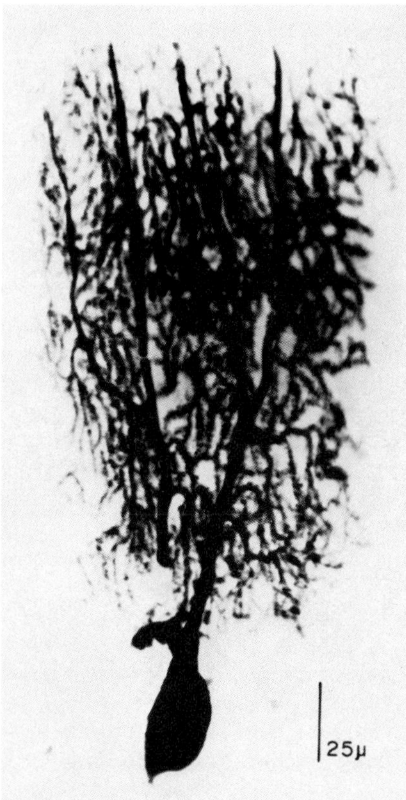

Figure 8-6. Photomicrograph of a single Purkinje cell labeled iontophoretically with horseradish peroxidase (HRP). This technic labels the dendritic arborization, the axon and axonal collaterals. (Courtesy of Dr. S. T. Kitai, School of Medicine, University of Tennessee.) (From Carpenter and Sutin, *Human Neuroanatomy*, 1983; courtesy of Williams & Wilkins.)

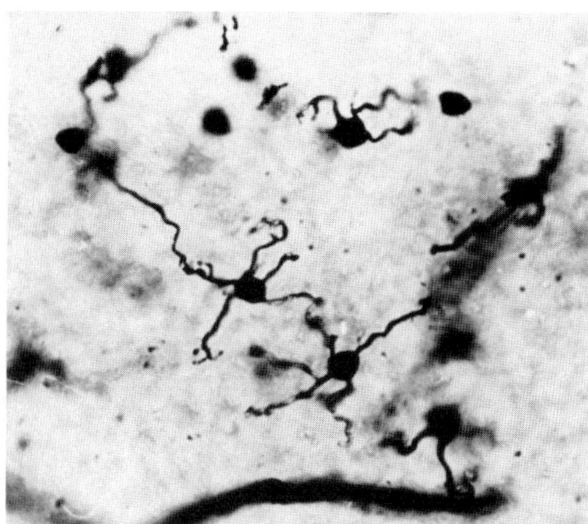

Figure 8-7. Photomicrograph of granule cells in the cerebellar cortex showing short dendrites with clawlike endings. (Golgi preparation; ×200.) (Courtesy of Dr. Donald B. Newman, Uniformed Services University.)

limeter) that residual space seems insufficient to accommodate their processes or other fibers of passage. These cells are round or oval, 5 to 8 μm in diameter, with aggregated chromatin granules near the nuclear membrane. Granule cell nuclei appear naked because of the thinness of the rimming cytoplasm and the absence of discrete Nissl granules. Each granule cell gives rise to four or five short dendrites which end in the "glomeruli" (Fig. 8-7). The so-called "cerebellar islands" or "glomeruli" are irregularly dispersed spaces free of granule cells (Figs. 8-2 and 8-3). Axons of granule cells are ummyelinated fibers that ascend vertically into the molecular layer and bifurcate into branches which run parallel to the long axis of the folium (Figs. 8-3 and 8-4). These fibers, referred to as *parallel fibers*, are found throughout the molecular layer where they are oriented perpendicular to the dendritic expansions of the Purkinje cells. In a descriptive sense, they resemble telegraph wires strung through the branches of a bushy tree. Granule cell axons make synaptic contacts with the spiny processes of Purkinje cells; this synaptic contact between the parallel fibers and the Purkinje cell dendrites is called the "crossover" synapse (Figs. 8-3 and 8-4).

Golgi type II cells, found mainly in the upper part of the granular layer, have vesicular nuclei and definite chromophilic bodies (Figs. 8-2, 8-3, and 8-4). Dendrites of these cells extend throughout all layers of the cerebellar cortex, and arborizations are not restricted in orientation (Figs. 8-3 and 8-4). Golgi cell dendrites are in contact with parallel fibers in the molecular layer, while axonal arborizations are dense within the granular layer beneath the cell body. Axons of these cells terminate within the "glomeruli."

Cortical Input. Afferent fibers to the cerebellum convey impulses primarily to the cerebellar cortex. These tracts enter the cerebellum mainly via the inferior and middle cerebellar peduncles and include the spinocerebellar, cuneocerebellar, olivocerebellar, vestibulocerebellar and pontocerebellar tracts, as well as numerous smaller bundles. Within the cerebellar cortex these

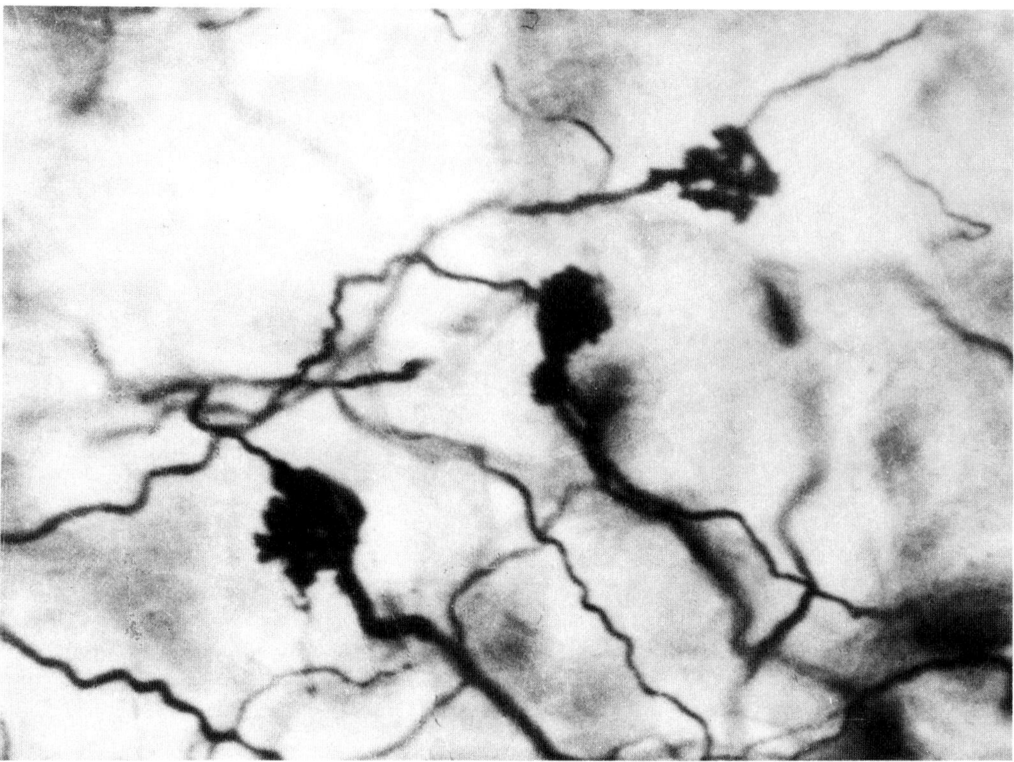

Figure 8-8. Mossy fiber rosettes in the granular layer of the monkey cerebellum as seen in a Golgi preparation. Although mossy fiber rosettes appear as solid structures under low magnifications, under oil immersion the rosettes appear as coiled convoluted fibers, (×850). (Courtesy of the late Dr. C. A. Fox, School of Medicine, Wayne State University.) (From Carpenter and Sutin, *Human Neuroanatomy*, 1983; courtesy of Williams & Wilkins.)

fibers lose their myelin sheath and end either as mossy fibers or climbing fibers.

Mossy fibers bifurcate repeatedly in the white matter, enter the granular layer and often provide branches to adjacent folia (Fig. 8-3). These fibers pass into the granular layer, lose their myelin sheath and give off many fine collaterals. Fine lobulated enlargements occur along the course of the branches and at their terminals; these are referred to as *mossy fiber rosettes*. A single mossy fiber may have as many as 44 mossy fiber rosettes along its many branches (Fox, et al., '67). Each mossy fiber rosette forms the center of a cerebellar glomerulus. In Golgi preparations under oil immersion, mossy fiber rosettes appear as coiled, convoluted fibers (Fig. 8-8; Fox et al., '67). Electron micrographs also reveal synaptic vesicles, concentrations of mitochondria, and a conspicuous core of neurofilaments and neurotubules (Mugnaini, '72).

A *glomerulus* is a complex synaptic structure contained within the "cerebellar islands" of the granular layer (Figs. 8-3, 8-4 and 8-9). A cerebellar glomerulus is a nodular structure formed by: (1) one mossy fiber rosette, (2) the dendritic terminals of numerous granule cells, (3) the terminals of Golgi cell axons, and (4) proximal parts of Golgi cell dendrites. The center of the glomerulus contains a single mossy fiber rosette (Fig. 8-8) with which dendrites of about 20 different granule cells interdigitate (Figs. 8-4 and 8-9). Axons of Golgi cells form a plexus on the outer surface of the granule cell dendrites. The entire structure is encased in a single glial lamella (Eccles et al., '67). In the glomerulus the mossy fiber-granule cell synapse is excitatory, while the Golgi axon-granule cell junction is inhibitory. Thus a cerebellar glomerulus is basically a synaptic cluster in which two types of presynaptic fibers enter into a com-

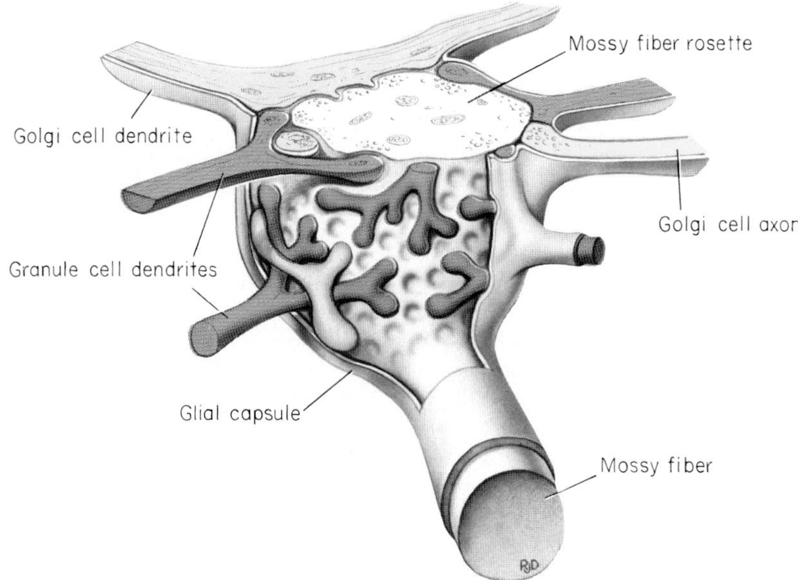

Figure 8-9. Schematic reconstruction of a cerebellar glomerulus based upon electron microscopic studies. A cerebellar glomerulus is formed by one mossy fiber rosette, the dendritic terminals of numerous granule cells (*red*), and terminals of Golgi cell axons (*yellow*). Proximal parts of Golgi dendrites (*blue*) also enter the glomerulus and establish broad synaptic contacts with the mossy fiber rosette. The entire nodular structure is ensheathed in a glial capsule. In this reconstruction the glomerulus is shown in horizontal section, and in a schematic three-dimensional view (based on Eccles et al., '67). (From Carpenter and Sutin, *Human Neuroanatomy*, 1983; courtesy of Williams & Wilkins.)

plex relationship with one postsynaptic element. The granule cell and its dendrites constitute the postsynaptic element. Golgi cells function as a negative feedback to the mossy fiber-granule cell relay.

Climbing fibers pass from the white matter through the granular and Purkinje cell layer to reach the dendrites of the Purkinje cells (Figs. 8-3 and 8-4). These non-myelinated fibers divide into numerous branches and climb the dendritic arborizations of the Purkinje cells. Climbing fibers contact only the smooth branches of Purkinje cell dendrites. Many climbing fibers form infraganglionic plexuses immediately beneath the Purkinje cell layer before turning toward the surface to be displayed over the dendritic arbor of a single Purkinje cell (Fig. 8-3). Golgi studies indicate that collaterals of climbing fibers may establish synaptic contact with adjacent Purkinje cells (Scheibel and Scheibel, '54), but these appear insignificant in comparison to the repeated synaptic contacts that a climbing fiber makes with dendrites of its own Purkinje cell (Eccles et al., '67). Although climbing fibers and basket cell axons partially overlap on portions of the Purkinje cell dendritic tree, there are no synaptic contacts between these fibers (Chan-Palay and Palay, '70).

Physiologically the climbing fiber system is remarkably specific. Each climbing fiber possesses an extensive all-or-none excitatory connection with Purkinje cell dendrites. When a climbing fiber discharges, the Purkinje cell also discharges. Stimulation of a climbing fiber not only excites a single Purkinje cell, but it also excites a number of granule cells whose axons (parallel fibers) in turn excite Purkinje cells arranged in the long axis of a folium.

The respective sources of mossy and climbing fibers have been difficult to determine. Mossy fibers constitute the principal mode of termination of most cerebellar afferent systems. The spinocerebellar, pontocerebellar, and vestibulocerebellar systems terminate as mossy fibers. Most climbing fibers are believed to be terminals of fibers arising from the inferior olivary nuclear complex (Szentágothai and Rajkovits, '59; Eccles et al., '67). Autoradiographic studies also conclude that the climbing fibers originate from the inferior olivary complex and are crossed (Batini et al., '76; Courville and Faraco-Cantin, '78). Olivocerebellar fibers terminate in a pattern of thin sagittal strips that interdigitate with unlabeled strips (Courville, '75). Because it has been shown that olivary neurons distribute fibers to different regions of the cerebellar cortex, it has been postulated that the empty strips receive climbing fibers from other unlabeled regions of the inferior olivary nucleus, rather than from extraolivary sources. This concept has been strengthened by data demonstrating that injections of [^{3}H]amino acids into the pons, reticulotegmental nucleus, the lateral reticular nucleus, the spinal trigeminal nucleus, the inferior vestibular nucleus and the accessory cuneate nucleus have labeled only mossy fibers (Courville and Faraco-Cantin, '78).

Fluorescence microscopy has revealed a hitherto unrecognized fiber system in the cerebellar cortex which contains norepinephrine (Hökfelt and Fuxe, '69). These fibers (Fig. 6-28), detectable by their green fluorescence, are present in all layers of the cortex, are not restricted to any particular plane, and are moderately concentrated in the Purkinje cell layer (Palay and Chan-Palay,'74). These fibers are considered to arise from the locus ceruleus (Figs. 6-26, 6-27, and 6-28) and establish synaptic contacts with Purkinje cells somata (Olson and Fuxe, '71; Bloom et al., '71; Pickel et al., '74). An HRP study in the cat indicates that cells in the caudal half of the locus ceruleus project to the entire cerebellar vermis, the flocculus, and the ventral paraflocculus (Somana and Walberg, '78). These authors found no evidence of a projection to the cerebellar cortex of the hemisphere.

The raphe nuclei which synthesize and transmit serotonin (5-hydroxytryptamine; 5-HT) to various parts of the central nervous system project fibers to the cerebellum, presumably via periventricular routes (Chan-Palay, '77). The largest number of serotonergic fibers appear to arise from the raphe nuclei of the pons and medulla (Taber-Pierce et al., '77; Gould, '80), although other raphe nuclei may make some contribution. All parts of the cerebellar cortex receive afferents from the raphe nuclei, with the most profuse projections passing to lobules VII and X of the vermis and to crus I and II (Gould, '80). Axons of raphe neurons: (1) terminate as mossy fiber rosettes in the granular layer, (2) terminate diffusely throughout all cortical layers without specialized junctions, and (3) pass directly to the molecular layer where they bifurcate like parallel fibers and establish synaptic contacts with cerebellar interneurons (Chan-Palay, '77). Serotonergic fibers differ from noradrenergic afferents in the molecular layer in that they do not synapse upon Purkinje cells.

Structural Mechanisms. Intricate geometric relationships of elements within the cerebellar cortex have furnished many hypotheses concerning the functions of individual neurons. Physiological studies indicate that: (1) climbing fibers exert powerful excitatory synaptic drives upon Purkinje cell dendrites (Eccles et al., '67), (2) parallel fiber systems excite Purkinje cells via "cross-over" synapses, and (3) outer stellate cells, basket cells, and Golgi type II cells are inhibitory interneurons in the cerebellar cortex. Outer stellate cells exert inhibitory influences on dendrites of Purkinje cells. Basket cell inhibition, effected by axo-somatic synapses on Purkinje cell somata, involves many Purkinje cells in a sagittal plane. Golgi type II cells inhibit afferent input to the cerebellar cortex at the mossy fiber-granule cell relay in the glomeruli. Because Golgi cell axons reach glomeruli throughout the depth of the cerebellar cortex, they can inhibit input via mossy fibers to parallel fibers for a considerable distance.

The cerebellar cortex has an elaborate structural and functional organization in which multiple interactions influence input, conduction, and synaptic articulations. The entire output of the cerebellar cortex is represented by the discharge of Purkinje cells. Every Purkinje cell is subject to two distinct excitatory inputs via: (1) climbing fibers and (2) mossy fibers. Climbing fibers have powerful, direct, all-or-none, excitatory action upon a single Purkinje cell

(Eccles et al., '66). The same climbing fiber has synaptic articulations with inhibitory interneurons, the Golgi type II, stellate, and basket cells. Excitation of basket cells results in inhibition of Purkinje cells on both sides of the single Purkinje cell receiving the main branches of a climbing fiber. A single basket cell theoretically could inhibit 7 rows of about 10 Purkinje cells. The excitation of Golgi cells via climbing fibers results in the inhibition of impulses through all glomeruli reached by the ramifications of the Golgi cell axon. This mechanism depresses the activity in Purkinje cells on both sides of the single Purkinje cell excited by the climbing fiber. The widespread inhibitory influence exerted by a single climbing fiber via interneurons appears to be a device to silence the background for a single Purkinje cell activated by a climbing fiber volley (Eccles et al., '67). Mossy fiber impulses exert their synaptic excitatory action solely within the cerebellar glomerulus, where they excite granule cells whose axons (the parallel fibers) excite all cells with dendrites in the molecular layer (i.e., Purkinje, basket, stellate and Golgi cells). Impulses conveyed to dendrites in the molecular layer by parallel fibers result in excitation of: (1) a narrow band of Purkinje and Golgi cells in the longitudinal axis of the folia, and (2) basket and outer stellate cells whose axons extend sagittally (transverse to the folia) on each side of the excited band of parallel fibers. This geometric configuration results in excitation of a narrow band of Purkinje cells, flanked on each side by Purkinje cells inhibited by basket and stellate cells (Eccles et al., '67).

The entire output of the cerebellar cortex, conveyed by Purkinje cell axons, is inhibitory (Eccles et al., '67; Ito et al., '64; Ito and Yoshida, '66). Thus, axons of Purkinje cells exert inhibitory influences upon cells with which they synapse, namely those of the deep cerebellar nuclei and portions of the vestibular nuclei. The neurotransmitter responsible for Purkinje cell inhibition is γ-aminobutyric acid (GABA) (Kuriyama et al., '66; Fonnum and Walberg, '73). Purkinje cell collaterals taking origin from proximal portions of the axon (Fig. 8-3) exert inhibitory influences upon Golgi cells that in turn inhibit granule cells; this disinhibition tends to release granule cells whose axons excite Purkinje cells.

DEEP CEREBELLAR NUCLEI

The corpus medullare is a compact mass of white matter, continuous from hemisphere to hemisphere and continuous with the three paired peduncles which connect the cerebellum with the brain stem. The four paired deep cerebellar nuclei are imbedded in the white matter of the cerebellum. From medial to lateral these nuclei are the fastigial, the globose, the emboliform and the dentate.

Dentate Nucleus. This nucleus, the largest of the deep cerebellar nuclei, lies in the white matter of the cerebellar hemisphere (Figs. 8-10 and 8-11). This large nucleus in section appears as a convoluted band of gray, having the shape of a folded bag with the opening or hilus directed medially. Its resemblance to the inferior olivary complex is obvious (Fig. 6-20). The nucleus is composed mainly of large multipolar neurons with branching dendrites. Axons of these cells acquire a myelin sheath within the nuclei and pass through the white matter to enter the superior cerebellar peduncle (Larsell and Jansen, '72).

Emboliform Nucleus. This is a wedge-shaped cell mass situated close to the hilus of the dentate nucleus. It is composed of cells similar to those found in the dentate nucleus and often is difficult to delimit from the latter (Figs. 6-20 and 8-11).

Globose Nucleus. This nucleus consists of one or more rounded cell groups lying medial to the emboliform nucleus and lateral to the fastigial nucleus (Figs. 6-20 and 8-11). His nucleus contains both large and small multipolar neurons.

In lower mammals the emboliform and globose nuclei appear continuous and collectively are referred to as the *nucleus interpositus*. However, cytological differences and distinctive connections make it possible to divide this complex into two parts: (1) the anterior interposed nucleus, considered to be the homologue of the emboliform nucleus, and (2) the posterior interposed nucleus which is homologous to the globose nucleus in man (Courville and Cooper, '70).

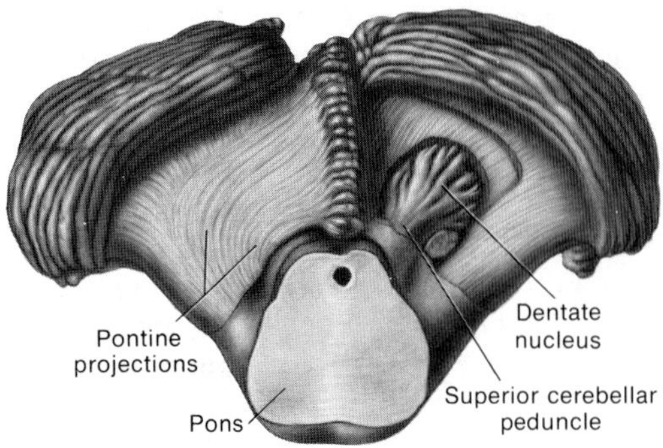

Figure 8-10. Drawing of a dissection of the superior surface of the cerebellum exposing the dentate nucleus (from Mettler's *Neuroanatomy*, 1948). (From Carpenter and Sutin, *Human Neuroanatomy*, 1983; courtesy of Williams & Wilkins.)

Fastigial Nucleus. The most medial of the deep cerebellar nuclei, the fastigial nucleus, lies near the mid-line in the roof of the fourth ventricle (Fig. 6-20). There are cytological differences within the fastigial nucleus, in that smaller cells are found in ventral regions. Cell strands emerging from the lateral border of the nucleus extend ventrolaterally toward the vestibular nuclei. Golgi studies indicate that both large and small cells have dendrites radiating in all directions which bear spines on distal branches (Matsushita and Iwahori, '71). Dendritic fields of neurons within the nucleus show extensive overlap, but there is no evidence of Golgi type II cells. Unlike the other deep cerebellar nuclei, cells of the fastigial nucleus give rise to both crossed and uncrossed axons; axons crossing to the opposite side are most numerous in rostral regions of the nucleus (Carpenter and Batton, '82).

CONNECTIONS OF THE DEEP CEREBELLAR NUCLEI

Corticonuclear Projections. The largest number of afferents to the deep cerebellar nuclei arise from Purkinje cells and have GABA as their neurotransmitter. All parts of the cerebellar cortex project fibers to the deep cerebellar nuclei. Cerebellar cortical projections to the deep cerebellar nuclei have been divided into three rostrocaudal longitudinal zones: (1) a medial or vermal zone projecting to the fastigial nucleus, (2) a paravermal zone projecting to the interposed nuclei, and (3) a lateral or hemispheric zone projecting to the dentate nucleus (Jansen and Brodal, '40; Eager, '63; Voogd, '64; Korneliussen, '72). Physiological studies appear consistent with the longitudinal zonal division of the cerebellum, particularly with respect to inputs (Oscarsson, '73). The medial cortical zone, constituting the vermis proper, projects to the fastigial nucleus and is strictly unilateral (Courville and Diakiw, '76; Haines, '76). Fibers from the cortical lobules of the vermis project to the nearest region of the fastigial nucleus so that this arrangement results in a sequential representation of the cerebellar vermis in the fastigial nucleus. HRP injections of one fastigial nucleus result in retrograde transport of the enzyme to Purkinje cells in a narrow longitudinal zone of the ipsilateral vermis in folia of lobules I through X (Ruggiero et al., '77; Carpenter and Batton, '82). Information concerning the paravermal and lateral longitudinal cerebellar zones is less precise, but the same principle appears to apply. Because the longitudinal zonal pattern, recognized during cerebellar corticogenesis, becomes distorted during later development, even small cortical lesions may involve more than one zone. Studies based upon anterograde transport of HRP and [^{3}H]amino acids provide more precise data concerning the longitudinal zonal cortical projections to the deep cerebellar nuclei (Dietrichs and Walberg, '79; Tolbert and Bantli, '79; Bishop et al., '79). These studies support the concept of three rostrocaudal zones projecting, respectively, to the fastigial, interposed and dentate nuclei. Other data indicate that nucleocortical fibers from the deep cerebellar nuclei project collaterals back to their specific cortical zones (Gould and Graybiel, '76; Tolbert et al., '76a, '77). Corticonuclear and nucleocortical fibers appear to have reciprocal relationships. Purkinje cell axons have a powerful monosynaptic inhibitory action upon cells of the deep cerebellar nuclei (Eccles et al., '67).

Nucleocortical Projections. The conceptional division of the cerebellum into three sagittal zones, each consisting of a

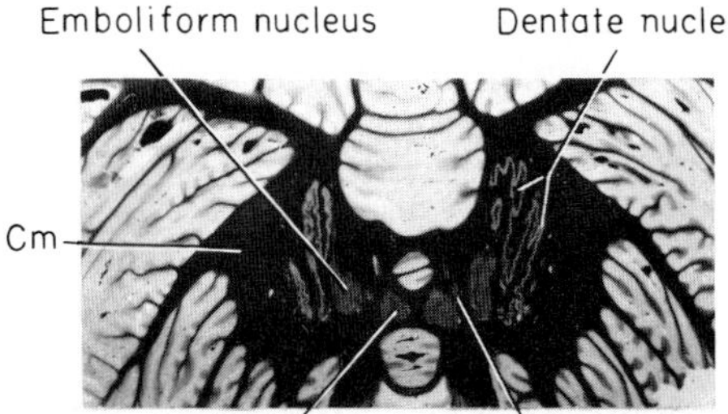

Figure 8-11. Horizontal section through adult cerebellum showing portions of the deep cerebellar nuclei and the corpus medullare (*Cm*). (Weigert's myelin stain; photograph.) (From Carpenter and Sutin, *Human Neuroanatomy*, 1983; courtesy of Williams & Wilkins.)

longitudinal strip of cerebellar cortex and the deep cerebellar nucleus to which its Purkinje cells project, has been strengthened by the observation that cells in the deep cerebellar nuclei project recurrent collaterals to the cortex in a specific manner (Gould and Graybiel, '76; Tolbert, Bantli and Bloedel, '77; Chan-Palay, '77; Gould, '79). HRP injected into a localized region of the cerebellar cortex results in retrograde transport of the enzyme to cells of a single deep cerebellar nucleus, and injections of [^{3}H]amino acids into the deep cerebellar nuclei can be traced autoradiographically into the cerebellar cortex. Nucleocortical and corticonuclear projections are reciprocally organized, so that neurons in the deep cerebellar nuclei project back to regions of the cerebellar cortex from which they receive input. Axons of the deep cerebellar nuclei projecting to the cerebellar cortex arise from a heterogenous population of cells, similar to those that project fibers to the thalamus and brain stem. Some cells in the dentate and interposed nuclei have collateral axons which project via the superior cerebellar peduncle to the thalamus and inferior olive, as well as to the cerebellar cortex (Tolbert, et al., '78). Nucleocortical collaterals terminate in the granular layer of the cerebellar cortex (Tolbert, et al., '77). Since the nucleocortical projection arises from axon collaterals of cerebellar efferent neurons,, the same signals projected to brain stem nuclei by the deep cerebellar nuclei are fed back to the cerebellar cortex. These projections from the deep cerebellar nuclei represent a major afferent system to the cerebellar cortex not previously recognized.

Extracerebellar Inputs. Although the Purkinje cells exert inhibitory influences upon the deep cerebellar nuclei, these nuclei maintain a high frequency excitatory discharge (Ito, et al., '64; Ito et al., '70). This observation implies that, unless the deep cerebellar nuclei are spontaneously active, they must receive excitatory inputs from extracerebellar sources. It is presumed that excitatory inputs from extracerebellar sources overcome the tonic inhibitory output from the cerebellar cortex. The current thesis is that extracerebellar inputs to the deep cerebellar nuclei provide the tonic facilitation which at times predominates over the cortical inhibition and maintains the discharge of impulses directed towards brain stem nuclei (Eccles et al., '67).

Retrograde transport studies indicate that the dentate nucleus receives afferents from: (1) the pontine nuclei, (2) the principal inferior olivary nucleus, (3) the trigeminal sensory nuclei, (4) the reticulotegmental nucleus, (5) the locus ceruleus, and (6) the raphe nuclei (Eller and Chan-Palay, '76; Chan-Palay, '77). The largest number of afferent fibers appear to arise from the pontine nuclei, the inferior olivary nucleus and the reticulotegmental nucleus. Both ipsilateral and contralateral pontine nuclei project to the dentate nucleus, but the larger number of fibers arise from the opposite side (Eller and Chan-Palay, '76). Olivocerebellar fibers pass to all parts of the cerebellar cortex and to the deep cerebellar nuclei (Brodal, '40). Afferent projections to the dentate nucleus are crossed and arise from cells of the principal inferior olivary nucleus (Courville et al., '77). The interposed nuclei receive crossed fibers from the medial and dorsal accessory olivary nuclei, and the fastigial nucleus receives fibers from the dorsomedial cell column and nucleus β, caudal subdivisions of the medial accessory olive (Brodal, '76). These projections to the deep cerebellar nuclei probably are collaterals of climbing fibers. The dentate nucleus and the interposed nuclei receive bilateral projections from the reticulotegmental nucleus (Eller and Chan-Palay, '76). The anterior interposed nucleus

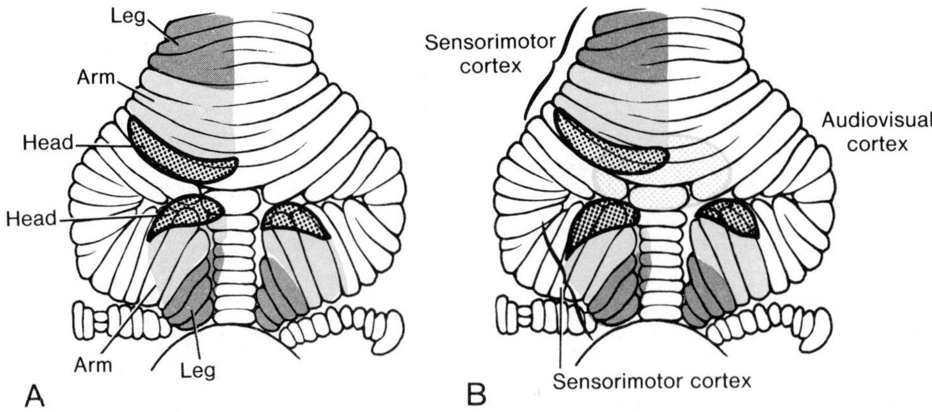

Figure 8-12. Schematic diagrams of somatotopic localization in the cerebellar cortex of the monkey. (*A*) Diagram of the tactile receiving areas of the cerebellum mapped by potentials recorded in response to movement of hairs on the left side of the body. (*B*) Diagram of cerebellar cortical areas responding to stimulation of the sensorimotor, auditory and visual cortex in the right hemisphere. The leg (*red*), arm (*blue*), and head (*black stipple*) are represented ipsilaterally in the anterior lobe and bilaterally in reversed fashion in the paramedian lobules. The auditory and visual cortex (*blue stipple*) are represented in the simple lobule, folium, tuber and adjacent cortex (based on Snider, '50). (From Carpenter and Sutin, *Human Neuroanatomy*, 1983; courtesy of Williams & Wilkins.)

(i.e., the emboliform nucleus) receives a projection from the red nucleus which is crossed (Courville and Brodal, '66), and is reciprocal to the major projection from this nucleus.

SOMATOTOPIC LOCALIZATION

The afferent fiber systems which convey sensory information to the cerebellum from receptors of various kinds in different parts of the body have been shown to be related to particular parts of the cerebellum. Electrophysiological studies have demonstrated in animals that exteroceptive impulses, such as tactile sense, audition and vision, give rise to action potentials in specific regions of the cerebellum (Adrian, '43; Snider and Stowell, '44; Snider, '50). The projection of exteroceptive impulses to the cerebellar cortex is somatotopically organized in a precise manner (Fig. 8-12). Tactile stimulation evokes potentials ipsilaterally in the anterior lobe and simple lobule, and bilaterally in the paramedian lobules. The leg area is represented in the central lobule, the arm in the culmen and the head and face in the simple lobule. The orientation was found to be reversed in the paramedian lobules with the leg representation caudally and the head represented rostrally. Responses in this pattern were most easily obtained from skin receptors or cutaneous nerves. The head area was found to partially overlap the middle region of the vermis (i.e., simple lobule, folium and tuber, and adjacent areas) where action potentials were recorded following auditory and visual stimuli (Fig. 8-12). The same somatotopic regions of the cerebellum can be activated by stimulating corresponding areas of the sensorimotor cortex contralaterally (Snider and Eldred, '52). Stimulation of the auditory and visual cortex in cerebrum likewise produced potentials in the audiovisual representation in the cerebellum (Hampson et al., '52). Many additional studies support in detail the somatotopic organization outlined above (Oscarsson, '73).

CEREBELLAR CONNECTIONS

Afferent Fibers. The cerebellum receives inputs generated in virtually all kinds of receptors in all parts of the body. Most afferents enter the cerebellum via the inferior and middle cerebellar peduncles. The number of afferent fibers exceeds efferent fibers by an estimated ratio of 40 to 1 (Heidary and Tomasch, '69).

The inferior cerebellar peduncle consists of a larger entirely afferent portion, the restiform body and a smaller medial juxtarestiform portion containing both afferent and efferent fibers. The juxtarestiform body (Fig. 6-20) contains primary and secondary vestibulocerebellar fibers (Carleton and Carpenter, '83, '84) and cerebellovestibular originating from the nodulus, uvula, and the fastigial nuclei. Most of the afferents to the cerebellar cortex are relayed by brain stem nuclei, such as the inferior olive and a number of smaller nuclei located in the medulla. Nuclei in the brain stem which project most of their fibers to the cerebellum are collectively referred to as *precerebellar nuclei.*

The pontine nuclei represent the most massive collection of precerebellar nuclei, and they constitute the most important relay in the conduction of impulses from the cerebral cortex to the cerebellum. Corticopontine fibers arise from all of the four major lobes of the cerebrum and terminate upon ipsilateral pontine nuclei. Cortical projections from the sensorimotor cortex project somatotopically upon two longitudinally oriented cell columns within the pontine nuclei (Brodal, '68). Studies in the monkey indicate that the motor area (area 4), the primary somatosensory area (areas 3, 1, 2), area 5, and portions of the visual cortex give rise to the major corticopontine fibers (Brodal, '78). Although projections from the motor and somatosensory areas are somatotopically organized they are separated from each other. All cells of the pontine nuclei project axons into the middle cerebellar peduncle. Projections to the cortex of the cerebellar hemisphere are crossed, while those to the vermal cortex are bilateral (Brodal, '81). The nodulus appears to be the only part of the cerebellum that does not receive a pontine projection. Pontocerebellar fibers terminate as mossy fibers (Mettler and Lubin, '42) and most cerebellar lobules receive afferents from two or more different sites within the pontine nuclei (Brodal and Hoddevik, '78; Hoddevik, '75). This pattern of cortical termination suggests a convergence of impulses from different regions of the pontine nuclei.

Efferent Fibers. Cerebellar efferent fibers arise from all of the deep cerebellar nuclei and from certain parts of the cerebellar cortex. Direct projections from the anterior and posterior vermis and from the vestibulocerebellum (i.e., regions of the cerebellar cortex receiving vestibular inputs) pass to the ipsilateral vestibular nuclear complex and collectively constitute the cerebellovestibular projection. The largest and most widely distributed efferent fibers from the cerebellum arise from the deep cerebellar nuclei. Cerebellar efferent fibers from the deep cerebellar nuclei are organized into two main systems contained in three separate bundles. The major efferent systems are the superior cerebellar peduncle and the fastigial efferent projection.

Superior Cerebellar Peduncle. The largest cerebellar efferent bundle, the superior cerebellar peduncle, is formed by fibers arising from cells in the dentate, emboliform, and globose nuclei (Figs. 2-20, 2-21, 6-20, and 6-25). This composite group of fibers emerges from the hilus of the dentate nucleus and passes rostrally into the upper pons where it forms a compact bundle along the dorsolateral wall of the fourth ventricle (Fig. 8-13). At isthmus levels, fibers of the superior cerebellar peduncle sweep ventromedially into the tegmentum (Fig. 6-25). All fibers of the superior cerebellar peduncle decussate at levels through the inferior colliculus. Most of these crossed fibers ascend to enter and surround the contralateral red nucleus. A relatively small part of the fibers from the dentate nucleus terminate in the rostral third of the red nucleus (Angaut and Bowsher, '65; Courville, '66); the bulk of these fibers project to the thalamus and end in parts of the ventral lateral and ventral posterolateral thalamic nuclei (Fig. 8-13). Degeneration and autoradiographic studies indicate that efferents from the deep cerebellar nuclei terminate in the ventral lateral (par oralis, VLo; pars caudalis, VLc), area "X," the central lateral (CL), the paralaminar part of the dorsomedial nucleus (DMpl), and the oral part of the ventral posterolateral (VPLo) thalamic nuclei (Chan-Palay, '77; Miller and Strominger, '77; Kalil, '81). Other investigators indicate that few, if any, fibers of the superior cerebellar peduncle terminate in VLo, long regarded as the major thalamic termination of this system (Kusama et al., '71; Percheron, '77; Thach and Jones, '79). This view is supported by retrograde transport studies which indicate that HRP injections

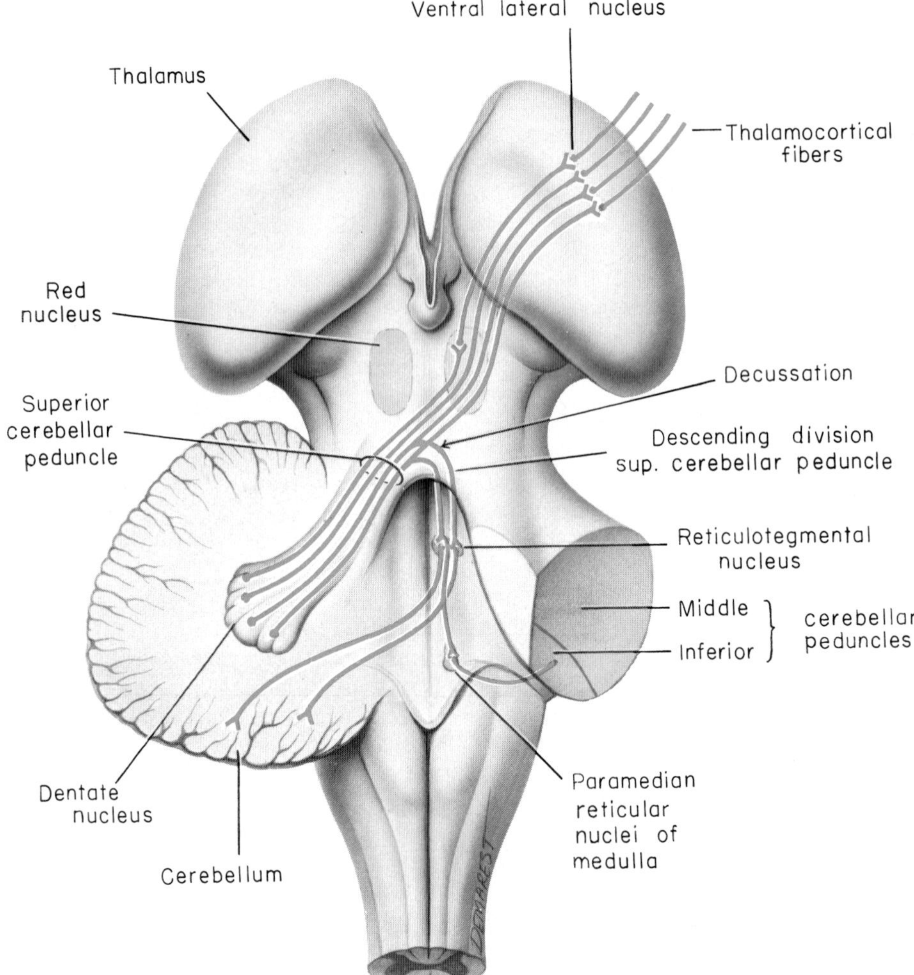

Figure 8-13. Diagram of the efferent fibers of the dentate nucleus. These fibers, contained in the superior cerebellar peduncle (*blue*), all decussate in the caudal mesencephalon. Ascending fibers project to the rostral part of the red nucleus and to the ventral lateral (VLc) and ventral posterolateral (VPLo) nuclei of the thalamus. Fibers of the descending division of the superior cerebellar peduncle project to the reticulotegmental nucleus, the paramedian reticular nuclei of the medulla, and to the inferior olivary nucleus (not shown). Descending fibers of the superior cerebellar peduncle constitute part of a cerebelloreticular system that conveys impulses back to the cerebellum. (From Carpenter and Sutin, *Human Neuroanatomy*, 1983; courtesy of Williams & Wilkins.)

confined to the VLo thalamic nucleus label only cells in the medial pallidal segment (Tracey et al., '80). Similar HRP injections in VLc and VPLo retrogradely label cells in the contralateral deep cerebellar nuclei. These studies suggest that pallidal and cerebellar efferent systems end upon different thalamic relay nuclei in the ventral tier.

A small number of fibers from the dentate nucleus project to the rostral intralaminar thalamic nuclei, mainly the central lateral (CL) nucleus. The ventral lateral nuclei of the thalamus project (VLc) and ventral posterolateral (VPLo) nuclei of the thalamus project upon the primary motor cortex. Thus impulses from the dentate nucleus are conveyed via contralateral thalamic nuclei to the motor cortex. In this manner, impulses from the dentate nucleus can influence activity of motor neurons in the cerebral cortex; impulses from the motor cortex are transmitted to spinal levels

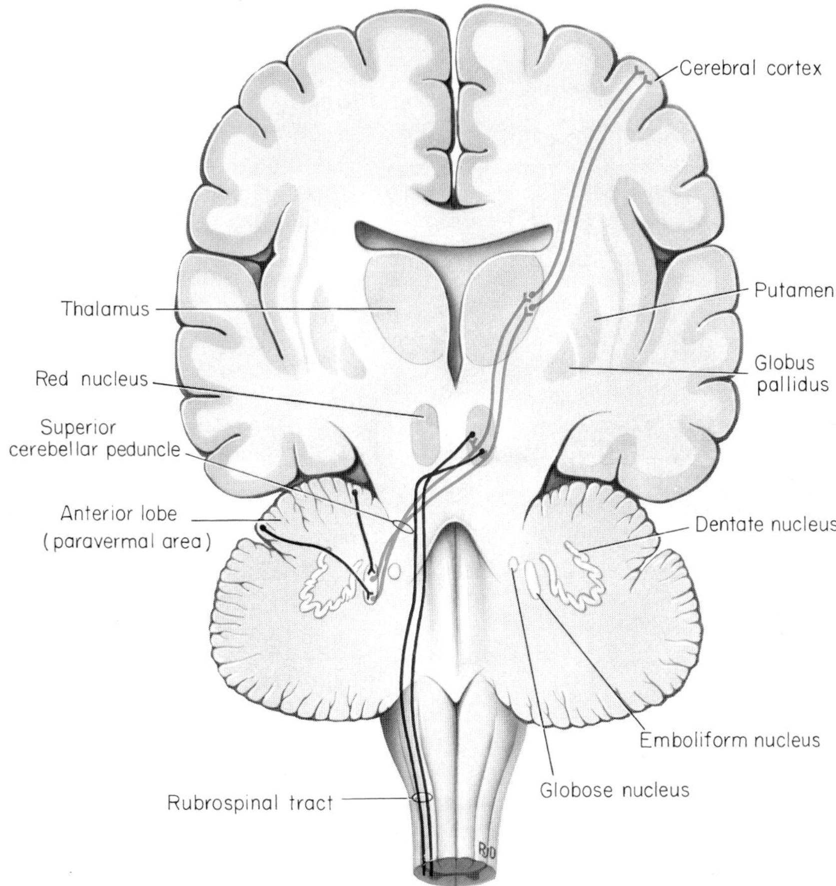

Figure 8-14. Schematic diagram of connections between the emboliform nucleus (anterior interposed nucleus) and the red nucleus. Axons of Purkinje cells (*black*) in the paravermal cortex of the anterior lobe of the cerebellum project somatotopically upon the emboliform nucleus. The most rostral cortical regions, concerned with the lower extremity (Figs. 8-12 and 8-17), project to the rostral part of the emboliform nucleus, while caudal regions, concerned with the upper extremity, project to caudal parts of this nucleus. Fibers from the emboliform nucleus (*blue*) project via the superior cerebellar peduncle to caudal portions of the contralateral red nucleus, and to the ventral lateral nucleus of the thalamus. Projections from the emboliform nucleus to the red nucleus terminate somatotopically. Rubrospinal fibers (*red*) arising from dorsomedial regions of the red nucleus project to cervical spinal segments, while fibers from ventrolateral parts of this nucleus project to lumbosacral spinal segments. Thus the somatotopic linkage is maintained from cerebellar cortex to spinal levels (Courville, '66; Massion, '67) (From Carpenter and Sutin, *Human Neuroanatomy*, 1983; courtesy of Williams & Wilkins.)

via the corticospinal tract. This system is concerned primarily with the coordination of somatic motor function.

A relatively small number of efferent fibers from the dentate nucleus decussate with those of the superior cerebellar peduncle and descend to reticular nuclei that in turn project back to the cerebellum (Fig. 8-13).

Fibers from the interposed nuclei (i.e., the emboliform nucleus) project primarily to cells in the caudal two-thirds of the red nucleus (Fig. 8-14); a smaller number of these fibers pass beyond the red nucleus to the ventral lateral nucleus of the thalamus (Angaut, '70; Appelberg, '60; Eccles et al., '67; Tolbert et al., '78). Fibers from the anterior interposed nucleus (i.e., emboliform nucleus in man) projecting somatotopically upon cells of the red nucleus form part of a somatotopic linkage extending from the paravermal cortex to spinal levels.

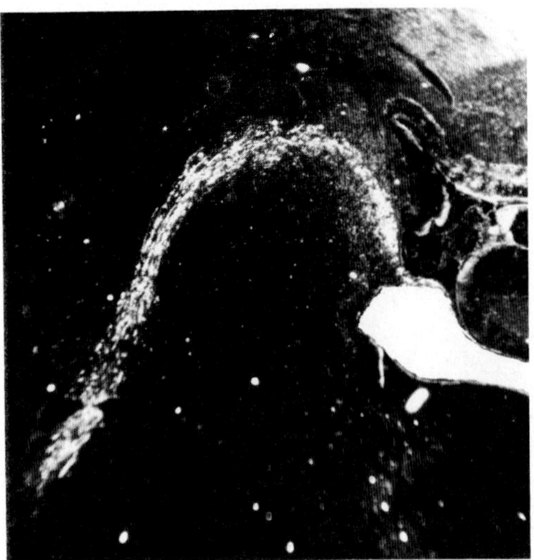

Figure 8-15. Dark-field photomicrogaph of [^{3}H]amino acids transported by fibers of the uncinate fasciculus as seen in an autoradiograph (Batton et al., '77). (From Carpenter and Sutin, *Human Neuroanatomy*, 1983; courtesy of Williams & Wilkins.)

In this pathway fibers from the paravermal cortex pass to the anterior interposed nucleus; fibers from the anterior interposed nucleus project via the superior cerebellar peduncle to the opposite red nucleus. Somatotopically organized rubrospinal fibers cross in the midbrain and descend to spinal levels. This small system involves two decussations, that of the superior cerebellar peduncle and that of the rubrospinal tract (Fig. 8-14). Thus, impulses conveyed from paravermal cortex to the spinal cord end on the same side. This system appears to be primarily concerned with mechanisms that facilitate ipsilateral flexor muscle tone.

Axoplasmic transport studies have shown that the deep cerebellar nuclei not only receive inputs from the contralateral inferior olivary nucleus, but these nuclei have reciprocal connections with specific parts of the inferior olivary nuclear complex (Martin et al., '76; Beitz, '76). The dentate nucleus projects primarily to the principal olive, while the anterior interposed nucleus (equivalent to the emboliform nucleus) projects to the dorsal accessory olive and the posterior interposed nucleus (equivalent to the globose nucleus) distributes fibers to the medial accessory olivary nucleus. These fibers reach parts of the contralateral inferior olivary nucleus via the descending limb of the superior cerebellar peduncle.

Fastigial Efferent Projections. The efferent projections of the fastigial nucleus are unique in that: (1) they do not emerge via the superior cerebellar peduncle, (2) a large part of the efferent fibers cross within the cerebellum, and (3) they project to nuclei at all levels of the brain stem (Carpenter and Batton, '82). Crossed fibers from the fastigial nucleus emerge from the cerebellum via the *uncinate fasciculus* (*Russell*) which arches around the superior cerebellar peduncle (Figs 8-15 and 8-16). Uncrossed fastigial efferent fibers project to the brain stem in the *juxtarestiform body* (Figs 6-20 and 8-16). Crossed efferent fibers contained in the uncinate fasciculus arise from cells in all parts of the fastigial nucleus and outnumber uncrossed efferents in the juxtarestiform body. Although data from degeneration studies suggested that fastigial efferent projections to vestibular nuclei are bilateral and differentially distributed (Thomas, et al., '56; Carpenter, '59; Walberg et al., '62), autoradiographic data indicate that these projections are bilateral and symmetrical only to ventrolateral portions of the lateral and inferior vestibular nuclei (Fig. 8-16) (Batton et al., '77). Fastigioreticular fibers arise predominantly from rostral parts of the nucleus, are mainly crossed and project to: (1) medial regions of the nucleus reticularis gigantocellularis, (2) parts of the caudal pontine reticular formation, (3) the dorsal paramedian reticular nucleus, and (4) portions of the lateral reticular nucleus (Walberg et al., '62a). Crossed fastigiopontine fibers separate from the uncinate fasciculus and pass ventrally to terminations in the dorsolateral pontine nuclei (Fig. 8-16). A small number of crossed fastigiospinal fibers descend ventral to the spinal trigeminal tract and enter the lateral funiculus of the spinal cord (Fig. 8-16). The largest number of crossed fastigiospinal fibers probably terminate in the C_2-C_3 segments (Fukushima et al., '77; Matsushita and Hosoya, '78). Antidromic stimulation of the upper cervical spinal cord and direct stimulation of the fastigial nucleus indicate that axons of fas-

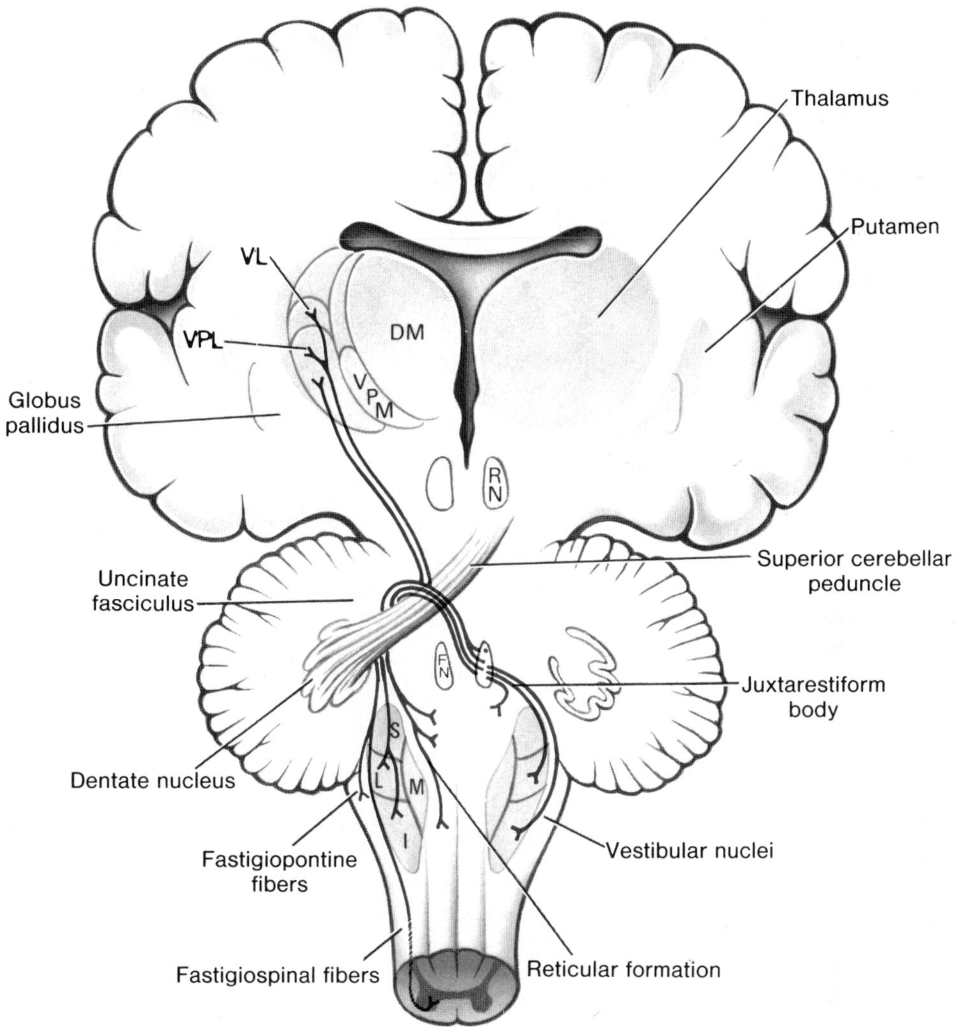

Figure 8.16. Schematic diagram of fastigial efferent projections. Crossed fastigial efferent fibers contained in the uncinate fasciculus arise from cells in all parts of the fastigial nucleus (*FN*) and outnumber uncrossed efferent fibers that emerge in the juxtarestiform body. Fastigiovestibular fibers project bilaterally and symmetrically upon ventral portions of the lateral (*L*) and inferior (I) vestibular nuclei. Fastigioreticular fibers arise predominantly from rostral parts of the nucleus. Crossed fastigiopontine fibers separate from the ucinate fasciculus and pass to the dorsolateral pontine nuclei. Crossed fastigiospinal fibers passing to upper cervical spinal segments exert excitatory effects upon motoneurons. Ascending fastigial projections originating from caudal parts of the nucleus, are entirely crossed and ascend in dorsolateral parts of the midbrain tegmentum. These fibers project to parts of the superior colliculus, the nuclei of the posterior commissure (not shown) and to the ventral posterolateral (*VPL*) and ventral lateral (*VL*) thalamic nuclei (Batton et al., '77; Carpenter and Batton, '82). Abbreviations: *DM*, dorsomedial nucleus; *FN*, fastigial nucleus; *RN*, red nucleus; *VL*, *VPL*, and *VPM*, ventral lateral, ventral posterolateral, and ventral posteromedial thalamic nuclei; vestibular nuclei: *I*, inferior, *L*, lateral, *M*, medial, and *S*, superior. (From Carpenter and Sutton, *Human Neuroanatomy*, 1983; courtesy of Williams & Wilkins.)

tigial neurons make monosynaptic excitatory contacts with motoneurons at the C_2-C_3 level (Wilson et al., '77; Wilson et al., '78).

A small number of fibers in the uncinate fasciculus ascend in dorsolateral parts of the brain stem and project fibers to thalamic nuclei (Angaut and Bowsher, '70; Batton et al., '77; Carpenter and Batton, '82). These fibers arise from caudal parts

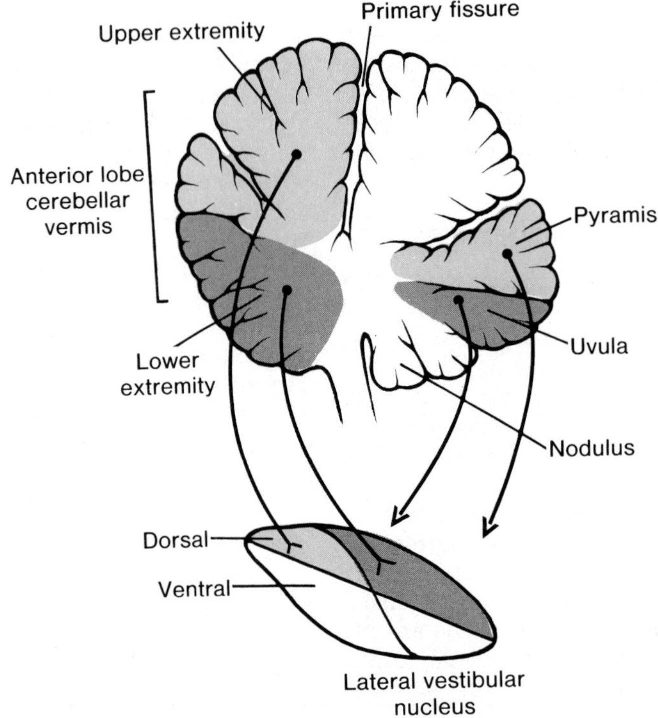

Figure 8-17. Schematic diagram of cerebellovestibular projections from the anterior and posterior vermis. Purkinje cell axons from the anterior lobe vermis project somatotopically upon dorsal regions of the lateral vestibular nucleus and exert inhibitory influences. Similar direct projections from the pyramis and parts of the uvula which are not somatotopically arranged are shown by arrows (modified from Brodal et al., '62). (From Carpenter and Sutin, *Human Neuroanatomy*, 1983; courtesy of Williams & Wilkins.)

of the fastigial nucleus, cross within the cerebellum and ascend contralaterally (Fig. 8-16). Fibers, or collaterals in this bundle, project bilaterally to rostral parts of the superior colliculus and the nuclei of the posterior commissure (Angaut, '69). Fibers projecting to the diencephalon terminate in the ventral posterolateral (VPLo) and ventral lateral (VLc) thalamic nuclei.

Cerebellovestibular Projections. Certain regions of the cerebellar cortex give rise to direct projections which pass to the vestibular nuclei (Fig. 8-17). These fibers, representing axons of Purkinje cells, arise (1) from the anterior and posterior cerebellar vermis and (2) from the vestibulocerebellum (i.e., the flocculonodular lobule). Thus, the vestibular nuclei receive cerebellar afferents bilaterally from the fastigial nucleus and ipsilaterally from specific cortical regions. Direct projections from lateral parts of the cerebellar vermis terminate in dorsal regions of the ipsilateral lateral and inferior vestibular nucleus and are somatotopically organized (Walberg and Jansen, '61; Walberg, '72; Haines, '76). Efferent fibers from the anterior lobe establish synaptic contacts on somata and dendrites of cells of all sizes in the lateral vestibular nucleus (Mugnaini and Walberg, '67). Fibers from the posterior part of the vermis also project to the lateral vestibular nucleus, but not in a somatotopical pattern (Fig. 8-17). Stimulation of the anterior lobe vermis of the cerebellum produces a monosynaptic inhibition of neurons of the lateral vestibular nucleus (Ito and Yoshida, '66).

The regions of the cerebellum which receive primary and secondary vestibular fibers constitute the "vestibulocerebellum" (Brodal and Høivik, '64; Carleton and Carpenter, '83, '84'). This designation includes ventral parts of the uvula in addition to the flocculonodular lobule. All parts of the "vestibulocerebellum" project fibers to the vestibular nuclei (Angaut and Brodal, '67).

The flocculus projects to the superior and medial vestibular nuclei; the nodulus and uvula projects fibers to the superior, medial, and inferior vestibular nuclei. All of these cerebellovestibular projections are ipsilateral.

CEREBELLAR ORGANIZATION

On the basis of cortical projections to the deep cerebellar nuclei and projections from the deep nuclei to the cerebellar cortex, the cerebellum has been divided into three sagittal zones of cortex and their connecting deep nuclei (Voogd, '64; Korneliussen, '72; Courville and Diakiw, '76; Haines, '76; Tolbert et al., '76a, '77; Bishop et al., '79; Tolbert and Bantli, '79; Dietrichs and Walberg, '79; Gould, '79). This concept provides an elementary view of the functional organization of the cerebellum. In this simplified scheme cerebellar efferent systems are related to three longitudinal (sagittal) zones referred to as vermal, paravermal and lateral.

The *vermal zone* is the midline, unpaired portion of the cerebellum related to the fastigial nuclei and concerned primarily with mechanisms that can modify muscle tone (Fig. 8-16). Direct projections from the anterior and posterior vermis exert inhibitory influences upon the vestibular nuclei which can result in a reduction of extensor muscle tone (Fig. 8-17). The projections of the fastigial nucleus, which receive strictly ipsilateral afferents from the vermis (Courville and Diakiw, '76), are to some extent bilateral, although crossed fibers are more numerous (Carpenter and Batton, '82). These fibers pass to terminations in the vestibular nuclei where they are excitatory, and to broad regions of the reticular formation of the pons and medulla (Fig. 8-16). A small number of crossed fastigiospinal fibers descending directly to the upper cervical spinal have excitatory influences upon motoneurons (Wilson et al., '78). Finally, some crossed fastigial efferents projecting to thalamic nuclei probably make a contribution to coordinated somatic motor activity. The vermal zone of the cerebellum is particularly concerned with control of posture, muscle tone, locomotion and equilibrium for the entire body (Chambers and Sprague, '55, '55a).

The *paravermal zone* relates the paravermal cortex with the emboliform and globose nuclei which have connections predominantly with the contralateral red nucleus. The emboliform nucleus (anterior interposed nucleus) projects somatotopically upon the caudal two-thirds of the contralateral red nucleus (Courville, '66; Flumerfelt et al., '73). This somatotopically organized system is concerned with mechanisms that can facilitate ipsilateral flexor muscle tone via the rubrospinal tract (Fig. 8-14). The red nucleus also recives some fibers from the globose nucleus (posterior interposed nucleus) which terminate in medial regions (Angaut, '70). Both of the interposed nuclei have modest projections to the contralateral ventral lateral (VL) nucleus of the thalamus.

The *lateral zone* relates the cortex of the cerebellar hemisphere with the dentate nucleus which has the most extensive thalamic projections. These efferent fibers project predominantly to VLc, VPLo, and area X (an area medial to VL) (Fig. 8-13). This, the largest of all cerebellar efferent systems, appears to be concerned with the coordination of ipsilateral somatic motor activity. Impulses conveyed to VLc, VPLo, and area X in the thalamus are relayed to the motor cortex where they modify activity of neurons projecting to the pontine nuclei and spinal levels.

FUNCTIONAL CONSIDERATIONS

The cerebellum is concerned with the coordination of somatic motor activity, the regulation of muscle tone and mechanisms that influence and maintain equilibrium. Afferent cerebellar pathways convey impulses from a wide variety of different receptors, including the organs of special sense. Among these afferent systems, the input from stretch receptors (i.e., muscle spindle and Golgi tendon organ) is especially large. These impulses are conveyed by the spinocerebellar and cuneocerebellar tracts. The principal function of stretch receptors appears to be the unconscious neural control of muscle tone. The cerebellum, which receives the major afferent input from stretch receptors, provides part of the neural mechanism that: (1) effects gradual alterations of muscle tensions for proper maintenance of equilibrium and posture, and (2) assures the smooth and orderly sequence of muscular contractions that characterize skilled voluntary movement.

Each movement requires the coordinated action (synergy) of a group of muscles. The agonist is the muscle which provides the actual movement of the part; the antagonist is the opposing muscle which must relax to permit movement. Other muscles must fix, or stabilize, certain joints in order to produce the desired movement. Such synergistic motor activity requires not only complex reciprocal innervation but coordinated control of muscle tone and movement. The cerebellum provides this control for the somatic motor system in an efficient, automatic manner without our being aware of it.

There are certain general principles that pertain to most of the disturbances resulting from cerebellar lesions. The principles are: (1) cerebellar lesions produce ipsilateral disturbances, (2) cerebellar disturbances occur as a constellation of intimately related phenomena, (3) cerebellar disturbances due to nonprogressive pathology undergo gradual attenuation with time, and (4) disturbances resulting from cerebellar lesions are the physiological expression of intact neural structures deprived of controlling and regulating influences. Lesions involving the dentate nucleus or the superior cerebellar peduncle produce the most severe and enduring cerebellar disturbances.

Neocerebellar Lesions. Lesions involving the cerebellar hemispheres and the dentate nucleus affect primarily skilled voluntary and associated movements (i.e., movements related to the corticospinal system). The muscles become *hypotonic* (flabby) and tire easily. The deep tendon reflexes tend to be sluggish and often have a pendular quality. There are severe disturbances of coordinated movement referred to as *asynergia* in which the range, direction and force of muscle contractions are inappropriate. Cerebellar asynergia can be demonstrated by many tests. Among these are tests of precise movements to a point; distances frequently are improperly gauged (*dysmetria*) and fall short of the mark or exceed it (*past-pointing*). Rapid successive movements, such as alternately, supinating and pronating the hands and forearms are poorly performed (*dysdiadochokinesis*). The patient is unable to adjust to changes of muscle tension. When the forearm is flexed at the elbow and held flexed against resistance, a sudden release of resistance causes the forearm to strike the chest. This is an example of the *rebound phenomenon.* These patients also demonstrate a *decomposition of movement* in which phases of complex movements are performed as a series of succesive single simple movements.

The *tremor* seen in association with neocerebellar lesions occurs primarily during voluntary and associated movements. This tremor is referred to as "*intention tremor*" because it is not present at rest. It involves especially the proximal appendicular musculature, but is transmitted mechanically to distal parts of the extremities.

Ataxia is an asynergic disturbance associated with neocerebellar lesions which results in a bizarre distortion of voluntary and associated movements. It involves particularly the axial muscles, and groups of muscle around the shoulder and pelvic girdles. This disturbance is evident during walking and is characterized by muscle contractions which are highly irregular in force, amplitude and direction, and which occur asynchronously in different parts of the body. There frequently is unsteadiness in standing, especially if the feet are close together. The gait is broadbased and the patient reels, lurches and stumbles.

Nystagmus commonly is seen in association with cerebellar disease; it is most pronounced when the patient deviates the eyes laterally toward the side of the lesion. This disturbance consists of an oscillatory pattern in which the eyes slowly drift in one direction and then rapidly move in the opposite direction to correct the drift. Although nystamus seen in association with cerebellar disease has been considered as an expression of asynergic phenomena in the extraocular muscles, many pathological processes which affect the cerebellum also involve the underlying brain stem and the vestibular nuclei located in the floor of the fourth ventricle.

Speech disturbances are common in association with cerebellar lesions of long standing. Speech often is slow, monotonous and some syllables are unnaturally separated. There is a slurring of speech and some words are uttered in an explosive manner.

Archicerebellar Lesions. Lesions involving portions of the posterior cerebellar vermis (i.e., nodulus and uvula) and probably portions of the flocculus produce what has been called the *archicerebellar syndrome.* These lesions produce disturbances of locomotion and equilibrium bilaterally. The patient is unsteady in the standing position and shows considerable swaying of the body. When attempts are made to walk, there is staggering and a tendency to fall to one side or backwards. The gait is jerky, uncoordinated and resembles that of a drunken individual. Muscle tone is not significantly altered and no tremor or asynergic disturbances are seen in the extremities. This syndrome is primarily a trunkal ataxia.

Anterior Lobe of the Cerebellum. There is no established paleocerebellar syndrome in man, but lesions of the anterior lobe of the cerebellum in the dog produce severe disturbances of posture and greatly increased extensor muscle tone. These animals exhibit many of the features seen in association with decerebration, but in time regain the ability to walk and perform voluntary movements.

Sherrington (1898) in a classic experiment demonstrated that electrical stimulation of the anterior lobe of the cerebellum could inhibit extensor muscle tone in a decerebrate animal. Subsequent studies showed that both inhibitory and facilitory effects upon muscle tone could be obtained by stimulating the anterior lobe of the cerebellum (Dow and Moruzzi, '58), depending upon the parameters of stimulation. Stimulation with low repetitive rates (2 to 10 cycles/sec) cause a slow increase in ipsilateral extensor muscle tone, while rapid stimulation (30 to 300 cycles/sec) produce a relaxation of muscle tone. Inhibitory influences obtained by stimulating the anterior lobe appear to be mediated by: (1) cerebelovestibular fibers of cortical origin which project to the lateral vestibular nucleus, and (2) fastigial efferent projections to the reticular formation. Facilitatory influences obtained from stimulating the anterior lobe of the cerebellum are mediated by projections from the fastigial nucleus acting upon the lateral vestibular nucleus (Brodal et al., '62).

Other cerebellar mechanisms which can influence muscle tone involve the paravermal cortex, the nucleus interpositus (i.e., emboliform nucleus) and the contralateral red nucleus (Massion, '67). All of the above structures are somatotopically organized and interconnected. Stimulation of the rostral part of the interposed nucleus in the cat produces flexion of the ipsilateral hindlimb; stimulation of the caudal part of this nucleus produces flexion in the ipsilateral forelimb (Pompeiano, '59; Maffel and Pompeiano, '62). These responses are ipsilateral because fibers of both the superior cerebellar peduncle and the rubrospinal tract are crossed. Crossed projections of the interposed nucleus excite rubral neurons which exert facilitatory influences upon flexor muscle tone via the rubrospinal tract.

Computer Functions. The functional organization of the cerebellar cortex suggest that the cerebellum may function as a special kind of computer in the regulation and control of movement. The cerebellum organizes and integrates information flowing to it via numerous neural pathways. The cerebellar output participates in the control of motor function by transmitting impulses to: (1) certain brain stem nuclei (i.e., the lateral vestibular and red nuclei) that in turn project to spinal levels, and (2) thalamic relay nuclei which can modify the activity of cortical neurons directly concerned with motor function.

Every part of the cerebellar cortex receives two different inputs, that of the mossy fibers and that of the climbing fibers. Although these inputs differ in structural characteristics, they appear to convey similar "sensory" information. The only output of the cerebellar cortex is conveyed by Purkinje cell axons. This output, entirely inhibitory, is exerted upon the deep cerebellar nuclei and the lateral vestibular nucleus. The output of the deep cerebellar nuclei is excitatory, which implies that both excitatory and inhibitory impulses must reach these nuclei. Excitatory input to the deep cerebellar nuclei, derived from extracerebellar sources, is conveyed by collaterals of climbing and mossy fibers.

The observation that the cerebellar cortex transforms all input into inhibition, suggests that there is probably no dynamic storage of information in the neuronal circuitry. Thus, the cerebellum processes its input information rapidly, conveys its output indirectly to specific brain stem nuclei, and has virtually no short-term dynamic memory. These qualities enhance the performance of the cerebellum as a special kind of computer in that it can provide a quick and clear response to any "sensory" input.

CHAPTER 9

The Diencephalon

The most rostral part of the brain stem, the diencephalon, is a nuclear complex composed of several major subdivisions. Most of these nuclear subdivisions are functionally related to the cerebral cortex. Although the entire diencephalon constitutes less than 2% of the neuraxis, it has long been regarded as the key to the understanding of the organization of the central nervous system.

The diencephalon extends from the region of the posterior commissure rostrally to the region of the interventricular foramen. Laterally it is bounded by the posterior limb of the internal capsule, the tail of the caudate nucleus and the stria terminalis (Figs. 9-1 and 9-6). The third ventricle separates the diencephalon into two symmetrical parts, except in the region of the interthalamic adhesion where the medial surfaces of the thalami may be in continuity (Fig. 9-9). The diencephalon is divisible into four major parts: the epithalamus, the thalamus, the hypothalamus, and the subthalamus or ventral thalamus (Fig. 2-25). The medial and lateral geniculate bodies, constituting the metathalamus, are partially separated from the more rostral parts of the thalamus by fibers of the internal capsule.

MIDBRAIN-DIENCEPHALIC JUNCTION

Several discrete nuclear masses of the caudal thalamus closely surround the posterior and lateral surfaces of the mesencephalon. These structures include the *medial* and *lateral geniculate bodies* and the *pulvinar*. External to all of these is the *retrolenticular* portion of the internal capsule (Fig. 9-2). The pineal body lies dorsally between the superior colliculi, while por-

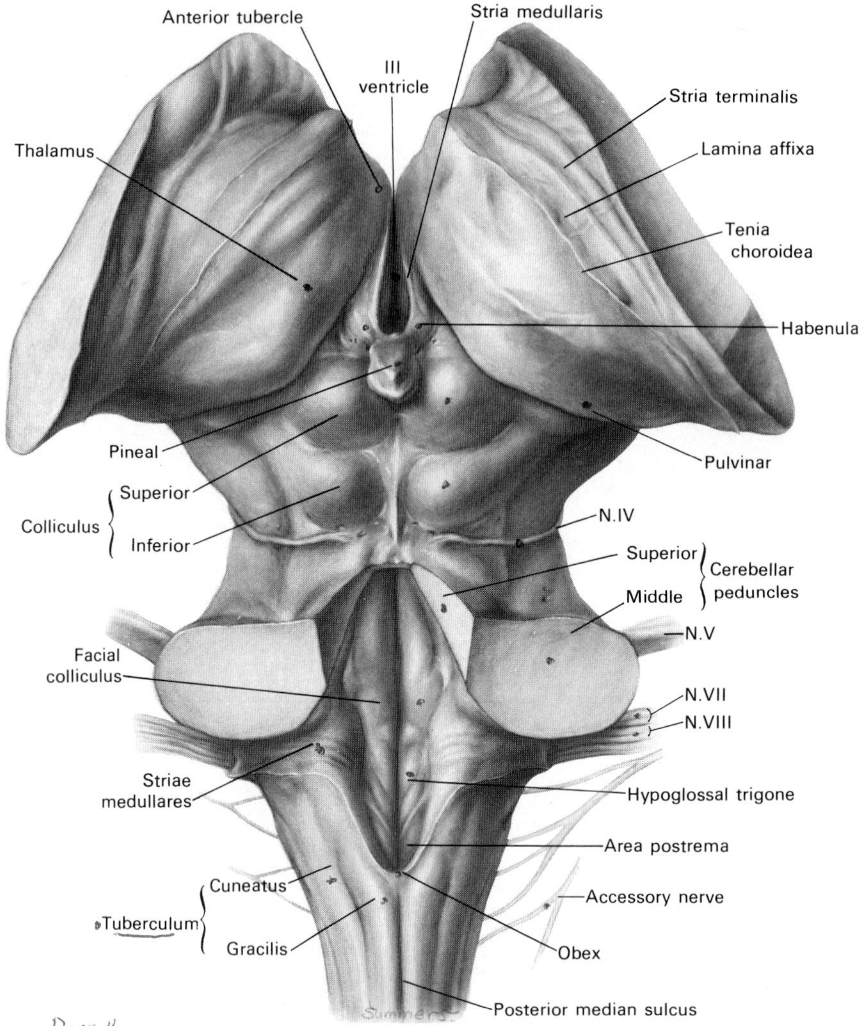

Figure 9-1. Posterior aspect of the brain stem with the cerebellum removed. This drawing shows the epithalamus and the pulvinar. (From Mettler's *Neuroanatomy*, 1948; courtesy of the C. V. Mosby Company.)

tions of the mammillary bodies can be seen in the interpeduncular fossa. Fibers from thalamic nuclei pass laterally into the internal capsule, through which they are distributed to various parts of the cerebral cortex. The internal capsule also contains corticofugal fibers projecting to thalamic nuclei (Fig. 9-21).

The pulvinar is a large nuclear mass dorsal to the medial and lateral geniculate bodies. Its dorsal surface is covered by a thin plate of fibers, the *stratum zonale*. Fibers passing laterally from the pulvinar contribute to the retrolenticular portion of the internal capsule (Figs. 9-2 and 9-3). The innermost portion of the internal capsule, wedged between the pulvinar and lateral geniculate body, forms a triangular area known as the *zone of Wernicke* (Fig. 9-2).

CAUDAL DIENCEPHALON

Transverse sections through the habenular nuclei and the mammillary bodies (Fig. 9-4) reveal the structural organization of the caudal diencephalon. The habenular nuclei are two small gray masses forming triangular eminences on the dorsomedial surface of the thalami. These nuclei receive fibers from the septal nuclei and the preoptic area via the striae medullares (Figs. 9-1 and 9-6) and from the medial pallidal seg-

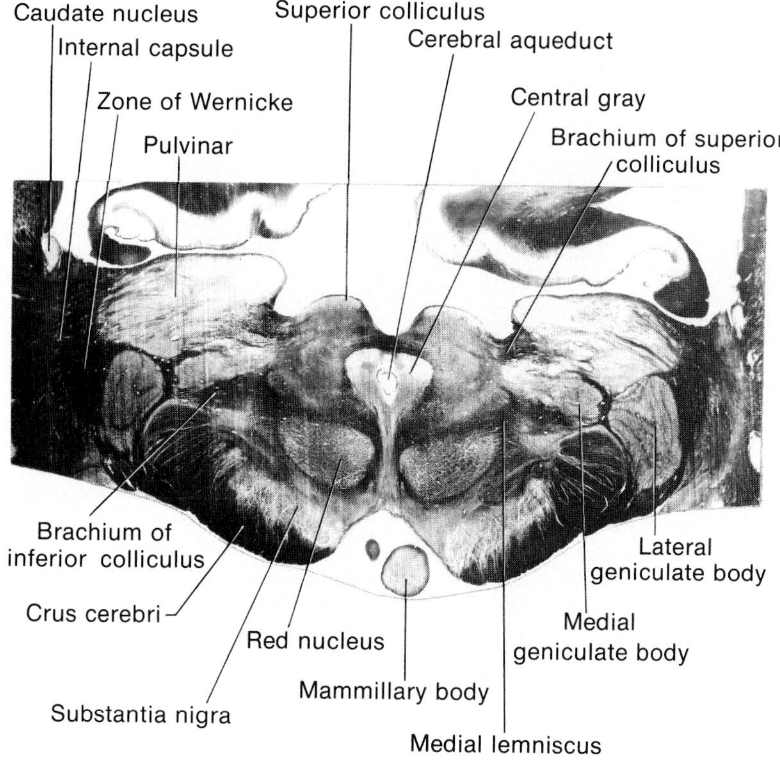

Figure 9-2. Transverse section through rostral midbrain demonstrating relationship of midbrain and caudal portions of the thalamus. (Weigert's myelin stain; photograph.) (From Carpenter and Sutin, *Human Neuroanatomy*, 1983; courtesy of Williams & Wilkins.)

ment. Some fibers cross to the opposite side in the *habenular commissure*. Axons from the habenular nuclei form the *fasciculus retroflexus*, which passes ventrally and caudally to terminate in the interpenduncular nuclei and certain midbrain nuclei. The fasciculus retroflexus passes through the rostromedial part of the red nucleus (Figs. 9-3 and 9-4).

The third ventricle appears enlarged, and parts of it are seen in two locations (Fig. 9-4). The main part of the third ventricle is present dorsally, where it is covered by a thin roof extending between the habenular nuclei and the striae medullares. The margins of this attachment (not shown in Fig. 9-4) on each side constitute the *tenia thalami*. A small part of the third ventricle, referred to as the infundibular recess, is present ventral to the mammillary bodies and dorsal to the infundibulum. The mammillary bodies, tuber cinereum, and infundibulum are parts of the hypothalamus.

Rostrally the thalamus progressively increases in size (Fig. 9-4). As the pulvinar reaches its maximum dimensions, the geniculate nuclei become smaller and several additional nuclear divisions appear ventrally and medially. Ventral to the pulvinar are parts of the ventral thalamic nuclei and the centromedian nucleus; the latter nucleus is delimited by a thin fibrous capsule.

EPITHALAMUS

The epithalamus comprises the pineal body, the habenular trigones, the striae medullares, and the epithelial roof of the third ventricle (Figs. 9-1 and 9-6). The habenula in man consists of a smaller medial and a larger lateral nucleus. These nuclei receive terminals of the stria medullaris (Figs. 9-1, 9-4, and 9-6) and give rise to the fasciculus retroflexus, which terminates in the interpeduncular nucleus and certain midline reticular nuclei. The *stria medul-*

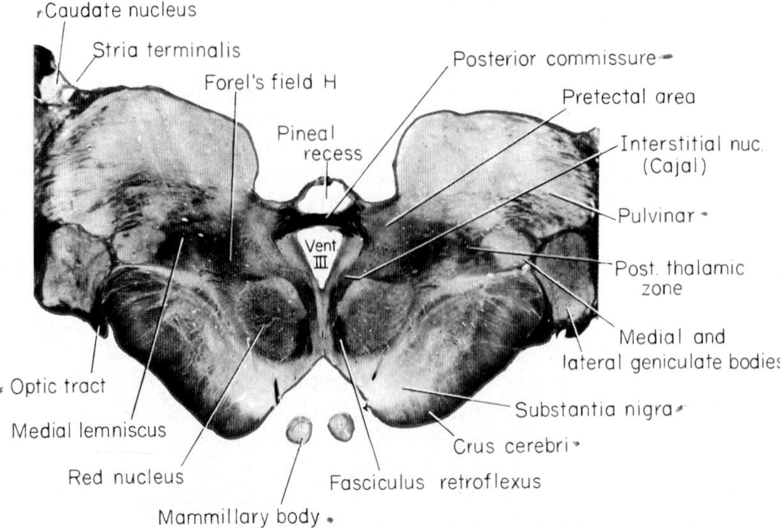

Figure 9-3. Transverse section of the brain stem at the junction of mesencephalon and diencephalon. The posterior thalamic zone, which receives collaterals from the spinothalamic tract, lies medial to the medial geniculate body (Fig. 9-15). This cell group lies caudal to the ventral posterior thalamic nucleus (Fig. 9-4). (Weigert's myelin stain; photograph.) (From Carpenter and Sutin, *Human Neuroanatomy*, 1983; courtesy of Williams & Wilkins.)

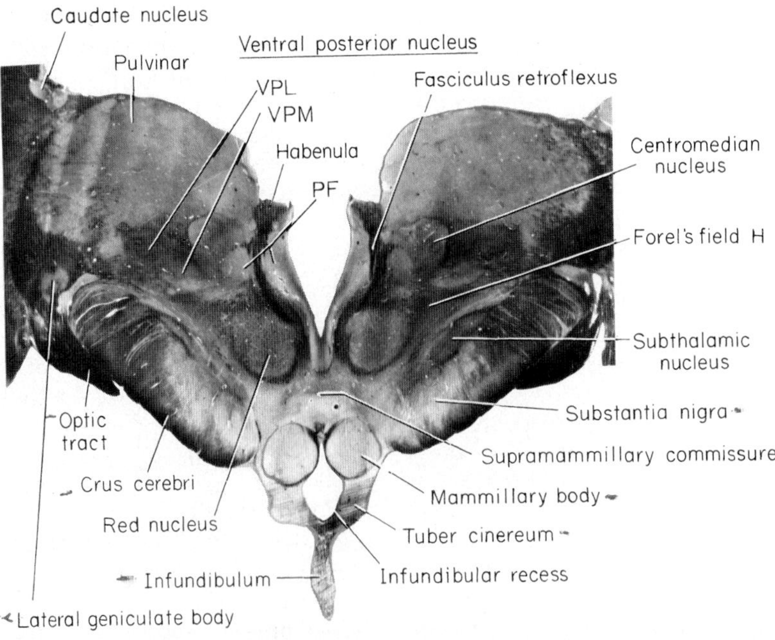

Figure 9-4. Transverse section of the diencephalon through the habenula, the fasciculus retroflexus, the mammillary bodies, and the infundibulum. *VPL* and *VPM* indicate the ventral posterolateral and ventral prosteromedial nuclei of the thalamus. PF indicates the parafascicular nucleus which surrounds the fasciculus retroflexus. (Weigert's myelin stain; photograph.) (From Carpenter and Sutin, *Human Neuroanatomy*, 1983; courtesy of Williams & Wilkins.)

laris is a complex bundle composed of fibers arising from: (1) the septal nuclei, (2) lateral preoptic region (Nauta, '58), (3) the anterior thalamic nuclei, and (4) certain basal forebrain structures (Kim et al., '76). Both the hippocampal formation and the amygdaloid nuclear complex project fibers to the septal nuclei.

The lateral habenular nucleus receives afferents from the globus pallidus, the lateral hypothalamus, the substantia innominata, and the lateral preoptic area, as well as from the ventral tegmental area and the midbrain raphe nuclei (Herkenham and Nauta, '77). The smaller medial habenular nucleus receives afferents from posterior parts of the septal nuclei and the midbrain raphe nuclei. Serotonergic projections from the raphe nuclei and adrenergic innervation from the superior cervical ganglion (Björklund et al., '72) reach the medial habenular nucleus. Although the habenular nuclei are adjacent to each other they do not appear to have connections. The habenular nuclei are sites of convergence of limbic pathways that convey impulses to rostral portions of the midbrain.

Pineal Gland. The pineal body or epiphysis is a small, cone-shaped body attached to the roof of the third ventricle in the region of the posterior commissure (Figs. 9-1 and 9-6). It appears to be a rudimentary gland whose function in the adult is only beginning to be understood. It consists of a network of richly vascular connective tissue trabeculae in the meshes of which are found glia cells and *pinealocytes* or *epiphysial cells*. Histofluorescent studies reveal that pinealocytes in the rhesus monkey have an intense yellow fluorescence characteristic of serotonin (Sheridan and Sladek, '75). Mammalian pinealocytes are phylogenetically related to the neurosensory photoreceptor elements which become predominantly secretory cells, but they remain indirectly photosensitive. The loss of central neural connections of the pineal is compensated for by the peripheral sympathetic system which provides innervation via the superior cervical ganglion. Each pinealocyte has one or more processes of variable length which from ultrastructural studies appear adapted for secretory function (Martin et al., '77). The club-shaped endings of these processes terminate close to perivascular spaces surrounding capillaries.

The best known pineal secretions are the biogenic amines serotonin, norepinephrine and melatonin, but the gland also contains significant concentrations of identified hypothalamic peptides such as thyrotropin-releasing hormone (TRH), luteinizing hormone-releasing hormone (LHRH), and somatostatin (Martin et al., '77). Serotonin is synthesized in the pinealocyte and released into the extracellular space. Norepinephrine is synthesized in sympathetic neurons which terminate on pineal parenchymal cells and in the perivascular space (Quay, '74).

The pineal gland synthesizes melatonin from serotonin by the action of two enzymes sensitive to variations of diurnal light, *N*-acetyltransferase and hydroxyindole-*o*-methyltransferase (Axelrod et al., '65; Klein and Weller, '70). Daily fluctuations in melatonin synthesis are rhythmic and directly related to the daily cycle of photic input. Light entrains the circadian rhythm to the environmental light cycle (Klein and Weller, '70; Moore and Klein, '74) and also acts by an unidentified pathway to rapidly block the transmission of neural signals to the pineal gland (Klein and Weller, '72). *N*-Acetyltransferase activity is elevated during the night, but exposure to light turns off the activity of the enzyme (Klein and Moore, '79). Bilateral lesions of the suprachiasmatic nucleus (Fig. 10-1) of the hypothalamus, which receives the retinohypothalamic tract, abolish the rhythm in pineal *N*-acetyltransferase activity and result in low levels of hydroxyindole-*o*-methyltransferase activity (Klein and Moore, '79). Such lesions abolish the circadian rhythms of spontaneous locomotor activity and of both feeding and drinking (Mosko and Moore, '79; van den Pol and Powley, '79). In female rats the normal estrous cycle is abolished by lesions of the suprachiasmatic nuclei. The photoregulation of pineal *N*-acetyltransferase and hydroxyindole-*o*-methyltransferase via the retinohypothalamic tract suggests that the suprachiasmatic nuclei are the endogenous sources of signals which generate the circadian rhythms in pineal *N*-acetyltransferase activity and tonically elevate hydroxyindole-*o*-methyltransferase activity (Klein and Moore, '79). The retinohypothalamic projection alters pineal function by directly interacting with structures in the suprachiasmatic nucleus. Environmental light can be regarded as having an entraining function and a transmission function. The effect of light in entraining the endogenous oscillator to the light cycle is slow, but the effect of light on signal transmission is rapid and probably accounts for the rapid "turn off" of *N*-acetyltransferase by light and the blocking of circadian rhythm by constant light.

Although a single neural pathway from the suprachiasmatic nucleus regulates both enzymes involved in the formation of melatonin by the pineal, details concerning these connections are not known. Localization injections of [^{3}H]amino acids in the suprachiasmatic nucleus in the rat have not revealed a projection to any well-defined cell mass in the hypothalamus (Swanson and Cowan, '75). On the basis of indirect evidence it is presumed that the pathway from the suprachiasmatic nucleus to the pineal involves relays to the tuberal region of the hypothalamus, the medial forebrain bundle and spinal pathways that reach the intermediolateral cell column and cells of the superior cervical ganglion. Lesions in the superior cervical ganglion, the medial forebrain bundle and the retrochiasmatic region of the hypothalamus block the stimulatory effects of the suprachiasmatic nucleus upon pineal enzymes (Moore and Rapport, '70; Klein et al., '71; Moore and Klein, '74). Thus the pineal gland appears to be a neuroendocrine transducer that converts neural signals received via sympathetic neurons into an endocrine output, melatonin.

Pineal secretions which alter hypothalamic functions do so after they enter the general circulation or the cerebrospinal fluid (Fraschini et al., '71; Martin et al., '77). Daily fluctuations in pineal serotonin and melatonin are rhythmic in response to the cycle of photic input. These rhythmic changes in pineal activity, suggest that this gland functions as a biological clock delivering signals that regulate both physiological and behavioral processes. These fluctuations, called *circadian rhythms*, have a period of exactly 24 hours in the presences of environmental cues, while in the absence of such cues they only approximate the 24-hour cycle (Binkley, '79).

Many observations suggest that parenchymatous pinealomas are associated with depression of gonadal function and delayed pubescence, while lesions which destroy the pineal frequently are associated with precocious puberty (Relkin, '76). These observations are consistent with experimental studies indicating that the pineal gland exerts an inhibitory influence on the gonads and the reproductive system (Fraschini et al., '71). Experimental data suggest that indoles and methoxyindoles synthesized in the pineal inhibit the secretions of pituitary gonadotropins. Melatonin which is a potent skin-lightening agent in amphibians, has no effect upon human skin, possibly because in man most melanin pigment is stored outside the melanocytes. After the age of 16, calcareous bodies frequently are present in the pineal body. These calcareous bodies form large conglomerations which often are visible in skull roentgenographs. Identification and measurements of the position of the pineal body in skull films can provide useful information, especially in the diagnosis of space-occupying intracranial lesions.

THALAMUS

Transverse sections through the central part of the diencephalon demonstrate three major divisions of the dincephalon: (1) the thalamus, (2) the hypothalamus, and (3) the subthalamic region (Fig. 2-25).

The narrow third ventricle, extending from the region immediately ventral to the striae medullares to the optic chiasm, completely separates the thalami. A shallow groove on the ventricular surface, the hypothalamic sulcus (Fig. 2-25 and 9-5), separates the dorsal thalamus from the hypothalamus. The dorsal surface of the thalamus is covered by the *stratum zonale.* At the junction of the dorsal and medial thalamic surfaces, fibers of the striae medullares are cut transversely and appear as small bundles of myelinated fibers (Fig. 9-5). The dorsal thalamus is divided into

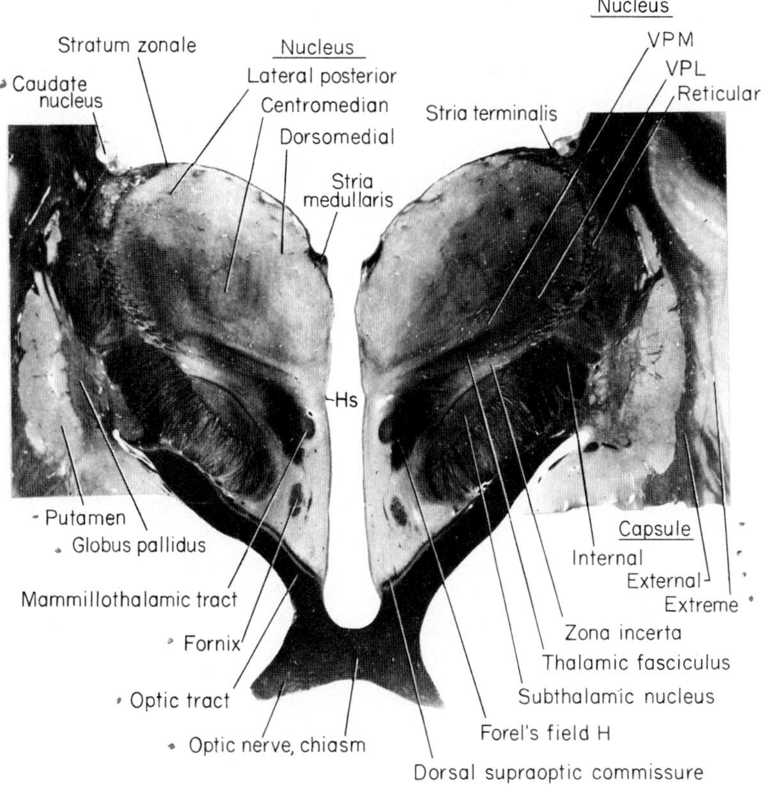

Figure 9-5. Transverse section through the diencephalon and corpus striatum at the level of the optic chiasm. *Hs* indicates the hypothalamic sulcus in the wall of the third ventricle. *VPM* and *VPL* refer to the ventral posteromedial and ventral posterolateral nuclei of the thalamus. (Weigert's myelin stain; photograph.) (From Carpenter and Sutin, *Human Neuroanatomy*, 1983; courtesy of Williams & Wilkins.)

medial and lateral nuclear groups by a band of myelinated fibers, the *internal medullary lamina* of the thalamus which contains several different cell groups (Figs. 2-25, 9-9, 9-10, and 9-11). The lateral nuclear group, between the internal and external medullary laminae, is further divided into ventral and lateral (dorsal) nuclear masses (Fig. 9-5). The ventral nuclear mass, extending nearly the entire length of the thalamus, is divisible into three separate nuclei: (1) a caudal, *ventral posterior nucleus*; (2) an intermediate, *ventral lateral nucleus*; and (3) a rostral, *ventral anterior nucleus*. The ventral posterior nucleus is subdivided into a ventral posterolateral nucleus, located laterally, and a ventral posteromedial nucleus, located medially (Figs. 2-25, 9-5, 9-10, and 9-11).

The lateral nuclear mass of the thalamus, located dorsal to the ventral nuclear mass discussed bove, also is divided into three separate nuclei: (1) a greatly expanded caudal part, the *pulvinar*, (2) an intermediate part, the *lateral posterior nucleus*, and (3) a smaller encapsulated rostral part, the *lateral dorsal nucleus* (Figs. 9-3, 9-4, 9-5, 9-6 and 9-11).

The medial nuclear group of the thalamus, located medial to the internal medullary lamina, contains the *dorsomedial nucleus*, a nuclear mass intimately related to the cortex of the frontal lobe. Wedged between the dorsomedial nucleus and the ventral nuclei caudally is the *centromedian nucleus*, the largest of the intralaminar thalamic nuclei (Figs. 9-4, 9-5, 9-10, and 9-11). The internal medullary lamina partially splits to surround this large nucleus.

Along the lateral border of the thalamus, near the internal capsule, is a narrow band of myelinated fibers, the *external medullary*

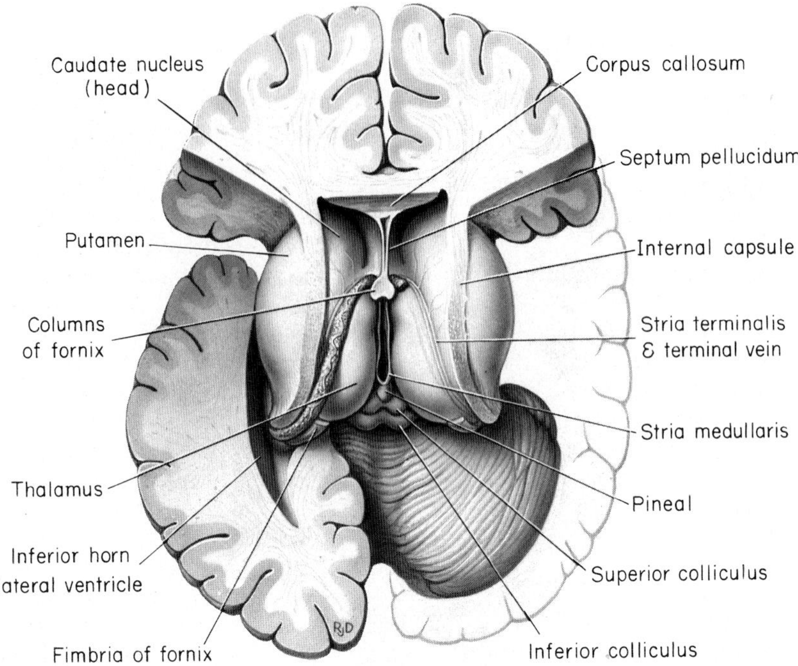

Figure 9-6. Drawing of a brain dissection showing gross relationships of the thalamus, internal capsule, corpus striatum and the ventricular system. (From Carpenter and Sutin, *Human Neuroanatomy*, 1983; courtesy of Williams & Wilkins.)

lamina of the thalamus. Cells located external to the lamina form a thin outer nuclear envelope, the *reticular nucleus* of the thalamus (Figs. 9-5, 9-9, 9-10, and 9-11). Ventrally the reticular nucleus becomes continuous with the zona incerta (Fig. 9-5).

The thalamic nuclei, many of which are microscopic subdivisions of a rich cellular matrix, are particularly difficult to visualize in three dimensions (Fig. 9-11). The nomenclature of the thalamus is complex, and in some instances the fiber connections and the significance of the smaller thalamic nuclei are unknown. In a general way, depending upon their fiber connections, most of the major thalamic nuclei can be classified either as specific relay nuclei (*R*), or as association nuclei (*A*). Specific relay nuclei project to, and receive fibers from, well defined cortical areas considered to be related to specific functions. Association nuclei of the thalamus do not receive direct fibers from ascending systems but project to association areas of the cortex. Other thalamic nuclei have predominantly, or exclusively, subcortical (*SC*) connections. Physiological and anatomical studies indicate that certain thalamic nuclei have diffuse cortical (*DC*) connections. The following classification of thalamic nuclei is based upon functional and morphological data drawn from many sources (Clark, '32; Olszewski, '52; Walker, '38, 38a, '66; Van Buren and Borke, '72). The major nuclear groups of the thalamus and the most important nuclei are in bold faced type. The abbreviations most frequently used to designate these nuclear subdivisions are in parentheses. Letters in italics indicate specific relay nuclei (*R*), association nuclei (*A*), and nuclei with subcortical (*SC*), or diffuse cortical (*DC*) projections.

A. **Anterior Nuclear Group**
   1. **Anteroventral nucleus** (AV) *R*
   2. Anterodorsal nucleus (AD) *R*
   3. Anteromedial nucleus (AM) *R*

B. **Medial Nuclear Group**
   Dorsomedial nucleus (DM)
   a. parvicellular part (DMpc) *A*
   b. magnocellular part (DMmc) *SC*
   c. paralaminar part (DMpl) *R*

C. **Midline Nuclear Group**
   1. Paratenial nucleus
   2. Paraventricular nucleus
   3. Reuniens nucleus
   4. Rhomboidal nucleus
D. **Intralaminar Nuclear Group**
   1. **Centromedian nucleus** (CM) *SC, DC*
   2. **Parafascicular nucleus** (PF) *SC, DC*
   3. Paracentral nucleus *SC, DC*
   4. Central lateral nucleus *SC, DC*
   5. Central medial nucleus *SC*
E. **Lateral Nuclear Group**
   1. **Lateral dorsal nucleus** (LD) *A*
   2. **Lateral posterior nucleus** (LP) *A*
   3. **Pulvinar** (P) *A*
      a. medial part
      b. lateral part
      c. inferior part *R*
F. **Ventral Nuclear Group**
   1. **Ventral anterior nucleus** (VA)
      a. parvicellular part (VApc) *R, SC, DC*
      b. magnocellular part (VAmc) *R, SC*
   2. **Ventral lateral nucleus** (VL)
      a. oral part (VLo) *R*
      b. caudal part (VLc) *R*
      c. medial part (VLm) *R*
   3. **Ventral posterior nucleus** (VP) *R*
      a. **ventral posterolateral** (VPL) *R*
         aa. oral part (VPLo) *R*
         bb. caudal part (VPLc) *R*
      b. **ventral posteromedial** (VPM) *R*
         aa. parvicellular part (VPMpc) *R*
      c. ventral posterior inferior (VPI) *R*
G. **Metathalamus**
   1. **Medial geniculate body** (MGB) *R*
      a. parvicellular part (MGpc) *R*
      b. magnocellular part (MGmc) *R*
   2. **Lateral geniculate body** (LGB) *R*
      a. dorsal part *R*
      b. ventral part *SC*
H. **Unclassified Thalamic Nuclei**
   1. Submedial nucleus
   2. Suprageniculate nucleus
   3. Limitans nucleus
I. **Thalamic Reticular Nucleus** (RN) *SC*

The gross appearance of the dorsal surface of the diencephalon is shown in different dissections in Figures 9-1 and 9-6. These figures illustrate the relationships of the thalamus and epithalamus to surrounding structures and the infratentorial brain stem. Two important levels of the thalamus in transverse section in Figures 9-9 and 9-10 show portions of major thalamic nuclei as they appear in Nissl stained sections. Major nuclear subdivisions of the thalamus are shown schematically together with established afferent and efferent connections in Figure 9-11. Cortical projection areas of major thalamic nuclei are represented diagrammatically in Figure 9-12. The same color coding is used in Figures 9-11 and 9-12. Several ascending thalamic afferent systems have been diagrammed in earlier chapters. Ascending spinal pathways are shown in Figures 4-1, 4-3, and 4-4, while pathways originating in the brain stem are diagrammed in Figures 6-10, 6-23, and 7-18. Cerebellar pathways projecting to the thalamus are shown in Figures 8-13, 8-14 and 8-16. These schematic diagrams and those in Chapter 11 (Figs. 11-15 and 11-20) supplement information contained in Figures 9-11 and 9-12.

Anterior Nuclear Group. The anterior nuclear group lies beneath the dorsal surface of the most rostral part of the thalamus, where it forms the anterior tubercle (Figs. 9-7, 9-9, and 9-11). It consists of a large principal nucleus, the *anteroventral* (AV), and accessory nuclei, the *anterodorsal* (AD) and *anteromedial* (AM). The round or polygonal cells composing these nuclei are of medium or small size; they have little chromophilic substance, a moderate amount of yellow pigment and are surrounded by a capsule of myelinated fibers. The anterior nuclei receive the mammillothalamic tract. Fibers from the medial mammillary nucleus project to the ipsilateral anteroventral and anteromedial nuclei, while the lateral mammillary nucleus projects bilaterally to the anterodorsal nucleus (Fry et al., '63). The lateral mammillary nucleus projects fibers to both AD and the midbrain tegmentum (van der Kooy et al., '78). The anterior nuclei of the thalamus are said to receive as many direct fibers from the fornix as from the mammillothalamic tract (Powell et al., '57). The cortical projections of the anterior nuclei are to the cingulate gyrus (areas 23, 24, and 32) via the anterior limb of the internal capsule

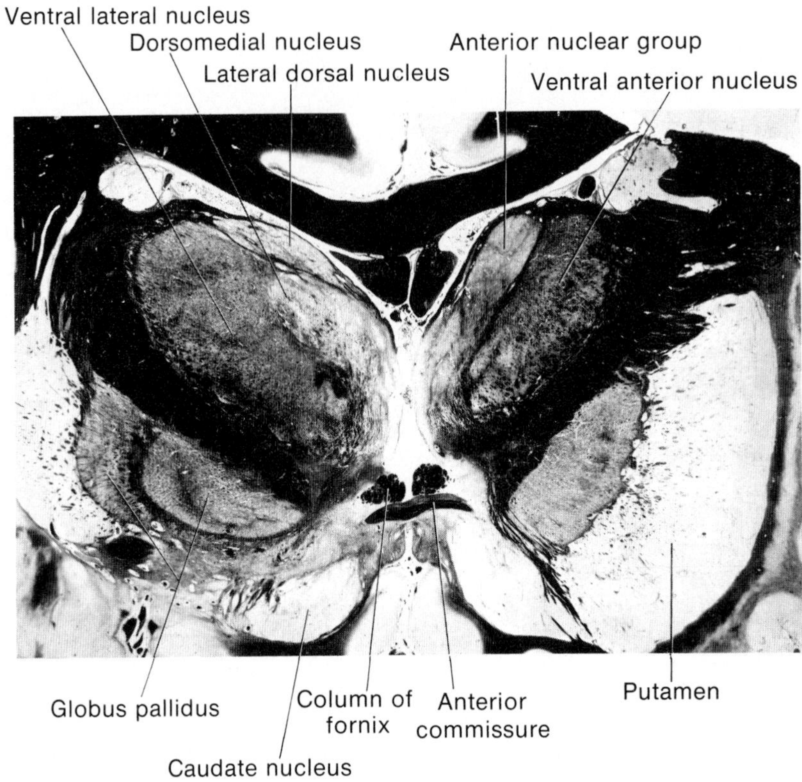

Figure 9-7. Photograph of an asymmetrical transverse section through rostral portions of the thalamus and corpus striatum. The right side reveals the anterior nuclear group and the ventral anterior nucleus. The more caudal level on the left is through the ventral lateral, dorsomedial and lateral dorsal thalamic nuclei. (Weigert's myelin stain.)

(Fig. 9-12). The anterodorsal nucleus sends fibers to the posterior cingulate gyrus including the retrosplenial area, while the anteroventral nucleus projects to the middle and posterior cingulate cortex (Niimi, '78). The anteromedial nucleus projects largely to the anterior cingulate cortex, but its diffuse projections extend to nearly the entire limbic cortex. Although there is considerable overlap, the cingulate cortex receives most of its input from the anteroventral and anteromedial nuclei (Niimi et al., '78). The bulk of the projections from these cortical areas are to the entorhinal cortex via the cingulum (Fig. 2-15) (Raisman et al., '65; Raisman, '66).

Dorsomedial Nucleus. The dorsomedial nucleus (DM), or mediodorsal nucleus, occupies most of the area between the internal medullary lamina and the periventricular gray (Figs. 9-5, 9-9, 9-10, 9-11, and 9-13). Three major regions of the nucleus are recognized: (1) a magnocellular portion (DMmc), located rostrally and dorsomedially, (2) a larger dorsolateral and caudal parvicellular portion (DMpc), and (3) a paralaminar portion (DMpl, pars multiformis) characterized by large cells forming a band adjacent to the internal medullary lamina (Olszewski, '52; Künzle and Akert, '77). The nucleus has extensive connections with intralaminar and lateral thalamic nuclear groups. The medial magnocellular division of the dorsomedial nucleus receives fibers from the amygdaloid complex, the temporal neocortex, the caudal orbitofrontal cortex, and possibly the substantia innominata via the inferior thalamic peduncle (Fig. 9-8) (Whitlock and Nauta, '56; Nauta, '62; Powell et al., '63, '65; Krettek and Price, '74; Mehler, '80). Most of these fibers constitute components of the *ansa*

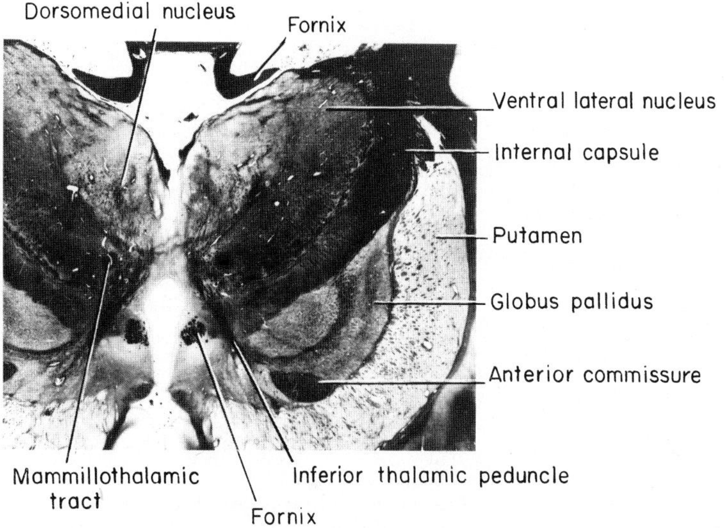

Figure 9-8. Transverse section through the diencephalon and corpus striatum demonstrating fibers of the inferior thalamic peduncle. The inferior thalamic peduncle consists of fibers from the amygdaloid complex, temporal neocortex, and possibly the substantia innominata which project to the dorsomedial nucleus of the thalamus. The inferior thalamic peduncle, plus amygdaloid projections to the hypothalamus and preoptic regions constitute the *ansa peduncularis.* (Weigert's myelin stain; photograph.) (From Carpenter and Sutin, *Human Neuroanatomy*, 1983; courtesy of Williams & Wilkins.)

peduncularis. The ansa peduncularis consists of the inferior thalamic peduncle, plus fibers interconnecting the amygdaloid complex and the preopticohypothalamic region (Nauta and Mehler, '66).

The larger parvicellular portion of this nucleus is connected by a massive projection with practically the entire frontal cortex rostral to areas 6 and 32 (Tobias, '75) (Fig. 9-12). After extensive prefrontal cortical lesions, or lesions interrupting fibers from this region (i.e., prefrontal lobotomy), nearly all small cells of the dorsomedial nucleus degenerate. Retrograde transport of horseradish peroxidase (HRP) indicates that no cells of the dorsomedial nucleus project to the precentral motor cortex (Kievit and Kuypers, '77). There are reciprocal connections between the dorsomedial nucleus and the granular frontal cortex (i.e., prefrontal cortex) and between the paralaminar subdivision and the premotor cortex (Kievit and Kuypers, '77; Akert and Hartmann-von Monakow, '80). Particularly profuse reciprocal connections exist between area 8 (frontal eye field) and the paralaminar part of the dorsomedial nucleus (Scollo-Lavizzari and Akert, '63; Künzle and Akert, '77). The paralaminar part of the dorsomedial nucleus also receives a substantial projection from the pars reticulata of the substantia nigra (Carpenter and Peter, '72; Carpenter et al., '76). It is of interest that although the magnocellular division of the dorsomedial nucleus receives projections from the amygdala, this connection is not reciprocal (Mehler, '80). The dorsomedial nucleus is thought to be concerned with integration of somatic and visceral impulses (Walker, '59). Impulses relayed to the prefrontal cortex may enter consciousness and influence various feeling tones. Psychosurgical studies (i.e., prefrontal lobotomy) suggest that the dorsomedial nucleus and large regions of the frontal association cortex may be concerned with aspects of affective behavior.

Midline Nuclei. The midline nuclei are less distinct cell clusters which lie in the periventricular gray matter of the dorsal half of the ventricular wall and in the interthalamic adhesion (Figs. 9-9 and 9-10). These nuclei are small and difficult to delimit in man. Efferent fibers from the paraventricular nucleus, the central nuclear complex, and the nucleus reuniens project

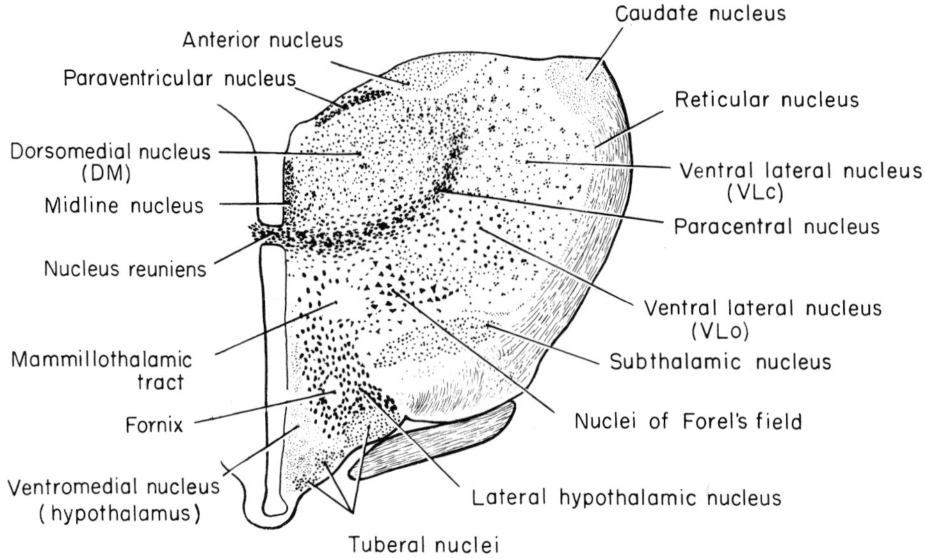

Figure 9-9. Drawing of a transverse Nissl section through the diencephalon at the level of the tuber cinereum showing nuclei of the thalamus and hypothalamus (modified from Malone, '10). (From Carpenter and Sutin, *Human Neuroanatomy*, 1983; courtesy of Williams & Wilkins.)

to the amygdaloid nuclear complex (Mehler, '80). Some of the midline thalamic nuclei may also project to the anterior cingulate cortex (Vogt et al., '79) and fine myelinated and unmyelinated fibers are thought to relate these nuclei to the hypothalamus. These nuclei are considered to be concerned with visceral functions.

Intralaminar Nuclei

The intralaminar nuclei (Figs. 9-4, 9-5, 9-9, 9-10, 9-11, and 9-13) are cell groups infiltrating the internal medullary lamina which separates the medial and the lateral subdivisions of the thalamus. Their cells vary in size in the different nuclei, are usually fusiform and dark staining, and resemble those of the midline nuclei.

Centromedian Nucleus. This, the largest and most easily identified of the intralaminar thalamic nuclei (Figs. 9-4, 9-5, 9-10, 9-11 and 9-13), is located in the middle third of the thalamus between the dorsomedial nucleus and the ventral posterior nucleus (Figs. 9-10, 9-11 and 9-13). It is almost completely surrounded by fibers of the internal medullary lamina, except along its medial border, where it merges with the parafascicular nucleus (Fig. 9-4). It is composed of ovoid or round cells containing a considerable amount of yellow pigment. Cells in the lateral portion of the nucleus are small, while those in more medial regions bordering the dorsomedial nucleus are larger and more densely arranged. There has been considerable controversy concerning precise delimitation of the centromedian nucleus (CM), particularly with respect to the border separating it from the parafascicular nucleus. According to Mehler ('66b) only the ventrolateral small-celled region should be identified as the centromedian nucleus.

Parafascicular Nucleus. This nucleus lies medial to the centromedian nucleus and ventral to the caudal part of the dorsomedial nucleus (Figs. 9-4 and 9-13). The most distinguishing feature of the parafascicular nucleus is that its cells surround the dorsomedial part of the fasciculus retroflexus. Portions of this nucleus medial and lateral to the fasciculus retroflexus show no cytological differences.

Rostral Intralaminar Nuclei. The paracentral, central lateral, and central medial nuclei are all associated with the internal medullary lamina of the thalamus (Figs. 9-9 and 9-10). The paracentral nucleus (PCN) lies in the internal medullary lamina

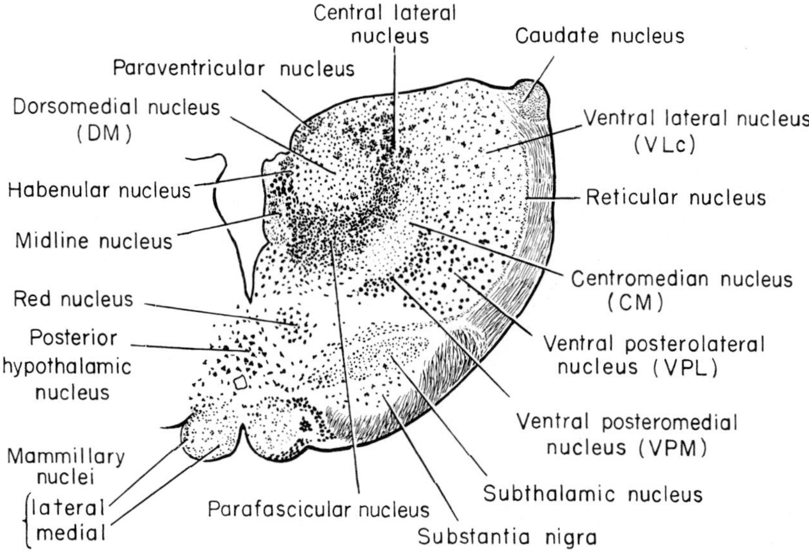

Figure 9-10. Drawing of a transverse Nissl section of the diencephalon at the level of the habenular nuclei and the mammillary bodies (modified from Malone, '10.) (From Carpenter and Sutin, *Human Neuroanatomy*, 1983; courtesy of Williams & Wilkins.)

adjacent to the rostral part of the dorsomedial nucleus. Cells are large, dark, and multipolar, and grouped into clusters between myelinated fiber bundles. Caudally the paracentral nucleus appears to fuse with the central lateral nucleus (CL) which lies dorsal to the centromedian nucleus and lateral to the dorsomedial nucleus (Figs. 9-9, 9-10, and 9-13). The central lateral nucleus is broader than the paracentral nucleus and composed of similar cells. The central medial nucleus lies adjacent to the medial part of the paracentral nucleus (Toncray and Krieg, '46; Olszewski, '52).

The brain stem reticular formation is regarded as one of the principal sources of afferent impulses to the intralaminar thalamic nuclei. Fibers from broad regions of the brain stem reticular formation ascend in the central tegmental tract (Figs. 6-1, 6-4, 6-25, 7-2, and 7-4). Ascending fibers in the central tegmental tract have been traced into: (1) the paracentral and central lateral nuclei and (2) the subthalamic region (Nauta and Kuypers, '58; Scheibel and Scheibel, '58). These projections are said to be chiefly ipsilateral. Because potentials in the brain stem reticular formation have been recorded following stimulation of virtually every type of receptor, it has been presumed that activation of the ascending reticular system was a consequence of "collateral" excitation derived from specific sensory pathways (Chapter 7).

As mentioned earlier with respect to the spinothalamic tract, anterolateral cordotomy (Mehler et al., '60) produces ascending degeneration which passes not only to the ventral posterolateral nucleus and the posterior thalamic nucleus, but also to the intralaminar thalamic nuclei. Unilateral anterolateral cordotomy produces bilateral degeneration in these nuclei which is greatest ipsilaterally, except in the intralaminar nuclei where it is bilateral and nearly equal. Within the intralaminar nuclei fibers are distributed to the paracentral and central lateral nuclei (Figs. 9-9, 9-10, and 9-13). Spinal afferents to parts of the intralaminar nuclei follow pathways in the brain stem that are independent of the classic spinothalamic pathway. Other afferents to the rostral intralaminar arise from the contralateral dentate nucleus. These fibers pass via the superior cerebellar peduncle and mostly terminate in the central lateral nucleus (Percheron, '77; Hendry et al., '79; Thach and Jones, '79).

The centromedian (CM) and parafascicular (PF) nuclei receive afferent fibers mainly from forebrain derivatives. Area 4 projects fibers which are distributed

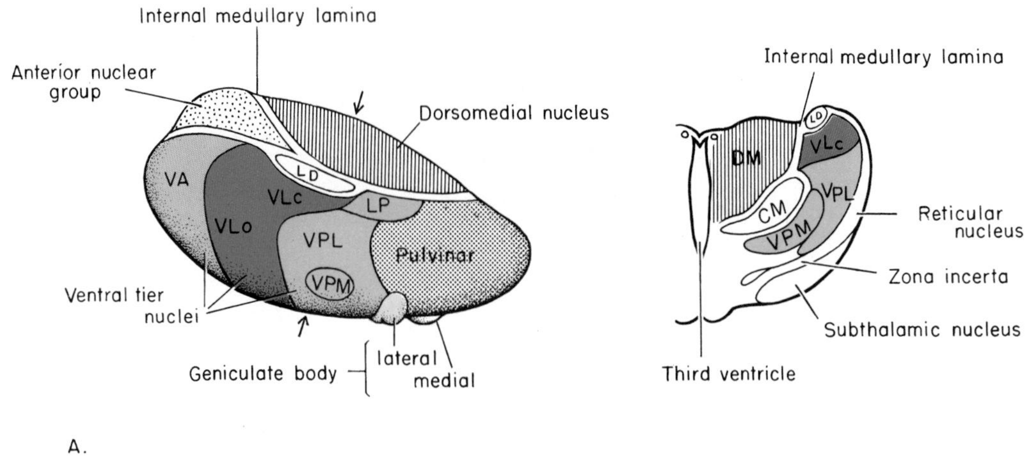

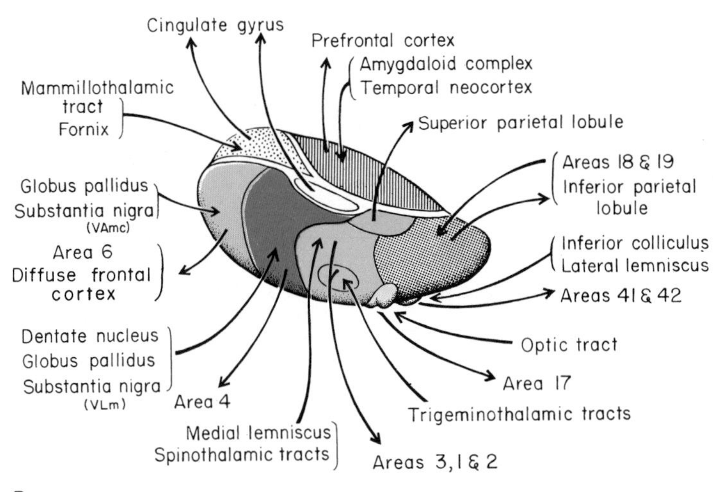

Figure 9-11. Schematic diagrams of the major thalamic nuclei. An oblique dorsolateral view of the thalamus and its major subdivisions is shown in *A*. A transverse section of the thalamus at level of arrows, shown on the right in *A*, indicates the relationships between VPM and VPL, and the location of CM with respect to the internal medullary lamina of the thalamus. In *B*, the principal afferent and efferent projections of major thalamic subdivisions are indicated. While most cortical areas project fibers back to the thalamic nuclei from which fibers are received, this generalization does not apply to the intralaminar nuclei or the reticular nucleus of the thalamus. (From Carpenter and Sutin, *Human Neuroanatomy*, 1983; courtesy of Williams & Wilkins.)

throughout the centromedian nucleus, while area 6 projects to the lateral part of the parafascicular nucleus (Petras, '64, '69; Mehler, '66b; Rinvik, '68). Autoradiographic studies indicate substantial cortical projections to the intralaminar thalamic nuclei which arise from broad regions of the frontal lobe (Künzle, '76, '78; Akert and Hartmann-von Monakow, '80). The precentral motor cortex (area 4) projects terminals to the paracentral, central lateral, and centromedian thalamic nuclei. The cortical projection to the centromedian nucleus is massive and some of these fibers cross the midline to corresponding parts of the same nucleus on the opposite side. The premotor area (area 6) sends afferents to parts of the central lateral nucleus and to the parafascicular nucleus. Only areas 8 and 9 of the prefrontal cortex project to the intralaminar nuclei; these fibers end in the parafascicular nucleus. Although most corticothalamic and thalamocortical projection systems are reciprocal, this generali-

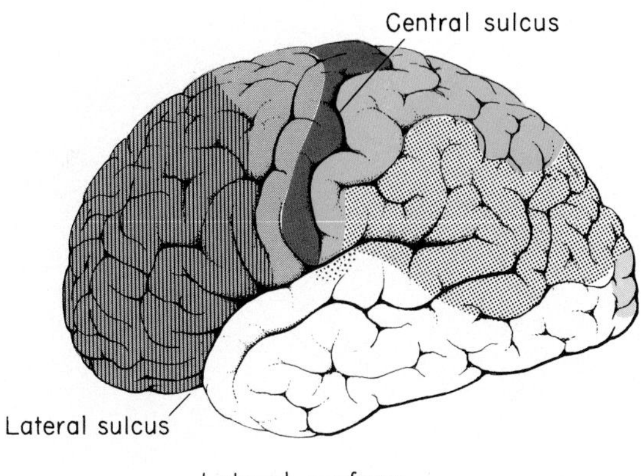

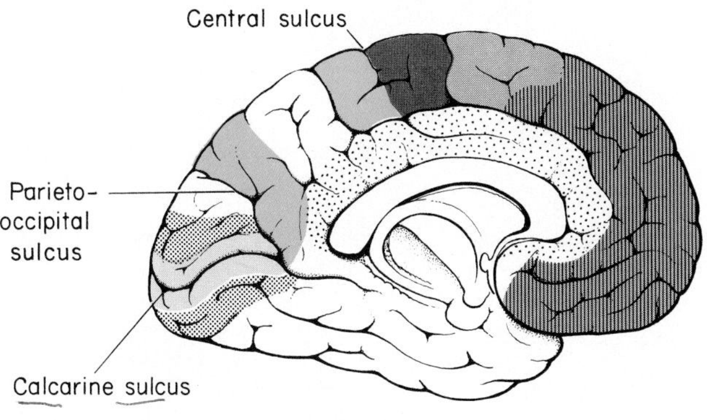

Figure 9-12. Diagram of the left cerebral hemisphere showing the cortical projection areas of thalamic nuclei. The color code is the same as in Figure 9-11. The diffuse projection of the ventral anterior nucleus (VApc) to the frontal lobe appears to largely overlap the projection of the dorsomedial nucleus (DM). Information concerning the cortical projections of some nuclear subdivisions are incomplete. (From Carpenter and Sutin, *Human Neuroanatomy*, 1983; courtesy of Williams & Wilkins.)

zation does not pertain to the intralaminar thalamic nuclei which have diffuse cortical projections that are in no sense reciprocal.

The centromedian nucleus (CM) also receives a large number of pallidal efferent fibers that separate from the thalamic fasciculus at nearly right angles (Nauta and Mehler, '66; Carpenter and Strominger, '67; Kuo and Carpenter, '73; Kim et al., '76). A considerable part of these fibers may be collaterals of pallidofugal fibers passing to the ventral anterior and ventral lateral thalamic nuclei (Figs. 11-19 and 11-20).

While all of the efferent projections of the intralaminar nuclei are not known, the principal projections of the centromedian-parafascicular complex is to the putamen (Powell and Cowan, '56, '67; Mehler, '66b; Kuo et al., '78); Jones and Leavitt, '74), where thalamostriate fibers terminate upon dendritic spines of spiny striatal neurons (Kemp, '68; Fox et al., '71). The smaller rostral intralaminar nuclei project fibers to the caudate nucleus.

Axoplasmic transport studies indicate that the centromedian-parafascicular complex (CM-PF) also projects to the rostral pole of the subthalamic nucleus (Sugimoto et al., '83; Sugimoto and Hattori, '83). Labeled neurons scattered throughout CM-PF participating in this projection are not numerous. These data suggest that CM-PF

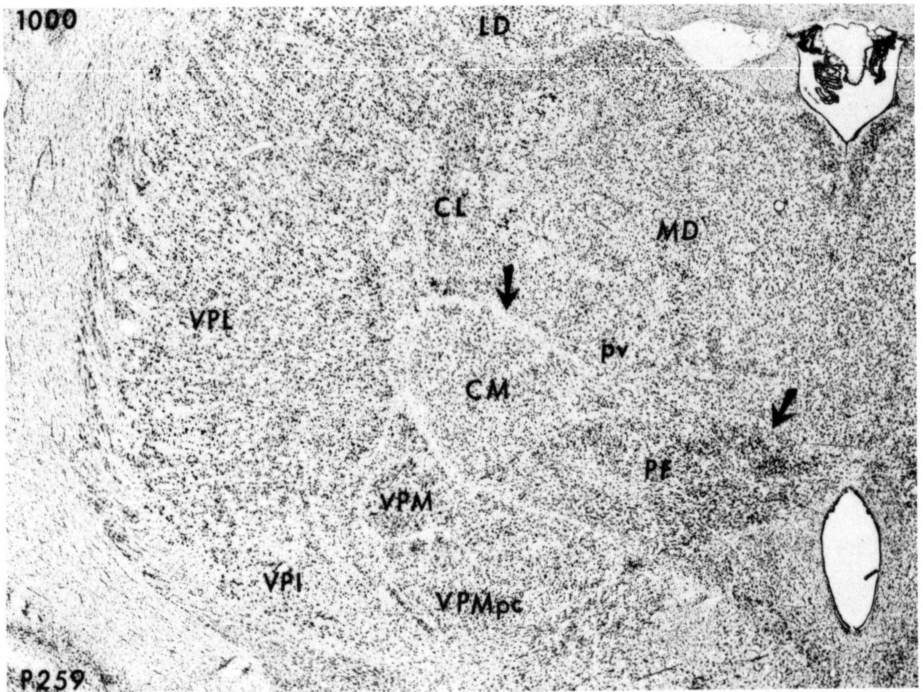

Figure 9-13. Photomicrograph of a transverse section of the thalamus through the ventrobasal complex and the intralaminar nuclei in the monkey. Abbreviations used: *CL*, central lateral nucleus; *CM*, centromedian nucleus; *LD*, lateral dorsal nucleus; *MD*, dorsomedial nucleus; *PF*, parafascicular nucleus; *pv*, ventral paralaminar part of dorsomedial nucleus; *VPI*, ventral posterior inferior nucleus; *VPL*, ventral posterolateral nucleus; *VPM*, ventral posteromedial nucleus; *VPMpc*, parvicellular part of *VPM*. *Arrows* on superior border of the internal medullary lamina define limits of *CM* and *PF*. Numbers refer to animal and sequential section. (Cresyl violet; ×22.) (From Roberts and Akert, '63, courtesy of Dr. Konrad Akert, Zürich.) (From Carpenter and Sutin, *Human Neuroanatomy*, 1983; courtesy of Williams & Wilkins.)

serves to regulate activities of both the putamen and the subthalamic nucleus.

The intralaminar nuclei of the thalamus have long been regarded as having no cortical projections. This conclusion was based upon the absence of retrograde cell changes in these nuclei following virtually complete decortication (Walker, '38a) and the absence of degeneration traceable from lesions in the centromedian nucleus to any part of the cortex. These observations have been difficult to reconcile with physiological evidence indicating that the intralaminar nuclei are of great importance in the control of electrocortical activity over broad regions of the cerebral cortex. Studies based upon the retrograde transport of the enzyme horseradish peroxidase (HRP) provide evidence that thalamostriate fibers from the intralaminar thalamic nuclei give rise to collateral systems which project diffusely to broad cortical regions (Jones and Leavitt, '74). These collaterals have overlapping cortical terminations with fibers from at least one cortical thalamic relay nucleus.

The more rostral intralaminar thalamic nuclei (central lateral and paracentral) contain cells which receive fibers from the midbrain reticular formation project directly to widespread cortical regions (Hendry et al., '79; Itoh and Mizuno, '77; Glen and Steriade, '82; Steriade and Glen, '82). These neurons in CL and PCN do not have bifurcating axons and conduction velocities of fibers projecting to cortex and to the striatum are different. In the cat, cells in these intralaminar thalamic nuclei project directly and mainly to the sensory motor cortex (Steriade and Glen, '82). Thus pathways from the midbrain reticular formation to the cerebral cortex are monosynaptic with relays in the central lateral and paracentral nuclei (CL-PCN). Monosynaptic relays in CL-PCN convey impulses from the midbrain reticular formation to many separate cortical areas, as well as to the caudate nucleus. It is hypothesized that cortical projecting intralaminar thalamic neurons that relay activity from the midbrain reticular formation to the cerebral cortex play an important role in processes that characterize wakefulness and desynchronized sleep.

The intralaminar thalamic nuclei show a striking development in primates and man, in relation to thalamic relay nuclei, suggesting that they constitute a complex intrathalamic regulating mechanism concerned with diverse functions. The intralaminar thalamic nuclei have been considered to serve as: (1) the thalamic pacemaker controlling electrocortical activities (Dempsey and Morrison, '42, '43; Jasper, '49; Purpura and Shofer, '63); (2) part of a nonspecific sensory system (Albe-Fessard and Rougeul, '58; Roudomin et al., '65); (3) a component of a central pain mechanism (Albe-Fessard and Kruger, '62; Lim et al., '69; Emmers, '76); and (4) a modulator of striatal activities (McGuinness and Krauthamer, '80). Anatomical evidence indicates the spinal, trigeminal, reticular and cerebellar projections to the intralaminar thalamic nuclei end in the central lateral nucleus (Nauta and Kuypers, '58; Mehler, '66b; McGuiness and Krauthamer, '80; Jones and Burton, '74; Boivie, '79). This nucleus may be particularly concerned with pain mechanisms and sensory integration. The large CM-PF nuclear complex appears closely related to motor functions in that it receives major projections from the motor and premotor cortex and from the globus pallidus; this nuclear complex projects mainly to the striatum. This evidence suggests that the unique functions may be related to particular nuclei of the intralaminar thalamic group.

Lateral Nuclear Group

The lateral nuclear group begins as an oblique narrow strip on the dorsomedial surface of the thalamus caudal to the anterior nuclear group (Fig. 9-11). This group consists of three nuclear masses arranged in rostrocaudal sequence, the lateral dorsal nucleus, the lateral posterior nucleus and the pulvinar (Figs. 9-3 and 9-11).

Lateral Dorsal Nucleus. This nucleus, which lies on the dorsal surface of the thalamus, extends along the upper margin of the internal medullary lamina and is surrounded by a myelin fiber capsule, similar to that of the anterior nuclear group (Figs. 9-7 and 9-11). The nucleus achieves its largest size dorsal to the paracentral (PCN) and central lateral nuclei (Fig. 9-7) and has been considered as a caudal extension of the anterior thalamic nuclei (Walker, '66). Projections from the lateral dorsal nucleus (LD) are mainly to the posterior parts of the cingulate gyrus, but it also sends fibers to the supralimbic cortex of the parietal lobe (Niimi and Inoshita, '71). The precuneal cortex has reciprocal connections with the lateral dorsal nucleus. Afferent fibers to this nucleus are poorly understood.

Lateral Posterior Nucleus. This nucleus lies caudal, lateral, and ventral to the lateral dorsal nucleus, and is composed of medium-sized cells evenly distributed (Fig. 9-11). The irregularly shaped nucleus lies dorsal to the ventral posterolateral nucleus and adjacent to the lateral medullary lamina. Caudally the nucleus merges with the oral and medial parts of the pulvinar, from which it is not easily distinguished (Olszewski, '52). Unlike the lateral dorsal nucleus it has no myelin capsule. The input to this thalamic nucleus is poorly understood but it may receive inputs from adjacent primary relay nuclei, especially the ventral posterior nucleus (Walker, '66). Degeneration studies in the cat indicate that the superior and inferior parietal lobules project upon the lateral posterior nucleus (LP) (Robertson and Rinvik, '73). Area 5 of the parietal cortex, constituting part of the superior parietal lobule, has been demonstrated to transport isotope to laminar arrays distributed throughout the lateral posterior nucleus (Jones et al., '79). Some of the these thalamic neurons appear to have reciprocal cortical connections. Retrograde transport studies indicate that the lateral posterior nucleus projects upon areas 5 and 7 (Pearson et al., '78). Cortical areas 5 and 7 in monkey respond to stimulation of peripheral receptors and both of these areas receive association fibers from the primary somesthetic cortex (Jones and Powell, '70a; Mountcastle et al., '75). Area 7 in the monkey, considered the equivalent of the greatly expanded inferior parietal lobule in man, is concerned with the integration of sensory modalities that serve important cognitive and symbolic functions and appears to have a heterogeneous afferent inputs (Divac et al., '77).

Pulvinar. The large nuclear mass, forming the posterior and dorsolateral portion of the thalamus, is known as the pulvinar. Caudally it overhangs the geniculate bodies and dorsolateral surface of the midbrain (Figs. 9-1, 9-3, 9-4, and 9-11). Because the pulvinar exhibits considerable cytological uniformity it is subdivided on a topographic basis into four parts: (1) a *pars oralis*, located between the ventral posterolateral and centromedian nuclei; (2) a *pars inferior*, located ventrally between the medial and lateral geniculate bodies; (3) a *pars medialis*, forming the medial half of the pulvinar; and (4) a *pars lateralis*, extending along the external medullary lamina (Olszewski, '52). The pulvinar is composed of lightly stained, medium-sized, multipolar cells, whose density and arrangement varies in the different subdivisions. Cells in the oral division of the pulvinar are small, light-staining, and loosely arranged. The pars inferior, separated from the main body of the pulvinar by fibers of the brachium of the superior colliculus, is composed of scattered dark-staining cells. The lateral pulvinar is traversed by oblique fiber bundles extending from the external medullary lamina. The medial nucleus contains medium-sized cells and few fibers.

The nuclei of the pulvinar do not receive inputs from long ascending sensory pathways, but the inferior division receives a projection from the superficial layers of the superior colliculus (Harting et al., '73; Benevento and Fallon, '75; Partlow et al., '77). Topographically this projection represents the contralateral visual hemifield. Both the inferior pulvinar and the adjacent portion of the lateral pulvinar have reciprocal connections with occipital cortex, including striate cortex (Ogren and Hendrickson, '76). The inferior pulvinar and the adjacent lateral pulvinar each contain a representation of the contralateral visual hemifield and project retinotopically upon: (1) cortical areas 18 and 19 where fibers end in layers IV, III, and I (Benevento and Rezak, '76), and (2) the striate cortex (area 17) where fibers terminate upon the supragranular layers (Rezak and Benevento, '79). These findings indicate three visuotopically organized inputs from the thalamus (lateral geniculate body, inferior pulvinar, and adjacent lateral pulvinar) to the primary visual cortex which terminate upon different layers. Projections from the inferior pulvinar to cortical areas 17, 18, and 19 constitute the final link in an extrageniculate visual pathway. The lateral pulvinar does not receive a visual input from the superior colliculus, but parts of this nucleus have reciprocal connections with all recognized areas of the visual cortex.

The lateral nucleus of the pulvinar (other than portions adjacent to the inferior pulvinar) projects to temporal cortex and receives reciprocal projections from the same region (Trojanowski and Jacobson, '75). The medial pulvinar appears to have more distant projections in that fibers project to parts of the frontal lobe (Bos and Benevento, '75; Trojanowski and Jacobson, '74).

Ventral Nuclear Mass

The ventral nuclear mass of the thalamus is divided into three nuclei: the *ventral anterior*, the *ventral lateral*, and the *ventral posterior*. The ventral anterior nucleus is the most rostral and the smallest subdivision (Figs. 9-7 and 9-11). The ventral posterior nucleus, the largest and most posterior nucleus of this group, is further subdivided into the *ventral posterolateral and ventral posteromedial* nuclei (Figs. 9-5 and 9-11). Although the *medial* and *lateral geniculate bodies* together constitute the *metathalamus*, these well-defined nuclear masses may be considered as a caudal continuation of the ventral nuclear mass. The ventral nuclear group and the metathalamus constitute the largest division of the thalamus concerned with relaying impulses from other portions of the neuraxis to specific parts of the cerebral cortex. Caudal parts of this complex are concerned with relaying impulses of specific sensory systems to cortical regions, while more rostral nuclei (ventral anterior and ventral lateral nuclei) relay impulses from the corpus striatum, the substantia nigra and the contralateral dentate nucleus.

Ventral Anterior Nucleus. This subdivision lies in the extreme rostral part of the ventral nuclear mass where it is bounded anteriorly and ventrolaterally by the reticular nucleus. Rostrally the ventral anterior nucleus (VA) occupies the entire thalamic region lateral to the anterior nuclear group (Figs. 9-7 and 9-11), but caudally it becomes restricted to a more medial region. The mammillothalamic tract passes through the ventral anterior nucleus but does not form its medial border. The nucleus is composed of large and medium-sized multipolar cells arranged in clusters. Thick myelinated fiber bundles course longitudinally within the nucleus.

Part of the nucleus adjacent to the mammillothalamic tract and along the ventral border of the nucleus is composed of large, dark, densely arranged cells. This subdivision, called the magnocellular part (VAmc) (Olszewski, '52), extends further caudally than the principal part of the ventral anterior nucleus (VApc). Thus, there are two distinctive cytological subdivisions of the ventral anterior nucleus. Each of these subdivisions receives fibers from different sources. Afferent fibers to the ventral anterior nucleus (VApc) arise from the medial segment of the globus pallidus (Nauta and Mehler, '66; Kuo and Carpenter, '73; Kim et al., '76) (Figs. 9-11 and 11-19). The magnocellular part of the ventral anterior nucleus (VAmc) receives fibers primarily from the pars reticulata of the substantia nigra (Carpenter and Peter, '72; Rinvik, '75; Carpenter et al., '76). These fibers pass medially and rostrally through Forel's field H and enter the thalamus from its medioventral aspect (Fig. 7-18).

Cortical projections to the ventral anterior nucleus have been described in autoradiographic studies. Cortical area 6, projects primarily to VApc while fibers from area 8 terminate in VAmc (Künzle and Akert, '77; Künzle, '78); fibers from primary motor area do not reach any part of the nucleus (Künzle, '76). Other afferent fibers, arising from the intralaminar and midline nuclei, may account for some of the characteristics of the nonspecific thalamic system exhibited by this nucleus (Scheibel and Scheibel, '66a).

Information concerning the efferent projections of the ventral anterior nucleus is incomplete and conflicting. Following hemispherectomy, over 50% of the cells in the nucleus remain (Powell, '52). According to Carmel ('70) efferent fibers from this nucleus are distributed intrathalamically to the intralaminar nuclei and to widespread areas of the frontal cortex (Fig. 9-12). Rostrally projecting fibers from VAmc have been described as terminating in localized regions of the caudal and medial orbitofrontal cortex (Scheibel and Scheibel, '66a; Carmel, '70), but many of these fibers may arise from the rostral midline thalamic nuclei (Kievit and Kuypers, '77). Retrograde transport studies using HRP indicate that obliquely oriented bands of cells in VApc project to frontal cortex rostral to the precentral gyrus (Kievit and Kuypers, '77). Finally fibers from VAmc project to VApc, although this connection is not reciprocal.

Physiological data indicate that the ventral anterior nucleus may be functionally related to the intralaminar nuclei of the thalamus, in that recruiting responses in widespread cortical areas can be evoked by repeated low frequency stimulation of the nucleus. The *recruiting response* is a surface negative response evoked by repetitive low frequency stimulation of the ventral anterior, the midline or the intralaminar thalamic nuclei that waxes and wanes and can be recorded over broad areas of the cerebral cortex. The ventral anterior nucleus appears to be the pre-eminent site among thalamic nuclei for the production of the recruiting response. The efferent projections from VA appear to constitute part of the pathway by which diffuse synchronous discharges reach broad regions of the frontal cortex. The projections of VAmc to the orbitofrontal cortex play a special role in "triggering" the recruiting response. The recruiting response is abolished by ablations of the orbitofrontal cortex (Velasco and Lindsley, '65) and is reversibly diminished by cryogenic blockade of this cortical region (Skinner and Lindsley, '67). It is of particular interest that the ventral anterior nucleus seems to exhibit characteristics of both the specific and the nonspecific thalamic nuclei.

Ventral Lateral Nucleus. This nucleus, caudal to the ventral anterior nucleus, is composed of small and large neurons that show considerable differences in various parts of the nucleus (Figs. 9-8, 9-9 and 9-11). The nucleus has been subdivided into three main parts: (1) pars oralis (VLo), (2) pars caudalis (VLc), and (3) pars medialis (VLm). The largest subdivision (VLo) consists of numerous deep staining cells arranged in clusters. The pars caudalis (VLc) is less cellular but formed of scattered large cells. The pars medialis (VLm) begins ventral to VA and extends caudally toward the subthalamic region. A crescent-shaped thalamic area in the monkey caudal to VAmc and medial to VLo, designated as "area x" (Olszewski, '52), appears on the basis of connectivity to be an integral part of the ventral lateral nuclear complex (Carmel, '70; Mehler, '71; Percheron, '77). Nuclear subdivisions designated as VLc, "area x" and the oral part of the ventral posterolateral nucleus (VPLo) have been referred to as the "cell-sparse" zone and cytologically are distinct from VLo, VLm, VPLc, and VPM (Asanuma et al., '83). On the basis of connectivity, nuclei of the "cell sparse" zone of the ventral lateral thalamic region have been considered as the cerebellar relay nuclei to the motor cortex.

Cerebellar efferent fibers contained in the superior cerebellar peduncle decussate in the mesencephalon and project profusely to the contralateral ventral lateral thalamic region (Fig. 8-13). While there is general agreement that cerebellar efferents to the thalamus terminate in regions rostral to those of the medial lemniscus, there have been differences of opinion concerning the precise nuclear subdivisions which receive these fibers. Cerebellar efferent fibers have been described as terminating in all subdivisions of the ventral lateral nucleus (VL), except for the medial part of VLm, in "area x" and portions of the ventral posterolateral nucleus (VPLo) (Chan-Palay, '77); Miller and Strominger, '77; Kalil, '81). Both degeneration and autoradiographic studies indicate that efferents from the contralateral dentate nucleus terminate in VLo, VLc, "area x", the central lateral nucleus (CL), and the oral parts of the ventral posterolateral nucleus (VPLo) (Chan-Palay, '77; Miller and Strominger, '77; Kalil, '81). Other investigators suggest that few, if any, cerebellar efferent fibers terminate in VLo, which has long been regarded as a major thalamic terminus of this system (Percheron, '77; Thach and Jones, '79; Asanuma et al., '83a). This view is supported by retrograde transport studies which indicate that HRP injections confined to VLo in the thalamus retrogradely label only cells in the medial pallidal segment (Tracey et al., '80). This same study has shown that HRP injections in VLc and VPLo retrogradely label cells in the contralateral dentate nuclei. Present evidence suggests that cerebellar efferent fibers end largely in VLc, "area x," CL, and in VPLo, and do not overlap terminations of pallidothalamic fibers (Asanuma et al., '83a).

Pallidofugal fibers arising from the medial pallidal segment project to the ventral lateral nucleus of the thalamus via the thalamic fasciculus. The major projection from the globus pallidus is to the pars oralis, VLo, and the lateral part of the pars medialis (VLm) (Nauta and Mehler, '66; Kuo and Carpenter, '73; Kim et al., '76). Pallidofugal fibers also project rostrally to ventral anterior nucleus (VApc) and give off collateral fibers to the centromedian nucleus (CM) (Figs. 11-19 and 11-20). These projections are topographically organized and have been confirmed by retrograde transport studies (Tracey et al., '80). The pars medialis of the ventral lateral nucleus (VLm) receives efferent projections from the medial pallidal segment and the pars reticulata of substantia nigra but these are not overlapping. The medial part of the VLm receives nigral efferents while the lateral part of this nucleus receives pallidal efferents (Carpenter and Peter, '72; Kuo and Carpenter, '73; Carpenter et al., '76; Kim et al., '76).

The ventral lateral nucleus of the thalamus receives a considerable number of fibers from the precentral cortex. Autoradiographic studies in the monkey demonstrate that area 4 projects to VLo, VLm, VLc, and VPLo as well as to CM, the paracentral nucleus (PCN) and the central lateral nucleus (CL) (Künzle, '76). The projection from area 4 to VLc is not as impressive as that from area 6, which also projects to "area x" (Künzle, '78). The cortical projections of area 4 upon VLo and

VPLo are topographically arranged. Connections of the ventral lateral nucleus with the precentral cortex are reciprocal and topically arranged. Medial parts of the nucleus send fibers to the face area, lateral parts send fibers to the leg area, and fibers from intermediate portions of the nucleus pass to cortical regions representing the arm and trunk (Walker, '38a, '49). Retrograde transport studies based upon multiple injections of HRP into the precentral cortex result in labeling of cells in VLo, VLc, and VPLo, indicating that these nuclei have reciprocal connections with the motor cortex (Strick, '76; Kievit and Kuypers, '77). Similar HRP injections of the postcentral gyrus do not label cells in the ventral lateral nucleus or in VPLo. A more recent analysis indicates that the "cell-sparse" zone of the ventral lateral thalamic region, consisting of VPLo and VLc, projects topographically upon area 4 (Jones et al., '79; Asanuma et al., '83a). Thus the thalamic termination zones for the dentate, interposed and fastigial nuclei are nearly identical and relay impulses to the primary motor area. The cortical projection zones for VLo and "area x" appear different in that VLo projects to the supplementary motor area and "area x" has projections to the arcuate premotor area (Schell and Strick, '84). The distinctive cytoarchitectural subdivisions of the ventral lateral thalamic region appear to project to cortical areas concerned with different aspects of motor function.

Ventral Posterior Nucleus. This nuclear complex, whose cells are among the largest in the thalamus, is composed of two main portions, the *posteromedial* and the *posterolateral* (Figs. 9-5, 9-10). The smallest subdivision of the ventral posterior nucleus is the *ventral posterior inferior nucleus* (VPI) which lies ventrally adjacent to the thalamic reticular nucleus beneath parts of both the ventral posteromedial and posterolateral nuclei (Fig. 9-13). The VP is the largest primary somatic sensory relay nucleus of the thalamus and is referred to as the ventrobasal complex.

Ventral Posterolateral Nucleus (VPL). This nucleus has been subdivided into a pars oralis (VPLo), characterized by very large cells sparsely distributed, and a pars caudalis (VPLc), containing large evenly dispersed cells and a high density of small cells. Both divisions of the nucleus contain medium-sized fiber bundles radiating in an oblique dorsal direction.

As described above VPLo constitutes a distinctive part of the "cell-sparse" zone of the ventral lateral thalamic region which receives inputs from the contralateral deep cerebellar nuclei and projects to the primary motor cortex (Asanuma et al., '83a). Thalamic inputs to VPLc convey somesthetic impulses from the spinal cord and somatosensory relay nuclei in the medulla via: (1) the medial lemniscus, (2) the spinothalamic tract, and (3) the cervicothalamic tract. The spinocervicothalamic system is particularly well developed in carnivores but also exists in primates. The two principal long ascending somesthetic pathways projecting to VPLc are the medial lemniscus and the spinothalamic tracts. Fibers of the medial lemniscus course through the brain stem, without supplying collateral or terminal fibers to the reticular formation, and terminate exclusively in the ventral posterolateral nucleus, pars caudalis (VPLc) (Fig. 4-1). Fibers arising from the nucleus gracilis terminate lateral to those of the nucleus cuneatus. Terminals of the medial lemniscus establish predominantly axodendritic contacts throughout VPLc. Small injections of HRP into VPLc result in retrograde labeling of cells in the nuclei gracilis and cuneatus, while similar HRP injections in VPLo retrogradely label cells in the deep cerebellar nuclei (Tracey et al., '80). In autoradiographic studies where [^{3}H]amino acids have been injected into the nuclei gracilis and cuneatus the distribution of silver grains in the thalamus was confined to VPLc (Tracey et al., '80; Kalil, '81; Asanuma et al., '83a). The distribution of individual medial lemniscus axons in VPLc suggest that all axons have terminal ramifications at one level, are focal and none are sufficiently long to occupy more than one half of the anteroposterior extent of the nucleus (Jones, '83). Terminal ramifications are compressed into sagittal slabs 200 to 300μm wide. Axonal ramification end in either an anterodorsal shell or in the central core of VPLc. Cells in the anterodorsal shell respond to stimulation of deep tissue and largely terminate in cortical areas 3a and 2, while neurons in the central core respond to cutaneous stimulation and largely project to cortical areas 3b and 1 (Jones, '83).

The spinothalamic tracts form a far less discrete ascending sensory pathway than the medial lemniscus and in the spinal cord they are intermingled with fibers destined for multiple sites in the brain stem. Most of our information concerning the course and terminations of the spinothalamic tracts has been based upon the study of degeneration following anterolateral cordotomy or hemisection of the spinal cord (Mehler et al., '60; Asanuma et al., '83a). The spinothalamic tract, and fiber systems ascending with it, contributes a large number of projections and collaterals to various portions of the brain stem reticular formation at all levels.

At the midbrain-diencephalic junction fibers of the spinothalamic tract enter the thalamus near the dorsomedial border of the medial geniculate nucleus. Fibers of the spinothalamic tract terminate mainly in three thalamic nuclei: (1) the medial part of the posterior thalamic nucleus, located medial and rostral to the magnocellular part of the medial geniculate nucleus (Fig. 9-15), (2) the ventral posterolateral nucleus (VPLc), and (3) the central lateral nucleus (CL) of the intralaminar group (Fig. 9-13) (Mehler et al., '60; Mehler, '62, '66a, '74; Kerr and Lippman, '74; Kerr, '75; Boivie, '79). Terminals in the posterior thalamic nucleus are most numerous ventromedially, while those in VPLc are distributed unevenly over the entire nucleus (Boivie, '79; Asanuma et al., '83a). Clusters of fine terminals occur within both of these nuclei. Terminal degeneration in VPLc extends rostrally into the VPLo nucleus, where it exhibits a similar pattern (Asanuma et al., '83a). The number of fibers reaching VPLo is small compared with those that end in VPLc. In the central lateral (CL) nucleus terminals are distributed about clusters of neurons. Ascending spinothalamic fibers are distributed bilaterally in VPLc, CL, and the medial part of the posterior thalamic nucleus, but contralateral terminations are less numerous (Mehler et al., '60; Boivie, '79). Fibers entering the contralateral thalamus cross in the commissure of the superior colliculus and at lower brain stem levels. There is no evidence that fibers of the lateral and ventral spinothalamic tracts have distinctive thalamic terminations.

The cervicothalamic tract, arising from the lateral cervical nucleus in the upper cervical spinal cord, is particularly well developed in carnivores, which lack a typical spinothalamic tract terminating in VPL. Fibers of the cervicothalamic tract cross in upper cervical spinal segments and ascend in association with the opposite medial lemniscus (Boivie, '70). These fibers terminate in VPL. The combined thalamic termination of the cervicothalamic and spinothalamic tracts in the cat resemble the total spinothalamic projection in the monkey (Boivie, '79).

Physiological studies (Poggio and Mountcastle, '60) indicate the precise and orderly fashion in which the contralateral body surface is represented in the ventral posterolateral nucleus (external portion of the ventrobasal complex). There is a complete, though distorted, image of the body; volume representation of a given part of the body is related to its effectiveness as a tactile organ (i.e., to its innervation density). Cervical segments are represented most medially and sacral segments most laterally. The thoracic and lumbar regions are represented only dorsally, while the regions concerned with the distal parts of the limbs extend ventrally. Each neuron of this complex is related to a restricted, specific and unchanging receptive field on the contralateral side of the body. Each neuron of the ventrobasal complex can be activated by either cutaneous tactile stimulation, or mechanical alteration of deep structures (especially joint rotation), but by only one of these. These neurons are regarded as place specific, modality specific, and concerned, almost exclusively, with the perception of tactile sense and position sense (kinesthesis). Few cells of the ventrobasal complex appear to be activated by noxious stimuli. Although the terminology used by these authors differs from that employed here, it is generally accepted that these superbly defined principles apply to man. The inner portion of the ventrobasal complex is known as the ventral posteromedial nucleus.

Ventral Posteromedial Nucleus (VPM). This crescent-shaped nucleus with a relatively light-staining neuropil lies medial to the ventral posterolateral nucleus and lateral to the curved boundary of the centromedian nucleus (Figs. 9-4, 9-5, 9-10, and 9-13). The ventral posteromedial nucleus (VPM) consists of two distinct parts: (1) a principal part composed of both small and large cells, designated simply as VPM, and (2) a small celled, lighter staining part which occupies the medial apex of this arcuate-shaped nucleus, referred to as the pars parvicellularis (VPMpc). The principal part of VPM receives somatic afferent fibers from receptors in the head, face and intraoral structures, while VPMpc is concerned with taste (Figs. 5-21, 9-13, and 9-14). Precise boundaries of VPM are defined best on the basis of its fiber connections. Ascending secondary trigeminal fibers terminating in VPM include: (1) crossed fibers from the spinal and principal sensory trigeminal nuclei, which ascend in association with the medial lemniscus, and (2) uncrossed fibers of the dorsal trigeminal tract (Fig. 6-23). Tactile impulses from the face and intraoral structures are transmitted bilaterally to parts of the ventral posteromedial nucleus.

Secondary gustatory fibers arising from the nucleus solitarius ascend ipsilaterally in the central tegmental tract to terminate in VPMpc (Figs. 5-21 and 9-14) (Beckstead et al., '80). VPMpc also receives ipsilateral gustatory fibers from the parabrachial nuclei, that also receive projections from the nucleus solitarius (Norgren and Pfaffman, '75). HRP injected into VPMpc retrogradely labels cells in the lateral division of the rostral part of the nucleus solitarius.

Ventral Posterior Inferior Nucleus (VPI). This smallest subdivision of the ventral posterior nucleus lies ventrally between VPL and VPM. The ventral border of the nucleus is adjacent to the reticular nucleus and the thalamic fasciculus. Cells of the nucleus are medium-sized and light-staining. Ascending afferents to VPLc traverse the nucleus, but do not end in it. Most evidence suggests that VPI receives ascending vestibular projections (Deecke et al., '73, '74, '77). The best anatomical data indicate that ascending vestibular fibers terminate bilaterally in small scattered regions of VPLo and to a lesser extent in VPI (Fig. 9-13) (Lang et al., '79).

Cortical Connections of the Ventral Posterior Nucleus. The ventral posterior nucleus has a precise topical projection to the cortex of the postcentral gyrus. Portions of the gyrus high on the lateral convexity receive fibers from VPLc while inferior portions of the gyrus near the lateral sulcus are supplied by fibers from VPM (Fig. 9-12). This thalamocortical projection forms a large part of the superior thalamic radiation and is precisely correlated with the termination of ascending somatosensory systems in the ventral posterior nuclear complex. VPMpc projects fibers upon the parietal operculum, area 43 (Benjamin and Akert, '59; Roberts and Akert, '63). Cells of VPL and VPM, which constitute the ventrobasal complex project ipsilaterally to the primary (S I) and secondary (SS II) somatosensory areas (Jones and Powell, '69). The second area (SS II) lies buried in the superior bank of the lateral sulcus (Fig. 13-8). Projections of the ventrobasal complex to both of these areas are somatotopic. Cortical areas 3, 1, and 2 receive the major projections from VPL and VPM, with the largest number of cells projecting to area 3.

Posterior Thalamic Nuclear Complex. Caudal to the ventral posterior nucleus there is a transitional diencephalic zone with a complex and varied cellular morphology (Fig. 9-15). The posterior nuclear complex lies caudal to VPLc, medial to the rostral part of the pulvinar, and dorsal to the medial geniculate body (Figs. 9-3 and 9-15). The nuclear complex consists of the *suprageniculate nucleus*, the *nucleus limitans*, and an ill-defined region of heterogeneous cell types caudal to VPLc, referred to as the *posterior nucleus* (Burton and Jones, '76). The posterior nucleus is comprised of small and medium-sized cells and is difficult to distinguish from overlying regions of the pulvinar and the suprageniculate nucleus (Fig. 9-15).

The posterior nucleus is of particular interest because it receives spinothalamic fibers and has been considered to be concerned with the perception of painful and noxious stimuli (Mehler et al., '60; Kerr and Lippman, '74; Kerr, '75; Boivie, '79). Some studies suggest that fibers of the medial lemniscus and cervicothalamic tract may terminate in this nucleus (Boivie, '70, '78). The medial part of the posterior nu-

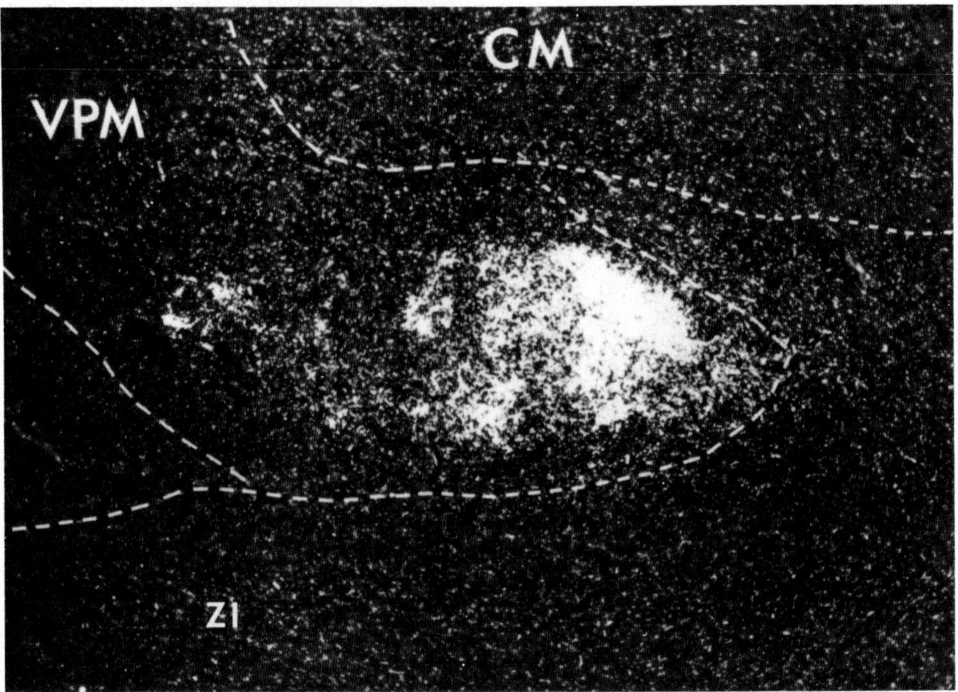

Figure 9-14. Photomicrograph of an autoradiograph demonstrating transport of isotope from the rostrolateral nucleus of the solitary fasciculus to the ipsilateral ventral posteromedial nucleus (pars parvicellularis). See diagrammatic drawing of taste pathways in Fig. 5-21. Abbreviations used: *CM*, centromedian nucleus; *VPM*, somatic part of the ventral posteromedial nucleus; *ZI*, zona incerta. (From Beckstead et al., '80; courtesy of Dr. Norgren and Allan R. Liss, Inc., New York.) (From Carpenter and Sutin, *Human Neuroanatomy*, 1983; courtesy of Williams & Wilkins.)

cleus also receives projections from the primary (S I) and the secondary (S II) somatosensory cortex (Jones and Powell, '68a, '69), as well as from the auditory cortex (Heath and Jones, '71).

Neurons in the region of the posterior thalamic nucleus originally were considered to project in a sustaining fashion to the second somatic area (SS II), a cortical sensory representation on the superior bank of the lateral sulcus (Rose and Woolsey, '58. Detailed studies in the cat and monkey indicate that cells in the medial division of the posterior thalamic nucleus (Fig. 9-15) project to the retroinsular cortex and cells in the lateral division of this nucleus project to postauditory cortex (Burton and Jones, '76). Neither of these cortical projections overlap recognized somatosensory or auditory areas. The retroinsular cortex which receives projections from the medial part of the posterior thalamic nucleus appears to respond to cutaneous stimuli from well-defined contralateral receptive fields located in the hand and foot (Robinson and Burton, '80). These findings raise questions concerning the notion that cells of the posterior thalamic nucleus and SS II are concerned with perception of pain and noxious stimuli.

Medial Geniculate Body. The medial geniculate body (MGB) lies on the caudal ventral aspect of the thalamus, medial to the lateral geniculate body (LGB) and dorsal to the crus cerebri (Figs. 9-2, 9-3, and 9-16). This nuclear mass, the thalamic auditory relay nucleus, receives fibers from the inferior colliculus and gives rise to the auditory radiation (Fig. 9-21). Unlike auditory relay nuclei at lower brain stem levels, there are no commissural connections between the medial geniculate bodies. The medial geniculate nucleus consists of several subdivisions with distinctive cytoarchitecture and connections (Morest, '64; Harrison and Howe, '74; Oliver and

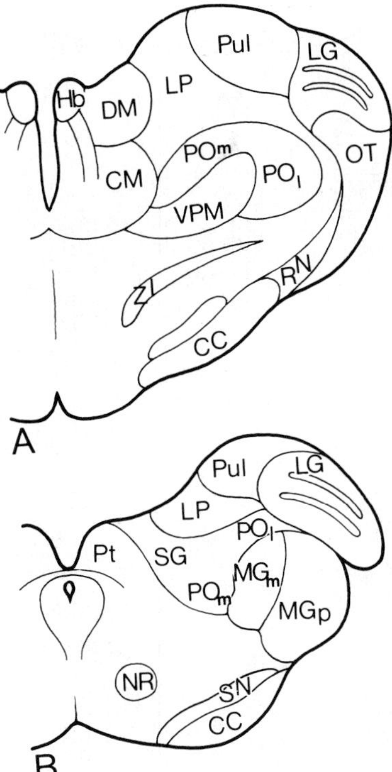

Figure 9-15. Outline drawing through two levels of the caudal thalamus in the cat showing relationships of the nuclei of the posterior thalamic complex to other thalamic nuclei. Two divisions of the posterior thalamic nuclei are recognized, medial (PO_m) and a lateral (PO_l). In *B*, the posterior thalamic nuclei lie medial and dorsal to the magnocellular part of the medial geniculate nucleus (MG_m); the medial nucleus, PO_m, appears continuous with the suprageniculate nucleus (*SG*). In *A*, PO_m and PO_l lie dorsal and lateral to the ventral posterior medial nucleus (*VPM*) and immediately caudal to the ventral posterolateral nucleus (*VPL*). Abbreviations used: *CC*, crus cerebri; *CM*, centromedian nucleus; *DM*, dorsomedial nucleus; *Hb*, habenula; *LG*, lateral geniculate body; LP, lateral posterior nucleus; MG_p, medial geniculate, parvicellular part; *NR*, red nucleus; *OT*, optic tract; *Pt*, pretectum; *Pul*, pulvinar; *RN*, reticular nucleus of the thalamus; *SN*, substantia nigra; *ZI*, zona incerta (modified from Jones and Powell, '71). (From Carpenter and Sutin, *Human Neuroanatomy*, 1983; courtesy of Williams & Wilkins.)

Hall, '78). According to Morest ('64) the medial geniculate body consists of three main divisions referred to as medial, dorsal and ventral (Fig. 9-16). These subdivisions of the medial geniculate nucleus are not easily distinguished in ordinary histological preparations, but become apparent in Golgi preparations (Morest, '64, '65, '65a).

The ventral nucleus extends throughout the rostrocaudal length of the MGB and is bounded medially by the brachium of the inferior colliculus. Unlike all other major subdivisions of the MGB the ventral nucleus has a distinct laminar organization. Cells of the ventral division are fairly constant in size and shape and have tufted dendrites. The lamination, produced by the dendritic pattern of tufted cells and fibers of the brachium of the inferior colliculus, is in the form of spirals or curved vertical sheets (Fig. 9-16). Afferent fibers from the inferior colliculus enter particular laminae and remain continuously associated with the same, or contiguous dendritic layers. The lamination in the ventral division of the MGB is similar to that in the lateral geniculate body (LGB), except the cellular laminae are not separated by bands of myelinated fibers. Physiological mapping of ventral division of the MGB reveals that the cellular laminae are related to the tonotopic organization, in which high frequencies are represented medially and low frequencies laterally (Aitkin and Webster, '72; Gross et al., '74). Neurons in the ventral division of the MGB give rise to the auditory radiation which terminates in the primary auditory cortex (Figs. 9-12 and 9-21), where there is a spatial representation of tonal frequencies. The primary auditory cortex gives rise to reciprocal corticothalamic fibers that terminate in the ventral division of the MGB (Oliver and Hall, '78a). Both geniculocortical and cortiogeniculate fibers are ipsilateral.

In man, the principal cortical projection of the medial geniculate body is to the superior temporal convolution (transverse gyrus of Heschl) via the geniculotemporal or auditory radiation (Figs. 2-4, 2-9, 6-10, 9-12 and 9-21). This cortical projection area (area 41) is presumed to have a tonotopic localization in which high tones are appreciated medially and low tones are represented laterally and anteriorly (Merzenich and Brugge, '73). Present evidence suggests that the tonotopic organization at the cortical level in man is similar to that in the monkey (Imig et al. '77).

The dorsal division of the MGB contains several nuclei, among which are the suprageniculate and the dorsal nuclei (Oliver and Hall, '78). The dorsal nucleus, prominent at caudal levels of the MGB (Fig. 9-16),

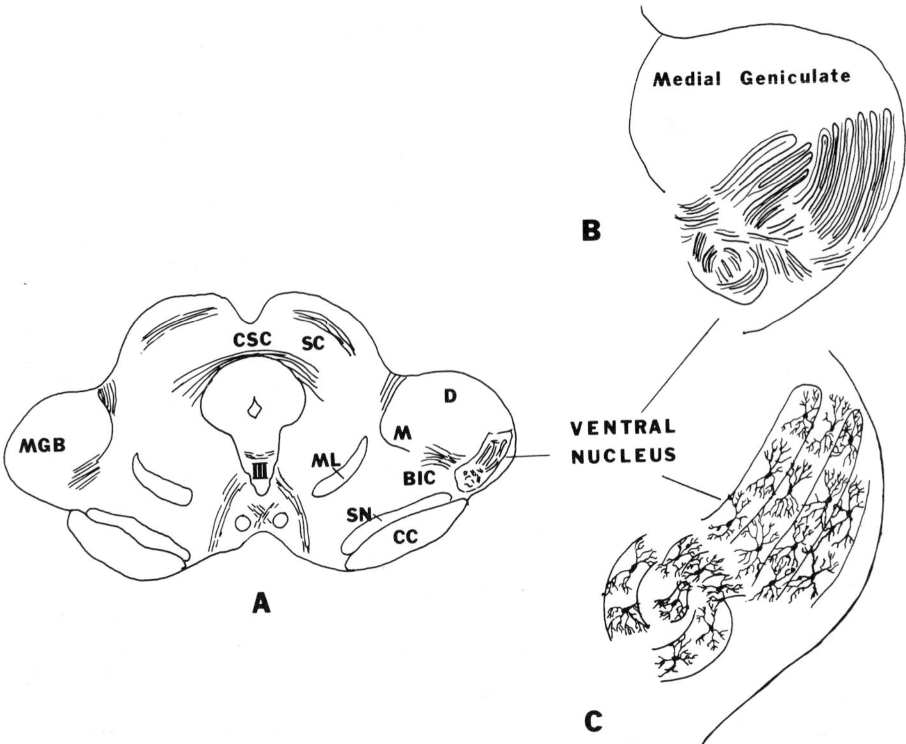

Figure 9-16. Transverse reconstructions of the fibrodendritic laminations in the ventral nucleus of the medial geniculate body in the cat based on Golgi preparations. (*A*) Transverse section of midbrain through the superior colliculus (*SC*) and medial geniculate body (*MGB*); *M* and *D* indicate the magnocellular and dorsal nuclei of the *MGB*. The lamination in the ventral nucleus of MGB (*A*, *B*, and *C*) is produced by the arrangement of dendrites of geniculate neurons and fibers of the brachium of the inferior colliculus and occurs in spirals and vertical sheets. Abbreviations used: *BIC*, brachium of the inferior colliculus; *CC*, crus cerebri; *CSC*, commissure of the superior colliculus; *SN*, substantia nigra; *III*, oculomotor nucleus (based upon Morest, '65.) (From Carpenter and Sutin, *Human Neuroanatomy*, 1983; courtesy of Williams & Wilkins.)

receives projections from the lateral tegmental area, broadly defined as a region extending from the deep layers of the superior colliculus to the area adjacent to the lateral lemniscus. The medial division, containing the largest cells in the MGB, is known as the magnocellular part (Fig. 9-15). This division of the MGB receives inputs from the inferior colliculus, the lateral tegmentum and spinal cord (Jones and Powell, '71; Casseday et al., '76; Oliver and Hall, '78). All nonlaminated portions of the MGB (i.e., the dorsal and medial divisions) send fibers ipsilaterally to at least five cytoarchitectonically distinct areas which form a cortical belt surrounding the primary auditory area (Raczkowski et al., '76; Winer et al., '77; Oliver and Hall, '78a).

Lateral Geniculate Body. The lateral geniculate body (LGB), the thalamic relay nucleus for the visual system, lies rostral and lateral to the medial geniculate body (MGB), lateral to the crus cerebri, and ventral to the pulvinar (Figs. 9-2, 9-3, 9-11, and 9-17). This thalamic nucleus has a laminated cellular structure which in transverse sections has a horseshoe-shaped configuration with the hilus directed ventromedially. Crossed and uncrossed fibers of the optic tract enter via the hilus and are distributed in precise pattern. In man and primates the lateral geniculate body consists of six cellular layers or laminae arranged in two major subdivisions (Clark, '41; Hickey and Guillery, '79). The six concentric cell layers, separated by intervening fiber bands, customarily are numbered from 1 to 6, beginning from the ventrome-

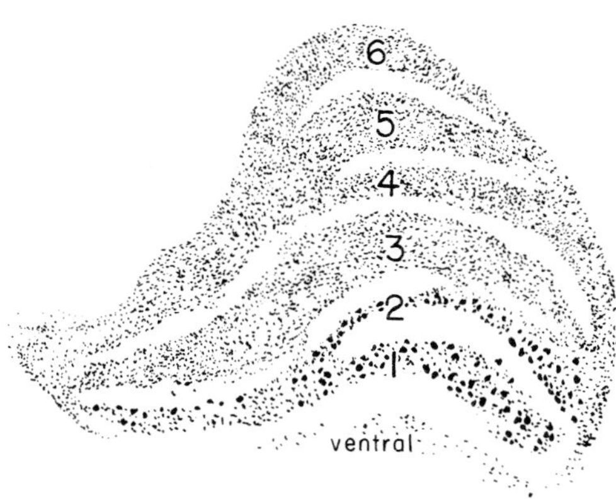

Figure 9-17. Drawing of the cellular lamination of the lateral geniculate body with laminae numbered from the hilus. The magnocellular laminae (*1* and *2*) constitute the ventral nucleus. Parvicellular laminae *3* through *6* are referred to as the dorsal nucleus. Crossed fibers of the optic tract terminate in laminae 1, 4, and 6; uncrossed optic fibers terminate on other laminae. Only cells in the dorsal nucleus project fibers to the visual cortex. (From Carpenter and Sutin, *Human Neuroanatomy*, 1983; courtesy of Williams & Wilkins.)

dial hilar region (Fig. 9-17). Subdivisions of the LGB are the ventral nucleus (layers 1 and 2), the magnocellular part, and the dorsal nucleus (layers 3 to 6), the parvicellular part. Both divisions of the lateral geniculate nucleus receive afferents from the ganglion cells of the retina (Sanides, '75). The ventral magnocellular part of the LGB projects to the pretectum, the superior colliculus, the suprachiasmatic nucleus of the hypothalamus and the zona incerta (Edwards et al. '74; Swanson et al., '74). Direct projections from the retina terminate in overlapping fashion in all of the structures receiving inputs from the ventral nucleus, except the superior colliculus; in the latter structure inputs from the retina and the ventral nucleus of LGB end in adjacent layers. The ventral nucleus, a derivative of the ventral thalamus, receives an input from the striate cortex (Garey et al., '68) and has been considered to play a role in visuomotor integration.

The parvicellular layers of LGB, consisting of layers 3, 4, 5, and 6 in ventrodorsal sequence, are most easily distinguished in the caudal half of the nucleus in man (Fig. 9-18). As these layers are traced laterally they fuse in pairs: layer 4 with layer 6, and layer 3 with layer 5 (Hickey and Guillery, '79). In rostral parts of the dorsal nucleus the individual layers are more difficult to identify. The projection from the retina onto the lateral geniculate body is precise and crossed and uncrossed fibers in the optic tract end upon separate layers. Crossed fibers of the optic tract end upon layers 1, 4, and 6, while uncrossed fibers terminate in layers 2, 3, and 5 (Fig. 9-17). This pattern of laminar termination in the LGB has been established by the studies of anterograde degeneration following enucleation or section of the optic nerve and by the study of transneuronal cell changes following similar lesions. These findings have been confirmed in studies in which one eye has been injected with tritiated amino acids and the retinofugal fibers have been traced in serial autoradiographs (Hendrickson et al., '70; Tigges and O'Steen, '74; Kaas et al., '77). Two unique features related to crossed retinogeniculate fibers are reflected in structure. The monocular crescent of the visual field is subserved by receptor elements in the most medial part of the contralateral nasal retina (Fig. 9-18). Ganglion cells in this part of the retina project crossed fibers to the bilaminar segment (Fig. 9-18) of opposite LGB, located laterally where parts of layers 4 and 6 fuse (Kaas et al., '72; Hickey and Guillery, '79). The optic disc, located in the nasal half of the retina and representing optic nerve fibers, has no photoreceptors; it is responsible for the blind spot detectable on perimetry. The optic disc is represented in the contralateral LGB by cellular discontinuities in layers 4 and 6 (Fig. 9-18). These cellular discontinuities in laminae 4 and 6 of the LGB are a constant feature (Hickey and Guillery, '79).

Nissl preparations through the human lateral geniculate nucleus reveal a linear cellular organization in which the long axis of the cells is oriented perpendicular to the axis of the laminae. Perikarya in the parvicellular layers parallel "lines of projection" which indicate isorepresentation of points in the visual field (Bishop et al., '62; Kaas et al., '72).

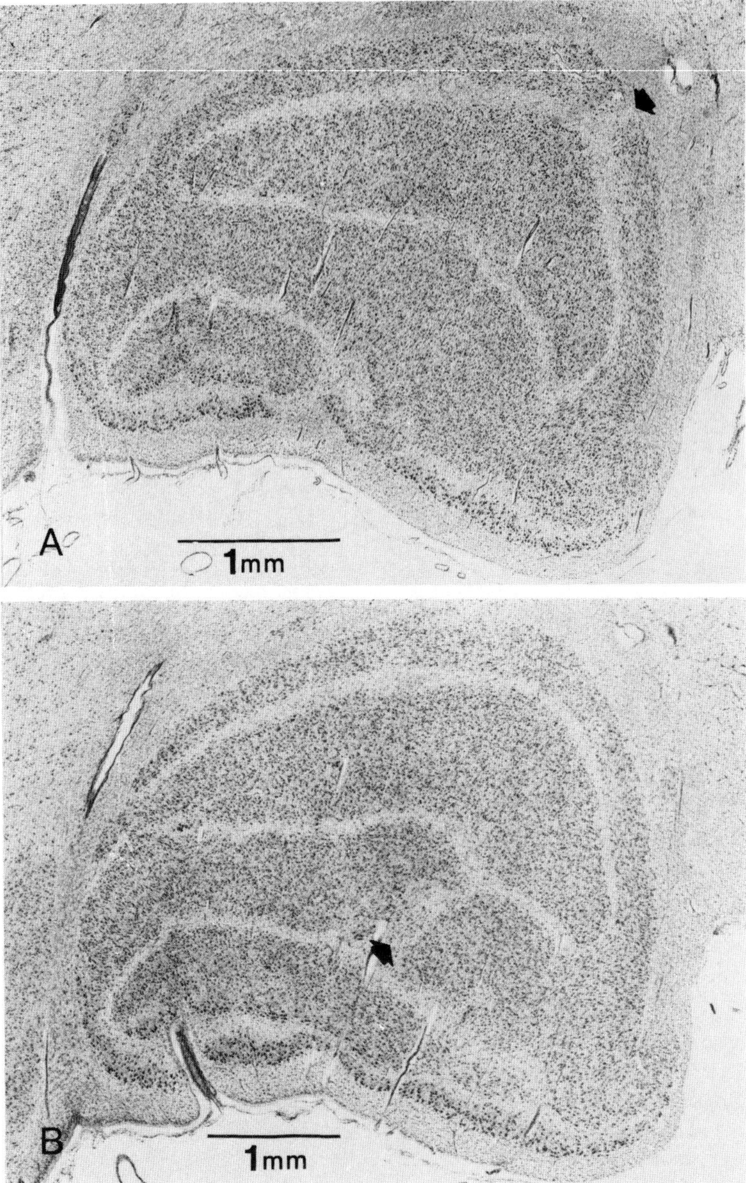

Figure 9-18. Photomicrographs of sections through the human lateral geniculate body. The blind spot is represented by discontinuities in layers 6 (*A*, *arrow*) and 4 (*B*, *arrow*). Layers 4 and 6 fuse laterally (right) in both *A* and *B* producing the bilaminar segment ventrally. The bilaminar segment receives an input from the most medial contralateral nasal retina that subserves the monocular visual field (i.e., the monocular crescent). (From Hickey and Guillery, '79; courtesy of the authors and The Wistar Institute Press.) (From Carpenter and Sutin, *Human Neuroanatomy*, 1983; courtesy of Williams & Wilkins.)

The topographic representation of the retinal surface within the LGB is highly organized and precise. The contralateral half of the binocular visual field is represented in all layers of the LGB, even though crossed and uncrossed fibers end in different layers. The projection locales in the six layers lie in perfect register so that any small area in the contralateral binocular visual field can be shown to correspond to a dorsoventral column of cells extending radially through all six layers parallel to the "lines of projection" (Figs. 9-18 and 9-19) (Kaas et al., '72). The LGB consists of six sheets of cells bent in a horseshoe configuration, but in exact registration, so that columns of cells in the "lines of projection" receive inputs from corresponding points in the retina of each eye related to the contralateral binocular visual field (Fig. 9-19). Binocular fusion does not occur in the LGB because retinogeniculate fibers end on different layers. Following section of the optic nerve anterograde degeneration or transneuronal degeneration (after long survivals) will occur in three layers of the LGB on each side. The layers in which degeneration of fibers or cells occur differs in accordance with the disposition of crossed (layers 1, 4 and 6) and uncrossed (layers 2, 3, and 5) retinal fibers. Small lesions of the retina produce transneuronal degeneration in localized clusters of cells in three different layers on each side aligned according to the "lines of projection." The contralateral monocular visual field (monocular crescent), related to receptor elements in the most medial nasal retina, is represented by only crossed fibers terminating in the bilaminar segment (Figs. 9-18 and 9-19).

The "lines of projection" in the lateral geniculate body also can be demonstrated by the study of retrograde cell degeneration in the LGB following a lesion in the striate cortex (Hickey and Guillery, '79). Since one half of the visual field is represented topographically in the striate cortex of each hemisphere, the zone of retrograde cell degeneration in the LGB would be bounded on each side by lines of projections. Cortical projection zones in geniculate segments would involve cells only in the dorsal nucleus of the LGB.

Information concerning the retinotopic organization of retinofugal fibers in the optic nerve, chiasm, tract, and lateral geniculate body in man and monkey is based upon extensive research (Brouwer and Zeeman, '26; Polyak, '57). Nonmacular fibers from the retina maintain their retinal topography throughout the optic nerve. Macular fibers pass through central and peripheral regions of the optic nerve, and after decussating in the chiasm, both crossed and uncrossed fibers occupy superior parts of the optic tract. Macular axons are fine fibers while those from nonmacular regions are large fibers. In the LGB the horizontal meridan of the visual field corresponds to an oblique dorsoventral plane that divides the nucleus into medial and lateral segments (Fig. 9-20). Fibers from superior retinal quadrants of both eyes project to the medial half of the LGB; the inferior retinal quadrants send fibers to the lateral half of the nucleus (Fig. 9-20). The retinal projection from the macula is represented in a broad wedgeshaped sector in the caudal part of the LGB on both sides of the plane representing the horizontal meridian. The macular representation accounts for about 12% of the total volume of the LGB and the caudal third of the nucleus represents the central 20% of vision. Retinal zones subserving the contralateral peripheral visual field are represented serially along the caudorostral axis of the LGB (Fig. 19-20) with retinal fibers related to the most peripheral part of the visual field, the monocular crescent, projecting to the oral pole (Malpeli and Baker, '75). The vertical meridian of the visual field, corresponding to the line separating temporal and nasal parts of the retina, is represented along the caudal margin of the nucleus from its medial to lateral borders (Fig. 9-20) (Kaas et al., '72); Malpeli and Baker, '75).

Physiological and anatomical evidence indicate at least three distinct classes of retinal ganglion cells and it is well known that retinofugal fibers provide inputs to several neural regions in addition to the LGB (Fukuda and Stone, '74; Stone and Fukuda, '74; Boycott and Wässale, '74).

Each neuron of the lateral geniculate body receives a direct input from the retina and projects directly to the visual cortex (striate cortex, area 17). Cells within this nucleus exhibit both convergence and divergence. A retinofugal fiber may synapse with several neurons in the LGB (divergence), and each neuron of the LGB may recive inputs from several retinofugal fibers (convergence). Retinofugal fibers from ganglion cells of the retina establish different types of synaptic articulations with LGB neurons. These fibers terminate axosomatically and axodendritically upon primary and secondary dendrites, in boutons *en passage*, and in complex glomerular endings.

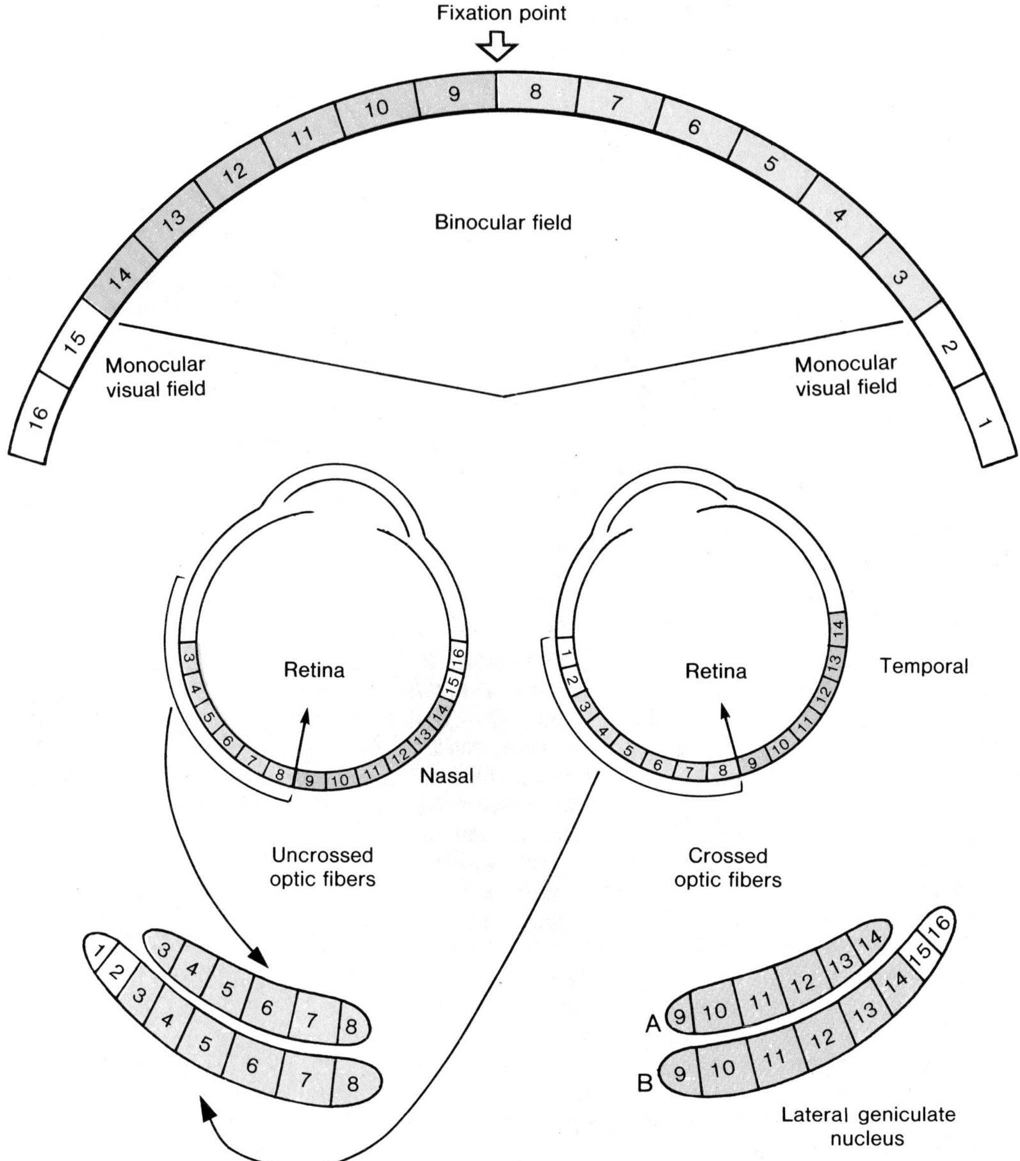

Figure 9-19. Schematic diagram showing the representation of the visual field in the retinae and in the layers of the lateral geniculate nucleus. Portions of the binocular visual field are shown in *red* (left) and *blue* (right), while the monocular visual fields are *white*. Light from numbered sectors of both the binocular and monocular visual fields falls upon corresponding number sectors of the retinae. Crossed and uncrossed retinofugal fibers project upon columns of cells in different laminae of the lateral geniculate nucleus which are in exact registration, represented here by corresponding numbers. *A*, represents laminae receiving uncrossed fibers (i.e., laminae 2, 3 and 5). *B* represents laminae receiving crossed fibers (i.e., laminae 1, 4 and 6). Light from the right monocular vision field (sectors 1 and 2) falls upon retinal receptors of the corresponding number in the most medial ipsilateral nasal retina. Crossed retinofugal fibers project to cell columns of the left lateral geniculate nucleus (1, 2). Cell columns 1 and 2 are best developed in laminae 4 and 6 which fuse to form the bilaminar segment (modified from Kaas et al., '72). (From Carpenter and Sutin, *Human Neuroanatomy*, 1983; courtesy of Williams & Wilkins.)

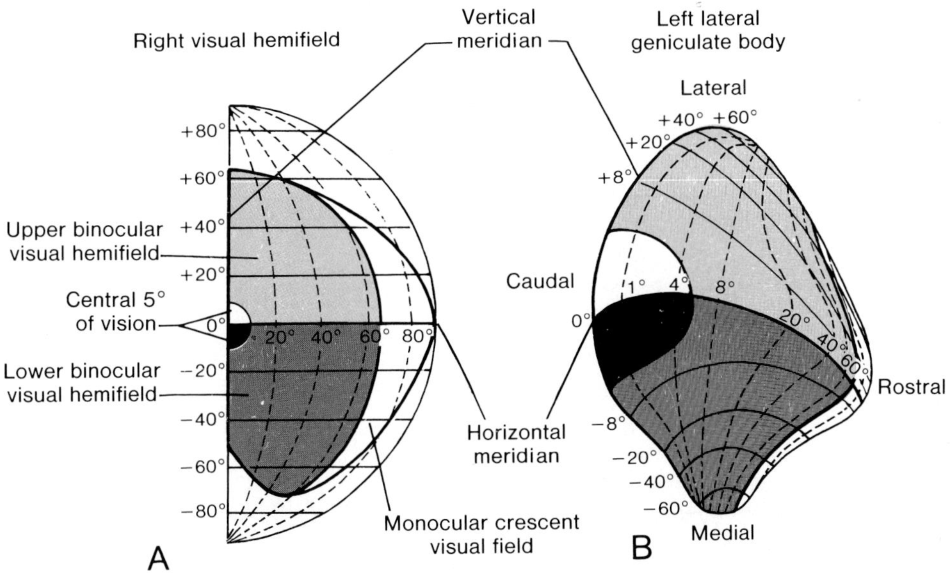

Figure 9-20. Schematic drawing of the right visual hemifield of the monkey (*A*) and its projection on to the dorsal surface of the unfolded left lateral geniculate body (LGB) (*B*). The vertical meridian is represented by the heavy *black* line on the left in both *A* and *B*; visual field zones of increasing eccentricity are represented serially in degrees of dashed lines. In the left lateral geniculate body visual field zones (dashed lines) are represented serially along the caudorostral axis of the nucleus in degrees. The horizontal meridian of the hemifield at 0° is represented by a *curved line* in the caudorostral axis of the LGB (*B*); thin lines above and below the horizontal meridian indicate positive or negative elevations in degrees. Upper (*blue*) and lower (*red*) portions of the binocular visual hemifield indicated in *A* are represented by the same colors in *B*. The central 5° of vision, a generous estimate of the angle subtended by the fovea centralis, are shown in *black* and *white* at the intersection of the vertical and horizontal meridians. The monocular crescent (*white*) in *A* is represented along the rostral border of the LGB (based on Malpeli and Baker, '75). (From Carpenter and Sutin, *Human Neuroanatomy*, 1983; courtesy of Williams & Wilkins.)

Glomeruli in the LGB constitute a synaptic complex of interlocking nerve processes of various origins which are arranged in a specific manner and separated from the environment by a capsule of glial processes (Szentágothai, '70) It is assumed that the synaptic arrangements within the glomeruli are effective in the versatile processing of information. The interpretation of the structural arrangements, within the LGB glomeruli suggests that optic afferents depolarize Golgi cell terminals, and thus presynaptically inhibit the inhibitory influence exerted by these cells upon geniculate body neurons (Szentágothai, '70). This concept of presynaptic disinhibition by retinal afferents appears attractive because LGB neurons exhibit less activity if the visual field is uniformly illuminated than if there is a sharp contrast of light and dark projected upon the retina.

The lateral geniculate nucleus is the main end station of the optic tract. It projects to the calcarine cortex (area 17) via the geniculocalcarine tract or visual radiation, and it receives corticogeniculate fibers from the same area (Figs. 2-9, 2-10, 9-21 and 9-23). Its internuclear connections are with the pulvinar.

Thalamic Reticular Nucleus. The thalamic reticular nucleus (RN) is a thin neuronal shell which surrounds the lateral, superior, and rostroinferior aspects of the dorsal thalamus (Figs. 9-7, 9-9, 9-10, and 9-11). This thalamic nuclear envelope is a derivative of the ventral thalamus which has migrated dorsally and lies between the external medullary lamina of the thalamus and the internal capsule. Cells in this nucleus are heterogeneous in type, ranging from very small cells in dorsal regions to quite large cells in ventral and caudal regions (Jones, '75). Golgi studies of the reticular formation reveal neurons similar to those of the brain stem reticular formation (Scheibel and Scheibel, '66). Dendrites of these cells are long and exhibit no specific orientation. The main axons of the majority of cells project medially into the principal thalamic nuclei, although some axons run entirely within the reticular nucleus.

Autoradiographic studies in the cat and monkey have shown that inputs to the reticular nucleus are derived from the principal thalamic nuclei and from the cerebral cortex (Carman et al., '64; Jones, '75). Fibers emanating from a nucleus of the dorsal thalamus and destined for a specific cortical area give collateral branches that terminate in a particular part of the reticular nucleus. Corticothalamic fibers passing towards a particular nucleus of the dorsal thalamus give collaterals to the same portions of the reticular nucleus as the target nucleus of the thalamus (Jones, '75). Cells of this restricted part of the reticular nucleus project back to the thalamic nucleus from which it receives an input. Both the intralaminar and relay nuclei of the dorsal thalamus project to the reticular nucleus and both receive fibers from it. The reticular nucleus is situated so as to sample neural activity passing between the cerebral cortex and nuclei of the dorsal thalamus, but it has no projection to the cerebral cortex (Carman et al. '64; Scheibel and Scheibel, '66; Jones, '75). Cortical projections to portions of the reticular nucleus arise from the entire cerebral cortex and are topographically ogranized. About one-fifth of the axons from cells in the reticular nucleus project caudally to enter the mesencephalic tegmentum. Since the major projections of the thalamic reticular nucleus are to specific and nonspecific thalamic nuclei, it may serve to integrate and "gate" activities of thalamic neurons.

CLAUSTRUM

This thin plate of gray matter lies in the white matter of the hemisphere between the lentiform nucleus and the insular cortex; it is separated from these structures by the external capsule medially and the extreme capsule laterally (Figs. 2-11, 2-16, 2-17, and 11-5). Although the claustrum is situated close to the striatum, its principal connections are with the cerebral cortex and it bears striking resemblances to the thalamus. Two distinct parts of the claustrum are recognized: (1) an insular part composed of large cells underlying the insular cortex and (2) a temporal part located between the putamen and the temporal lobe (Narkiewicz, '64). Although the claustrum has widespread reciprocal connections with the cerebral cortex (Norita, '77; Riche and Lanoir, '78), it also receives inputs from the lateral hypothalamus, the centromedian nucleus of the thalamus and the locus ceruleus (LeVay and Sherk, '81). However, the sensory nuclei of the thalamus do not project to the claustrum. The major afferents to claustrum arise from the cerebral cortex; corticoclaustral projections arise from pyramidal cells in layer VI, a layer whose principal subcortical projections are to the thalamus (Carey et al., '80). Fibers from numerous cortical areas each terminate in a distinct zone within the claustrum. Observations in the cat indicate discrete visual, somatosensory and auditory zones in the claustrum (Jayaraman and Updyke, '79; Olson and Graybiel, '80).

Studies in the cat indicate that the dorsocaudal claustrum receives a retinotopic projection from several visual cortical areas, which arises from cells that are separate from those projecting to the lateral geniculate body. The visual claustrum projects back to the areas of the visual cortex from which it receives inputs (LeVay and Sherk, '81). The return projection is mainly ipsilateral and ends largely in layers IV and VI. The claustrum has no subcortical projections. The claustrum contains a single orderly map of the contralateral visual hemifield (LeVay and Sherk, '81a). Claustral neurons respond to appropriately oriented bars of light, and moving stimuli are more effective than stationary ones (Sherk and LeVay, '81). Cells in the claustrum show little spontaneous activity. Although data are incomplete, they suggest that different regions of the claustrum have specific interconnections with corresponding sensory areas of the cortex and that each is topographically organized.

THALAMIC RADIATIONS AND THE INTERNAL CAPSULE

Fibers which reciprocally connect the thalamus and the cortex constitute the thalamic radiations. These thalamocortical and corticothalamic fibers form a continuous fan that emerges along the whole lateral extent of the caudate nucleus. Fiber bundles, radiating forward, backward, upward, and downward, form large portions of various parts of the internal capsule (Figs. 2-11, 2-16, 2-17, 9-2, 9-5, 9-7, 9-8, and 9-21). Though the radiations connect with practically all parts of the cortex, the richness of connections varies in different cortical areas. Most abundant are the projections to the frontal granular cortex, the precentral and postcentral gyri, the calcarine area, and the gyrus of Heschl. The posterior parietal region and adjacent portions of the temporal lobe also have rich thalamic connections, but relatively scanty radiations go to other cortical areas.

The thalamic radiations are grouped into four subradiations designated as the thalamic peduncles (Fig. 9-21). The *anterior* or *frontal peduncle* connects the frontal lobe with the medial and anterior thalamic nuclei. The *superior* or *centroparietal peduncle* connects the Rolandic area and adjacent portions of the frontal and parietal lobes with the ventral tier thalamic nuclei. The fibers, carrying general sensory impulses from the body and head, form part of this radiation and terminate in the postcentral gyrus (Figs. 9-12 and 9-21). The *posterior* or *occipital peduncle* connects the occipital and posterior parietal convolutions with the caudal portions of the thalamus. It includes the optic radiation from the lateral geniculate body and claustrocortical projections to the calcarine cortex (Le Vey and Sherk, '81). The *inferior* or *temporal peduncle* is relatively small and includes the scanty connections of the thalamus with the temporal lobe and the insula (Fig. 9-8). Included in this peduncle is the auditory radiation from the medial geniculate body to the transverse temporal gyrus of Heschl (Fig. 9-21).

The cerebral hemisphere is connected with the brain stem and spinal cord by an extensive system of projection fibers. These fibers arise from the whole extent of the cortex, enter the white substance of the hemisphere, and appear as a radiating mass of fibers, the *corona radiata*, which converges toward the brain stem (Fig. 2-10). On reaching the latter they form a broad, compact fiber band, the *internal capsule*, flanked medially by the thalamus and caudate nucleus and laterally by the lentiform nucleus (Figs. 2-11, 2-16, 2-17 9-6 and 9-21). Thus the internal capsule is composed of all the fibers, afferent and efferent, which go to, or come from, the cerebral cortex. A large part of the capsule is composed of the thalamic radiations described above. The rest is composed mainly of efferent cortical fiber systems (i.e., corticofugal fibers), which descend to lower portions of the brain stem and to the spinal cord. These include the corticospinal, corticobulbar, corticoreticular and corticopontine tracts, as well as a number of smaller bundles.

The internal capsule, as seen in a horizontal section, is composed of *anterior* and *posterior limbs*, which meet at an obtuse angle; the junctional zone is known as the *genu* (Figs. 2-11 and 9-21). The anterior limb lies between the lentiform and caudate nuclei. The posterior limb of the internal capsule (*lenticulothalamic portion*), lies between the lentiform nucleus and the thalamus. A *retrolenticular* part of the internal capsule extends caudally behind the lentiform nucleus for a short distance (Fig. 9-2). In this caudal region, fibers passing beneath the lentiform nucleus to reach the temporal lobe collectively form the *sublenticular* portion of the internal capsule.

The *anterior limb* of the internal capsule contains the anterior thalamic radiation and the prefrontal corticopontine tract. The *genu* contains corticobulbar and corticoreticular fibers.

The *posterior limb* of the internal capsule contains: (1) corticospinal fibers, (2) frontopontine fibers, (3) the superior thalamic radiation, and (4) relatively smaller numbers of corticotectal, corticorubral and corticoreticular fibers. Corticospinal fibers in man classically have been considered to lie in the posterior limb of the internal capsule relatively close to the genu (Déjérine, '01). This traditional localization of cortico-

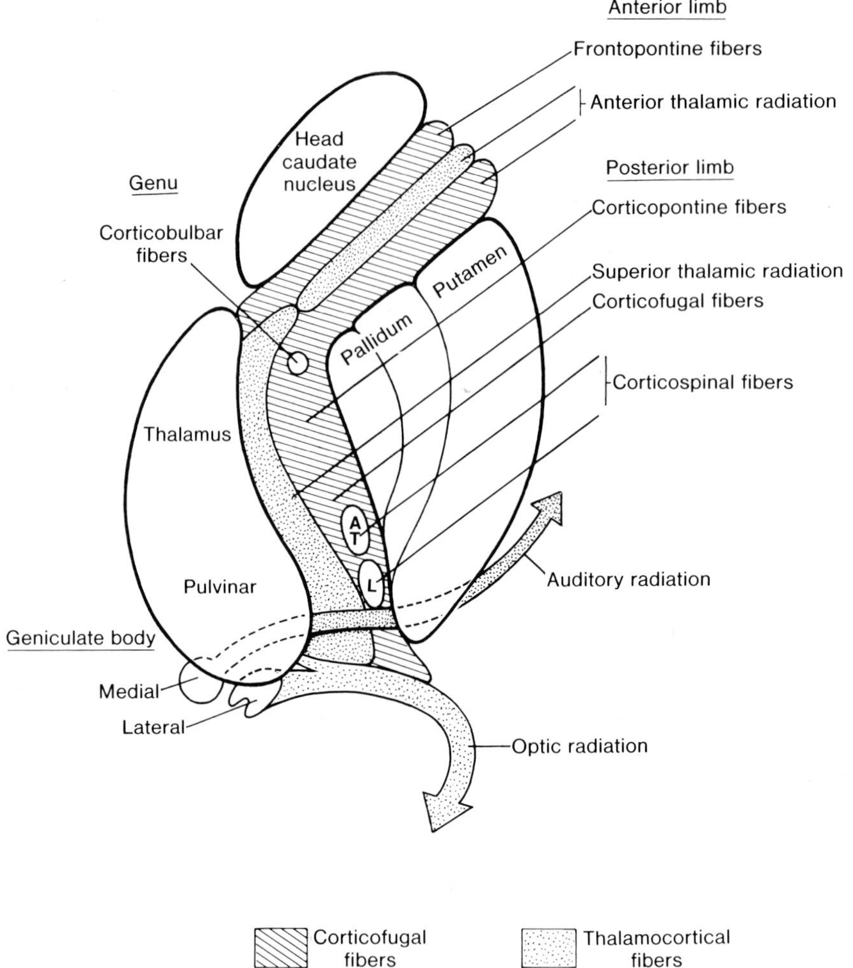

Figure 9-21. Schematic diagram of the right internal capsule as seen in a horizontal section similar to that shown in Figure 2-11. Corticospinal fibers in man occupy the caudal third of the posterior limb of the internal capsule. (From Carpenter and Sutin, *Human Neuroanatomy*, 1983; courtesy of Williams & Wilkins.)

spinal fibers in the internal capsule has been challenged by explorations using electrical stimulation and by careful pathological studies. More recent data suggest that corticospinal fibers are largely confined to compact region in the posterior half of the posterior limb of the internal capsule (Gillingham, '62; Bertrand et al., '65; Smith, '67; Englander et al., '75; Hanaway and Young, '77). Fibers of the corticospinal tract are somatotopically arranged in this part of the internal capsule, with those destined for cervical, thoracic, lumbar, and sacral spinal arranged in a rostrocaudal sequence. The classic view that corticospinal fibers occupy the medial three-fifths of the crus cerebri and are somatotopically organized appears unreasonable on the basis of the number of fibers in the crus cerebri. The somatotopic arrangement of corticospinal fibers in the crus cerebri is much less precise than commonly depicted. Fibers of the superior thalamic radiation, located caudal to the corticospinal fibers, project impulses concerned with general somatic sense to the postcentral gyrus (Fig. 9-21).

The *retrolenticular portion* of the posterior limb contains the posterior thalamic radiations, including the optic radiation, parietal and occipital corticopontine fibers, and fibers from the occipital cortex to the superior colliculi and pretectal region (Figs. 9-2 and 9-3). The *sublenticular* portion, difficult to separate from the retrolenticular, contains the *inferior thalamic peduncle* (Fig 9-8). the auditory radiation, and corticopontine fibers from the temporal and the parieto-occipital area.

Thalamocortical and *corticofugal* fibers within the internal capsule occupy a small, compact area (Fig. 9-21). Lesions in this area produce more widespread disturbances than lesions in any other region of the nervous system. Thrombosis or hemorrhage of the anterior choroidal, striate, or capsular branches of the middle cerebral arteries (Figs. 14-9) and 14-10) are responsible for most of the lesions in the internal capsule. Vascular lesions in the posterior limb of the internal capsule result in contralateral hemianesthesia due to injury of thalamocortical fibers en route to the sensory cortex. There is also a contralateral hemiplegia due to injury of corticospinal fibers. If the genu of the internal capsule is included in the injury, corticobulbar fibers may be destroyed. Lesions in the most posterior region of the posterior limb may include the optic and auditory radiations. In such instances there may be a contralateral triad consisting of hemianesthesia, hemianopsia, and hemihypacusis.

VISUAL PATHWAY

Retina. The rods and cones of the retina are visual receptors which react specifically to physical light (Fig. 9-22). The cones have a higher threshold of excitability and are stimulated by light of relatively high intensity. They are responsible for sharp vision and for color discrimination in adequate illumination. The rods react to low intensities of illumination and subserve twilight and night vision. Close to the posterior pole of the eye, the retina shows a small, circular, yellowish area, the macula lutea. The macula represents the retinal area for central vision, and the eyes are fixed in such a manner that the retinal image of any object is always focused on the macula. The rest of the retina is concerned with paracentral and peripheral vision. In the macular region the inner layers of the retina are pushed apart, forming a small central pit, the *fovea centralis*, which constitutes the point of sharpest vision and most acute color discrimination. Here the retina is composed entirely of closely packed slender cones.

The rods and cones are composed of an outer segment, a narrow neck, an inner segment, a cell body, and a synaptic base (Fig. 9-22). Photopigments are present in the outer segments, where the photochemical reactions to light take place that give rise to the generator potential. The outer segment is composed of a series of laminated discs derived from the infolding of the plasma membrane. The photopigments, bound to the membranes of the discs, are constantly renewed. Rhodopsin is the photopigment of the rods in primates, and three pigments with maximum absorptions for blue, green, and red are present in the cones (Wald, '68). The synaptic base of the cone is called a pedicle, while that of the rod is referred to as a spherule. Each cone pedicle has several invaginations which contain terminals of horizontal, midget bipolar, and flat bipolar cells in a specific arrangement. Rod spherules have a single invagination containing multiple processes of horizontal and rod bipolar cells (Fig. 9-22). Each midget ganglion cell makes several synaptic contacts with a single bipolar cell. Diffuse ganglion cells establish synaptic contacts with all types of bipolar cells (Dowling and Boycott, '66). Horizontal cells and amacrine cells constitute retinal interneurons. It is difficult to determine whether processes of horizontal cells are axons or dendrites, and it is possible that each process may be capable of both receiving and transmitting signals. Amacrine cells in the inner plexiform layer have no axon, but make synaptic contacts with all types of bipolar cells, other amacrine cells, and the dendrites and somata of ganglion cells. The axons of ganglion cells, at first unmyelinated, are arranged in fine radiating bundles which run parallel to the retinal surface and converge at the optic disc to form the optic nerve. On emerging from the eyeball, the fibers at once acquire a myelin sheath.

Retinal ganglion cells are of different sizes, project to different sites and form at least three functional classes (Boycott and Wässle, '74; Fukuda and Stone, '74; Stone and Fukuda, '74; Bunt et al., '75; Kelly and Gilbert, '75). Distinct classes of ganglion

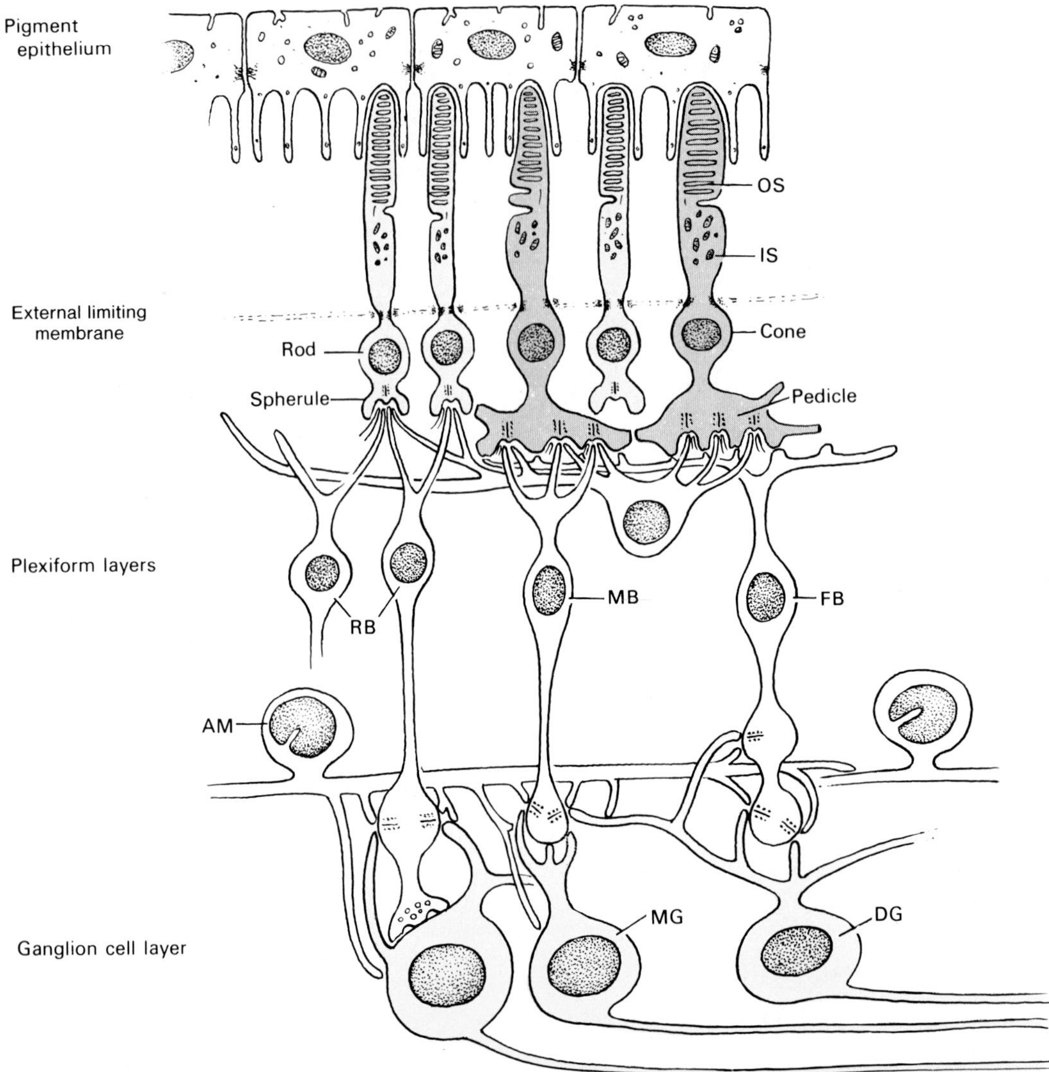

Figure 9-22. Schematic diagram of the ultrastructural organization of the retina. Rods (*blue*) and cones (*red*) are composed of an outer segment (*OS*), an inner segment (*IS*), a cell body and a synaptic base. Photopigments are present in the outer segments (*OS*) which are composed of laminated discs. The synaptic base of the rod is called a spherule, while the synaptic base of the cone is called a pedicle. In the plexiform layers *RB* indicates rod bipolar cells, *MB* a midget bipolar cell and *FB* a flat bipolar cell. *AM* indicates an amacrine cell. Ganglion cells (*MG*, midget ganglion cell; *DG*, diffuse ganglion cell) and retinal afferents are in *yellow* (modified from Dowling and Boycott, '66). (From Carpenter and Sutin, *Human Neuroanatomy*, 1983; courtesy of Williams & Wilkins.)

cells are referred to as *X*, *Y*, and *W* cells. The *X* class cells have slower conduction velocities than *Y* cells, exhibit sustained or tonic responses and project to the dorsal nucleus of the LGB and the pretectum. The *Y* cells have rapid conduction, exhibit transient or phasic responses and project to the dorsal nucleus of the LGB and the superior colliculus. The *W* ganglion cells have either tonic or phasic responses, very slow axonal conduct velocities and project to the superior colliculus and the pretectum. It has been suggested that: (1) the largest ganglion cells correspond to the *Y* cells, (2) medium-sized cells with narrow dendritic arborizations correspond to the *X* cells, and (3) the smallest ganglion cells with the widest dendritic arborizations correspond to the *W*

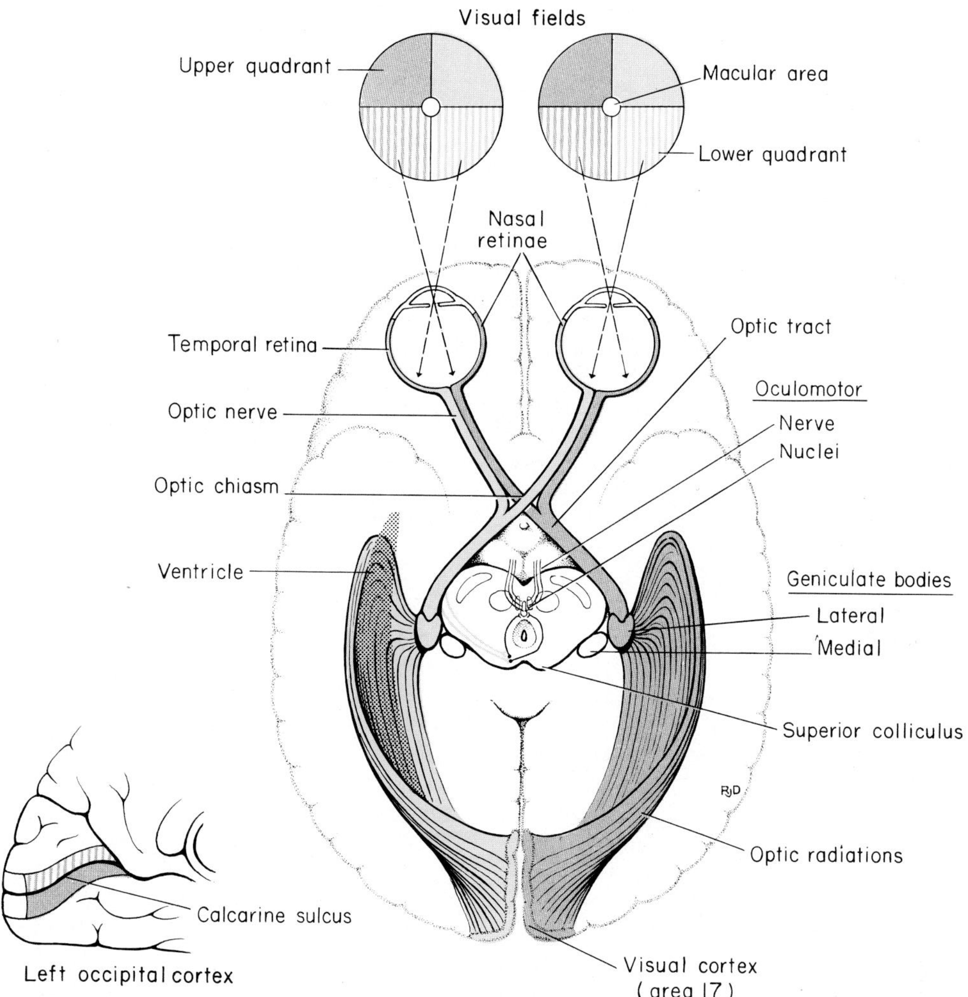

Figure 9-23. Diagram of the visual pathways viewed from the ventral surface of the brain. Light from the upper half of the visual field falls on the inferior half of the retina. Light from the temporal half of the visual field falls on the nasal half of the retina, while light from the nasal half of the visual field falls on the temporal half of the retina. The visual pathways from the retina to the striate cortex are shown. The plane of the visual fields has been rotated 90° toward the reader. The *insert* (*lower left*) shows the projection of the quadrants of the right visual field upon the left calcarine (striate) cortex. The macular area of the retina (white) is represented nearest the occipital pole. Fibers mediating the pupillary light reflex leave the optic tract and project to the pretectal region; other fibers relay impulses indirectly to the visceral nuclei of the oculomotor complex. (From Carpenter and Sutin, *Human Neuroanatomy*, 1983; courtesy of Williams and Wilkins.)

cells. Because the central projections of these classes of retinal ganglion cells differ, it is presumed that their functional roles also differ. The *Y* cells are present in much smaller numbers than either *X* or *W* cells. The retinal density of *X* and *W* cells is maximal in the area centralis. Since *W* cells do not project to the dorsal nucleus of the LGB, it is presumed that *X* type ganglion cells must be concerned with central vision (Fukuda and Stone, '74).

Optic Nerves. These nerves enter the cranial cavity through the optic foramina and unite to form the optic chiasm, beyond which they are continued as the optic tracts (Figs. 2-7, 2-8, 9-5, and 9-23). Within the chiasm a partal decussation occurs, the fibers from the nasal halves of the retina crossing to the opposite side, and those from the temporal halves of the retina remaining uncrossed (Figs. 9-19 and 9-23). In binocular vision each visual field, right and left, is projected upon portions of both retinae. Thus the images of objects in the right field of vision (red in Fig. 9-23) are projected on the right nasal and the left temporal halves of the retina. The right monocular crescent of the visual field (not shown in Fig. 9-23) projects upon retinal receptors only in the most medial part of the right nasal retina (Fig. 9-19). In the chiasm the fibers from these two retinal portions are combined to form the left optic tract. By this arrangement the whole right field of vision is projected upon the left hemisphere, and the left visual field upon the right hemisphere.

Optic Tracts. Each optic tract partially encircles the hypothalamus and the rostral portions of the crus cerebri. Most of its fibers terminate in the lateral geniculate body, though small portions continue as the brachium of the superior colliculus to the superior colliculus and pretectal area (Fig. 9-23). The lateral geniculate body gives rise to the geniculocalcarine tract, which forms the last relay of the visual path. The pretectal area (Figs. 7-11 and 9-3) is concerned with the light reflex, and the superior colliculi with reflex movement of the eyes and head and tracking of visual stimuli. Retinohypothalamic fibers terminate bilaterally in the suprachiasmatic nucleus of the hypothalamus in a variety of mammals (Moore and Lenn, '72; Moore, '73) (Fig. 10-1). This direct retinal projection is functionally relevant to neuroendocrine regulation.

Geniculocalcarine Tract. This tract arises from cells in the parvicellular part of the LGB, passes through the retrolenticular portion of the internal capsule, and forms the optic radiation (Fig. 9-21). These fibers terminate on both sides of the calcarine sulcus in the striate cortex (Figs. 9-23 and 9-24). All fibers of the radiation do not reach the cortex by the shortest route. The most dorsal fibers pass almost directly backward to the striate area. More ventral fibers first turn forward and downward into the temporal lobe, and spread out over the rostral part of the inferior horn of the lateral ventricle; these fibers then loop backward, and run close to the outer wall of the lateral ventricle (external sagittal stratum) to reach the occipital cortex. The most ventral fibers make the longest loop (Figs. 9-23 and 9-24).

The retinal areas have a precise point-to-point relationship with the lateral geniculate body, each portion of the retina projecting on a specific and topographically limited portion of the lateral geniculate. The fibers from the upper retinal quadrants (representing the lower visual field) terminate in the medial half, those from the lower quadrants terminate in the lateral half of the geniculate body (Fig. 9-20). The macula is represented by a wedge-shaped sector in the caudal part of the LGB on both sides of the plane representing the horizontal meridian (Malpeli and Baker, '75). The peripheral field, including the monocular crescent, is represented rostrally in the LGB and is continuous across the horizontal meridian (Fig. 9-20). A similar point-to-point relation exists between the geniculate body and the striate cortex. The medial half of the lateral geniculate body, representing the upper quadrants (lower visual field) projects to the superior lip of the calcarine sulcus, and the fibers form the superior portion of the optic radiation (Fig. 9-23). The lateral half of the lateral geniculate body, representing the lower retinal quadrants (upper visual field) projects to the inferior lip of the calcarine sulcus. These fibers occupy the inferior portion of the optic radiation. The macular fibers, which constitute the intermediate part of the optic radiation, terminate in the caudal third of the calcarine cortex. Those from the paracentral and peripheral retinal areas end in respectively more rostral portions.

Experimental studies (Kuffler, '53) with stationary spots of light indicate that the receptive fields of ganglion cells in the retina are organized into concentric zones with either an "on" or "off" type of discharge in the center and the reverse in the periphery (Fig. 13-10). In the retina the receptive field is related to those receptors, rods and cones, and other retinal neurons which influence the excitability of a single ganglion cell. The retina is a composite of as many receptive fields as there are ganglion cells. Each receptive field is organized into two zones: (1) a small circular central zone, and (2) a surrounding concentric zone referred to as the periphery, or surround. These two zones are functionally antagonistic. Two general types of receptive fields have been described: (1) those with an "on" center and an "off" surround and (2) those

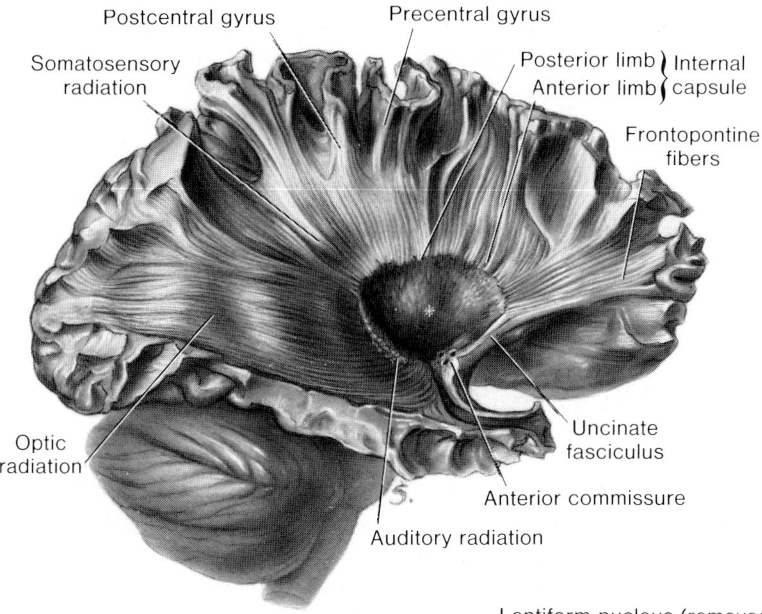

Figure 9-24. Drawing of brain dissection showing the corona radiata. The lentiform nucleus has been removed and its position marked by an asterisk. The visual, auditory and somatosensory radiations are identified. (From Mettler's *Neuroanatomy*, '48; courtesy of the author and The C. V. Mosby Company.) (From Carpenter and Sutin, *Human Neuroanatomy*, 1983; courtesy of Williams & Wilkins.)

with an "off" center and an "on" surround. If a light stimulus illuminates an "on" center, or an "on" surround, the ganglion cell will fire vigorously (Fig. 13-10). If the light stimulus illuminates both "on" and "off" zones, which exhibit mutual inhibition, the stimuli cancel each other. Retinal connections account for the concentric circular receptive fields at the ganglion cell level (Dowling and Boycott, '66). Impulses from the central zone are said to be mediated by direct connections between receptor cells, bipolar cells, and ganglion cells, while the antagonistic surround zone has interposed connections with amacrine cells (i.e., between bipolar and ganglion cells). The receptive fields of neurons in the lateral geniculate body appear similar with stationary spots of light, but LBG neurons show a greater suppression of the receptive field periphery (Hubel and Wiesel, '61). Cells in different laminae of the lateral geniculate body are driven from receptive fields in one eye, either ipsilaterally or contralaterally. Few, if any, cells in the LGB are influenced binocularly. However, single unit studies of the receptive field properties of cells in the striate cortex show that those cells are sensitive to "slits" of light, or moving visual patterns oriented in certain directions (Figs. 13-10 and 13-11). The transformation which occurs in the striate cortex is based upon columns of cortical cells of different functional types that encode a variety of variables in vertical and horizontal systems.

Clinical Considerations. Injury to any part of the optic pathway produces visual defects whose nature depends on the location and extent of the injury. During examination each eye is covered in turn as the retinal quadrants of the opposite eye are tested. Visual defects are said to be *homonymous* when restricted to a single visual field, right or left, and *heteronymous* when parts of both fields are involved. It is evident that homonymous defects are caused by lesions on one side anywhere behind the chiasm (i.e., optic tract, lateral geniculate body, optic radiations, and visual cortex). Complete destruction of any of these structures results in a loss of the whole opposite field of vision (*homonymous hemianopsia*, Fig. 9-25); partial injury may produce *quadrantic homonymous* defects. Lesions of the temporal lobe, destroying the looping fibers in the lower portion of the optic radiation, are likely to produce such quadrantic defects in the upper visual field. Injury to the parietal lobe may involve

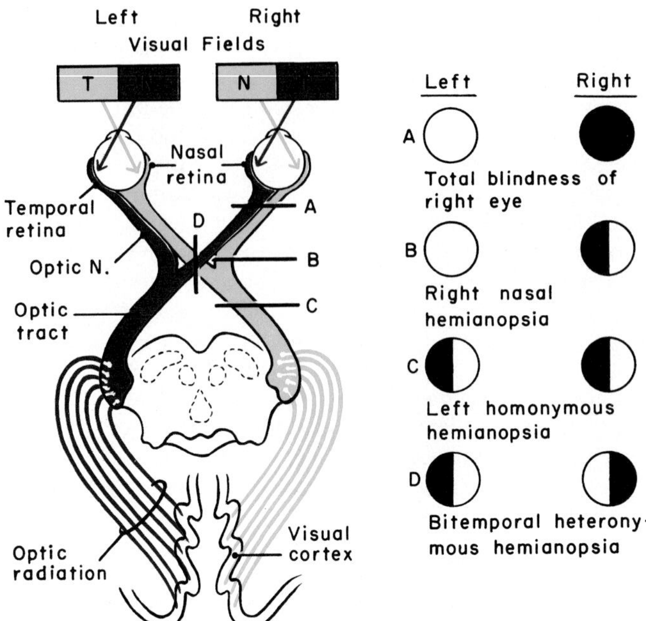

Figure 9-25. Diagram of common lesions within the visual pathway. On the *left*, *A* through *D* indicate the locations of lesions in the visual pathways. Corresponding visual field defects are shown on the *right* (modified from Haymaker, '56). (From Carpenter and Sutin, *Human Neuroanatomy*, 1983; courtesy of Williams & Wilkins.)

the more superiorly placed fibers of the radiation and cause similar defects in the lower field of vision.

Lesions of the chiasm may cause several kinds of heteronymous defects. Most commonly, crossing fibers from the nasal portions of the retina are involved, with consequent loss of both temporal fields of vision (*bitemporal hemianopsia*; Fig. 9-25). Rarely, both lateral angles of the chiasm may be compressed; in such cases the non-decussating fibers from the temporal retinae are affected, and the result is loss of the nasal visual fields (*binasal hemianopsia*). Injury of one optic nerve naturally produces blindness in the corresponding eye with loss of the pupillary light reflex (Fig. 9-25). The pupil will, however, contract consensually to light entering the other eye, since the pretectal reflex center is related to both Edinger-Westphal nuclei. The pupillary reflex will not be affected by lesions of the visual pathway above the brachium of the superior colliculus (Fig. 9-25).

FUNCTIONAL CONSIDERATIONS OF THE THALAMUS

All sensory impulses, with the sole exception of the olfactory ones, terminate in the gray masses of the thalamus, from which they are projected to specific cortical areas by the thalamocortical radiations. While portions of the dorsal thalamus serve as primary relay nuclei in various sensory pathways in which impulses are projected to specific regions of the cerebral cortex, the structure and organization of the thalamus indicate that its function is more complex and elaborate than that of a simple relay station. It seems certain that the thalamus is the chief sensory integrating mechanism of the neuraxis, but its functions are not limited to this. There is abundant evidence that specific parts of the thalamus play a dominant role in the maintenance and regulation of the state of consciousness, alterness, and attention, through widespread functional influences upon the activity of the cerebral cortex. The thalamus is concerned not only with general and specific types of awareness, but with certain emotional conotations that accompany most sensory experiences. Other data suggest that some thalamic nuclei serve as integrative centers for motor functions, since they receive the principal efferent projections from the deep cerebellar nuclei and the corpus striatum.

Physiologically the thalamus and related

neuronal subsystems are concerned with high-fidelity transmission of sensory information, input selection, output tuning, synchronization and desynchronization of cortical activity, parallel processing of information, signal storing and signal modification (Purpura, '70).

Specific Sensory Relay Nuclei. These thalamic nuclei are in the ventral tier of the lateral nuclear group. They include the medial and lateral geniculate bodies and the two divisions of the ventral posterior nucleus, known as the ventrobasal complex. The medial geniculate body receives fibers from the inferior colliculus. The laminated, tonotopically organized parvicellular part of this nucleus projects fibers via the geniculotemporal radiation to the transverse temporal gyrus of Heschl, the *primary auditory area* (Figs. 6-10 and 9-12). The lateral geniculate body, receiving both crossed and uncrossed fibers of the optic tract, gives rise to the geniculocalcarine fibers, which project in a specific way to the cortex surrounding the calcarine sulcus; cortex surrounding the calcarine sulcus represents the *primary visual area* (Figs. 9-12 and 9-23).

The divisions of the ventral posterior nucleus (VPLc, VPM, and VPMpc) project to the cortex of the postcentral gyrus. In the postcentral gyrus all parts of the body are represented in a definite sequence; this cortical region is referred to as the *primary somesthetic area* (somatic sensory area I). The sensory representation of the body in somatic sensory area I (S I) is duplicated in a different sequence in the second somatic area (SS II) which lies buried along the superior bank of the lateral sulcus (Penfield and Boldrey, '37; Woolsey, '58; Robinson and Burton, '80). Somatic sensory area II receives fibers ipsilaterally from VPLc and bilaterally from S I (Friedman et al., '80). This cortical area has a representation of different body regions in obliquely oriented cortical strips parallel to the lateral sulcus (Friedman et al., '80; Robinson and Burton, '80) (Fig. 13-8). Cell columns respond to cutaneous stimulation mainly on contralateral body surface (Robinson and Burton, '80). Ablation experiments indicate that somatic area II is not essential for somatic discrimination.

The relatively simple impulses from peripheral receptors do not pass through the thalamus without modification. Many of the impulses become synthesized and integrated at a thalamic level before being projected to specific cortical areas. In certain lesions of the thalamus, or of the thalamocortical connections, after a brief initial stage of complete contralateral anesthesia, pain, crude touch, and some thermal sense return. However, tactile localization, two-point discrimination, and the sense of position and movement remain severely impaired. The sensations recovered are poorly localized and are accompanied by a great increase in "feeling tone," most commonly of an unpleasant character. Though the threshold of excitability is raised on the affected side, tactile and thermal stimuli, previously not unpleasant, evoke disagreeable sensations.

There are two aspects to sensation: the discriminative and the affective. In the former, stimuli are compared with respect to intensity, locality, and relative position in space and time. These impulses are integrated into perceptions of form, size and texture; movements are judged as to direction, amplitude and sequence. These aspects of somatic sensation are related to VPLc and VPM and their cortical projection areas. VPLc and VPM represent a complete though distorted image of the body, and the relationship between the periphery and portions of this complex is precise. These neurons are modality specific, being concerned mainly with tactile and position sense, and respond to either superficial mechanical stimulation of the skin, mechanical distortion of deep tissues, or joint rotation, but not to more than one of these. Physiological data indicate that some impulses arising from primary endings in muscle spindles (group Ia fibers) are conveyed via relays to the cerebral cortex (Jones and Porter, '80). Short latency cortical responses can be evoked by stimulation of group I muscle afferents in a transitional cortical zone designated as 3a (Oscarsson and Rosen, '66), Area 3a is considered to lie in the depths of the central sulcus between areas 4 and 3. These short latency responses from muscle spindles are considered to reach the thalamus via the posterior column nuclei and VPLc (Asanuma et al., '83).

The visual and auditory thalamic nuclei likewise are organized in a very specific manner in which point-for-point relationships exist between the receptor organ, thalamic nuclei and the projections of thalamic nuclei to cortex. Columns of cells in all layers of the LGB receive inputs from corresponding points in the retina of each eye related to the contralateral binocular visual field. Cell columns in the dorsal nucleus of the LGB (parvicellular laminae) project to the striate cortex in a precise retinotopic fashion. No binocular fusion occurs in the LGB. This visual input to the striatal cortex is transformed in a complex manner that gives individual cortical neurons properties different from geniculate neurons, but better suited to detect shapes, patterns and provide binocular vision. The auditory thalamic relay nuclei are organized in a similar specific manner. The cellular laminae of the ventral nucleus of the medial geniculate body (MGB), evident only in Golgi preparation, forms the basis for the tonotopic organization. Neurons in the ventral division of the MGB project to the primary auditory cortex, while those in other cytological subdivisions of the MGB project to a belt of secondary auditory cortex surrounding the primary auditory area.

The "affective" side of sensation is concerned with pain, agreeableness and disagreeableness. Pain is a subjective sensation with considerable affective quality that often is difficult to describe and almost impossible to measure. The localization of different types of pain is often inexact and clinical judgment of its intensity must take into account the personality of the patient. Temperature and many tactile sensations likewise have a marked affective tone. This is especially true for visceral sensation, in which the discriminative element is practically absent.

Cortical Relay Nuclei. These thalamic nuclei receive impulses from specific subcortical structures and project to well-defined cortical regions. These include: (1) the anterior nuclei, (2) the ventral posterolateral nucleus, pars oralis (VPLo), (3) the ventral lateral nucleus (VLo, VLc, area X and VLm), and (4) the ventral anterior nuclei (in part). The anterior nuclei of the thalamus receive the largest efferent fiber bundle from the hypothalamus—the mammillothalamic tract (Figs. 9-8, 10-6, and 10-7) and direct projections from the hippocampal formation via the fornix (Figs. 9-7, 10-6, 10-7 and 12-9). These nuclei in turn project to the cingulate gyrus, a cortical area demonstrated to be concerned with a variety of visceral responses (Fig. 9-12).

The contralateral deep cerebellar nuclei project most of their ascending fibers to nuclei in the ventral lateral thalamic region (VPLo, VLc, "area x"), which collectively are called the "cell sparse" zone (Percheron, '77; Thach and Jones, '79; Tracey et al., '80; Asanuma et al., '83a). These thalamic afferents come from all deep cerebellar nuclei with the largest number arising from the dentate nucleus. VPLo also receives, along with VPI, ascending vestibular projections which terminate bilaterally in small islands (Lang et al., '79). The major part of this "cell sparse" zone in the ventral lateral thalamic region projects topographically upon the primary motor cortex, area 4 (Jones et al., '79; Tracey et al., '80; Asanuma et al., '83a; Schell and Strick, '84). The medial segment of the globus pallidus projects topographically upon the ipsilateral VLo, VLm, and VApc, and none of its terminations overlap fiber systems arising from the deep cerebellar nuclei or pars reticulata of the substantia nigra (Nauta and Mehler, '66; Kuo and Carpenter, '73; Carpenter et al., '76; Kim et al., '76; Tracey et al., '80). The cortical projection zone of VLo is to the supplementary motor area (Schell and Strick, '84). "Area x" projects to other parts of the premotor cortex on the lateral convexity of the hemisphere while VApc has broad connection with frontal cortex, including the premotor region. The pars reticulata of the substantia nigra projects ipsilaterally to medial parts of VLm, VAmc and the paralaminar parts of DM. The cortical projection zone for these thalamic nuclei are not established, although DMpl has reciprocal connections with the frontal eye field (Künzle and Akert, '77). Even though evidence is incomplete, it strongly suggests that the distinctive subdivisions of the ventral lateral thalamic region which receive inputs from the deep cerebellar nuclei, the medial segment of the globus pallidus and the pars reticulata of the substantia nigra project to cortical areas concerned with unique and different aspects of motor function.

As a group the cortical relay nuclei of the

thalamus possess common features, although the ventral anterior nucleus presents certain exceptions: (1) all receive substantial projections from specific parts of the neuraxis, (2) all, except for parts of VA, project to well-defined cortical areas, and (3) all, except VA, undergo extensive cell change following ablation of their cortical projection areas. These nuclei, with the exception of parts of VA, constitute the *specific thalamic nuclei*. Low frequency electrical stimulation of individual specific sensory relay nuclei, and certain cortical relay nuclei (e.g., the ventral lateral nucleus) evokes a primary surface potential followed by an augmenting sequence which is limited to the cortical projection area. This response is called the augmenting response. Characteristically, *augmenting responses*: (1) have a short latency, (2) are diphasic and increase in magnitude during the initial four or five stimuli of a repetitive train, and (3) are localized to the primary cortical projection area of the specific thalamic nucleus stimulated (Dempsey and Morison, '42).

Association Nuclei. The association nuclei of the thalamus receive no direct fibers from the ascending systems, but have abundant connections with other diencephalic nuclei. They project largely to association areas of the cerebral cortex in the frontal and parietal lobes and, to a lesser extent, in the occipital and temporal lobes. The principal association nuclei include the dorsomedial nucleus (DM), the lateral dorsal nucleus (LD), the lateral posterior nucleus (LP), and the pulvinar (P). The dorsomedial nucleus, the most prominent gray mass of the medial thalamus, is highly developed in primates, especially man (Figs. 9-8 and 9-9). It is connected with the lateral thalamic nuclei, the amygdaloid nuclear complex and the temporal neocortex, and has reciprocal connections with the frontal granular cortex. Large bilateral injuries to the frontal lobes are likely to cause defects in complex associations, as well as certain changes in behavior, expressed by loss of acquired inhibitions and more direct emotional responses. Similar alterations in emotional behavior are produced when the pathways between the dorsomedial nucleus and the frontal cortex are severed (e.g., in frontal lobotomy).

The lateral dorsal nucleus projects upon portions of the limbic and precuneal cortex. The larger lateral posterior nucleus has extensive connections with the association cortex of the superior and inferior parietal lobules, concerned with cognitive and symbolic functions. The pulvinar, considered as an outgrowth of the lateral posterior nucleus, develops into a huge nuclear mass concerned with the integration of somatic and special senses, particularly vision and audition.

Intralaminar and Midline Nuclei. These nuclei of the dorsal thalamus for a long time have constituted an unexplored and poorly understood region. Phylogenetically these nuclei are older than the specific relay nuclei which develop *pari passu* with the cerebral cortex. Although the midline thalamic nuclei show a progressive regression in ascending phylogeny, the intralaminar thalamic nuclei continue to develop in primates and man (Niimi et al., '60). Most of these nuclei have been regarded as having no cortical projections, though they appear to have established connections with other thalamic nuclei and with the striatum. Afferent projections to parts of the intralaminar nuclei are derived from the spinal cord, the reticular formation, the cerebellum and from forebrain derivatives (i.e., the globus pallidus and broad cortical areas).

Stimulation of the ascending reticular activating system and various kinds of sensory stimuli result in a generalized desynchronization and activation of the electroencephalogram, and behavioral arousal. It seems accepted that the electroencephalographic (EEG) arousal response, which produces dramatic effects upon cortical activity, is mediated, at least in part, by the intralaminar nuclei. Physiological studies suggest that impulses producing these changes in cortical activity reach the cortex via a diffuse, nonspecific thalamic projection system. Studies utilizing retrograde axonal transport of the enzyme horseradish peroxidase indicate that many of the diffuse, nonspecific cortical projections are collaterals of thalamostriate fibers from the intralaminar thalamic nuclei, principally CM-PF (Jones and Leavitt, '74). The more rostral intralaminar thalamic nuclei (CL and PCN) which receive fibers from the midbrain reticular formation project directly to widespread cortical regions (Glen and Steriade, '82; Steriade and Glen, '82).

The classical studies of Dempsey and Morison ('42, '43) and of Morison and Dempsey ('42) showed that stimulation of the so-called nonspecific thalamic nuclei, and the basal diencephalic region, produced widespread and pronounced effects upon electrocortical activity. The *nonspecific*, or *diffuse*, thalamic nuclei include the intralaminar and midline nuclei and, in part, the ventral anterior nucleus of the ventral tier. Repetitive stimulation of these thalamic nuclei alters spontaneous electrocortical activity over large areas and, under certain conditions, resets the frequency of brain waves by eliciting responses that are time-locked to the thalamic stimulus. The most characteristic effect of stimulating the nonspecific thalamic nuclei is the *recruiting response*. When the frequency of stimulation is in the range of 6 to 12 cycles per second, predominantly surface negative cortical responses rapidly increase to a maximum (by the fourth to sixth stimulus of the train) and then decrease over a broad area; continued stimulation causes the evoked responses to wax and wane. Stimulation of one of the nonspecific thalamic nuclei causes all others to be activated in a mass excitation (Starl and Magoun, '51). Bilateral cortical responses do not depend upon transmission of impulses across the midline by the corpus callosum or anterior commissure, nor does spread from one cortical area to another depend upon intracortical propagation.

The observation of Moruzzi and Magoun ('49) that cortical recruiting responses induced by low frequency stimulation of the nonspecific thalamic nuclei could be reduced, or blocked, by stimulation of the bulbar reticular formation appears to provide experimental evidence that the nonspecific thalamic nuclei are within the sphere of influence of the ascending reticular formation.

The largest component of the intralaminar nuclei, the centromedian-parafascicular nuclear complex (CM-PF) receives its input mainly from forebrain derivatives. The precentral and premotor cortex project profusely upon these nuclei (Künzle, '76, '78; Akert and Hartmann-von Monakow, '80) and CM also receives pallidofugal fibers. The principal projection of CM-PF is to the striatum suggesting that this nuclear complex must play an important role in motor function. The intralaminar thalamic nuclei also have been considered as components of a nonspecific sensory system and part of a central mechanism concerned with pain (Albe-Fessard and Kruger, '62; Emmers, '76).

It has been suggested that the nuclei of the posterior thalamic complex should be grouped with the intralaminar nuclei (Jones and Powell, '71). The posterior thalamic nuclei are hypothesized to constitute a posterior extension of the intralaminar thalamic nuclei related to cortex on the lateral surface of the hemisphere caudal to area 4, with the exception of areas 17, 18, and 19. All cortical areas within this region project fibers to: (1) their respective principal nucleus, (2) parts of the reticular nucleus, and (3) either a part of the intralaminar or posterior thalamic nuclei. The visual cortex appears unique in that it does not send or receive fibers from either the intralaminar or posterior thalamic nuclei.

The thalamus is played upon by two great streams of afferent fibers: the peripheral and the cortical. The former brings sensory impulses from all parts of the body concerning changes in the external and internal environment. The cortical connections link the thalamus with the associative memory mechanism of the pallium and bring it under cortical control. The thalamus has subcortical efferent connections with the hypothalmus and striatum(i.e., caudate nucleus and putamen) through which the thalamus can influence visceral and somatic effectors. The functional nature of these subcortical efferent thalamic pathways is unknown, but they are considered to serve primarily affective reactions. These pathways, like the thalamus itself, are under the control of the cerebral cortex.

CHAPTER 10

The Hypothalamus

The hypothalamus is the part of the diencephalon most concerned with visceral, autonomic and endocrine functions. All of these functions are intimately related to affective and emotional behavior. This structure lies in the walls of the third ventricle below the hypothalamic sulci and is continuous across the floor of this ventricle (Figs. 10-1, 10-2, and 10-3). On the ventral surface of the brain the *infundibulum*, to which the hypophysis is attached, emerges posterior to the optic chiasm (Figs. 9-4, 10-1, and 10-10). A slightly bulging region posterior to the infundibulum is the *tuber cinereum* (Fig. 10-6). The *mammillary bodies* are found posteriorly near the interpeduncular fossa.

The ventral external hypothalamus is bounded anteriorly by the optic chiasm, laterally by the optic tracts and posteriorly by the mammillary bodies (Figs. 1-8, 2-7 and 2-8). This region is roughly diamond shaped and its surface is irregular because of several small protuberances, identified as eminences. The zone forming the floor of the third ventricle is called the *median eminence* of the tuber cinereum. The portion rostral to the infundibular stem is the *anterior median eminence*; the portion posterior to the infundibular stem forms the *posterior median eminence*, which is better developed in man (Figs. 2-7 and 2-8). Paired lateral eminences form well defined landmarks. The ventral protrusion of the hypothalamus and the third ventricular recess form the infundibulum (Fig. 9-4). The most distal portion of the infundibular process is the neurohypophysis; tissue joining the infundibular process to the median eminence is called the infundibular stem. The median eminence represents the final point of convergence of pathways from the central nervous system upon the peripheral endocrine system (Knigge and Silverman, '74). The median eminence is the anatomical site of the interface between brain and the anterior pituitary. Primary capillaries of the hypophysial portal vessels vascularize the median eminence (Porter et al., '74). Ependymal cells lining the floor of the third ventricle have processes that traverse the width of the median eminence and terminate near the portal perivascular space. These cells, called tanycytes, provide a structural and functional link between the cerebrospinal fluid (CSF) and the perivascular space of the pituitary portal vessels.

The hypothalamus can be described as extending from the region of the optic chiasm to the caudal border of the mammillary bodies. Anteriorly it passes without sharp demarcation into the basal olfactory area (diagonal gyrus of the anterior perforated substance) (Fig. 12-2). The region immediately in front of the optic chiasm, extending to the lamina terminalis and the anterior commissure, is known as the preoptic area (Fig. 10-1). The preoptic area, classically regarded as a forebrain derivative, is considered by Kuhlenbeck ('69) to arise from a rostral hypothalamic anlage and to be structurally and functionally a part of the hypothalamus. Caudally the hypothalamus merges imperceptibly into the central gray and tegmentum of the midbrain. The thalamus lies dorsal to the hypothalamus; the subthalamic region is lateral and caudal (Figs. 9-4 and 9-5).

HYPOTHALAMIC NUCLEI

Pervading the whole area is a diffuse matrix of cells constituting the central gray substance, in which are found a number of more or less distinct nuclear masses. A sagittal plane passing through the anterior pillar of the fornix roughly separates the medial and the lateral hypothalamic areas (Figs. 10-2, 10-5 and 10-6).

Lateral Hypothalamic Area. This area is bounded medially by the mammillothalamic tract and the anterior column of the fornix (Figs. 10-2 and 10-3); the lateral boundary is the medial margin of the internal capsule and the subthalamic region (Fig. 10-2). Rostrally this area is continuous with the lateral preoptic nucleus, while caudally it merges with the midbrain tegmentum (Fig. 10-3). This area contains scattered groups of large, darkly staining cells—the *lateral hypothalamic nucleus*—and two or three sharply delimited circular cell groups known as the tuberal nuclei (nuclei tuberales), which often produce small visible eminences on the basal surface of the hypothalamus. They consist of small, pale, multipolar cells surrounded by a delicate fiber capsule about which are found the large cells of the lateral hypothalamic nucleus (Figs. 10-2 and 10-3).

Preoptic Region. This region constitutes the periventricular gray of the most

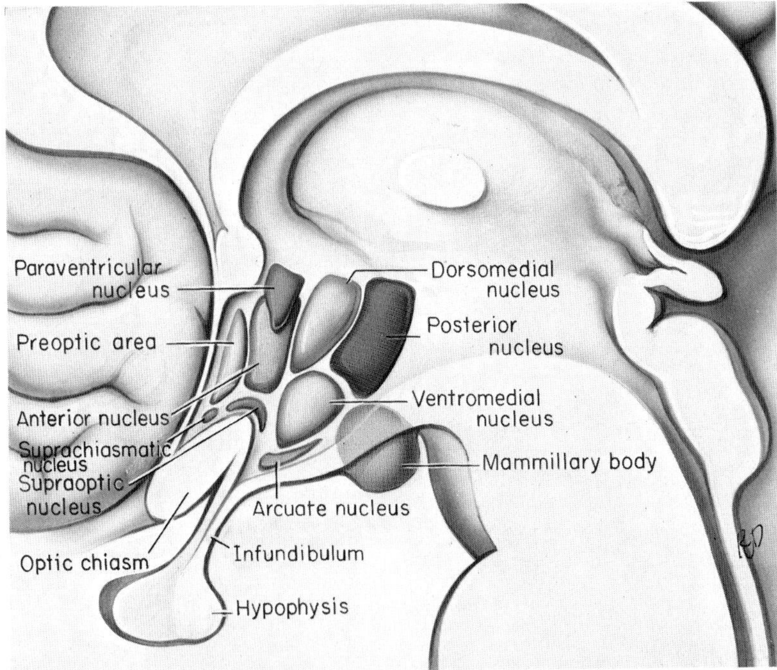

Figure 10-1. Schematic diagram of the medial hypothalamic nuclei. Nuclei in the supraoptic region are in *blue*. The paraventricular and supraoptic nuclei are *dark blue*; the suprachiasmatic and anterior nuclei of the hypothalamus are *light blue*. Nuclei of the middle or tuberal region of the hypothalamus are *yellow*. Nuclei of the caudal or mammillary region are shades of *red*. The preoptic area lies rostral to the anterior hypothalamic region and classically is regarded as a forebrain derivative functionally related to the hypothalamus. (From Carpenter and Sutin, *Human Neuroanatomy*, 1983; courtesy of Williams & Wilkins.)

rostral part of the third ventricle (Figs. 10-1, 10-2 and 10-3). The *preoptic periventricular nucleus* surrounds the walls of the third ventricle in the region of the preoptic recess. The diffusely arranged small cells are poorly differentiated from the ependymal lining. The *medial preoptic nucleus*, composed of predominantly small cells, lies lateral to the preoptic periventricular nucleus and extends ventrally to the optic chiasm (Fig. 10-2). The *lateral preoptic nucleus*, rostral to the lateral hypothalamic area, is composed of diffusely dispersed medium-sized cells (Figs. 10-2 and 10-3) and is regarded as the interstitial nucleus of the median forebrain bundle (Kuhlenbeck, '69).

Caudal to the preoptic area three hypothalamic regions are recognized: (1) an anterior or *supraoptic region*, lying above the optic chiasm and continuous rostrally with the preoptic area; (2) a middle, or *tuberal region*; and (3) a caudal, or *mammillary region* which is continuous caudally with the central gray of the cerebral aqueduct (Fig. 10-1).

Supraoptic Region. This region contains two of the most striking and sharply defined hypothalamic nuclei, the *paraventricular nucleus* and the *supraoptic nucleus*. Cells of the paraventricular nucleus form a vertical plate of densely packed cells immediately beneath the ependyma of the third ventricle, while cells of the supraoptic nucleus straddle the optic tract (Figs. 10-2, 10-3 and 10-4). Cells in both of these nuclei are similar. They are larger than cells in the surrounding central gray and stain deeply. The Nissl substance is distributed peripherally and cytoplasmic inclusions of colloidal material are regarded as the neurosecretory product of these cells. Both of these nuclei send fibers to the posterior lobe of the hypophysis.

The less differentiated central gray in the supraoptic region constitutes the *anterior hypothalamic nucleus* (Fig. 10-1). This nucleus merges imperceptibly with the preoptic area.

The *suprachiasmatic nucleus* forms a group of small round cells immediately dorsal to the optic chiasm and close to the third ventricle. This small nucleus receives direct projections from the retina (Moore and Lenn, '72; Moore, '73; Pierson and Carpenter, '74) and an indirect input from the ventral nucleus of the lateral geniculate body (Swanson et al., '74).

Tuberal Region. In this region, the hypothalamus reaches its widest extent; the fornix separates the medial and the lateral hypothalamic areas (Figs. 10-2, 10-3, and 10-6).The medial portion forms the central gray substance of the ventricular wall, in which there may be distinguished a ventromedial and a dorsomedial nucleus.

The *ventromedial nucleus*, the largest cell group in the tuberal region, has a round or oval shape and is surrounded by a cell-poor zone that helps to delineate its boundaries (Figs. 10-1, 10-2, 10-3, and 10-5). Neurons of the ventromedial nucleus typically have dendrites that extend beyond the borders of the nucleus (Millhouse, '79). The cell-free capsular zone around the nucleus is formed by a dense ring of axons and terminals (Fig. 10-5). The *dorsomedial nucleus* is a less distinct aggregation of cells that borders the third ventricle (Fig. 10-3). The *arcuate nucleus* (infundibular nucleus) is located in the most ventral part of the third ventricle near the entrance to the infundibular recess and extends into the median eminence (Figs. 10-1 and 10-15). The small cells of this nucleus are in close contact with the ependyma lining the ventricle. In coronal sections the nucleus has an arcuate shape (Nauta and Haymaker, '69). In the caudal part of the tuberal region many large oval or rounded cells are scattered in a matrix of smaller ones; collectively they constitute the *posterior hypothalamic nucleus* (Figs. 10-1, 10-2 and 10-3). The large cells, especially numerous in man, extend caudally over the mammillary body to become continuous with the central gray of the midbrain.

Mammillary Region. This region consists of the mammillary bodies and the dorsally located cells of the posterior hypothalamic nucleus (Fig. 10-2, 10-3, 10-6, and 10-7). In man the mammillary body consists almost entirely of the large, spherical medial *mammillary nucleus*, composed of relatively small cells invested by a capsule of myelinated fibers. Lateral to this is the small *intermediate (intercalated) mammillary nucleus* composed of smaller cells.

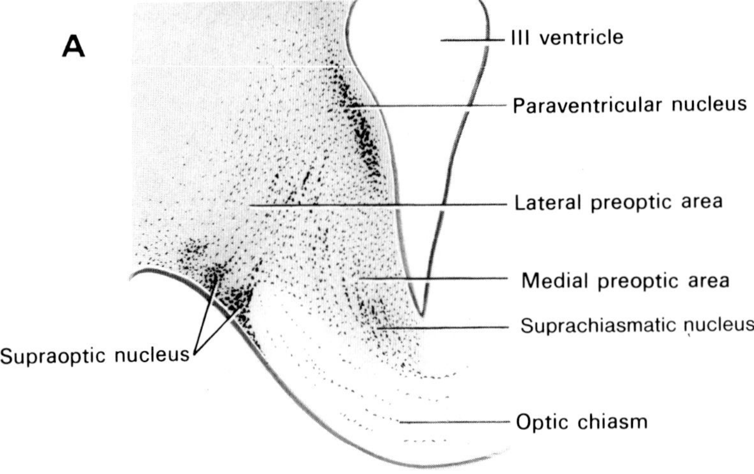

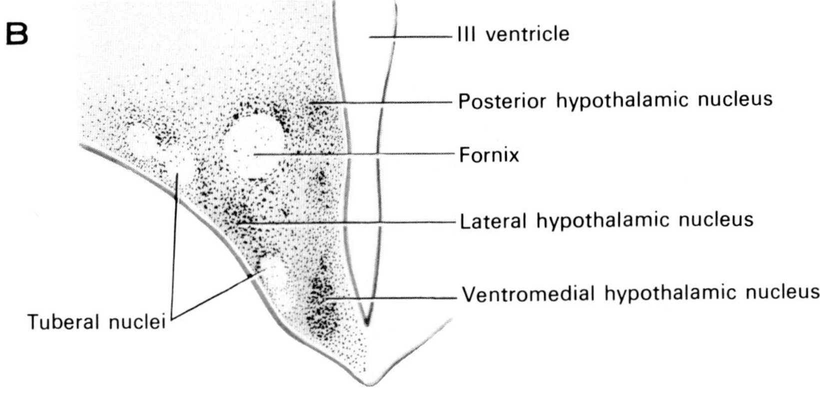

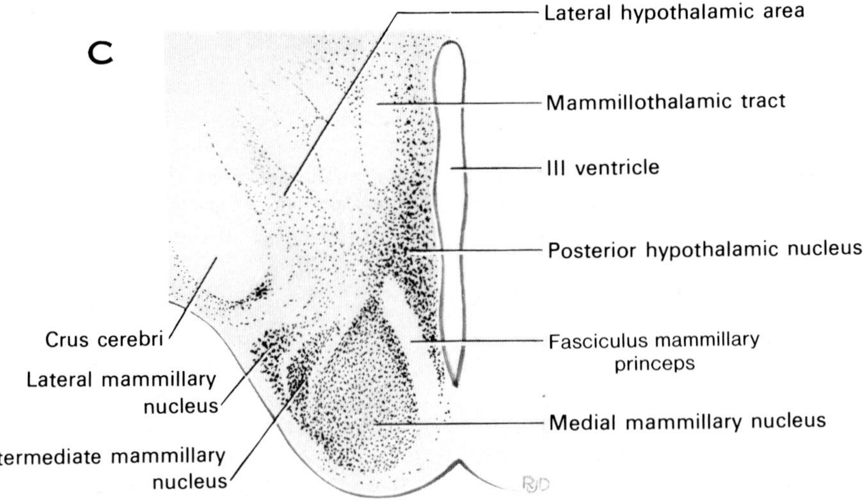

Figure 10-2. Drawings of transverse sections through portions of the human hypothalamus: (*A*) supraoptic region, (*B*) infundibular region, and (*C*) mammillary region (after Clark et al., '38). (From Carpenter and Sutin, *Human Neuroanatomy*, 1983; courtesy of Williams & Wilkins.)

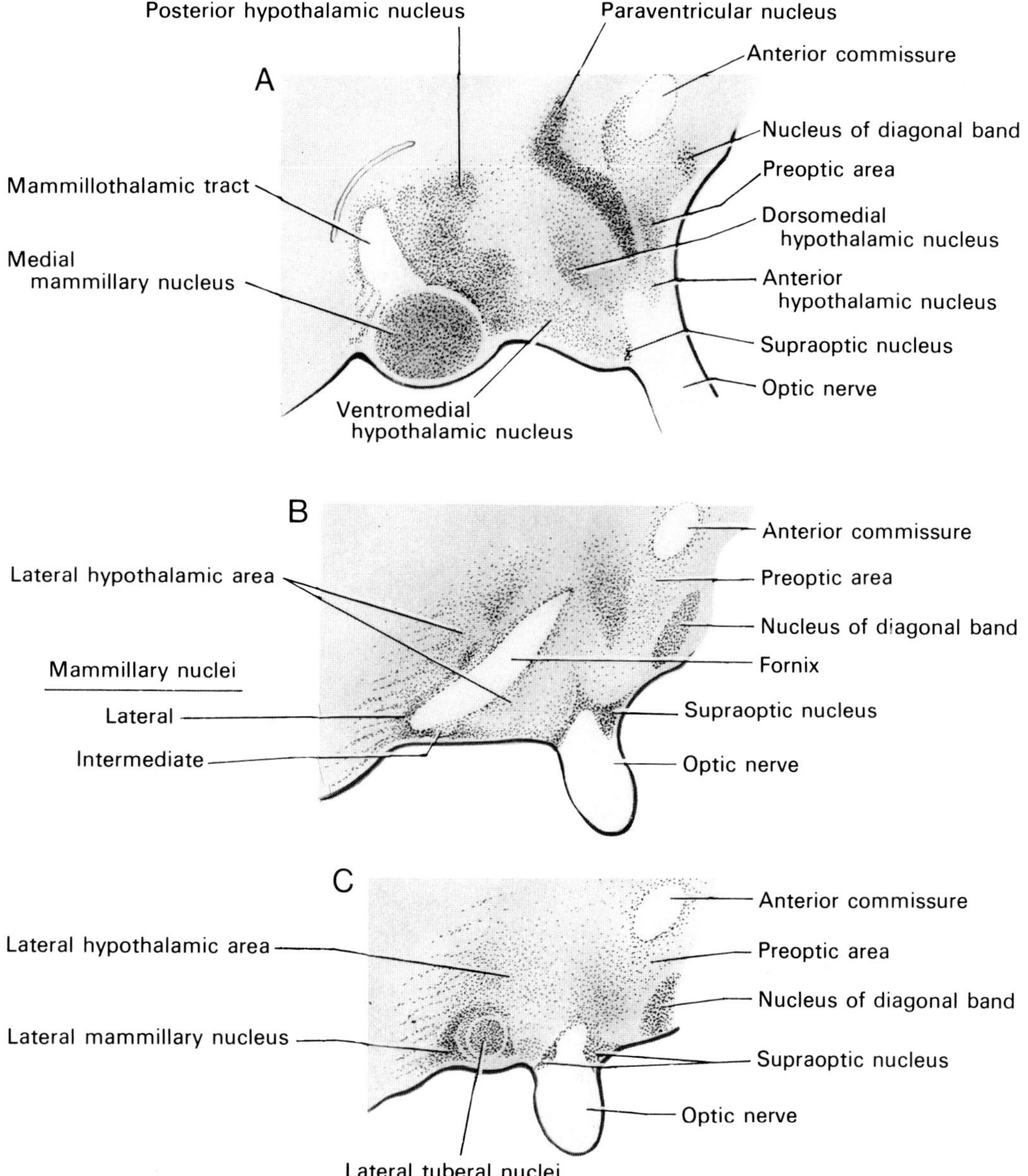

Figure 10-3. Sagittal drawings of the human hypothalamus: (*A*) medial, near ventricular surface, (*B*) through the anterior column of the fornix, and (*C*) near lateral border of hypothalamus (after Clark et al., '38). (From Carpenter and Sutin, *Human Neuroanatomy*, 1983; courtesy of Williams & Wilkins.)

Even further lateral is a well-defined group of large cells, the *lateral mammillary nucleus*, which probably represents a condensation of cells from the posterior hypothalamic nucleus (Fig. 10-2). The most characteristic features of the human hypothalamus are the sharply circumscribed tuberal nuclei, the large size of the medial mammillary nuclei, and the extensive distribution of the large cells in the posterior and lateral hypothalamic areas. Synthetic descriptions may suggest that all hypothalamic nuclei are sharply circumscribed, but the cellular matrix of the hypothalamus is broadly continuous with the surrounding gray matter. Tissue continuities with the surrounding gray matter contain the major afferent and efferent hypothalamic pathways.

Rostrally and laterally the hypothalamus

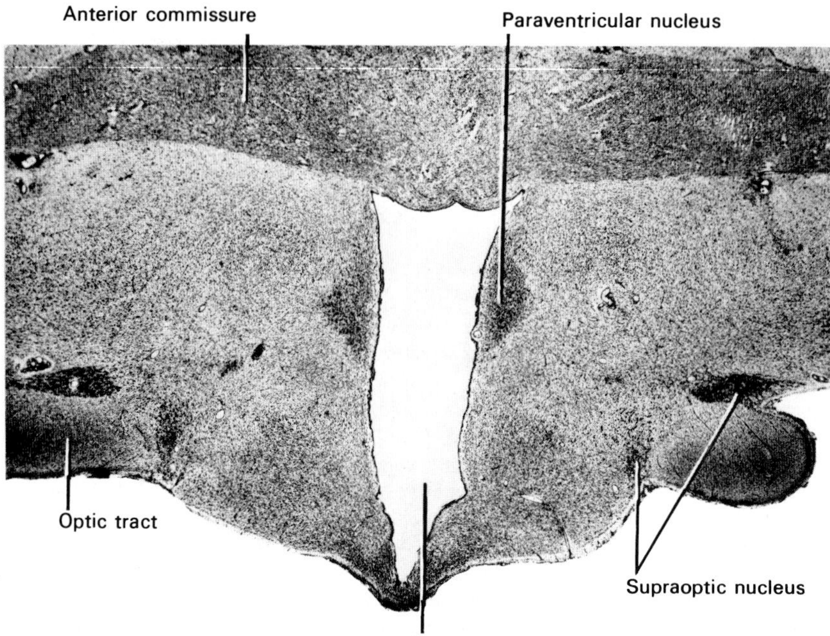

Figure 10-4. Photograph of human hypothalamus at the level of the anterior commissure demonstrating the paraventricular and supraoptic nuclei. (Nissl stain). (From Carpenter and Sutin, *Human Neuroanatomy*, 1983; courtesy of Williams & Wilkins.)

is continuous with the *basal olfactory region*, a large gray mass beneath the rostral part of the lentiform nucleus and the head of the caudate nucleus (Figs. 10-2 and 10-3). Near the median plane this region extends dorsally, rostral to the anterior commissure, where it becomes the *septal region*. Beneath the lentiform nucleus the gray mass extends toward the amygdaloid complex and contains groups of large cells, referred to as the substantia innominata on the nucleus basalis (Fig. 12-16). The base of the septal region is continuous with the substantia innominata laterally and with the preoptic region caudally. The septal region contains the *medial septal nucleus*, the *lateral septal nucleus*, and the *nucleus accumbens septi* (Figs. 12-6 and 12-16).

CONNECTIONS OF THE HYPOTHALAMUS

The hypothalamus, in spite of its small size, has extensive and complex connections. Some fibers are organized into definite and conspicuous bundles, while others are diffuse and difficult to trace.

Afferent Connections of the Hypothalamus. The afferent connections of the hypothalamus which have been established are:

The *medial forebrain bundle* is a complex group of fibers arising from the basal olfactory regions, the periamygdaloid region, and the septal nuclei, that passes to, and through, the lateral preoptic and hypothalamic regions (Fig. 10-8). The bundle is formed, at levels rostral to the anterior commissure, mainly of fibers from the septal region. In its parasagittal course it receives contributions from the substantia innominata and the amygdaloid complex. This tract is well developed in lower vertebrates, but in man it is small. The bundle is a loosely textured fiber system, in part composed of short fibers, although longer axons continue caudally into the midbrain tegmentum.

Hippocampo-hypothalamic fibers originating from the hippocampal formation form the fornix (Figs. 10-2, 10-3, 10-6, and 12-9), and the medial corticohypothalamic tract (Fig. 10-9). In transverse section the medial corticohypothalamic tract appears

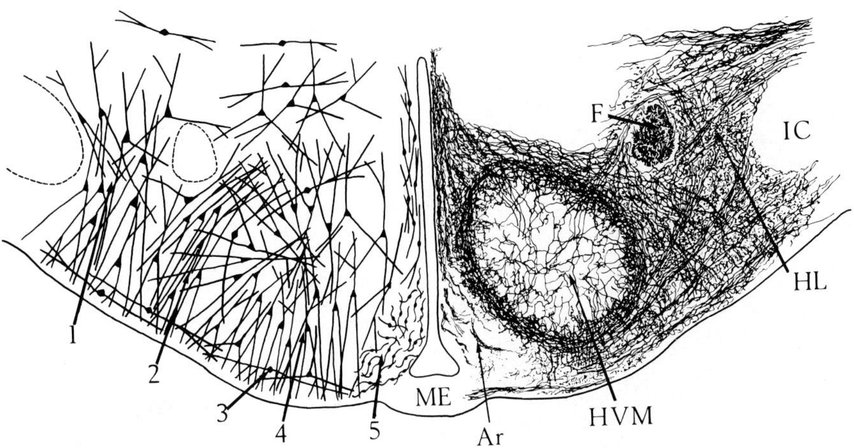

Figure 10-5. Drawings of the tuberal region of rodent hypothalamus based upon Golgi preparations. The general arrangement of dendrites and axons is shown on the left: (*1*) Dendrites of HL radiate in mediolateral and dorsoventral directions. (*2*) There is a compression of dendritic fields of neurons located between F and HVM. (*3*) The dendritic fields of neurons along the hypothalamic surface are generally parallel with the pia. (*4*) The long dendrites of HVM extend in all directions from the nucleus. (*5*) Small bipolar neurons of the Ar nestle against the ventricle, adjacent to ME. Abbreviations used: Ar, arcuate nucleus; *F*, fornix; *HL*, lateral hypothalamic area; *HVM*, hypothalamic ventromedial nucleus; *IC*, internal capsule; *ME*, median eminence. (Reproduced with permission from O. E. Millhouse: *Handbook of the Hypothalamus*, *Vol. 1. Anatomy of the Hypothalamus*, edited by P. Morgane and J. Panksepp, Marcel Dekker, New York, 1979.) (From Carpenter and Sutin, *Human Neuroanatomy*, 1983; courtesy of Williams & Wilkins.)

as a group of myelinated fibers coursing medial to the fornix (Fig. 12-8). The hippocampal formation projects to the hypothalamus via both the fornix and the medial corticohypothalamic tract. Axoplasmic transport studies indicate that fibers arising from the subiculum project via the fornix to the septum and the medial and lateral mammillary nuclei (Nauta, '56; Raisman et al., '66; Meibach and siegel, '77; Swanson and Cowan, '77). Pyramidal cells from all regions of the hippocampal formation project to the septum, but not to the hypothalamus. Fibers in the medial corticohypothalamic tract originate from the subiculum and terminate in a cell-free zone surrounding the ventromedial hypothalamic nucleus (Fig. 10-5). The distribution of these fibers corresponds to the location of hypothalamic neurons which concentrate tritiated estradiol (Stumpf, '72).

In the septal region fibers of the fornix form two distinct bundles: (1) a compact fornix column, or postcommissural fornix, which arches caudal to the anterior commissure, and (2) a more diffuse precommissural fornix.

Precommissural fibers of the fornix are distributed to the septal nuclei, the lateral preoptic region, the nucleus of the diagonal band, and the dorsal hypothalamic area. *Postcommissural fibers* of the fornix project to the medial mammillary nucleus, except for those which leave this bundle and terminate in thalamic nuclei.

Amygdalo-hypothalamic fibers follow two pathways to the hypothalamus: (a) the stria terminalis (Fig. 9-6 and 12-6), and (b) a course ventral to the lentiform nucleus. The stria terminalis arises mainly from the corticomedial part of the amygdaloid complex, and distributes fibers to the medial preoptic nucleus, the anterior hypothalamic nucleus, and the ventromedial and arcuate nuclei (Heimer and Nauta, '67; Nauta and Haymaker,'69). Ventral amygdalofugal fibers arise from the basolateral amygdaloid nuclei and the pyriform cortex and spread medially and rostrally under the lentiform nucleus to reach the lateral hypothalamic nucleus and the medial forebrain bundle (Raisman, '66).

Brain stem reticular afferents ascend to the hypothalamus via the mammillary pe-

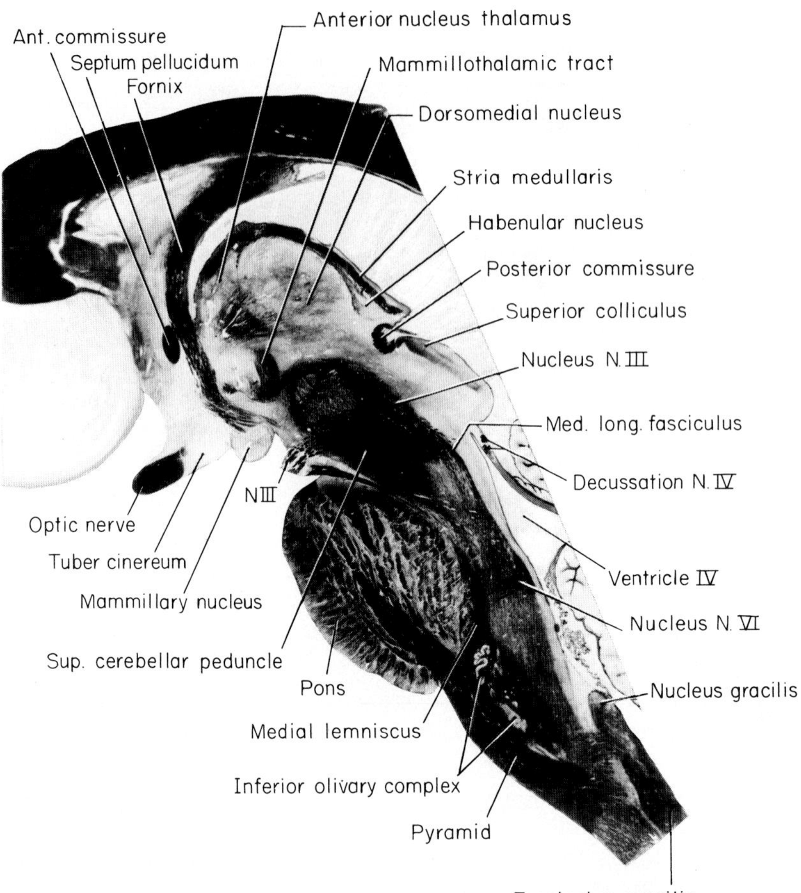

Figure 10-6. Sagittal section of brain stem through the pillar of fornix, the mammillothalamic tract and the stria medullaris. (Weigert's myelin stain; photograph.) (From Carpenter and Sutin, *Human Neuroanatomy*, 1983; courtesy of Williams & Wilkins.)

duncle and the dorsal longitudinal fasciculus. The *mammillary peduncle* arises from the dorsal and ventral tegmental nuclei of the midbrain and projects mainly to the lateral mammillary nucleus (Fig. 10-8). A few fibers of this bundle pass beyond the hypothalamus. The ascending component of the *dorsal longitudinal fasciculus* is formed from cells in the central gray of the midbrain (Fig. 10-8). Fibers in this bundle spread out over caudal and dorsal regions of the hypothalamus where they become part of the periventricular system.

Brain stem afferents to the hypothalamus also arise from neurons in the raphe nuclei of the midbrain (Fig. 5-11), the lateral parabrachial nuclei in the pons (Fig. 5-21) and from the locus ceruleus (Figs. 6-27 and 6-28). Ascending serotonergic fibers arise mainly from the medial (superior central nucleus) and dorsal nuclei of the raphe, ascend in the medial forebrain bundle to, and through the lateral hypothalamus (Bobillier et al., '75; Bobillier et al., '76; Moore et al., '78); terminals are distributed to the preoptic region, the suprachiasmatic nucleus and the mammillary bodies (Aghajanian et al., '69; Bobillier et al., '75; Geyer et al., '76). The parabrachial nuclei receive afferents from different parts of the nucleus solitarius and projections from the medial and lateral parabrachial nuclei can be correlated with these inputs (Fulwiler and Saper, '84). The general visceral afferent

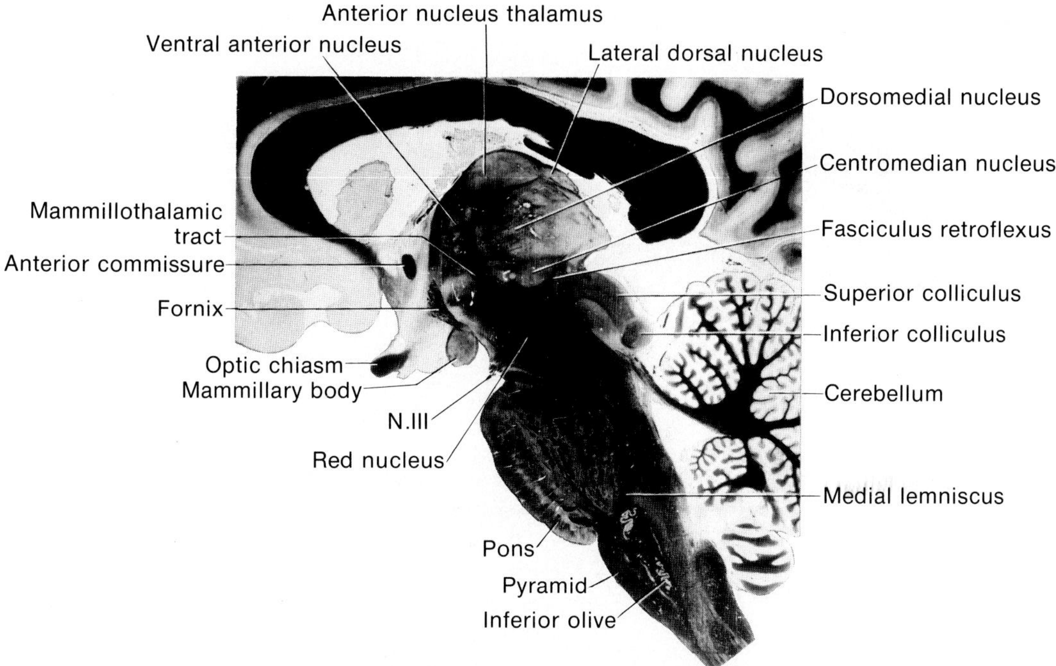

Figure 10-7. Sagittal section of the brain stem demonstrating the mammillothalamic tract and thalamic nuclei lateral to those shown in Figure 10-6. (Weigert's myelin stain; photograph.) (From Carpenter and Sutin, *Human Neuroanatomy*, 1983; courtesy of Williams & Wilkins.)

part (located caudally) of the nucleus solitarius projects primarily to the lateral parabrachial nuclei (Fig. 5-21). Subnuclei of the lateral parabrachial complex innervate the medial preoptic region, the paraventricular and dorsomedial hypothalamic nuclei and the lateral hypothalamic area. The medial parabrachial nuclei which receive afferents from the special visceral afferent part (located rostrally) of the nucleus solitarius project to several areas of cortex, the substantia innominata, the central nucleus of the amygdala and posterior lateral regions of the hypothalamus (Fulwiler and Saper, '84). Ascending noradrenergic fibers originate in the locus ceruleus and ascend in a dorsal tegmental bundle which distributes dense terminals in the dorsomedial, supraoptic and paraventricular hypothalamic nuclei (Lindvall and Björklund, '74; Knigge and Silverman, '74). Afferent fibers to the hypothalamus from the brain stem and other sources are shown in Figures 10-9 and 10-11.

Retinohypothalamic fibers arise from ganglion cells of the retina and project bilaterally to the suprachiasmatic nuclei via the optic nerve and chiasm (Hendrickson et al., '72; Moore, '73; Tigges and O'Steen, '74). Retinal axons also extend into the medial preoptic neuropil and project bilaterally near the third ventricle to the level of the paraventricular nuclei (Pickard and Silverman, '81). In addition this nucleus receives an indirect input from the retina via the ventral nucleus of the lateral geniculate body (Swanson et al., '74). The suprachiasmatic nucleus is concerned with light entraining mechanisms that control circadian rhythms and daily fluctuations in melatonin synthesis (Klein and Weller, '72; Klein et al., '81). This nucleus is the pacemaker for circadian rhythms (Ibuka et al., '77). Nearly a third of the cells in the suprachiasmatic nucleus are immunoreactive for vasopressin (Sofroniew and Weindl, '80).

Opinions vary concerning corticohypothalamic fibers which are usually described as arising from the posterior orbital cortex.

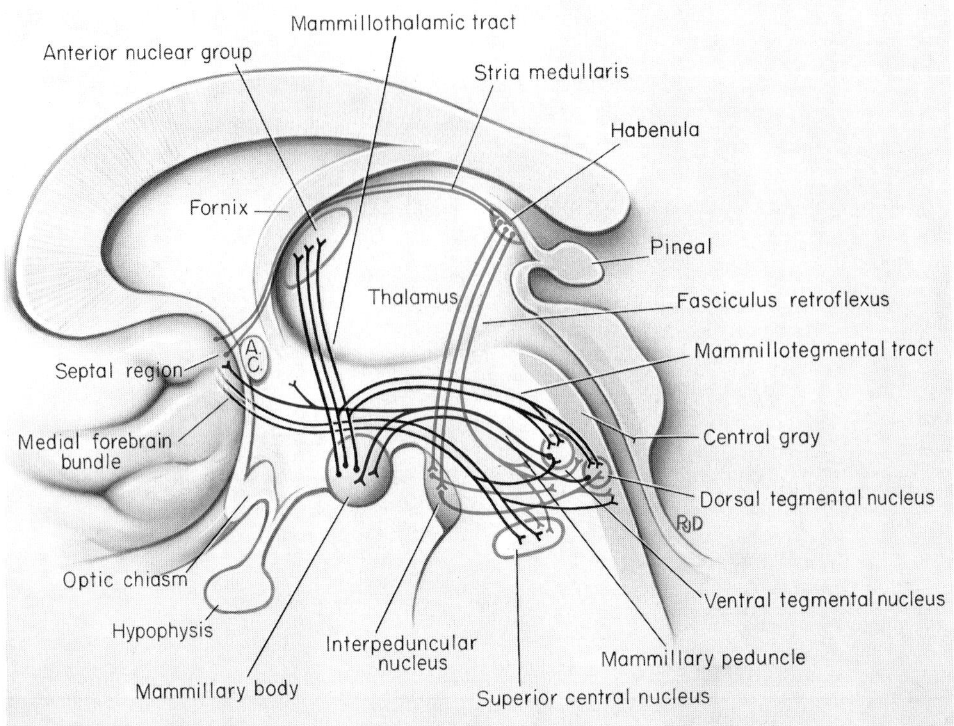

Figure 10-8. Semischematic diagram of limbic pathways interrelating the telencephalon and diencephalon with medial midbrain structures. The medial forebrain bundle and efferent fibers of the mammillary body are shown in *black*. The *medial forebrain bundle* originates from the septal and lateral preoptic regions, traverses the lateral hypothalamic area and projects into the midbrain tegmentum. The *mammillary princeps* divides into two bundles, the *mammillothalamic tract* and the *mammillotegmental tract*. Ascending fibers of the *mammillary peduncle*, arising from the dorsal and ventral tegmental nuclei, are shown in *red*; most of these fibers pass to the mammillary body, but some continue rostrally to the lateral hypothalamus, the preoptic region and the medial septal nucleus. Fibers arising from the septal nuclei project caudally in the medial part of the *stria medullaris* (*blue*) to terminate in the medial habenular nucleus. Impulses conveyed to the habenular nucleus are distributed to midbrain tegmental nuclei via the *fasciculus retroflexus* (based on Nauta, '58). (From Carpenter and Sutin, *Human Neuroanatomy*, 1983; courtesy of Williams & Wilkins.)

Direct thalamohypothalamic pathways also are regarded as sparse.

Broadly stated, the principal forebrain afferents to the hypothalamus arise from the two phylogenetically oldest cortical areas, the pyriform cortex and the hippocampal formation (Fig. 10-11). In each instance the cortical projection is reinforced by a corresponding subcortical projection, the amygdala in the case of the pyriform cortex, and the septum in the case of the hippocampal formation (Raisman, '66). Each of these subcortical nuclei is reciprocally connected with the overlying cortical area. Of the phylogenetically newer cortical areas the cingulate gyrus appears particularly favored to influence the hypothalamus indirectly through the entorhinal cortex and the hippocampal formation. The cingulate cortex can in turn be influenced by hypothalamic projections to the anterior nuclear group of the thalamus. Both the sense of taste and olfaction are directly involved in arousal and phases of consumatory behavior. Gustatory pathways to the hypothalamus are multisynaptic and complex, while olfactory projections to the hypothalamus are relatively direct.

Efferent Connections of the Hypothalamus. The efferent connections of the hypothalamus appear, in part, to be reciprocal to the afferent systems. There are

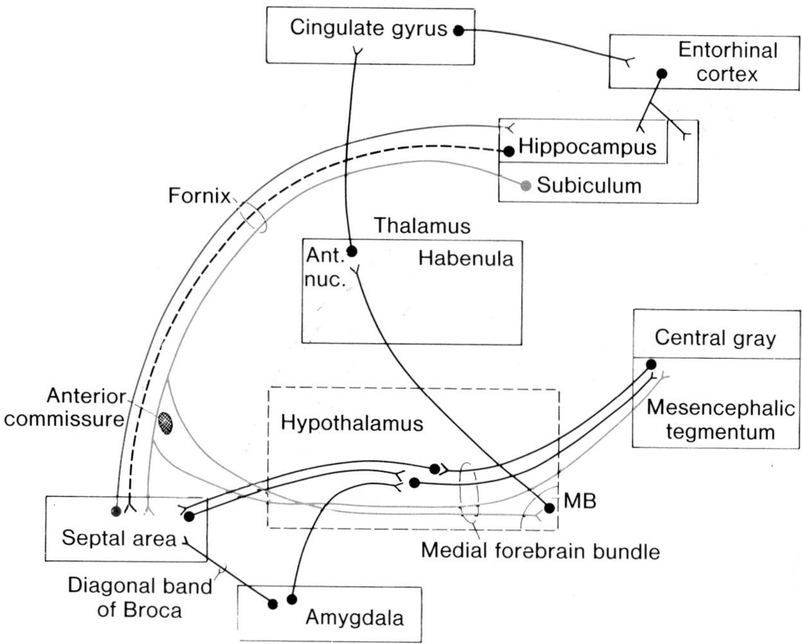

Figure 10-9. Schematic block diagram of major interconnections of structures comprising the "limbic system." Projections arising from the subiculum (*blue*) pass via the fornix to the septal area, hypothalamus and mesencephalic tegmentum. Fibers projecting in the fornix from the hippocampal formation are shown in *black*-dashed lines. Projections from the septal area to the hippocampal formation are shown in *red*. *MB* indicates the mammillary body. (From Carpenter and Sutin, *Human Neuroanatomy*, 1983; courtesy of Williams & Wilkins.)

reciprocal connections in the medial forebrain bundle which provide indirect connections between the lateral hypothalamus and the hippocampal formation (Raisman, '66a). In addition there are hypothalamic projections to the amygdaloid nuclear complex via both the stria terminalis and the ventral pathway (Figs. 10-9 and 10-11). Reciprocal connections with the midbrain tegmentum and central gray are conducted by the dorsal longitudinal fasciculus and via pathways projecting to and from the mammillary bodies (Figs. 10-8 and 10-10). In addition, there are several efferent hypothalamic pathways which have no counterpart among afferent systems.

The *medial forebrain bundle* (Fig. 10-8) conveys impulses from the lateral hypothalamus rostrally to the nuclei of the diagonal band (Fig. 10-3) and to the medial septal nuclei which in turn send fibers to the hippocampal formation via the fimbria of the fornix (Daitz and Powell, '54). Descending hypothalamic efferents in the medial forebrain bundle project through the ventral tegmental region to the superior central nucleus, the ventral tegmental nucleus and to parts of the central gray (Fig. 10-8). Hypothalamic efferents to the amygdaloid nuclear complex pass via both the stria terminalis and the ventral pathway (Cowan et al., '65; Szentágothai et al., '68). Fibers from the lateral hypothalamic region follow the ventral pathway through the substantia innominata to the amygdala, while those that pass via the stria terminalis arise from more medial cells (Nauta and Haymaker, '69).

The *dorsal longitudinal fasciculus* contains descending fibers from medial and periventricular portions of the hypothalamus distributed to the central gray of the midbrain and the tectum. Some descending fibers in this system may extend to the

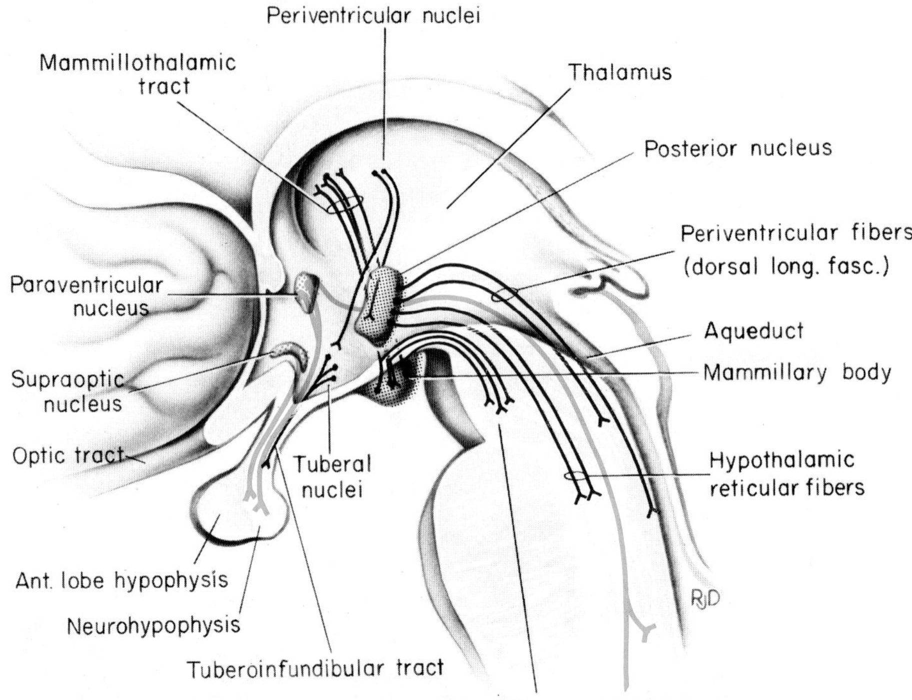

Figure 10-10. Diagram of some of the efferent hypothalamic pathways. Color code is the same as in Figure 10-1. Terminations of the mammillotegmental tract are shown in Figure 10-8. (From Carpenter and Sutin, *Human Neuroanatomy*, 1983; courtesy of Williams & Wilkins.)

dorsal tegmental nucleus (Fig. 10-10). The pathways by which impulses originating in the hypothalamus are relayed to nuclei in the medulla and spinal cord have been poorly understood. Previously it was presumed that hypothalamic impulses transmitted to cells in the reticular formation were relayed by reticular neurons to the medulla and spinal levels (Fig. 10-10). Studies using the enzyme marker horseradish peroxidase (HRP) indicate direct projections from the hypothalamus to spinal levels. Thus both direct and indirect pathways from the hypothalamus may convey impulses to spinal levels (Fig. 4-15).

Mammillary efferent fibers, arising from the medial mammillary nucleus, and to a lesser extent from the lateral and intermediate mammillary nuclei, form a well-defined bundle, the *fasciculus mammillaris princeps* (Figs. 10-6, 10-7 and 10-8). This bundle passes dorsally for a short distance and divides into two components: the *mammillothalamic tract* and the *mammillotegmental tract* (Figs. 10-6, 10-7, and 10-8). The mammillothalamic tract contains fibers from the medial mammillary nucleus that project to the ipsilateral anteroventral and anteromedial thalamic nuclei, and fibers from the lateral mammillary nucleus that pass bilaterally to the anterodorsal nuclei (Fry et al., '63). Superimposed upon this hypothalamic relay to the anterior nuclei of the thalamus are direct projections from the hippocampal formation via the fornix (Guillery, '56; Valenstein and Nauta, '59). Each of the anterior thalamic nuclei in turn project to subdivisions of the cingulate cortex (Figs. 2-6 and 12-17). The cingulate cortex projects back to the hippocampal formation via the entorhinal cortex, forming a closed anatomical circuit (Fig. 10-11).

The *mammillotegmental tract* arches caudally into the midbrain tegmentum where fibers terminate in the dorsal and ventral tegmental nuclei (Fig. 10-8).

Hypothalamospinal Fibers. Although at one time no projections from the hypothalamus were thought to descend caudal

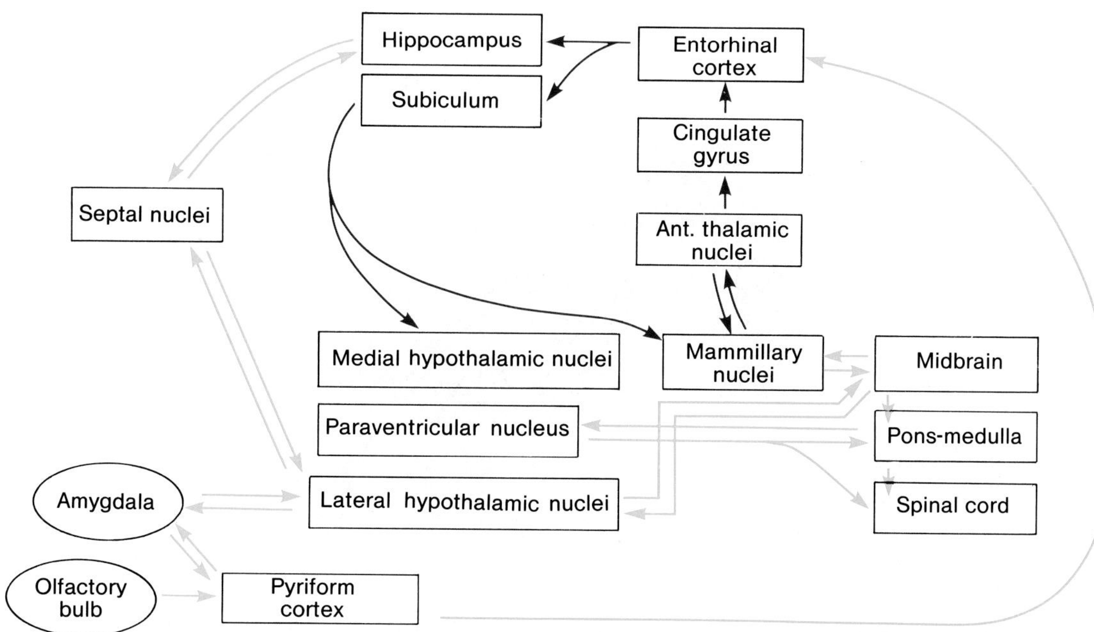

Figure 10-11. A schematic diagram of the principal fiber connections of the hypothalamus. The principal afferents to the hypothalamus from the forebrain arise from two phylogenetically older cortical areas, the *pyriform cortex* and the *hippocampal formation*. Each of these projections is reinforced by a second projection from a related subcortical nuclear mass; this secondary projection arises from the *amygdaloid complex* in the case of the pyriform cortex, and from the *septal nuclei* in the case of the hippocampal formation. Reciprocal connections exist between the hypothalamus and these subcortical nuclei. The cingulate gyrus and the pyriform cortex can exert influences upon the hypothalamus via the entorhinal area and the hippocampal formation. The mammillary nuclei and the hippocampal formation project to the anterior thalamic nuclei which in turn influence activities in the cingulate gyrus. Pathways from the mammillary nuclei to the cortex and from the hippocampal formation and subiculum to the hypothalamus are indicated in *red*. All other connections are shown in *blue* (modified from Raisman, '66). (From Carpenter and Sutin, *Human Neuroanatomy*, 1983; courtesy of Williams & Wilkins.)

to the midbrain, axoplasmic transport technics have revealed direct hypothalamic pathways to the lower brain stem and spinal cord (Kuypers and Maisky, '75; Saper et al., '76). Hypothalamic neurons projecting to spinal levels arise primarily from: (1) the paraventricular nucleus, (2) dorsal parts of the lateral hypothalamic nucleus, and (3) posterior hypothalamic regions dorsal to the mammillary bodies. Fluorescent retrograde double labeling methods indicate that parvicellular divisions of the paraventricular nucleus give rise to predominantly descending projections, while magnocellular divisions of this nucleus project to the neurohypophysis (Swanson and Kuypers, '80). Approximately 15% of the cells in the parvicellular division of the paraventricular nucleus send divergent axon collaterals to the dorsal motor nucleus of the vagus and to spinal cord. Cells in the lateral hypothalamic area also project to both dorsomedial medulla and spinal cord; about 15% of these cells project collaterals to both locations. Fibers from these sources descend in the lateral funiculus of the spinal cord and terminate in relation to cells of the intermediolateral cell column in thoracic, lumbar and sacral levels (Fig. 4-15). These direct descending autonomic fibers influence preganglionic sympathetic and parasympathetic neurons at different levels. Paraventricular nucleus neurons projecting to the lower brain stem and spinal cord arise from different cells (parvicellular) than those (magnocellular) which project to the neurohypophysis (Ono et al., '78; Hosoya and Matsushita, '79; Swanson and Kuypers, '80).

Supraoptic Hypophysial Tract. This term is used to designate the fibers from the supraoptic and paraventricular nuclei

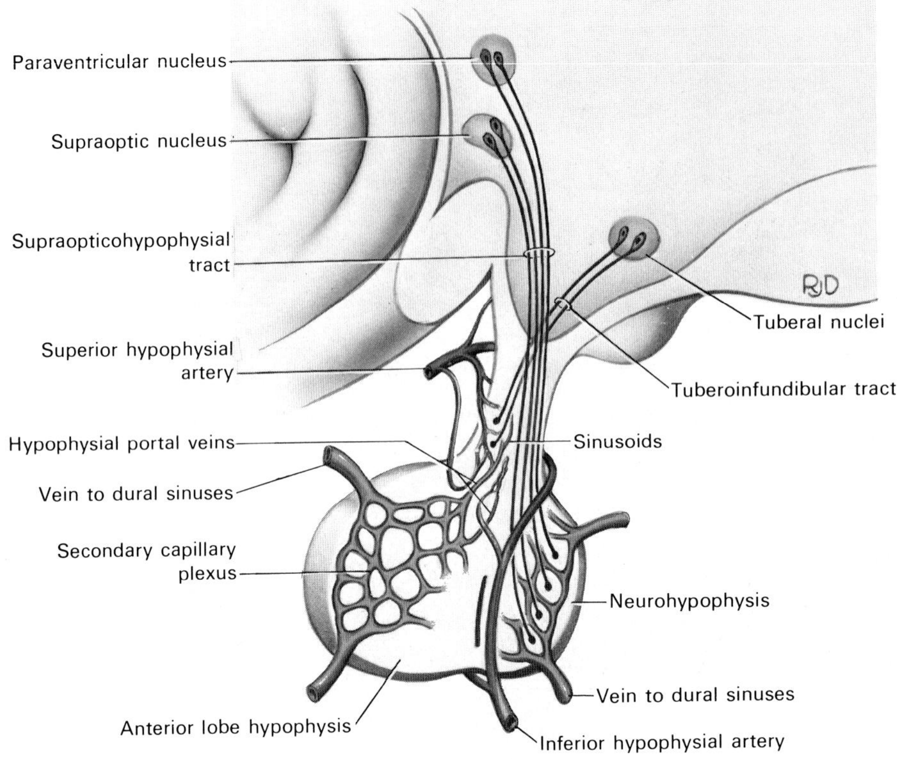

Figure 10-12. Diagram of the hypophysial portal system, the tuberoinfundibular tract and the supraopticohypophysial tract. The hypophysis is supplied by the *superior* and *inferior hypophysial arteries.* Branches of these arteries form sinusoidal capillaries about the infundibulum. Blood from the sinusoids passes to the anterior lobe of the hypophysis via the portal vessels which give rise to a second capillary plexus in the anterior lobe. The tuberoinfundibular tract ends in the sinusoids of the infundibular stem and transports neurosecretory substances, called *releasing hormones*, which enter the sinusoids. The *supraopticohypophysial tract* contains fibers from the *supraoptic* and *paraventricular nuclei* which pass to the neurohypophysis. Neurosecretory products of cells in these hypothalamic nuclei are conveyed directly to the neurohypophysis. Cells in the supraoptic and paraventricular nuclei produce both vasopressin and oxytocin. (From Carpenter and Sutin, *Human Neuroanatomy*, 1983; courtesy of Williams & Wilkins.)

that project to the posterior lobe of the hypophysis (neurohypophysis) (Figs. 10-4 and 10-10). Cells of the supraoptic and paraventricular nuclei are *neurosecretory* and transmit colloid droplets (peptides) which are liberated at their endings in the neurohypophysis. Following transection of the hypophysial stalk, stainable neurosecretory substance accumulates above the cut, while it disappears distally. Electron microscopic studies reveal that the neurosecretory material consists of granular aggregates 5 to 200 nm in diameter. The neurosecretory substance, which consists of a carrier protein and a peptide hormone, is liberated into the blood of the neurohypophysis (Fig. 10-12). While some evidence suggests that the supraoptic nucleus is related mainly to vasopressin (antidiuretic hormone) and the paraventricular nucleus to oxytocin, both hormones are found in each nucleus (Olivecrona, '57; Heller, '66; Pickford, '69; Vandesande and Dierickx, '79). Immunocytochemical data show that these peptides are nearly equally distributed in both nuclei (Gainer, '81). In the magnocellular parts of these nuclei individual cells are associated with only one peptide. Cells associated with oxytocin and vasopressin show regional separations within these nuclei (Fig. 10-4). The newly synthesized hormone is packaged in dense granules within membranous vesicles and is bound to carrier proteins known as neu-

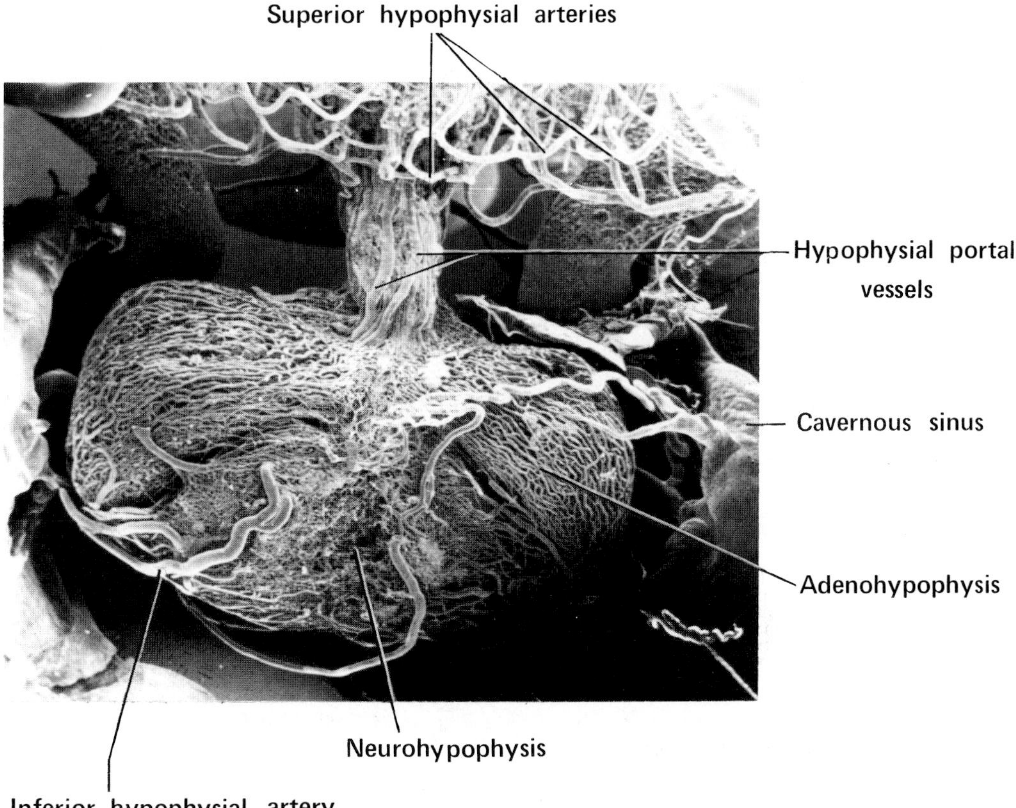

Figure 10-13. Scanning electron micrograph of vascular casts of the pituitary gland, infundibular stem and median eminence in the monkey. The pituitary is viewed from its posterior aspect. The hypophysial arteries and the portal system shown here should be compared with the schematic diagram shown in Figure 10-12 (from Page and Bergland, '77). (From Carpenter and Sutin, *Human Neuroanatomy*, 1983; courtesy of Williams & Wilkins.)

rophysins. Neurosecretory cells retain their capacity to conduct electrical impulses. Stimulation of the cell bodies in the hypothalamus gives rise to action potentials conducted in axons which trigger the release of the hormones.

Recent studies utilizing radioimmunoassays indicate that vasopressin and its binding protein, neurophysin, also are released into the hypophysial portal system (Zimmerman et al., '73; Zimmerman, '81). Thus vasopressin and neurophysin also reach the anterior lobe of the pituitary where they may have a potentiating influence upon adrenocorticotrophic hormone releasing factor.

Tuberohypophysial Tract. The tuberohypophysial or tuberoinfundibular tract arises from the tuberal region, mainly from the arcuate nucleus (Fig. 10-1), and can be traced only to the median eminence and the infundibular stem (Figs. 10-10 and 10-12) (Szentágothai et al., '68; Haymaker, '69). Although these fibers accompany those of the supraoptic hypophysial tract in part of their course, they end upon capillary loops near the sinusoids of the hypophysial portal system (Figs. 10-12 and 10-13). These are fine fibers, but secretory granules can be demonstrated in their axons (provided tissues are not fixed in formalin). Fibers of the tuberoinfundibular tract convey "releasing" hormones which are transported via the hypophysial portal vessels to the anterior lobe of the hypophysis where they modulate the synthesis and release of adenohypophysial hormones. Functionally, the tuberoinfundibular tract and the hypophysial portal system establish the neurohumoral link between the hypothalamus and the anterior pituitary. Under stressful conditions neurosecretory granules disappear from nerve fibers and adrenocorticotrophic hormone (ACTH) releasing factor is present in the plasma obtained from portal vessels (Porter and Jones, '56). The infundibulum also contains high concentrations of acetylcholine (Haymaker, '69), and the cell bodies and fibers of the tuberoinfundibular system contain dopamine (Fuxe and Hökfelt, '70). Increases in dopamine in the arcuate nucleus occur in pregnancy, pseudopregnancy and during lactation.

Hypothalamic efferent projections fall into five main categories: (1) those that emerge via the medial forebrain bundle, (2) those concerned with neurosecretion which convey hormones to the neurohypophysis, (3) those concerned with releasing hormones liberated by the tuberoinfundibular tract into the hypophysial portal system, (4) those that arise from the mammillary nuclei which project to the anterior nuclear group of the thalamus and to nuclei in the midbrain tegmentum, and (5) those that project to the lower brain stem and spinal cord.

HYPOPHYSIAL PORTAL SYSTEM

The hypophysis is supplied by two sets of arteries, both of which arise from the internal carotid artery (Figs. 10-12 and 10-13). The superior hypophysial artery forms an arterial ring around the upper part of the hypophysial stalk; the inferior hypophysial artery forms a ring about the posterior lobe and gives branches to the lower infundibulum. Both of these arteries enter the hypophysial stalk and break up into a number of sinusoids. Blood from these sinusoids collects into vessels which pass into the anterior lobe of the hypophysis. The anterior lobe of the pituitary receives almost all of its blood supply via these vessels. These vessels are referred to as the hypophysial portal vessels. There is considerable anatomical evidence that hypothalamic influences upon the anterior lobe of the hypophysis are conveyed by humoral substances transported along the tuberoinfundibular tract to the sinusoids and reach the anterior lobe via the portal system. Blood flow from the hypophysial stalk and median eminence to the anterior lobe of the hypophysis has been demonstrated in living animals (Green and Harris, '49).

Ependymal cells lining the floor of the third ventricle in the region of the median eminence (i.e., tanycytes) appear to form a functional link between the CSF and the perivascular spaces of the hypophysial portal system. Processes of these cells extend to the basement membrane of the perivascular spaces of both capillary loops and portal vessels. Suggestions as to the functional role of tanycytes in the median eminence have included secretion into the CSF, absorption of substances from portal blood and a receptor action for feedback influences.

The hypothalamus appears intimately concerned with mechanisms that influence the hormonal activity of the anterior lobe and cause the secretion of gonadotrophic, adrenocorticotrophic (ACTH) and thyrotrophic (TSH) hormones (Fig. 10-14). Electrical stimulation of the hypothalamus can increase the discharges of gonadotrophic hormone and ACTH. Stimulation of the tuberal region in the rabbit has produced ovulation. Direct stimulation of the anterior lobe does not elicit these responses, presumably because the humoral part of this pathway is not electrically excitable. The neurosecretory substances acting upon cells of the anterior lobe are called *releasing hormones* and are named according to the hormone they release.

The *hypophysiotrophic agents*, called releasing hormones, have most of the attributes of hormones and most appear to be neuropeptides (Saffran, '74). The neuropeptide nature of releasing hormones has made their synthesis possible. These studies indicate that the luteinizing-hormone releasing hormone (LHRH) stimulates the release of follicle-stimulating hormone (FSH) and luteinizing hormone (LH), which suggest that a distinct hypothalamic hormone for FSH may not exist. Both a growth hormone-releasing hormone (GHRH) and a growth inhibiting hormone-releasing factor, named *somatostatin*, have been identified (Fig. 10-14). While many studies have suggested that the ventromedial nucleus of the hypothalamus was the

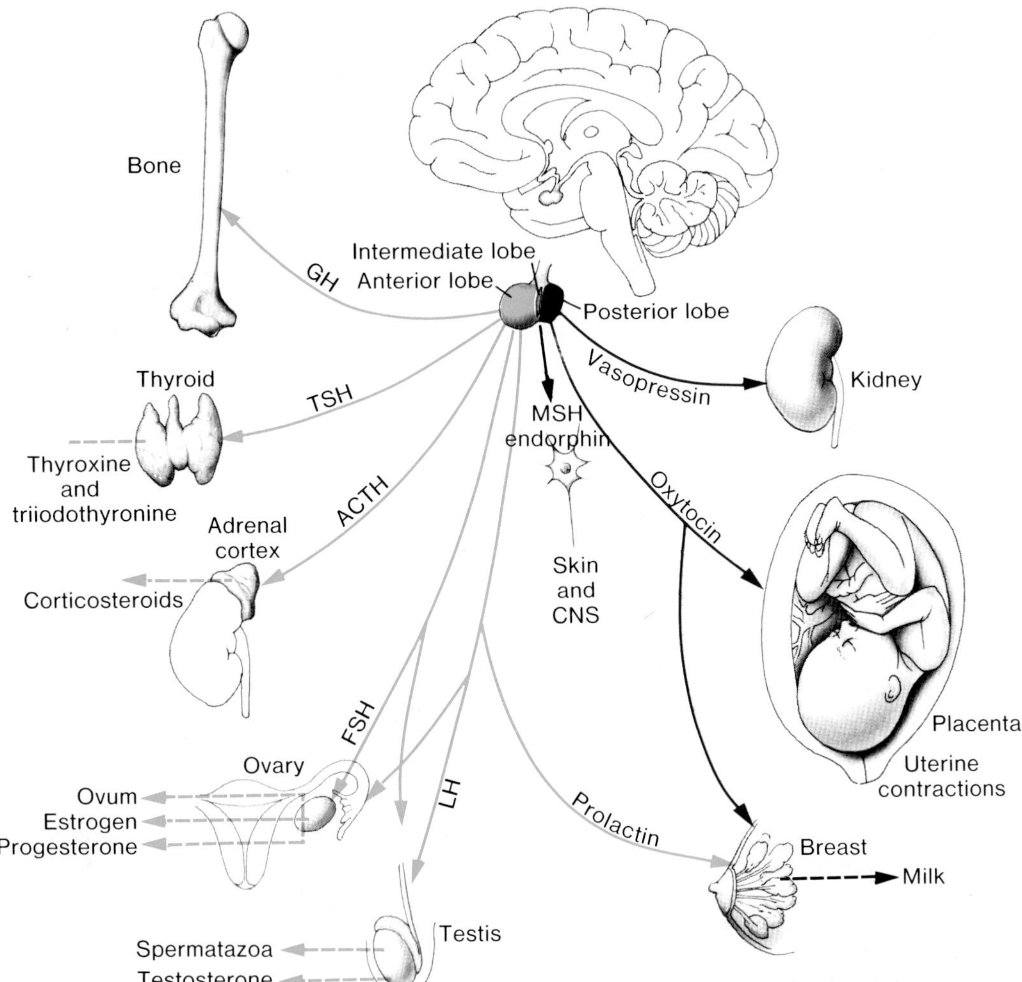

Figure 10-14. Schematic diagram of the target organs upon which pituitary hormones act. Pituitary hormones are secreted by, or controlled by, hypothalamic neurons. Hormones secreted by cells in the anterior (*blue*) and intermediate (*black*) lobes of the pituitary are regulated by hypothalamic hypophysiotrophic peptides conveyed by the hypophysial portal system. Hormones of the anterior lobe include: (1) growth hormone (*GH*), (2) thyrotropin (*TSH*), (3) corticotrophin (*ACTH*), (4) follicle stimulating hormone (*FSH*), (5) luteinizing hormone (*LH*), and (6) prolactin. The neurohypophysis (posterior lobe, *red*) contains vasopressin and oxytocin secreted by cells of the supraoptic and paraventricular hypothalamic nuclei. These hormones act upon the kidney tubules (vasopressin), the smooth muscle of the uterus and glandular tissue of the breast (oxytocin). Melanocyte stimulating hormone (*MSH*) is derived from cells of the intermediate lobe (*black*) of the pituitary (modified from Schally et al., '77). (From Carpenter and Sutin, *Human Neuroanatomy*, 1983; courtesy of Williams & Wilkins.)

center for regulation of growth hormone (GH), the concentration of somatostatin has been found to be much higher in the arcuate nucleus and the median eminence (Palkovits, et al., '76). The release of ACTH from the pituitary is stimulated by vasopressin (Saffran, '59, '74) but evidence suggests that vasopressin is not the corticotropin-releasing hormone.

Many of the hormone releasing hormones have been found in measurable amounts by radioimmunoassay in the so-called circumventricular organs (i.e., the subfornical organ, the subcommissural organ and the area postrema (Fig. 1-16). The so-called circumventricular organs which are relatively rich in biogenic amines have been demonstrated to contain LH, TSH and somatostatin (Palkovits et al., '76).

CHEMICALLY DEFINED NEURONS AND NEUROTRANSMITTERS

Many peptides and neurotransmitters can be localized with immunohistochemical and histochemical technics which permit determination of the location of cell bodies, the course of axonal projections and the sites of synaptic terminations. Noradrenergic neurons are not found in the hypothalamus, but terminals arising from cells in the pons and medulla are widely distributed with the most dense plexus in the periventricular zone (Hökfelt et al., '76; Palkovits, '81). Noradrenergic axons originating from the locus ceruleus (Fig. 6-28) form a dorsal bundle projecting to dorsal hypothalamic nuclei. A ventral noradrenergic bundle arises from medullary neurons with some contribution from pontine catecholaminergic (CA) neurons (Fig. 5-13). At rostral midbrain levels dorsal and ventral ascending bundles largely fuse. Most CA axons continue rostrally in the medial forebrain bundle, while others ascend in the periventricular zone. A particularly prominent plexus of CA terminals is found in the parvicellular portions of the paraventricular and supraoptic nuclei (McNeill and Sladek, '80).

Hypothalamic influence on the release of prolactin from the anterior pituitary is inhibited by dopamine (Thorner and Login, '81). Dopamine is synthesized by tuberoinfundibular dopaminergic neurons (DA) with cell bodies in the arcuate and periventricular nuclei of the mediobasal hypothalamus and terminals located near the hypophysial portal system at the median eminence (Hökfelt, '67; Hökfelt et al., '76). Tyrosine is a precursor of both dopamine and norepinephrine; tyrosine hydroxylase converts tyrosine to dopa which is decarboxylased to form dopamine (Fig. 10-15). Dopamine is both a neurotransmitter and the precursor of norepinephrine, formed by the β-hydroxylation of dopamine. Dopaminergic neurons in the hypothalamus secrete dopamine into the hypophysial capillaries which transmit it to cells in the anterior pituitary. Dopamine binds to dopamine receptors and activates mechanisms which inhibit prolactin release (Fig. 10-14). Prolactin increases as the effective dopamine concentration at the receptor site is reduced. The tuberoinfundibular dopaminergic system controlling prolactin release is unique in that it is controlled by circulating prolactin levels rather than feedback through dopamine autoreceptors. Clinical evidence indicates that large prolactin secreting pituitary tumors can be reduced by administration of dopamine agonists, particularly bromocriptine (Thorner and Login, '81).

Brain tryptophan, the precursor of serotonin, is derived from plasma tryptophan and both fluctuate in relation to plasma tryptophan (Frohman, '80). Tryptophan is hydroxylated to 5-hydroxytryptophan in a manner analogous to tryosine hydroxylation and then rapidly decarboxylated to serotonin (5-hydroxytryptamine, 5-HT). As a neurotransmitter serotonin operates in a manner similar to that described for norepinephrine and dopamine. The correlation of receptor distribution with the distribution of endogenous serotonin and tryptophan is not strong. The arcuate nucleus has the highest serotonin content in the brain, but only a moderate receptor density (Biegon et al., '82). Like dopamine, serotonin also serves as a precursor, being converted to melatonin in the pineal gland. Serotonin is considered to be involved in neuroendocrine function and steroid hormones can modulate the actions of serotonin-containing neurons, but its precise role is poorly defined. Serotonin has been implicated in disorders of mood and affect.

The naturally occurring opioid peptide β-endorphin is found in rat anterior and intermediate lobes of the pituitary. Radioimmunoassays and immunocytochemical technics indicate that cells in the arcuate nucleus of the hypothalamus contain a common 31,000 Dalton precursor of ACTH, β-lipotrophin and β-endorphin, which is cleaved in the anterior and intermediate lobes (Mains and Eipper, '76; Watson and Akil, '81). β-Endorphin has 5 to 10 times

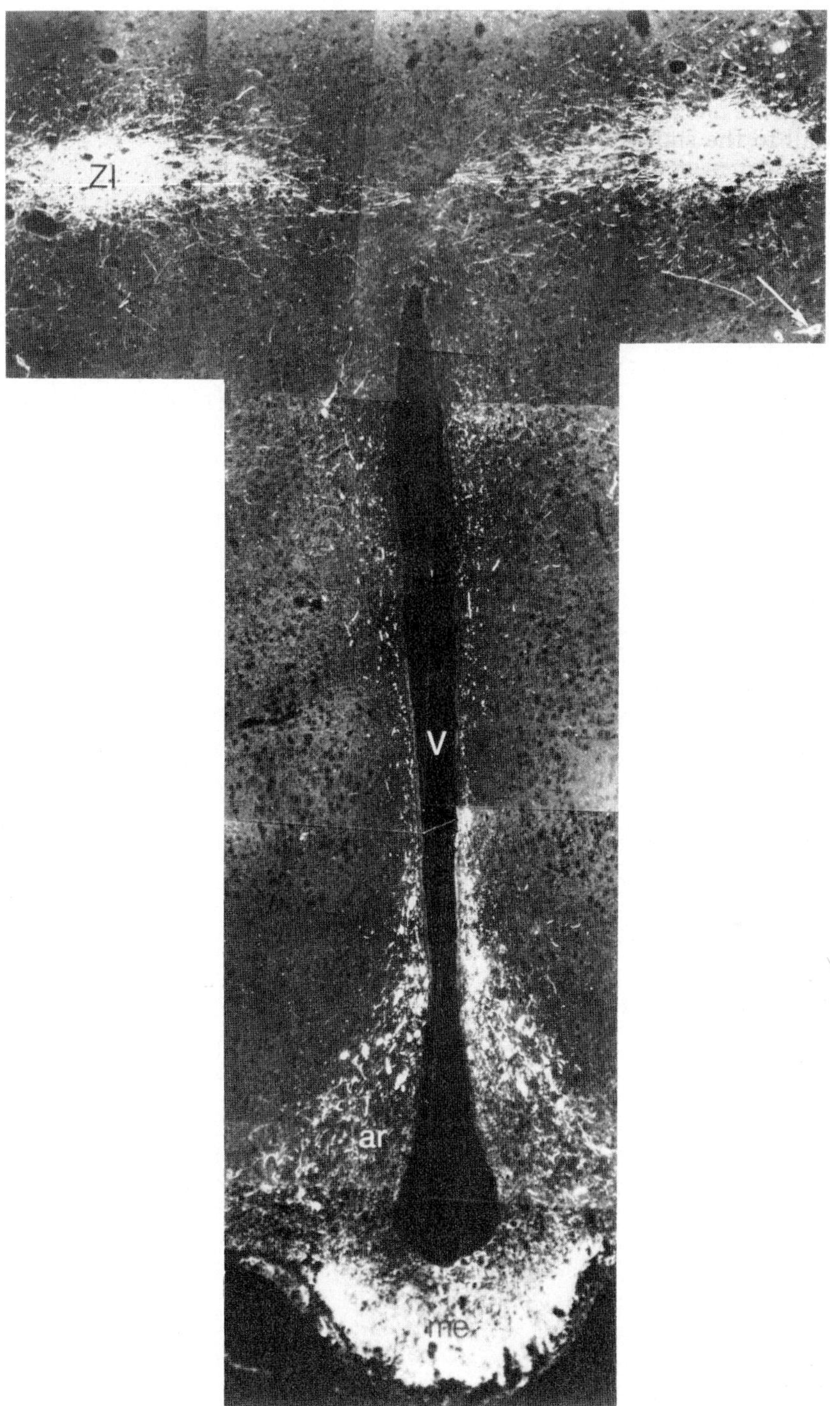

Figure 10-15. Frontal section through the hypothalamus and part of the subthalamic region showing the immunohistochemical localization of tyrosine hydroxylase (TH). Section is taken obliquely so that ventral region is more rostral. Fluorescent cell bodies are seen in the arcuate nucleus (*ar*) and in the zona incerta (*ZI*). The median eminence (*me*) contains a dense plexus of TH-positive fibers in its external part. *V* indicates third ventricle. Tyrosine hydroxylase is the enzyme which converts tyrosine to dopa which is decarboxylated to form dopamine (from Hökfelt et al., '76). (From Carpenter and Sutin, *Human Neuroanatomy*, 1983; courtesy of Williams & Wilkins.)

the analgesic potency of morphine, but its effects are seen only after intracerebral administration (Guillemin, '80). β-Endorphin labeled axons are distributed along the ventricular wall to the supraoptic, periventricular, paraventricular, and suprachiasmatic nuclei and some may reach the thalamus (Bloom et al., '78). There are suggestions that the β-endorphin system may be involved in maintaining behavioral homeostasis and that subtle disturbances in the regulation of the system might lead to mental illness. There is no evidence that the enkephalins are derived from β-lipotrophin or β-endorphin and the cells and fibers labeled for β-endorphin are distinct from those labeled by antisera specific for enkephalins.

FUNCTIONAL CONSIDERATIONS

Experimental evidence and clinical observations have demonstrated that the hypothalamus and immediately adjoining regions are related to all kinds of visceral activities. The most diverse disturbances of autonomic functions, involving water balance, internal secretion, sugar and fat metabolism, and temperature regulation, all can be produced by stimulation or destruction of hypothalamic areas. Even the mechanism for normal sleep may be altered profoundly by such lesions. It is established that the hypothalamus is the chief subcortical center for the regulation of both sympathetic and parasympathetic activities. These dual activities are integrated into coordinated responses which maintain adequate internal conditions in the body. It is highly improbable that each of the autonomic activities has its own discrete center in view of the small size of the hypothalamus and the complex nature of these activities. However, a specific function has been established for the supraoptic and paraventricular nuclei. There is also a fairly definite topographical organization with regard to the two main divisions of the autonomic system. Control of parasympathetic activities is related to the anterior and medial hypothalamic regions (supraoptic and preoptic areas) and the ventricular portion of the tuber cinereum. Stimulation of this region results in increased vagal and sacral autonomic responses, characterized by reduced heart rate, peripheral vasodilation, and increased tonus and motility of the alimentary and vesical walls.

The lateral and posterior hypothalamic regions are concerned with the control of sympathetic responses. Stimulation of this region, especially the posterior portion from which many descending efferents arise, activates the thoracolumbar outflow. This results in increased metabolic and somatic activities characteristic of emotional stress, combat or flight. These responses are expressed by dilatation of the pupil, piloerection, acceleration of the heart rate, elevation of blood pressure, increase in the rate and amplitude of respiration, somatic struggling movements, and inhibition of the gut and bladder. All these physiological correlates of emotional excitement can be elicited when the hypothalamus is released from cortical control. Removal of the cortex, or interruption of the cortical connections with the hypothalamus, induces many of the above visceral symptoms collectively designated as "sham rage" (Fulton and Ingraham, '29; Bard, '39). On the other hand, destruction of the posterior hypothalamus produces emotional lethargy, abnormal sleepiness, and a fall in temperature due to a general reduction of visceral and somatic activities.

The coordination of sympathetic and parasympathetic responses is strikingly shown in the regulation of body temperature. This complex function, involving widespread physical and chemical processes, is mediated by two hypothalamic mechanisms, one concerned with the dissipation of heat and the other with its production and conservation. There is considerable experimental evidence that the anterior hypothalamus is sensitive to increases in blood temperature, and sets in motion the mechanisms for dissipating excess heat. In man this consists mainly of profuse sweating and vasodilatation of the cutaneous blood vessels. These actions permit the rapid elimination of heat by convection and radiation from the surface of the engorged blood vessels, and by the evaporation of sweat. In animals with fur this is supplemented to a considerable degree by rapid, shallow respiratory movements (panting); the heat loss is effected mainly by the rapid warming of successive streams of inspired air. Lesions involving the anterior part of the hypothalamus abolish the neural control of mechanisms concerned with the dissipation of heat and result in hyperthermia. Thus, hyperthermia (hyperpyrexia) may result from tumors in, or near, the anterior hypothalamus.

The posterior hypothalamus, on the other hand, is sensitive to conditions of decreasing body temperature and controls mechanisms for the conservation and increased production of heat. The cutaneous blood vessels are constricted and sweat secretion ceases, so that heat loss is reduced. Simultaneously there is augmentation of visceral activities, and the somatic muscles exhibit shivering. All these activities tremendously increase the processes of oxidation, with a consequent production and conservation of heat. Bilateral lesions in posterior regions of the hypothalamus usually produce a condition in which body temperature varies with the environment (poikilothermia), since such lesions effectively destroy all descending pathways concerned with both the conservation and dissipation of heat.

These two intrinsically antagonistic mechanisms do not function independently but are continually interrelated and balanced against each other to meet the changing needs of the body; the coordinated responses always are directed to the maintenance of a constant optimum temperature.

The supraoptic nuclei are specifically concerned with the maintenance of body water balance (Figs. 10-2, 10-3, 10-4, 10-10, and 10-12). Destruction of these nuclei, or their hypophysial connections, invariably is followed by the condition known as *diabetes insipidus*, in which there is increased secretion of urine (polyuria) without an increase in the sugar content. The antidiuretic hormone, vasopressin, is secreted directly by the cells of the supraoptic nuclei. The peptide, vasopressin, is conjugated to a carrier protein, neurophysin, and transported by the unmyelinated axons of the supraopticohypophysial tract (Fig. 10-12). The antidiuretic hormone is stored in the posterior lobe of the pituitary. The production of antidiuretic hormone varies in accordance with changes in the osmotic pressure of the blood. An increase in the osmotic pressure of the blood which supplies the supraoptic nuclei increases the activity of these neurons and the release of antidiuretic hormone. In states of experimental dehydration there is a depletion of the hormone in the posterior lobe and increased secretory activity in the supraoptic nuclei. After reestablishment of water balance, there is a re-accumulation of the hormone in the posterior lobe (Hild, '56). The antidiuretic hormone is considered to act specifically on the kidneys, although the exact mechanism by which vasopressin brings about the reabsorption of renal water is not clear (Fig. 10-14). Reabsorption of sodium chloride and bicarbonate ions is followed by passive reabsorption of water. This hormone also appears to alter the osmotic permeability of water in the distal and collecting tubules of the kidney.

There is evidence that a region of the hypothalamus is responsible for the regulation of water intake. Electrical stimulation of anterior regions of the hypothalamus in goats creates fantastic "thirst" and results in consumption of large volumes of water. This is probably part of a more extensive system which regulates the consumption of both food and water. An increase in the osmotic pressure of body fluids may be an effective stimulus for water intake. According to Verney ('47), osmoreceptors probably are situated close to the cells of the supraoptic nucleus which have an abundant blood supply. Localized lesions in the lateral hypothalamus at the level of the ventromedial nucleus in rats cause a reduction in water intake without affecting food intake (Stevenson, '69), but larger lesions in the lateral hypothalamus may cause adipsia as well as aphagia. According to Emmers ('73), the lateral hypothalamic area can excite cells of the supraoptic nucleus which in turn inhibit the lateral hypothalamic area in a negative feedback circuit.

The paraventricular and supraoptic nuclei also produce a monopeptide, oxytocin, which chemically is related closely to the antidiuretic hormone, but causes contractions of uterine muscle and myoepithelial cells surrounding the alveoli of the mammary gland (Fig. 10-14).

The important role of the hypothalamus in maintaining and regulating the activity of the anterior lobe of the hypophysis has been described in relation to the hypophysial portal system. It should be emphasized that this is a humoral control mechanism in which releasing hormones are transmitted via the portal system (Harris and George, '69). There are no hypothalamic efferent fibers that reach the anterior lobe of the pituitary. The anterior pituitary stands in marked contrast to other endocrine organs, such as the ovary, testis, thyroid and adrenal cortex, which may be transplanted to distant sites and still retain their endocrine functions. The anterior lobe of the pituitary cannot be transplanted to distant locations and retain its function, because it is dependent upon its close relationships with the hypothalamus. The essential hypothalamic connections are the tuberoinfundibular tract and the hypophysial portal system (Figs. 10-12 and 10-13).

The hypothalamus is considered the site of elaboration of releasing hormones related to gonadotrophic, adrenocorticotrophic (ACTH), thyrotrophic (TSH) and growth hormones (Harris and George '69; Sawyer, '69). Attempts to determine the loci within the hypothalamus concerned with particular releasing factors suggest that the neural area related to TSH appears to lie on either side of the midline between the paraventricular nucleus and the median eminence (Greer and Erwin, '56). Electrical stimulation of the anterior median eminence also results in increased thyroid activity (Harris and Woods, '58). Similarly, electrical stimulation of the hypothalamus in the rabbit can cause the discharge of gonadotrophic hormone (Markee et al., '46; Harris, '48) and of ACTH (de Groot and Harris, '50). While bilateral lesions in almost any region near the base of the hypothalamus will reduce ACTH release, the median eminence-tuberal region was found to have the most important controlling influence (Brodish, '64).

The brain plays an important role in the initiation and coordination of reproductive functions and these functions are different in the two sexes. The tuberal region of the hypothalamus appears essential for the maintenance of basal levels of gonadotrophic hormone, but the integrity of the preoptic area is necessary for the cyclic surge of gonadotropin which precedes ovulation (Sawyer, '59; Everett, '64; Raisman and Field, '73). Electrical stimulation of the preoptic area, or the corticomedial nuclear group of the amygdaloid complex, produces ovulation in rabbits and cats. The effects of preoptic stimulation are abolished by lesions separating this area from the tuberal region of the hypothalamus; the effects of amygdaloid stimulation are blocked by section of the stria terminalis. These observations suggest a functional linkage between the amygdala and the medial preoptic area via the stria terminalis, and fiber systems from the medial preoptic area to the tuberal region of the hypothalamus. However, the amygdaloid input to the preoptic area is not essential for ovulation, for bilateral destruction of the stria terminalis does not prevent ovulation (Brown-Grant and Raisman, '72).

Tumors and other pathological processes involving the hypothalamus frequently modify sexual development. Such lesions may be associated with precocious puberty or hypogonadism associated with underdevelopment of secondary sex characteristics. Although hypergonadism has been attributed to tumors of the pineal, most tumors of the brain associated with precocious puberty actually involve, or impinge upon, the hypothalamus. These lesions frequently destroy the posterior hypothalamus and leave the anterior hypothalamus intact; the intact hypothalamic regions functioning in the absence of inhibitory influences from posterior regions leads to increased pituitary function (Weinberger and Grant, '41).

The preoptic region plays an important role in regulating the release of gonadotrophic hormones from the anterior lobe of the hypophysis. In the female, pituitary gonadotropins are released in a cyclic manner, the duration of the cycle corresponding to the menstrual period. In the male, the gonadotropins are released topically without regularly occurring fluctuations. Therefore it is not surprising that there are differences in the functional organization of the preoptic region in the male and female. A morphological expression of this difference has been observed in the preoptic region of the rat, where a nucleus of densely stained cells is larger in the male (Gorski et al., '80). This nucleus has been termed the "sexually dimorphic nucleus of the preoptic area." The full ontogenetic development of this nucleus, as well as the male pattern of tonic gonadotrophic release, depends upon the presence in the circulation of testosterone during the first week of life. If the testes are removed from the newborn animal, the genetic male will fail to develop the sexually dimorphic nucleus of the preoptic region and will also show a female pattern of gonadotropin release. Conversely, a newborn female given exogenous testosterone will, as an adult, show the male pattern of gonadotropin release.

Tumors of the adenohypophysis may produce symptoms due to their increasing size or because they result in alterations of pituitary functions. Expanding tumors cause a ballooning of the sella turcica, may compress fibers in the optic chiasm or optic tract and frequently produce headaches due to traction on the meninges. The most typical visual field defect is a bitemporal hemianopsia due to involvement of the decussating fibers in the optic chiasm (Fig. 9-25), but visual field defects take many forms dependent upon the growth pattern of the tumor. Endocrinopathy may take the form of hypersecretion or hyposecretion depending upon the type of tumor. The pituitary syndrome may be associated with excess prolactin (amenorrhea-galactorrhea), growth hormones (acromegaly), and adrenocorticotrophic hormone (Cushing's syndrome). Patients with prolactin secreting tumors have been successfully treated with dopamine agonists, particularly bromocriptine (Thorner and Login, '81). Dopamine synthesized in the arcuate and periventricular nuclei of the hypothalamus and transported via the portal system inhibits prolactin release. Modern neuroradiographic evaluations and serum hormone radioimmunoassays make possible early diagnosis and treatment.

It has been known for a long time that certain lesions near the base of the brain are associated with obesity. Localized bilateral lesions in the hypothalamus involving primarily, or exclusively, the ventromedial nucleus in the tuberal region produce *hyperphagia*. Such animals eat voraciously, consuming two or three times the usual amount of food. Obesity appears to be the direct result of increased food intake. Lesions destroying portions of the lateral hypothalamic nucleus bilaterally impair, or abolish, the desire to feed in hyperphagic and normal animals. These data suggest that the ventromedial nucleus of the hypothalamus is concerned with *satiety*, while the lateral hypothalamic nucleus may be regarded as a *feeding center*. Most animals with hyperphagia due to hypothalamic lesions exhibit savage behavior and rage reactions.

The hypothalamus is regarded as one of the principal centers concerned with emotional expression. Since it is acknowledged that the physiological expression of emotion is dependent, in part, upon both sympathetic and parasympathetic components of the autonomic nervous system, it is evident that the hypothalamus, intimately relating both of these, probably is involved directly or indirectly in most emotional reactions. As mentioned above, lesions in the ventromedial nucleus of the hypothalamus produce savage behavior and extreme rage reactions. Stimulation of the hypothalamus in unanesthetized cats with implanted electrodes (Masserman, '43; Hess, '54; Glusman, '74) provokes responses resembling rage and fear which can be increased by graded stimuli of different intensities. These reactions, referred to by some as "pseudo-affective," are "stimulus-bound" in that they are present only during the period of stimulation. Different types of responses are elicited from different parts of the hypothalamus; flight responses are most readily evoked from lateral regions of the anterior hypothalamus, while aggressive responses characterized by hissing, snarling, baring of teeth, and biting are seen most commonly with stimulation of the region of the ventromedial nucleus. Because the emotional reactions provoked by electrical stimulation of the hypothalamus are directed, it seems likely that the cerebral cortex and thalamus play important roles in these responses. In these reactions the hypothalamus cannot be regarded as a simple efferent mechanism influencing only lower levels of the neuraxis.

Observations that selective stimulation and lesions of the ventromedial nucleus of the hypothalamus both produce aggressive behavior raise questions concerning the mechanism. Savage behavior after bilateral lesions of the ventromedial nucleus cannot be assumed to result from release of inhibitory influences (Glusman, '74). Because animals with such lesions never show spontaneous outburst of aggressive behavior and this hyperirritable state develops slowly, it has been postulated that destruction of these nuclei leads to a state of supersensitivity, as described by Cannon and Rosenblueth ('49). Further secondary lesions involving the central gray and the reticular formation may have a "taming" effect upon this savage behavior. Hypothalamic induced rage reactions may be blocked by midbrain lesions, indicating that structures at this level are essential for the expression of savage and aggressive behavior (Chi and Flynn, '71).

It is generally accepted that morphophysiological substrates of abnormal and aggressive behavior involve, in some differential and selective fashion, predominantly brain structures rostral to the rhombencephalon. This part of the central nervous system contains the neural structures concerned with goal-directed behavior, and the motivational and emotional concomitants that make such behavior possible. Impulses generated in sensory systems, the cerebral cortex and still undetermined neural structures may trigger mechanisms that excite visceral and somatic systems whose activities in concert provide the physiological expression of aggressive behavior.

CHAPTER 11

Corpus Striatum and Related Nuclei

In close relationship to parts of the diencephalon, but separated from it by the internal capsule, are nuclear masses that constitute the corpus striatum (Figs. 11-1 and 11-2). The corpus striatum represents the largest component of the basal ganglia. The basal ganglia are large subcortical nuclei classically considered to be derived from the telencephalon. The major divisions of the basal ganglia are: (1) the corpus striatum, considered to be concerned primarily with somatic motor functions, and (2) the amygdaloid nuclear complex, functionally related to the hypothalamus and regarded as an integral part of the limbic system. The corpus striatum consists of the putamen, the caudate nucleus, and the globus pallidus. Although the corpus striatum (neostriatum and paleostriatum) and the amygdala (archistriatum) have been considered to have separate and distinctive functions, recent evidence indicates a significant projection from the amygdala to parts of the putamen and caudate nucleus (i.e., the neostriatum) (Kelley et al., '82). Thus, some functions of the basal ganglia may not be easily segregated and the neostriatum may consist of limbic and nonlimbic subdivisions. Because the terms designating components of the basal ganglia are used in various ways, it is appropriate to clarify them at the outset.

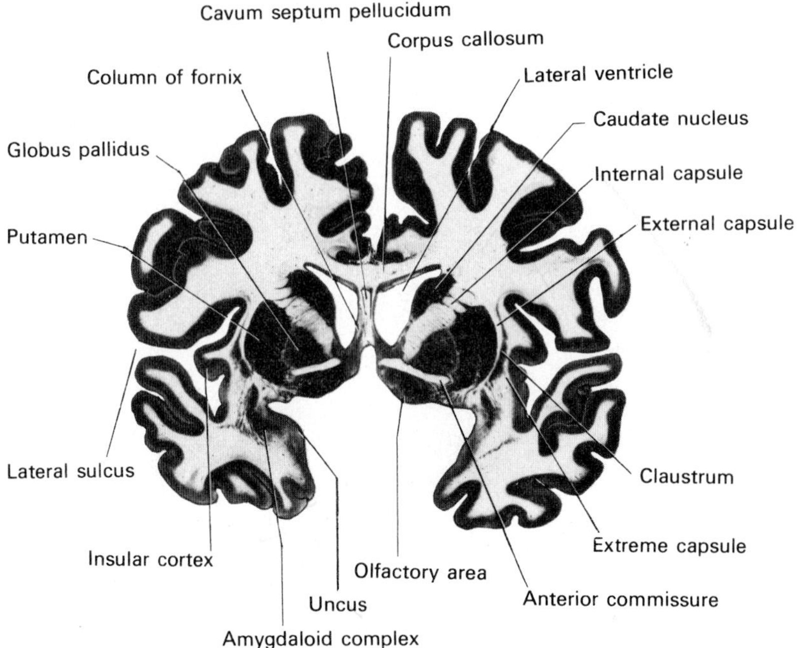

Figure 11-1. Photograph of a frontal section of the brain passing through the columns of the fornix and the anterior commissure. At this level the putamen and the lateral pallidal segment lie beneath the insular cortex. (From Carpenter and Sutin, *Human Neuroanatomy*, 1983; courtesy of Williams & Wilkins.)

The *amygdaloid nuclear complex*, phylogenetically the oldest part of the basal ganglia, is known as the *archistriatum*. This structure is located internal to the uncus in the temporal lobe (Figs. 2-8 and 11-2). Because the amygdaloid nuclear complex has primarily olfactory inputs and is concerned with visceral functions, it is considered in detail in Chapter 12.

CORPUS STRIATUM

The *corpus striatum* consists of two distinctive parts, the *neostriatum* (caudate nucleus and putamen) and the *paleostriatum* (globus pallidus). The two components of the corpus striatum lie adjacent to each other but have different embryological origins. The caudate nucleus and putamen are derived from different parts of striatal ridge in the telencephalic vesicle, but separate migratory paths in their development give each a distinctive configuration in the adult (Hamilton and Mossman, '72). Continuity between the caudate nucleus and the putamen is preserved rostrally and ventrally (Fig. 11-3). The globus pallidus, consisting of two segments, lies medial to the putamen and lateral to the internal capsule (Fig. 11-4). Medullary laminae separate the two segments of the globus pallidus from each other and the lateral segment from the putamen (Fig. 11-13). Both segments of the globus pallidus and the subthalamic nucleus are diencephalic derivatives arising from a dorsolateral hypothalamic cell column (Kuhlenbeck, '48; Kuhlenbeck and Haymaker, '49; Richter, '65). The caudate nucleus and putamen together form the newest and largest component of the basal ganglia (Figs. 11-1, 11-2, 11-3, 11-4, and 11-5); these components of the neostriatum are commonly called the striatum. The putamen plus the globus pallidus are together referred to as the lentiform nucleus.

The two components of the corpus striatum, the neostriatum (caudate nucleus and putamen) and the paleostriatum (globus pallidus), appear to serve distinct and separate functions. The neostriatum, considered the receptive component, receives the massive inputs which originate from: (1) broad regions of the telencephalon, (2) the phylogenetic older thalamic nuclei, (3) the basal lateral amygdala, and (4) more than

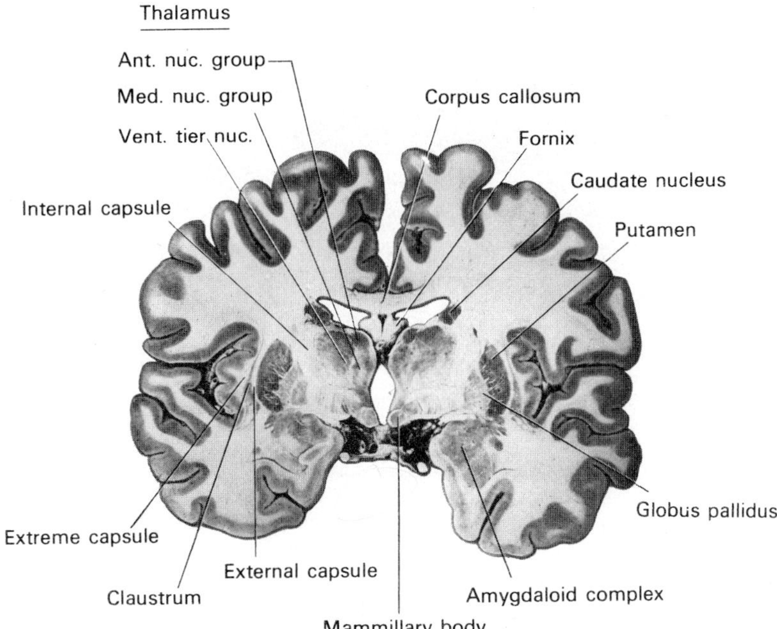

Figure 11-2. Photograph of a frontal section of the brain at the level of the mammillary bodies. In this section the main nuclear groups of the thalamus are identified and portions of all components of the basal ganglia are present. The amygdaloid nuclear complex lies in the temporal lobe internal to the uncus and ventral to the lentiform nucleus. (From Carpenter and Sutin, *Human Neuroanatomy*, 1983; courtesy of Williams & Wilkins.)

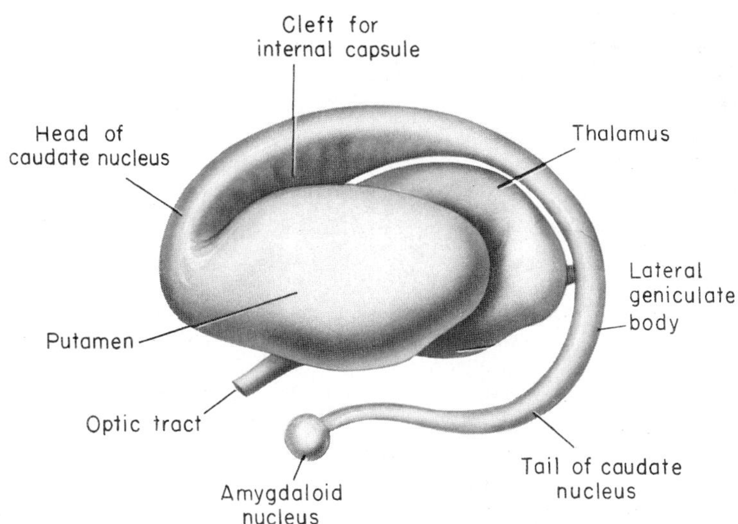

Figure 11-3. Semischematic drawing of the isolated striatum, thalamus, and amygdaloid nucleus showing: (1) the continuity of the putamen and head of the caudate nucleus rostrally, and (2) the relationships between the tail of the caudate nucleus and the amygdaloid nucleus. The cleft occupied by fibers of the internal capsule is indicated. The anterior limb of the internal capsule is situated between the caudate nucleus and the putamen (Figs. 9-21, 11-4, and 11-5), while the posterior limb of the internal capsule lies between the lentiform nucleus and the thalamus. (From Carpenter and Sutin, *Human Neuroanatomy*, 1983; courtesy of Williams & Wilkins.)

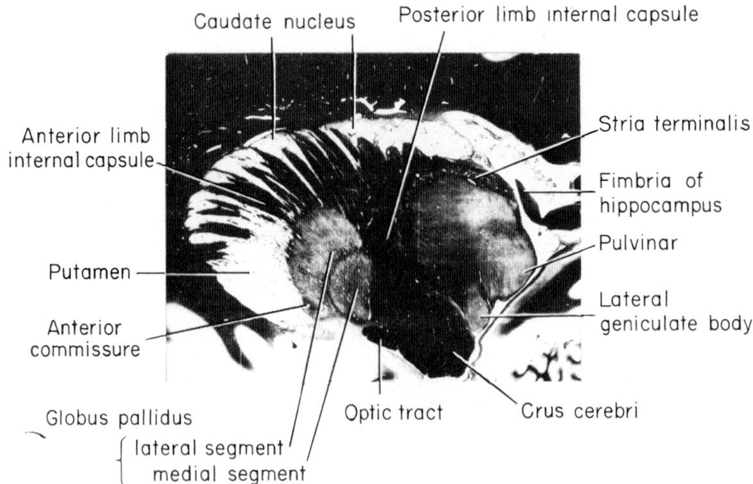

Figure 11-4. Sagittal section through the basal ganglia, internal capsule, and thalamus. Note the relationships of the caudate nucleus to the fibers of the anterior limb of the internal capsule. (Weigert's myelin stain; photograph.) (From Carpenter and Sutin, *Human Neuroanatomy*, 1983; courtesy of Williams & Wilkins.)

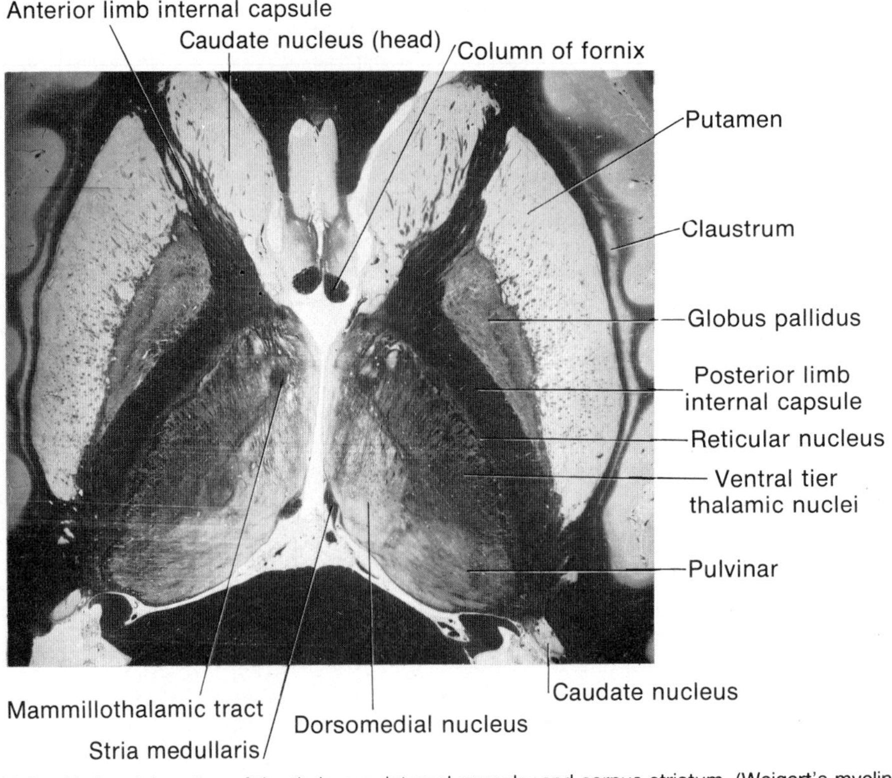

Figure 11-5. Horizontal section of the thalamus, internal capsule, and corpus striatum. (Weigert's myelin stain; photograph.) (From Carpenter and Sutin. *Human Neuroanatomy*, 1983; courtesy of Williams & Wilkins.)

one mesencephalic structure. Most of the striatal afferent systems are associated with distinctive neurotransmitters. The neural activities of the neostriatum involve the largest number of distinctive cell types and the largest number of different neurotransmitters, which include acetylcholine, monamines, peptides, and amino acids

(Dahlström and Fuxe, '64; Andén et al., '66; Pasik et al., '79; Graybiel and Ragsdale, '79; Pickel et al., '80; Graybiel et al., '81a; Haber and Elde, '81; DiFiglia et al., '82; Fibiger, '82; Haber and Nauta, '83). The striatum has a form of reciprocal connections with the distinctive cytological subdivisions of the substantia nigra in which fibers arise from and terminate on different cell populations. Specific alterations of complex interrelationships between different neurotransmitters involved in striatal activities constitute one of the most critical aspects of the metabolic disturbances that underlie two forms of dyskinesia, namely, parkinsonism and Huntington's disease (Hornykiewicz, '66; Bird and Iversen, '74).

The globus pallidus forming the smaller, most medial part of the lentiform nucleus consists of two cytologically similar segments that have input systems with both common and distinctive neurotransmitters (Figs. 11-4, 11-5, and 11-10). Each pallidal segment gives rise to an output system distributed differently in the brain stem. The projections of the medial pallidal segment are to ipsilateral thalamic nuclei which in turn have access to motor regions of the cerebral cortex (Nauta and Mehler, '66; Kuo and Carpenter, '73). The lateral pallidal segment, with a greater volume and cell density, projects primarily to portions of the subthalamic nucleus (Carpenter et al., '68, '81a). A form of reciprocal connections interrelate the lateral pallidal segment and the subthalamic nucleus. The output systems of the corpus striatum arise from the medial pallidal segment and from the pars reticulata of the substantia nigra.

STRIATUM

Caudate Nucleus. The caudate nucleus is an elongated, arched gray mass related throughout its extent to the surface of the lateral ventricle (Figs. 9-6, 11-1, 11-2, 11-3, 11-4, and 11-5). Its enlarged anterior portion, or *head*, lies rostral to the thalamus and bulges into the anterior horn of the lateral ventricle (Figs. 2-11, 2-12, and 11-5). The head of the caudate nucleus and the putamen are separated by fibers of the anterior limb of the internal capsule, except rostroventrally where continuity is maintained. The *body* of the caudate nucleus extends along the dorsolateral border of the thalamus, from which it is separated by the stria terminalis and the terminal vein (Fig. 9-6). This part of the caudate nucleus is regarded as suprathalamic (Szabo, '70). The *tail* of the caudate nucleus is the long, attenuated caudal portion which sweeps into the temporal lobe in the roof of the inferior horn of the lateral ventricle and comes into relationship with the central nucleus of the amygdaloid complex (Figs. 2-11, 9-6, 11-2, 11-3, and 12-14).

Putamen. The putamen, the largest and most lateral part of the basal ganglia, lies between the external capsule and the lateral medullary lamina of the globus pallidus (Figs. 11-1, 11-2, 11-3, 11-4, and 11-5). Most of the putamen is situated deep to the insular cortex and is separated from it by the extreme capsule, the claustrum and the external capsule. In transverse sections it appears lightly stained and is traversed by numerous fascicles of myelinated fibers directed ventromedially toward the globus pallidus. The caudate nucleus and putamen are continuous rostroventrally, beneath the anterior limb of the internal capsule, and in dorsal regions where slender gray cellular bridges pass across the posterior limb of the internal capsule (Figs. 11-3 and 11-4). At levels through the septum pellucidum the nucleus accumbens lies adjacent to ventromedial portions of the striatum (Fig. 12-16). The nucleus accumbens is ontogenetically more closely related to the caudate nucleus and putamen than to the septal nuclei and has projections to both the globus pallidus and the substantia nigra (Swanson and Cowan, '75).

Cytologically the caudate nucleus and the putamen appear identical and are composed of enormous numbers of small cells with scant cytoplasm, small numbers of large cells with chromatic cytoplasmic granules, and variable numbers of medium-sized cells which exhibit no lamination or special arrangements (Fox et al., '71, '71/'72; Kemp and Powell, '71; Pasik et al., '79). Morphometric data indicate that small and medium-sized cells (11,000 cells/mm^3) outnumber large cells (65 cells/mm^3) by ratios ranging from 130:1 to 258:1 (Schröder et al., '75). The striatum may not be as uniform as it appears because in the developing striatum cells of different types migrate in clusters (Brand and Rakic, '79), histochemical activity seems to have a patchy distri-

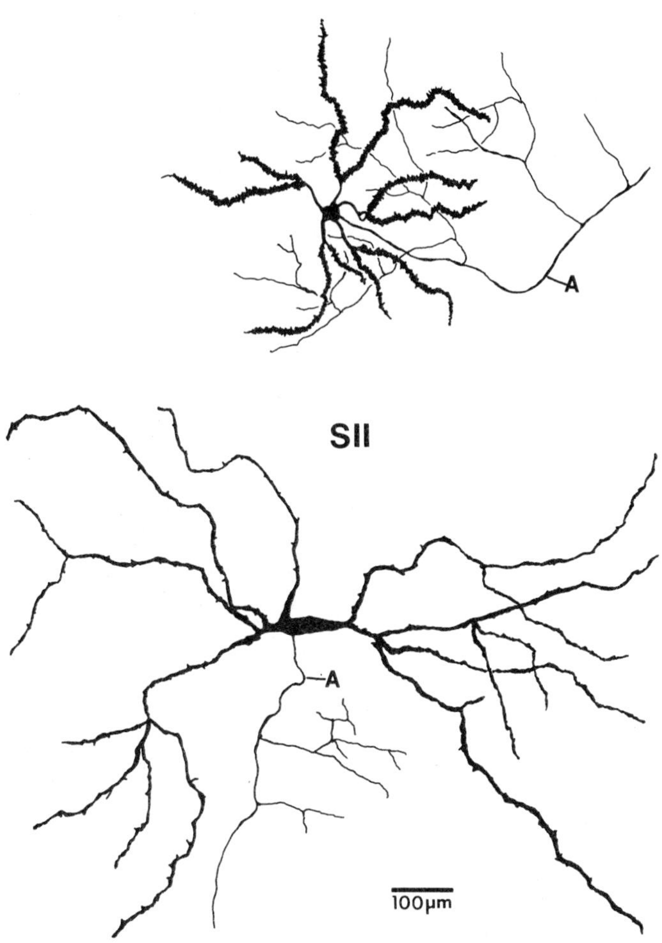

Figure 11-6. Drawings of spiny I (*SI*) and spiny II (*SII*) striatal efferent neurons. Spiny II neurons vary in size and shape and have dendrites that extend 600 μm from the somata. Spiny I neurons have dendrites that radiate into a spheroid domain of about 200 μm, but the first 20 μm of the dendritic stems are free of spines. GABA and enkephalin are considered to be the neurotransmitters of spiny I neurons (Ribak et al., '79; Pasik et al., '79; DiFiglia et al., '82). *A* indicates axons.

bution (Graybiel and Ragsdale, '80; Graybiel et al., '81, '81a) and efferent neurons are grouped into geometrical configurations (Graybiel et al., '79).

Golgi and electron microscopic studies indicate that striatal neurons fall into two categories: (1) those with spiny dendrites and (2) those with smooth dendrites (Fox et al., '71, '71/'72; Kemp and Powell, '71; DiFiglia et al., '76; Pasik et al., '76, '79). Spiny neurons, considered the most numerous striatal neuron, are round or oval, have relatively large nuclei, emit seven or eight primary dendrites which are covered with spines, and have long axons (Fig. 11-6). Two types of spiny striatal neurons are recognized (DiFiglia et al., '76; Pasik et al., '76, '79). Type I spiny neurons, present in enormous numbers, have smooth somata and proximal dendrites, but at about 20 μm from the soma the dendrites abruptly become laden with dendritic spines; dendrites radiate into spherical space of about 200 μm (Kemp and Powell, '71; Fox et al., '71; Pasik et al., '79). Axons of these cells arise from the somata or proximal dendrites and

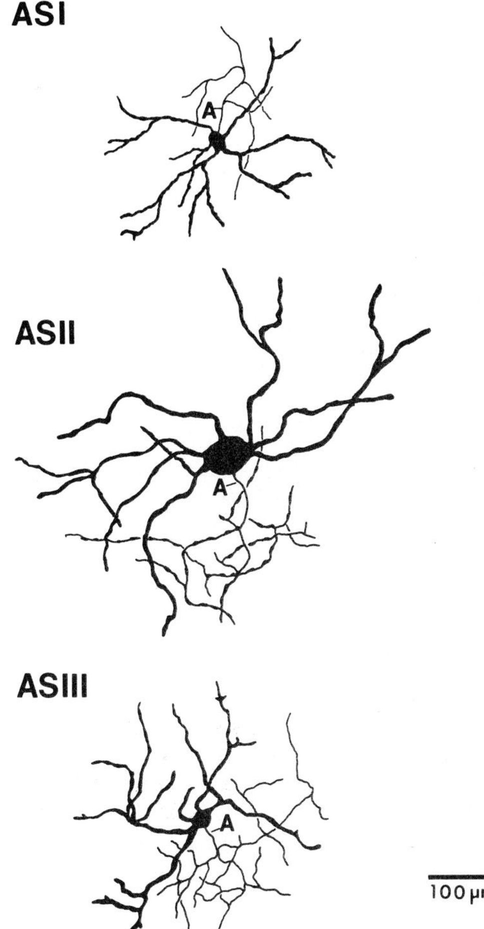

Figure 11-7. Drawings of aspiny striatal neurons whose processes are contained within the striatum. Aspiny I (*ASI*) neurons are the most frequently impregnated striatal cell in Golgi preparations; this local circuit neuron probably has GABA as its neurotransmitter (Ribak et al., '79). Aspiny II (*ASII*) neurons correspond to a population of giant neurons considered to have acetylcholine as their neurotransmitter (Kimura et al., '80; Henderson, '81). The neurotransmitter of aspiny III (*ASIII*) has not been identified (based on Pasik et al., '79). *A* indicates axons.

give rise to collateral networks which may be coextensive with the dendritic field. Retrograde labeling technics indicate that the main axons of type I spiny neurons, reach both the globus pallidus and the substantia nigra (Grofová, '75, '79; Bak et al., '78; Preston et al., '80; Chang et al., '81; Somogyi et al., '81). Immunocytochemical localization of glutamic acid decarboxylase (GAD) in the soma of type I spiny neurons and in synaptic endings in the globus pallidus and substantia nigra provide convincing evidence that large numbers of these neurons contain γ-aminobutyric acid (GABA) which acts as their neurotransmitter (Jessell et al., '78; Ribak et al., '79, '80, '81; Ribak, '81). Light and electron microscopic study of the localization of immunoreactive Leu-enkephalin, in the basal ganglia of the monkey, indicates that striatal neurons also contain this opioid pentapeptide (DiFiglia et al., '82). At the electron microscopic level striatal neurons immunoreactive for Leu-enkephalin have the morphological features of type I spiny neurons. Thus, spiny type I striatal neurons may be associated with two different neurotransmitters (Figs. 11-6, 11-8, and 11-10).

Spiny type II striatal neurons vary in size and shape but commonly are large neurons with spiny dendrites that extend 600 μm from the somata (Figs. 11-6, 11-9, and 11-10). Spiny processes tend to be stubby and less dense than those on spiny I neurons (Pasik et al., '79; Groves, '83). The main axons of spiny II neurons are long and give off collaterals near the somata (Fig. 11-6). While the neurotransmitter of spiny II neurons has not been established, it seems likely that substance P, contained in spiny II neurons, may act as their neurotransmitter (Gale et al., '77; Hong et al., '77; Kanazawa et al., '77; Ljundahl et al., '78; DiFiglia et al., '81).

Three short-axoned Golgi type II striatal neurons are referred to as aspiny neurons (Pasik et al., '79). The aspiny type I neuron is distinguished by its small size, varicose and recurring dendrites, a short, highly arborized axon (Fig. 11-7 and 11-10), and immunoreactivity to GAD, the enzyme that synthesizes GABA (Ribak et al., '79). In Golgi preparations aspiny I neurons are the most frequently impregnated striatal cell (Pasik et al., '79). Aspiny type II neurons have large cell bodies, eccentric nuclei, and dendrites extending 250 μm or more. These cells correspond to a subpopulation of giant striatal neurons seen in Nissl preparations. Immunohistochemical methods demonstrate that aspiny II neurons (Figs. 11-7 and 11-10) stain for choline acetyltransferase (Kimura et al., '80), and acetylcholinesterase has been localized within these neurons in ultrastructural studies (Hender-

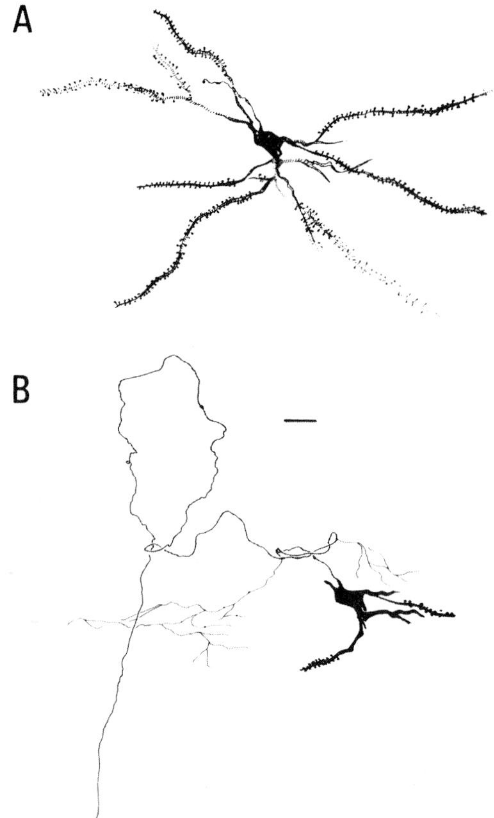

Figure 11-8. Drawing of a single spiny striatal neuron injected iontophoretically with horseradish peroxidase to produce a Golgi-like picture of the soma and dendrites. Unlike the usual Golgi preparation the axon can be followed beyond the proximal segment. (*A*) Reconstruction of the soma, dendrites, and the proximal portion of the axon. (*B*) A reconstruction of the soma and part of the axon. The axon follows a coiled and circuitous course and gives rise to two collaterals. This axon was followed for a total distance of 1.5 mm (Kocsis et al., '77). (Calibration in *B* is 20 μm.) (Courtesy of Dr. S. T. Kitai, School of Medicine, University of Tennessee and Elsevier Scientific Publishing Co., Amsterdam.)

son, '81). Aspiny type III striatal neurons have centrally placed nuclei, a thin rim of cytoplasm, rather straight, smooth dendrites, and a short axon with extensive arborizations (Figs. 11-7 and 11-10). The neurotransmitter of this interneuron has not been identified.

On the basis of cytological data available

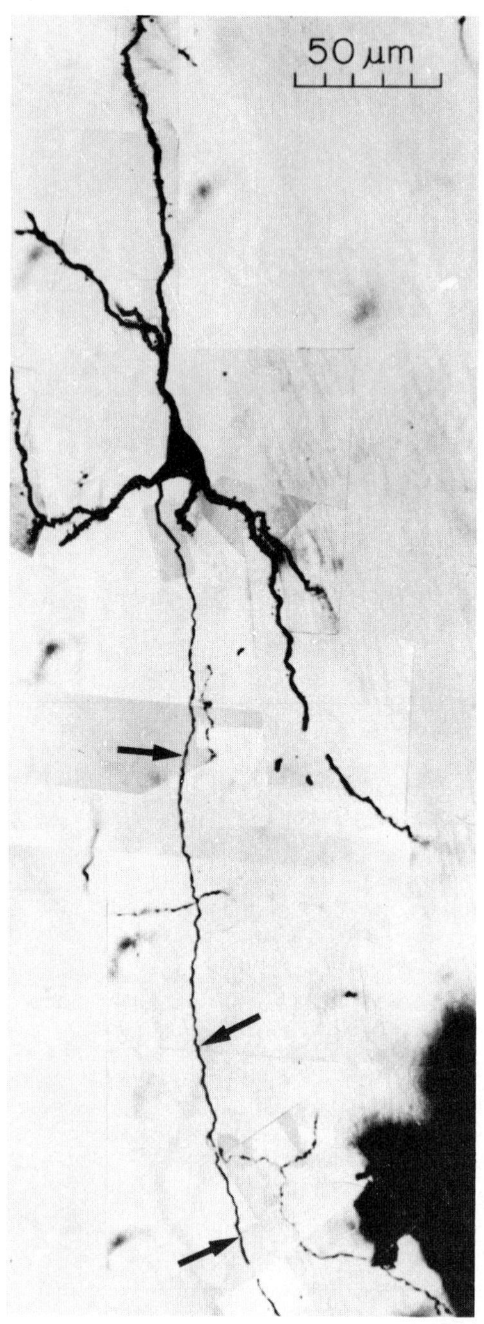

Figure 11-9. Photomontage of a *spiny type II* striatal neuron in a Golgi preparation of the monkey. These cells are pyramidal in shape, give rise to 4 to 6 primary dendrites with relatively low spiny densities and have an axon which emerges from the soma or a proximal dendrite. Axons of these neurons take a straight course and have been followed for 300 μm without narrowing or forming terminal arborizations. The axon (*arrows*) is directed toward the globus pallidus and appears to give rise to collaterals (DiFiglia et al., '76). (Full scale; 50 μm.) (Courtesy of Dr. M. DiFiglia, Harvard Medical School and Elsevier Scientific Publishing Co., Amsterdam.)

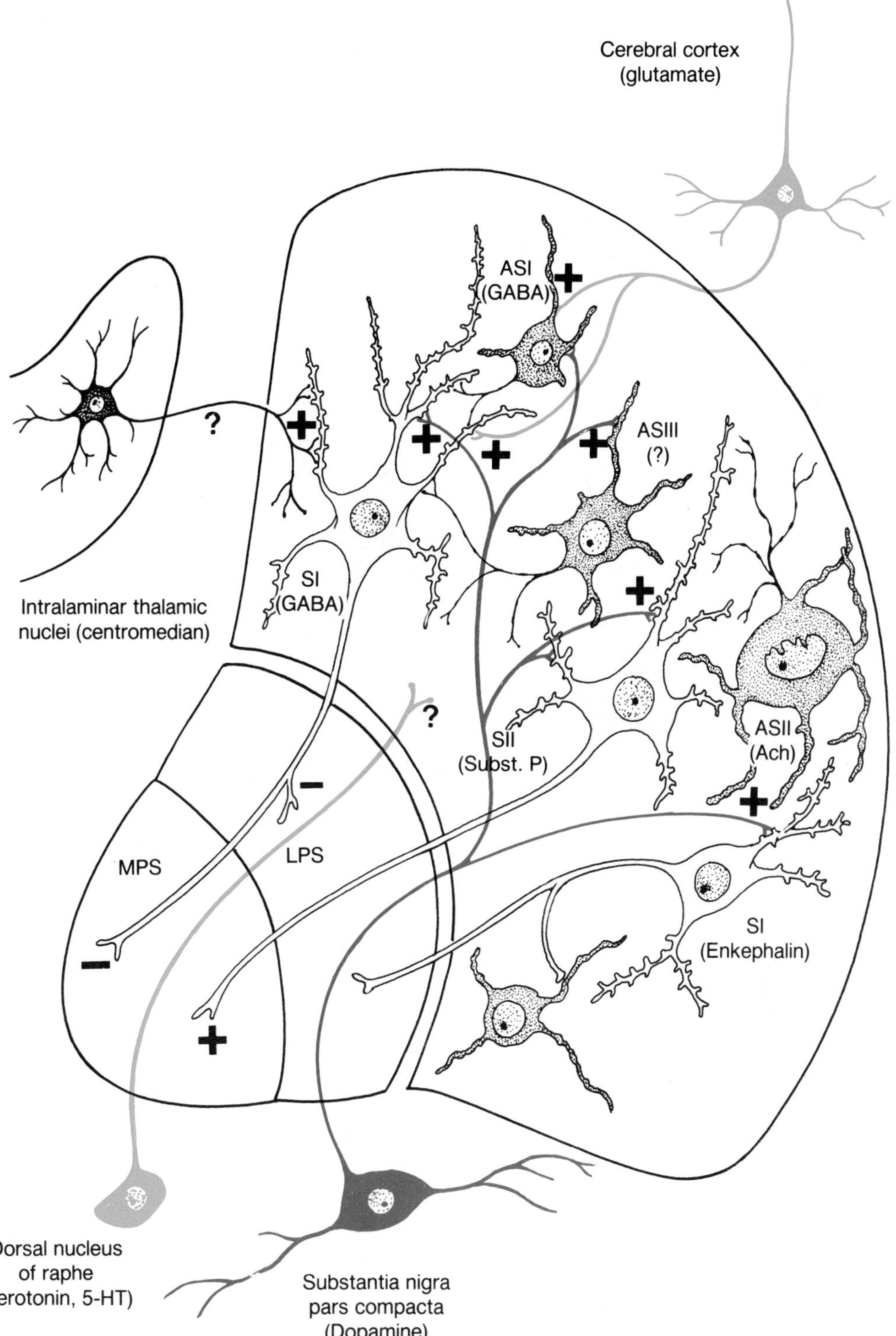

Figure 11-10. Schematic drawing of striatal neurons with inputs and outputs, tentative indications of excitatory (+) or inhibitory (−) action and suspected neurotransmitters. Striatal inputs arise from: (1) the cerebral cortex (glutamate, *blue*); (2) the intralaminar thalamic nuclei (glutamate?); (3) the pars compacta of the substantia nigra (dopamine, *red*); and (4) the dorsal nucleus of the raphe (5-HT, serotonin, *green*). Striatal outputs arise from spiny striatal neurons (*yellow*) and project to both pallidal segments and the pars reticulata of the substantia nigra. Spiny I (SI) neurons have GABA and enkephalin as neurotransmitters. Spiny II (SII) probably have substance P as their neurotransmitter. Aspiny I (ASI) and aspiny II (ASII) (*gray*) local circuit neurons are considered to be GABA-ergic and cholinergic neurons, respectively. The neurotransmitter associated with the aspiny III (ASIII) (*gray*) has not been identified (based upon Pasik et al., '79 and DiFiglia et al., '82).

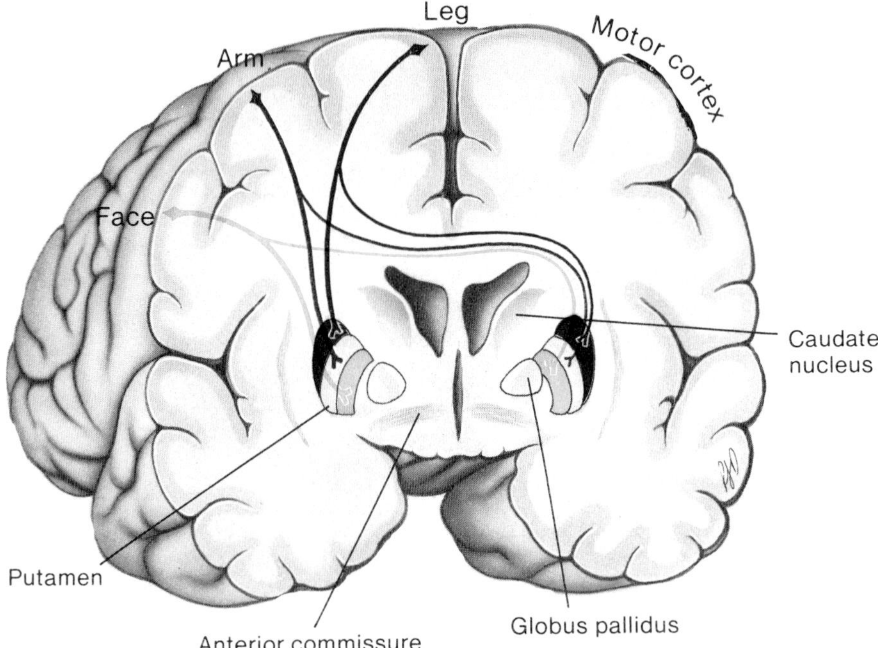

Figure 11-11. Schematic diagram of bilateral somatotopically arranged corticostriate projections from the primary motor area (area 4) to the putamen in the monkey. The ipsilateral projection is much greater than the contralateral projection. Projections from the leg area of the motor cortex are in *red*, while those from the arm and face areas are *black* and *blue*, respectively. The premotor cortex projects ipsilateral to both the caudate nucleus and the putamen; the prefrontal cortex projects fibers to all parts of the caudate nucleus (based on Künzle, '75, '78).

it is not possible to provide a complete interpretation of the neuronal organization and synaptic articulations within the striatum, although there is impressive evidence that the afferent systems arising from cortex, thalamus, and various midbrain nuclei terminate upon spiny neurons (Kemp, '68, '70; Kemp and Powell, '70, '71). It is widely accepted that spiny neurons also constitute the striatal output neuron (Pasik et al., '79; Ribak, '81; DiFiglia et al., '82). The role of interneurons (Golgi type II) with short axons, represented by aspiny striatal neurons, is unknown, but it seems certain they are involved in modulating activities related to both striatal inputs and outputs (Fig. 11-10).

STRIATAL CONNECTIONS

Striatal Afferent Fibers. The caudate nucleus and the putamen receive the principal afferent systems projecting to the corpus striatum. Afferent fibers arise from the cerebral cortex, parts of the amygdala, the intralaminar thalamic nuclei, the substantia nigra, and the dorsal nucleus of the raphe (Figs. 11-11 and 11-12).

Corticostriate Fibers. Virtually all regions of the neocortex project fibers to the striatum and all parts of the striatum receive fibers from the cortex (Carman et al., '63, '65; Kemp and Powell, '70). No part of the striatum is under the sole influence of one neocortex area. The projection to the striatum from the sensorimotor cortex is substantial while that from the visual cortex is small. Corticostriate fibers from the association cortex of the frontal and parietotemporal lobes in the monkey are greater than in other mammals.

Degeneration studies suggested that different regions of cortex projected to specific parts of the striatum, although overlap of corticostriate projections was a common feature (Kemp and Powell, '70, '71a). Autoradiographic studies have revealed observations undetected by degeneration studies, namely that: (1) corticostriate terminals form mosaic-like patterns in the striatum, (2) many cortical areas have widespread

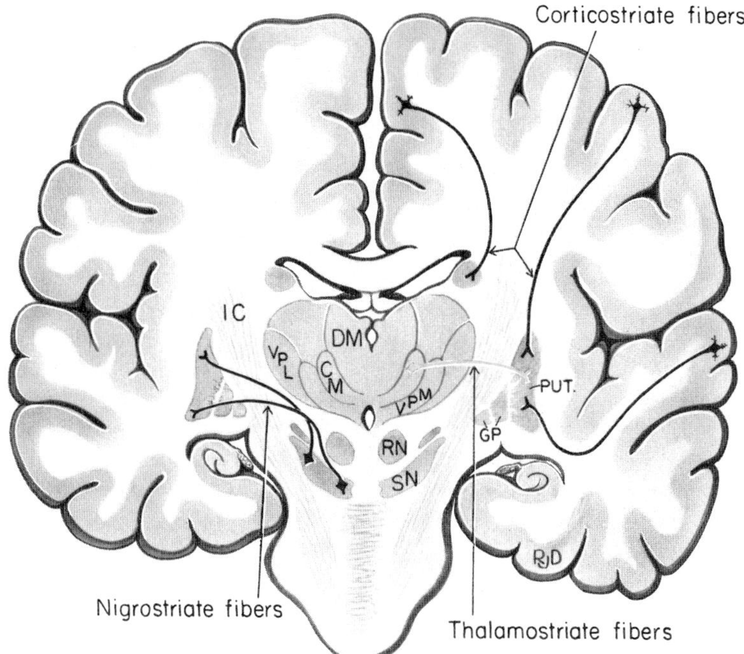

Figure 11-12. Semischematic diagram of the major striatal afferent systems. *Corticostriate projections* (*black*) arise from broad regions of the cerebral cortex, are topographically organized, and are distributed to both the caudate nucleus and the putamen. Corticostriate fibers arise from pyramidal cells in the upper half of lamina V, and those from area 4 project bilaterally and somatotopically upon the putamen (Fig. 11-11). These projections have glutamate as their neurotransmitter. *Nigrostriatal fibers* (*red*) arise from cells of the pars compacta of the substantia nigra and convey dopamine to terminals in the caudate nucleus and putamen. *Thalamostriate fibers* (*blue*) arise largely from the centromedian-parafascicular nuclear complex. Not shown in this diagram are striatal afferents from mesencephalic indolamine cell groups in the median raphe. Cells in the dorsal nucleus of raphe have serotonin as their neurotransmitter and project to both the putamen and the substantia nigra. Abbreviations used: *CM*, centromedian nucleus; *DM*, dorsomedial nucleus; *GP*, globus pallidus; *IC*, internal capsule; *PUT*, putamen; *RN*, red nucleus; *SN*, substantia nigra; *VPL* and *VPM*, ventral posterolateral and ventral posteromedial thalamic nuclei. (From Carpenter and Sutin, *Human Neuroanatomy*, 1983; courtesy of Williams & Wilkins.)

projections in several parts of the striatum, and (3) widely separated cortical areas give rise to overlapping terminal fields in portions of the striatum (Künzle, '75, '78; Goldman and Nauta, '77; Jones et al., '77; Yeterian and van Hoesen, '78; van Hoesen et al., '81). The terminal distribution of corticostriate fibers is extensive and characterized by a series of strips or clusters that separate from each other and then become confluent in other regions. The strips and clusters of striatal terminals arising from different cortical areas not only overlap each other, but also may overlap terminal projection zones of other striatal afferent systems. Cortical areas reciprocally connected via cortico-cortical fibers have their own unique corticostriate projection area and one shared by both cortical areas (Yeterian and van Hoesen, '78; van Hoesen et al., '81).

Corticostriate fibers arising in the primary motor area (area 4) project bilaterally and somatotopically upon the putamen (Fig. 11-11) where patchlike terminations are greatest in lateral regions and extend nearly the length of putamen (Künzle, '75). The premotor area projects ipsilaterally to both the caudate nucleus and the putamen, while fibers from the prefrontal cortex pass via an intranuclear trajectory to all parts of the caudate nucleus (Goldman and Nauta, '77; Künzle, '78).

The laminar origins of the corticostriate system, the most massive projection system to the striatum, have been determined by retrograde transport of horseradish peroxidase (HRP). In the monkey, these fibers, both ipsilateral and contralateral, arise from smaller pyramidal cells in the upper half of lamina V in all areas (Jones et al., '77; Jones and Wise, '77). The implication is that these fibers constitute a distinct projection, rather than collaterals of other descending systems. Other evidence suggests that the corticostriate fibers may arise from both supragranular (laminae II and III) and infragranular (laminae V and VI) layers of the cortex (Kitai et al., '76; Royce, '82). Striatal afferents from the cerebral cortex end principally upon the dendritic spines of spiny I and spiny II cells (Kemp, '68; Kemp and Powell, '71b; Frotscher et al., '81; Somogyi et al., '81). Corticostriate fibers are excitatory and have glutamate as their neurotransmitter (Fegér et al., '79; Hattori et al., '79; Dray, '80; Kitai, '81; Fonnum et al., '81).

Amygdalostriate Fibers. Although axoplasmic transport studies have indicated a modest projection from the amygdala to the striatum (Krettek and Price, '78; Royce, '78a), recent data suggest a widespread amygdalostriate projection to the striatum caudal to the anterior commissure (Kelley et al., '82). Rostral to the anterior commissure this striatal projection is dense only in ventromedial regions. A modest symmetrical contralateral distribution reaches the striatum via the anterior commissure. The amygdalostriatal projection originates mainly from the basal lateral amygdaloid nucleus. A division of the striatum into "limbic" and "nonlimbic" parts has been suggested. The smaller "nonlimbic" striatum occupies an anterodorsolateral region. This parcellation of the striatum into distinctive regions on the basis of amygdaloid projections suggests that the "limbic" striatum may be concerned with behavioral phenomenon.

Thalamostriate Fibers. Degeneration studies clearly indicate that the centromedian-parafascicular nuclear complex (CM-PF) projects to both the caudate nucleus and the putamen (Mehler, '66b; Powell and Cowan, '67). Retrograde HRP studies show that injections of the putamen produce intense labeling of cells in the CM-PF and some labeling in cells of the central lateral nucleus (CL) (Jones and Leavitt, '74; Royce, '78a); HRP injections in various cortical areas label corresponding thalamic relay nuclei intensely and lightly label portions of the intralaminar thalamic nuclei. These results were interpreted to mean that the intralaminar thalamic nuclei project profusely to the striatum and sparsely and diffusely, via collaterals, to broad cortical regions (Fig. 11-12). Autoradiographic studies in monkey and cat show that thalamostriate fibers from CM terminate, like corticostriate fibers, in mosaic disk-shaped aggregates or hollow rings in the caudate nucleus and putamen (Kalil, '78; Royce, '78). Cells in the central lateral (CL) and paracentral (PCN) thalamic nuclei contain two populations of neurons, one projecting to cortex and one projecting to the caudate nucleus; these distinct neuronal populations have different conduction velocities (Steriade and Glenn, '82). Monosynaptic relays in CL and PCN from the midbrain reticular formation conduct impulses separately to cortical areas and the caudate nucleus. Thalamostriate fibers terminate upon spiny type I neurons (Fox et al., '71; Kemp and Powell, '71a; Groves, '83) and are thought to be excitatory (Dray, '80; Kitai, '81). The neurotransmitter utilized by thalamostriate fibers is not known, but has been postulated to be glutamate (Fonnum et al., '81).

Nigrostriatal Fibers. Fluorescent histochemical studies not only provided evidence that cells of the pars compacta of the substantia nigra projected to the striatum but indicated that these cells conveyed dopamine to their terminals (Anden et al., '64; Dahlström and Fuxe, '64; Fuxe and Andén, '66; Bédard et al., '69; Moore et al., '71; Ungerstedt, '71). Dopamine, stored in varicosities in nerve terminals, is concentrated mainly in three forebrain areas: (1) the striatum, (2) the nucleus accumbens septi, and (3) the olfactory bulb (Fuxe and Andén, '66). In the striatum dopaminergic fibers form a matrix of terminal varicosities around striatal neurons of all types and sizes (Fig. 11-10) and exhibit a diffuse green fluorescence (Siggins et al., '76).

Studies of the organization of ascending striatal afferents based upon retrograde enzyme transport suggest cells in the rostral two-thirds of the pars compacta of the substantia nigra are related to the head of the caudate nucleus (Figs. 11-12, 11-21, and 11-22), while those projecting to the putamen are in more posterior regions (Szabo, '80, '80a). An inverse dorsoventral relationship exists between the substantia nigra and the caudate nucleus, so that cells in the ventral pars compacta project to the dorsal regions of the caudate nucleus, and vice versa. Lateral and posterior parts of the substantia nigra are related to dorsal and lateral parts of the putamen. Significant overlap in the projection fields of nigrostriatal fibers may be due to differences in the size of these structures. In autoradiographs of nigrostriatal fibers the distribution of silver grains in the striatum differs from that described for corticostriate and thalamostriate fibers in that they are spread evenly without forming clusters or patches (Carpenter et al., '76).

Although the major nigrostriatal neurotransmitter is acknowledged to be dopamine (Fig. 11-10), a consensus regarding its postsynaptic action has not emerged (Groves, '83). The inference that dopamine is excitatory is based upon: (1) intracellular recordings which show that electrical stimulation of the substantia nigra typically produces EPSPs or EPSP-IPSP sequences in striatal neurons and only rarely IPSPs (Kitai et al., '76; Kitai, '81; Wilson et al., '82), and (2) anatomical data indicating asymmetrical synaptic contacts of dopaminergic terminals on dendritic spines of what are thought to be spiny type I neurons (Groves, '83). The inference that dopamine is inhibitory is based upon extracellular recordings of striatal activity following application of dopamine or related agonists (Connor, '70; Gonzalez-Vegas, '74). Not all nigrostriatal fibers are considered dopaminergic (Fibiger et al., '72). It has been postulated that some 20% of nigrostriatal fibers are nondopaminergic, but their cells of origin are uncertain. Nondopaminergic nigrostriatal fibers are considered to form symmetrical synapses on spiny striatal neurons (Hattori et al., '73).

Striatal Afferents from the Raphe Nuclei. Histofluorescent technics have demonstrated several ascending pathways originating from mesencephalic indolamine cell groups in the median raphe (Dahlström and Fuxe, '64; Ternaux et al., '77). Anatomical, physiological and biochemical investigations suggest that the dorsal (B7) and median (B8) raphe nuclei provide two distinct, but partially overlapping ascending serotonergic (5-hydroxytryptamine, 5-HT) systems (Ungerstedt, '71; Conrad et al., '74; Miller et al., '75; Bobillier et al., '76; Dray et al., '76; Ternaux et al., '77; Royce, '78a). Pathways originating from the dorsal and median raphe nuclei, traced by a variety of technics, ascend in the medial forebrain bundle through the hypothalamic region, but the specific projection of each nucleus differs (Parent et al., '81). Serotonergic projections arising from the dorsal nucleus of the raphe terminate mainly in ventrocaudal regions of the striatum (Bobillier et al., '75; Ternaux et al., '77; Dray et al., '78; Dray, '80). Fluorescent retrograde double labeling technics demonstrate that the majority of neurons in the dorsal nucleus of the raphe project collaterals to both the striatum and the substantia nigra (Fig. 11-10), although populations of cells within the nucleus have single targets (van der Kooy and Hattori, '80). Stimulation of the dorsal nucleus of the raphe produces a strong, long-lasting inhibition of striatal neurons (Olpe and Koella, '77). The type of striate neuron receiving projections from the raphe is unknown. Identification of serotonergic neurons in the dorsal nucleus of the raphe with [^{3}H]serotonin in the rat revealed an estimate of 11,500 neurons, but twice this number of neurons in the nucleus are nonserotonergic (Descarries et al., '82).

Striatal Efferent Fibers. These fibers project to the globus pallidus and the substantia nigra.

Striopallidal Fibers. These fibers are topographically organized in both dorsoventral and rostrocaudal sequences and radiate into various parts of the pallidum like spokes of a wheel (Figs. 2-11, 9-7, 11-4, 11-5, and 11-13). Studies in the monkey (Nauta and Mehler, '66; Szabo, '67) indicate that putaminopallidal fibers terminate in both pallidal segments. According to Szabo ('67), the precommissural part of the putamen appears to project exclusively to the globus pallidus, while other regions of the striatum project to both globus pallidus

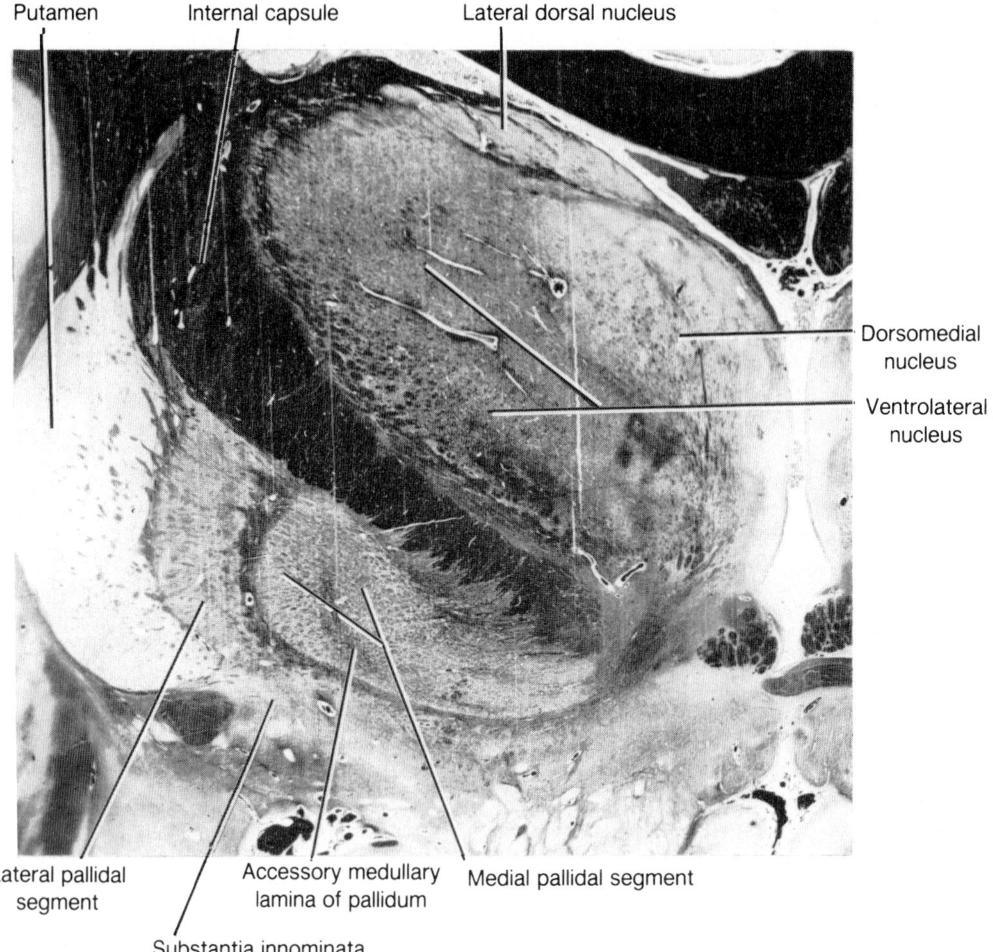

Figure 11-13. Photomicrograph of a transverse section of the human brain through the corpus striatum, internal capsule and thalamus. Segments of the globus pallidus are separated by the medial medullary lamina and the accessory medullary lamina divides the medial pallidal segment into inner and outer parts. The substantia innominata lies ventral to the globus pallidus and extends rostrally.

and substantia nigra. Striopallidal fibers from the caudate nucleus pass ventrally through the internal capsule, while fibers from the putamen project medially to the globus pallidus. The bundles of myelinated fibers which are most numerous in medial parts of the putamen are collections of striopallidal fibers. Large numbers of striopallidal fibers are considered to have γ-aminobutyric acid (GABA) as their neurotransmitter (McGeer et al., '71; Hattori et al., '73; Pycock et al., '76). The globus pallidus is particularly rich in glutamic acid decarboxylase (GAD), the enzyme that synthesizes GABA (Fonnum et al., '78; Ribak et al., '79). GABA is conveyed to the globus pallidus via axons of spiny I striatal neurons (Fig. 11-10) (Jessell et al., '78; Pasik et al., '79; Ribak, '81). Immunohistochemical studies also reveal striopallidal fibers immunoreactive for enkephalin and substance P which are distributed in a specific pattern (Hughes et al., '75; Elde et al., '76; Cuello and Kanazawa, '78; Wamsley et al., '80). Immunoreactive striatal neurons containing enkephalin are considered to be spiny type I neurons (Fig. 11-10) (Pickel et al., '80; DiFiglia et al., '82). Spiny type II are thought to be the source of substance P-like immunoreactive fibers in the globus pallidus (Fig. 11-10) (Hong et al., '77; Gale et al., '77; Pasik et al., '79; Haber and Nauta, '83).

Strionigral Fibers. Experimental studies have convincingly demonstrated that strionigral fibers are topographically organized and end upon cells of the pars reticulata (Szabo, '62, '67, '70). Fibers from the head of the caudate nucleus project to rostral parts of the nigra. Putaminonigral fibers pass to more caudal parts of the nigra and are arranged so that dorsal parts of the putamen project to lateral parts of the nigra and ventral parts of the putamen are related to medial parts of the nigra (Fig. 11-22).

Almost all strionigral fibers terminate in the pars reticulata of the substantia nigra (Grofová and Rinvik, '70; Kemp, '70; Schwyn and Fox, '74; Hattori et al., '75). Retrograde transport studies confirm the topographical projection from the striatum to the substantia nigra (Bunney and Aghajanian, '76). Strionigral projections arise from medium-sized spiny striatal neurons (Grofová, '75) that have GABA, enkephalin, and substance P as their neurotransmitters (Ribak et al., '76; Gale et al., '77; Hong et al., ;77; Kanazawa et al., '77; Jessell et al., '78; Ribak et al., '80; Emson et al., '80; DiFiglia et al., '81, '82). Spiny type I striatal neurons appear related to two distinctive neurotransmitters, GABA and enkephalin (Fig. 11-22) (DiFiglia et al., '82). Spiny type II striatal neurons appear to have substance P as their neurotransmitter (Pasik et al., '79; Groves, '83); fibers from these neurons have a course similar to those of the spiny type I but may arise from different locations within the striatum. Electrical stimulation of the caudate nucleus leads to a marked increase in the release of [^{3}H]GABA into the ipsilateral substantia nigra and some increases in the contralateral nigra (Kemel et al., '83).

It has been demonstrated that the highest concentrations of GAD and GABA in the mammalian central nervous system are found in the substantia nigra (Fahn, '76). The distribution of GAD in the substantia nigra is uneven, and is greatest in the pars reticulata (Fonnum et al., '74).

The striatum contains high concentrations of dopamine, considered to be present in terminal varicosities of nigrostriatal fibers (Andén et al., '64; Poirier and Sourkes, '65; Hornykiewicz, '66; Dahlström, '71; Ungerstedt, '71). Terminal varicosities in the striatum are fine, form a matrix about both large and small striatal neurons, and exhibit a diffuse green fluorescence (Fig. 11-10). In the developing striatum, the glyoxylic acid histofluorescence method reveals a patchwork of dopamine "islands" strikingly similar to the compartmentalization of acetylcholinesterase (Graybiel et al., '81a). In addition the striatum contains glutamate conveyed by corticostriate fibers (Spencer, '76; Fonnum and Storm-Mathisen, '77) and serotonin (5-HT) transmitted from the raphe nuclei of the midbrain (Fig. 11-10) (Miller et al., '75; Olpe and Koella, '77; Ternaux et al., '77). Striatal efferent neurons contain GABA, substance P, and enkephalin which are transmitted to both the globus pallidus and the substantia nigra (McGeer et al., '71; Gale et al., '77; Pasik et al., '79; Haber and Elde, '81; Ribak, '81; DiFiglia et al., '82; Haber and Nauta, '83). The different striatal neurons and some of the known input and output systems with their tentatively identified neurotransmitter are shown schematically in Figure 11-10.

GLOBUS PALLIDUS

This nucleus forms the smaller and most medial segment of the lentiform nucleus. Throughout most of its extent the pallidum lies medial to the putamen; the internal capsule forms its medial border (Figs. 2-11, 11-1, 11-2, 11-4, 11-5, and 11-13). A thin *lateral medullary lamina* is found on the external surface of the pallidum at its junction with the putamen. A *medial medullary lamina* divides the globus pallidus into medial and lateral segments (Figs. 11-5, 11-13, 11-14, and 11-15). A less distinct *accessory medullary lamina* (Kuo and Carpenter, '73) divides the medial pallidal segment into outer and inner portions which appear to give rise to efferent fibers that have distinctive courses (Fig. 11-13). The globus pallidus, phylogenetically older than the striatum, is well developed in lower vertebrates. Bundles of myelinated fibers traverse the globus pallidus, which in fresh preparations give it a paler appearance

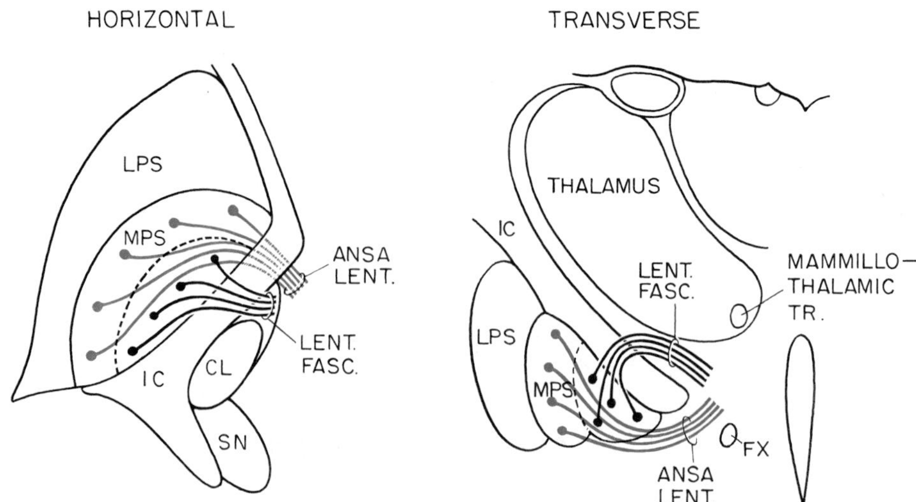

Figure 11-14. Diagrammatic representation of origin and course of pallidal efferent fibers forming the *ansa lenticularis* and *lenticular fasciculus*. Fibers of the ansa lenticularis (*red*) arise from the outer portion of the medial pallidal segment (lateral to the accessory medullary lamina, *dashed line*) and course rostrally, ventrally and medially. Fibers of the lenticular fasciculus (*black*) arise from the inner portion of the medial pallidal segment (medial to the accessory medullary lamina, *dashed line*) and course dorsally and medially through the fibers of the internal capsule (Kuo and Carpenter, '73). (From Carpenter and Sutin, *Human Neuroanatomy*, 1983; courtesy of Williams & Wilkins.)

than the putamen or caudate nucleus. Cells of the globus pallidus are predominantly large fusiform neurons with long, relatively smooth dendrites which are contacted by plexuses of afferent fibers that establish longitudinal axodendritic connections (Fox et al., '74). There are no apparent cytological differences between the medial and lateral pallidal segments. Large pallidal neurons intracellularly injected with HRP are of two subtypes: (1) medially located neurons with dorsoventral dendritic fields and (2) laterally situated neurons with disc-shaped dendritic fields extending both dorsoventrally and rostrocaudally (Park et al., '82). In man the lateral pallidal segment constitutes 70% of the total pallidal and has the highest cell density (Thörner et al., '75).

PALLIDAL CONNECTIONS

Pallidal Afferent Fibers. Major afferent fibers to the globus pallidus arise from the striatum and the subthalamic nucleus. Unlike the striatum, the globus pallidus does not receive afferents from the cerebral cortex, the thalamus or the substantia nigra. Autoradiographic studies in the monkey have revealed no projections to the globus pallidus from cortical areas 4, 6, 8, and 9 or from the somatosensory cortex (Künzle, '75, '78; Künzle and Akert, '77).

Striopallidal Fibers. These fibers which arise from spiny striatal neurons have GABA, enkephalin, and substance P as their neurotransmitters and are distributed in an organized manner to both segments of the globus pallidus (Fig. 11-10). Large numbers of striopallidal fibers considered to have GABA as their neurotransmitter are distributed to both pallidal segments (McGeer et al., '71; Hattori et al., '73; Pycock et al., '76; Jessell et al., '78; Ribak, '81; Groves, '83). GABA is conveyed to the globus pallidus via axons of spiny type I striatal neurons. Immunohistochemical studies indicate that striopallidal fibers immunoreactive for enkephalin and substance P are distributed in a specific pattern within the globus pallidus (Elde et al., '76; Haber and Elde, '81; Haber and Natua, '83). In the monkey, striopallidal fibers immunoreactive for enkephalin are dense in the lateral pallidal segment, while fibers immunoreactive for substance P are dense throughout the medial pallidal segment. The regional differences in the distribution

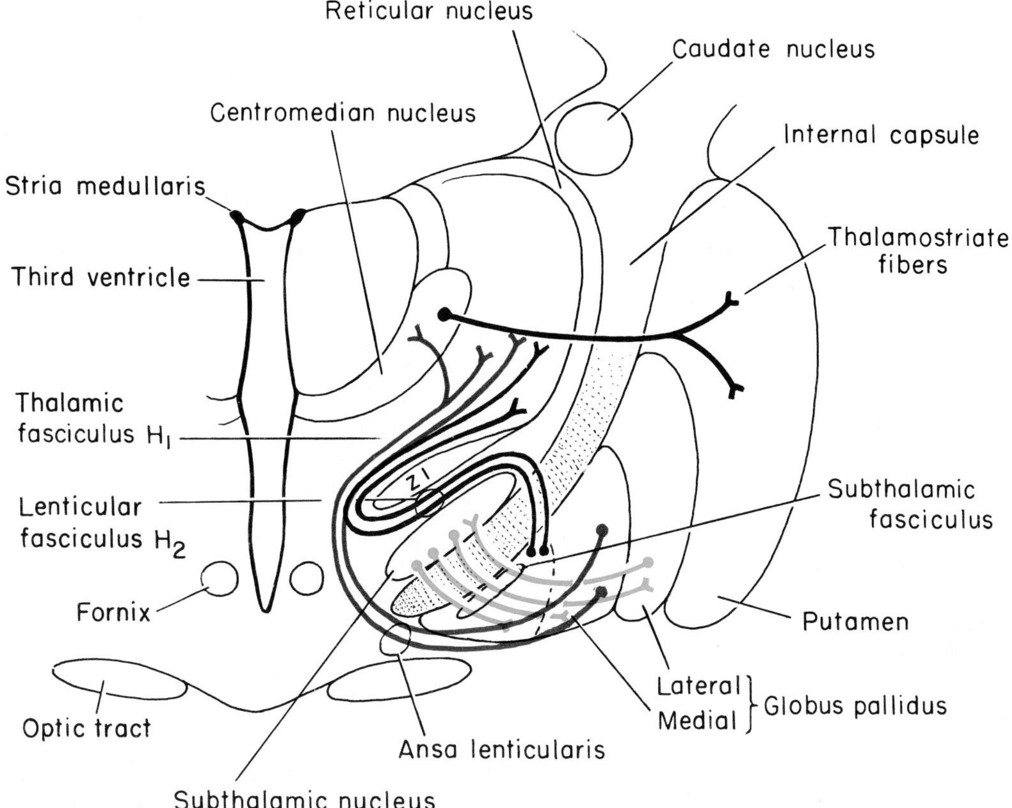

Figure 11-15. Schematic diagram of pallidofugal fiber systems in a transverse plane. Fibers of the ansa lenticularis (*red*) arise from the outer portion of the medial pallidal segment, pass ventrally, medially and rostrally around the internal capsule and enter the prerubral field. Fibers of the lenticular fasciculus (H_2, *black*) issue from the dorsal surface of inner part of the medial pallidal segment, traverse the posterior limb of the internal capsule, and pass medially dorsal to the subthalamic nucleus to enter the prerubral field. The ansa lenticularis and the lenticular fasciculus merge in the prerubral field (Field H of Forel, not labeled here), and project dorsolaterally as components of the thalamic fasciculus (H_1). Fibers of the thalamic fasciculus pass dorsal to the zona incerta (*ZI*). The subthalamic fasciculus (*blue*) consists of pallidosubthalamic fibers arising from the lateral pallidal segment, and subthalamopallidal fibers that terminate in arrays parallel to the medullary lamina in both pallidal segments. Both components of the subthalamic fasciculus traverse the internal capsule. Thalamostriate fibers from the centromedian nucleus (*black*) project to the putamen, as part of a feedback system. Compare with Figs. 11-14, 11-16, 11-17, and 11-18. (From Carpenter and Sutin, *Human Neuroanatomy*, 1983; courtesy of Williams & Wilkins.)

and concentration of these two peptides in the globus pallidus, as defined by immunocytochemical methods, may be related to specific pallidal efferent systems (Kuo and Carpenter, '73; Haber and Elde, '81). In immunoreacted preparations the cell bodies and dendrites of unstained pallidal elements (called "woolly" fibers) are enmeshed in a dense plexus of enkephalin or substance P-positive striopallidal fibers (Haber and Nauta, '83). Morphologically immunoreactive neurons containing enkephalin appear to be type I spiny neurons (Pickel et al., '80; DiFiglia et al., '82). Spiny type II neurons are thought to be the source of substance P-like immunoreactive fibers in the globus pallidus (Hong et al., '77; Kanazawa et al., '77; Gale et al., '77; Pasik et al., '79). Enkephalin-like and substance P-like immunoreactive striopallidal fibers arise from both "limbic" and "nonlimbic" regions of the striatum (Kelley et al., '82). Comparisons of normal human brains with those from patients with Huntington's disease indicate substantial reductions of substance P and enkephalin in the globus pal-

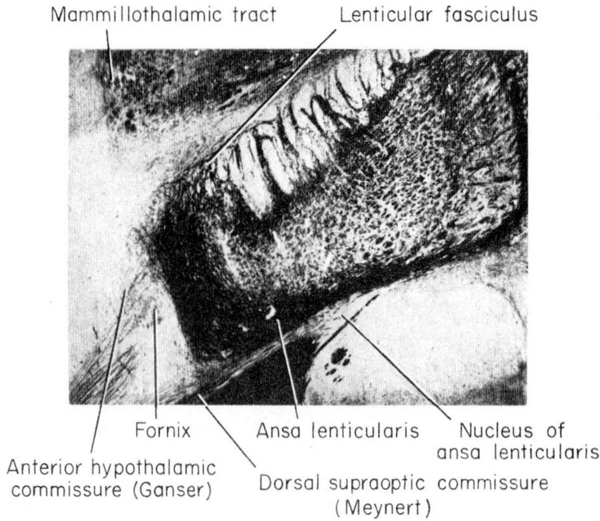

Figure 11-16. Photograph demonstrating the ansa lenticularis in a decorticate monkey. All fibers of the internal capsule have degenerated so that pallidofugal fibers sweeping medially around the internal capsule are especially prominent. (Weigert's myelin stain.) (Reproduced with permission from F. A. Mettler: *Neuroanatomy*, C. V. Mosby Company, St. Louis, 1948.)

lidus and substantia nigra (Emsen et al., '80).

Subthalamopallidal Fibers. Subthalamopallidal fibers are topographically organized and project to both segments of the pallidum in arrays parallel to the medullary lamina (Nauta and Cole, '78; Carpenter et al., '81a). The largest number of terminals appear in the medial pallidal segment. Studies of the subthalamic nucleus based on the retrograde transport of HRP from various regions of individual pallidal segments indicate: (1) cells in mediocaudal parts of the nucleus project mainly to the medial pallidal segment, (2) cells in medial parts of the middle third of the nucleus project to the rostral part of the lateral pallidal segment, and (3) cells in central parts of the rostral two-thirds of the nucleus project to the largest part of lateral segment adjacent to the putamen (Fig. 11-26, *C* and *D*) (Carpenter et al., '81). Cells in the lateral third of the subthalamic nucleus project few fibers to any part of the globus pallidus. An inverse dorsoventral topographical relationship exists between cells in the subthalamic nucleus and the lateral pallidal segment which is similar to that described for the substantia nigra and the head of the caudate nucleus (Szabo, '80, '80a). Retrograde fluorescent double labeling technics in the rat suggest that virtually all neurons of the subthalamic nucleus project to both the globus pallidus and the substantia nigra (Fig. 11-23) (van der Kooy and Hattori, '80a). Physiological studies in the rat also suggest that subthalamic neurons have branched axons reaching both the pallidum and the nigra, but different responses are recorded in each branch (Hammond et al., '83). Stimulation of the subthalamic nucleus produces short latency inhibition of spontaneous activity in the pallidum and short latency excitation in the substantia nigra. These dual responses are thought to involve local interneurons. Retrograde transport of [^{3}H]GABA from pallidum to subthalamic nucleus neurons, suggest that GABA may be the neurotransmitter of subthalamopallidal fibers (Nauta and Cuenod, '82).

Pallidofugal Fibers. Although cells in the medial and lateral pallidal segments appear cytologically identical and their inputs originate from the same sources, there are similarities (GABA) and differences (enkephalin and substance P) in the neurotransmitters conveyed by striopallidal fibers; each pallidal segment projects fibers to different brain stem nuclei. Fibers arising from cells of the medial pallidal segment project to thalamic nuclei, the lateral

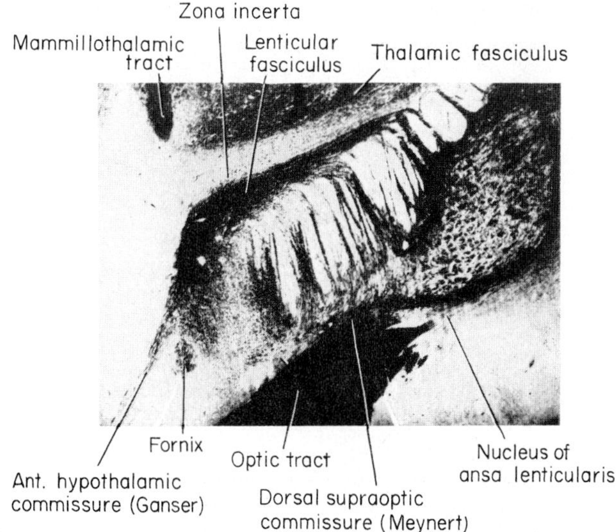

Figure 11-17. Photograph demonstrating the lenticular fasciculus in a decorticate monkey. Fibers of the lenticular fasciculus pass dorsally through the degenerated internal capsule and form a bundle between the zona incerta and the internal capsule. (Weigert's myelin stain.) (Reproduced with permission from F. A. Mettler: *Neuroanatomy*, C. V. Mosby Company, St. Louis, 1948.)

habenular nucleus, and via a descending tegmental bundle to a cell group in midbrain reticular formation (Figs. 11-20 and 11-24). Cells in the lateral pallidal segment project primarily to the subthalamic nuclei (Fig. 11-20). Some fibers from both pallidal segments end in parts of the substantia nigra. Pallidal efferent fibers can be divided into four main bundles: (1) the *ansa lenticularis*, (2) the *lenticular fasciculus*, (3) the *pallidotegmental fibers*, and (4) the *pallidosubthalamic fibers*. The first three of these arise exclusively from the medial pallidal segment (Nauta and Mehler, '66; Carpenter and Strominger, '67; De Vito and Anderson, '82). Pallidosubthalamic fibers arise exclusively from the lateral pallidal segment (Kim et al., '76; Carpenter et al., '81a). Pallidofugal fibers are arranged in a rostrocaudal sequence with the ansa lenticularis most rostral, the lenticular fasciculus in an intermediate position, and pallidosubthalamic fibers most caudal.

Ansa Lenticularis. These fibers arise from lateral portions of the medial segment of the globus pallidus and form a well-defined bundle on the ventral surface of the pallidum (Figs. 11-14, 11-15, and 11-16). This bundle sweeps ventromedially and rostrally around the posterior limb of the internal capsule, and then courses posteriorly to enter Forel's field H.

Lenticular Fasciculus. These fibers arise from inner portions of the medial pallidal segment, issue from the dorsomedial margin of the pallidum slightly caudal to the ansa lenticularis, and traverse the ventral parts of the internal capsule in a number of small fascicles (Figs. 11-14, 11-15, 11-17, and 11-18). Fibers cross through the internal capsule immediately rostral to the subthalamic nucleus and form a relatively large and discrete bundle ventral to the zona incerta. Although most of the lenticular fasciculus lies rostral to the subthalamic nucleus, some fibers of this bundle course along the dorsal border of this nucleus. Fibers of the lenticular fasciculus are referred to as Forel's field H_2. While fibers of the lenticular fasciculus pursue a distinctive course through the internal capsule, they pass medially and caudally to join fibers of the ansa lenticularis in Forel's field H (prerubral field). The major part of the fibers of the lenticular fasciculus (H_2) and the ansa lenticularis which merge in Forel's field H ultimately enter the thalamic fasciculus (Fig. 11-18).

Investigations of the origin of pallidothalamic fibers in the monkey indicate that

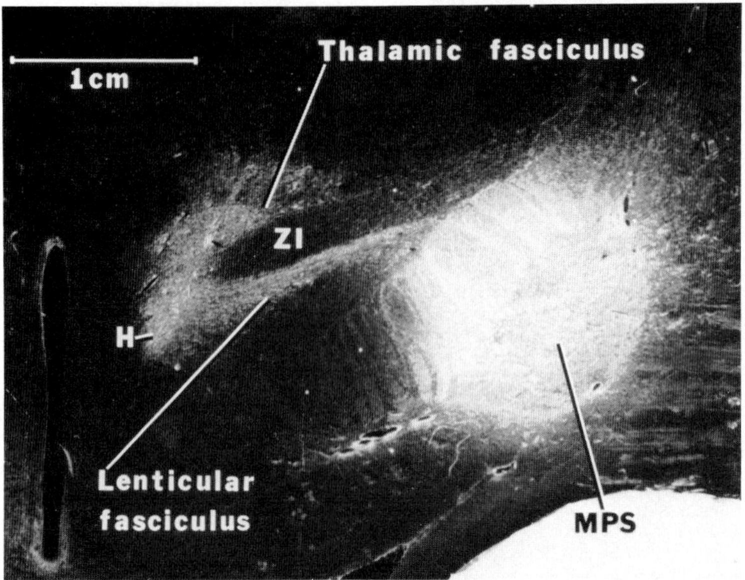

Figure 11-18. Autoradiograph of isotope transport from the medial pallidal segment (*MPS*) through the internal capsule and into the lenticular fasciculus. Continuity between the lenticular fasciculus and the thalamic fasciculus is seen in Forel's field H (*H*), medial to the zona incerta (*ZI*). (Dark-field photomicrograph from a rhesus monkey; ×16.)

fibers emerging via the ansa lenticularis and the lenticular fasciculus arise from specific portions of the medial pallidal segment (Kuo and Carpenter, '73). Fibers of the ansa lenticularis arise predominantly from the outer part of the medial pallidal segment (i.e., from that part of the medial pallidal segment lateral to the accessory medullary lamina). Fibers of the lenticular fasciculus arise mainly from the inner pallidal segment (i.e., from the portion medial to the accessory medullary lamina, Fig. 11-14).

Thalamic Fasciculus. Pallidofugal fibers from Forel's field H pass rostrally and laterally along the dorsal surface of the zona incerta where they form part of the thalamic fasciculus (Figs. 9-5, 11-15, 11-17, and 11-18). Some of the fibers of the lenticular fasciculus merely make a C-shaped loop around the medial part of the zona incerta and enter the thalamic fasciculus. The thalamic fasciculus is a complex bundle containing pallidothalamic fibers, as well as ascending fibers from the contralateral deep cerebellar nuclei. Fibers of this composite bundle project dorsolaterally over the zona incerta to terminate in specific nuclear subdivisions of the rostral ventral tier thalamic nuclei. In the region dorsal to the zona incerta, where fibers of this bundle are distinct and separate from those of the lenticular fasciculus (Figs. 11-15 and 11-18), the thalamic fasciculus is designated as bundle H_1 of Forel.

Pallidothalamic Projections. Fibers emerging from the medial pallidal segment via the ansa lenticularis and the lenticular fasciculus follow distinctive courses but merge in Forel's field H; from this area they pass rostrally and laterally as a component of the thalamic fasciculus (Figs. 11-15 and 11-18). Pallidothalamic fibers project to the ventral anterior (VApc, pars principalis) and ventral lateral (VLo, pars oralis and VLm, pars medialis) thalamic nuclei and give off collaterals which terminate in the centromedian (CM) nucleus (Figs. 11-19 and 11-20) (Nauta and Mehler, '66; Kuo and Carpenter, '73; Kim et al., '76; DeVito and Anderson, '82). Pallidal projections to the rostral ventral tier thalamic nuclei are topographically organized so that: (1) neurons in caudal and inner parts of the medial pallidal terminate mainly in VLo, and (2) neurons in outer portions of the medial pallidal segment project primarily to VApc via the ansa lenticularis (Kuo and Carpenter, '73).

There is increasing evidence that pallid-

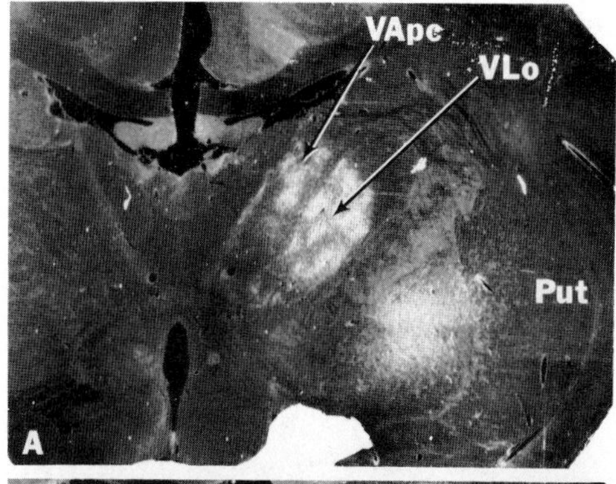

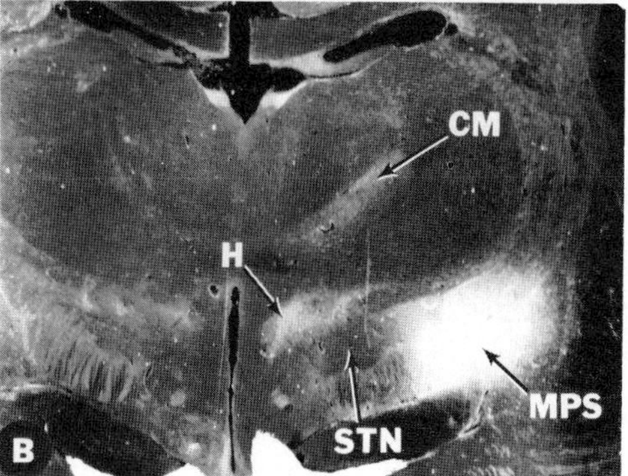

othalamic terminations do not overlap the crossed projections from the deep cerebellar nuclei (Nauta and Mehler, '66; Kuo and Carpenter, '73; Kim et al., '76; Percheron, '77; Tracey et al., '80; Asanuma et al., '83a, '83b). Cerebellothalamic projections terminate in the so-called cell-sparse zone which includes the ventral posterolateral nucleus (VPLo, pars oralis), the ventral lateral nucleus (VLc, pars caudalis), and area x of Olszewski ('52). The so-called cell-

Figure 11-19. Dark-field photomicrographs of sections through the diencephalon in a monkey demonstrating transport of [^{3}H]amino acids from the medial pallidal segment (*MPS*) to thalamic nuclei. (*A*) Transported radioactive label is distributed in a patchy fashion to the pars oralis of the ventral lateral (*VLo*) and to the principal part of the ventral anterior nuclei (*VApc*) of the thalamus. (*B*) Central region of the injection in the medial pallidal segment (*MPS*) and modest transport of the label to the centromedian nucleus (*CM*) of the thalamus. Radioactive label also is seen in Forel's field H and in lateral parts of the subthalamic nucleus (STN). (Cresyl violet; ×3.5.) (From Carpenter and Sutin, *Human Neuroanatomy*, 1983; courtesy of Williams & Wilkins.)

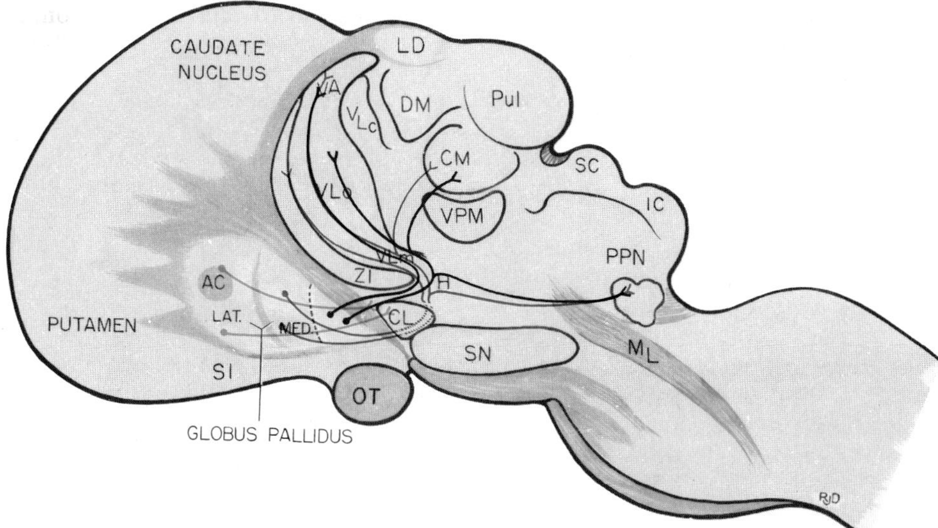

Figure 11-20. Schematic diagram of the efferent projections and terminations of pallidofugal fibers arising from the medial and lateral pallidal segments shown in a sagittal plane. Fibers of the ansa lenticularis (*red*) and lenticular fasciculus (*black*) merge in a field H of Forel. The bulk of these fibers pass in the thalamic fasciculus to the ventral lateral (*VLo* and *VLm*) and ventral anterior (*VA*) thalamic nuclei. Some fibers separating from the thalamic fasciculus project to the centromedian (*CM*) nucleus (Fig. 11-15). Descending pallidotegmental fibers from the medial pallidal segment terminate upon cells of the pedunculopontine nucleus (PPN; Fig. 11-24). Pallidosubthalamic fibers arising from the lateral pallidal segment (*blue*) project mainly to the subthalamic nucleus (CL). Other abbreviations are: *AC*, anterior commissure; *DM*, dorsomedial nucleus; *H*, Forel's field H; *IC*, inferior colliculus; *LD*, lateral dorsal nucleus; *ML*, medial lemniscus; *OT*, optic tract; *Pul*, pulvinar; *SC*, superior colliculus; *SI*, substantia innominata; *SN*, substantia nigra; *VLc*, ventral lateral nucleus, pars caudalis; *VPM*, ventral posteromedial nucleus; *ZI*, zona incerta. (From Carpenter and Sutin, *Human Neuroanatomy*, 1983; courtesy of Williams & Wilkins.)

sparse thalamic zone projects to area 4; VLo which receives pallidothalamic fibers projects to the premotor cortex (area 6) and the supplementary motor area (Asanuma et al., '83a; Schell and Strick, '84). Stimulation of the equivalent of the medial pallidal segment (i.e., entopeduncular nucleus) in the cat produces only monosynaptic inhibitory postsynaptic potentials (IPSPs) in the VA-VL nuclear complex (Uno and Yoshida, '75).

Pallidohabenular Fibers. Fibers from the medial pallidal segment projecting to the lateral habenular nucleus separate from the ansa lenticularis and the lenticular fasciculus in Forel's field H and follow a course through and around the medial part of the internal capsule to enter the stria medullaris (Nauta and Mehler, '66; Carpenter and Strominger, '67; Kim et al., '76). Double labeling studies indicate that pallidohabenular fibers arise from a different cell population than pallidothalamic fibers; most of these cells are located in a peripallidal zone which encroaches upon the lateral hypothalamus (Parent and De Bellefeuille, '82).

Pallidotegmental Fibers. The search for a descending pallidal projection in the brain stem has revealed one small pathway in which fibers could be followed only to caudal midbrain levels (Nauta and Mehler, '66; Kim et al., '76; Carpenter et al., '81; DeVito and Anderson, '82). These fibers descend from field H of Forel, ventral and lateral to the red nucleus and terminate in the compact portion of the pedunculopontine nucleus (PPN) (Figs. 11-20, 11-24, and 11-25). This nucleus is partially embedded in fibers of the superior cerebellar peduncle. Physiological and double fluorescent labeling studies in the monkey indicate that cells in the central core of the medial pallidal segment project dichotomizing axons with the same signal to thalamic nuclei and to the PPN (Harnois and Filion, '80; Parent and De Bellefeuille, '82).

The PPN in addition receives inputs from : (1) the motor cortex (Kuypers and Lawrence, '67; Hartman-von Monakow et al., '79), (2) the substantia nigra (Beckstead et al., '79; Carpenter et al., '81a; Moon Edley and Graybiel, '83), and (3) the subthalamic nucleus (Nauta and Cole, '78; Jackson and Crossman, '81; Moon Edley and Graybiel, '83). Data concerning the projections of PPN indicate it distributes fibers to the medial pallidal segment, the subthalamic nucleus, the substantia nigra, and possibly to the intralaminar thalamic nuclei (Graybiel, '77; DeVito et al., '80; Nomura et al., '80; Carpenter et al., '81, '81a; Moon Edley and Graybiel, '83). The major projection of PPN is to the ipsilateral substantia nigra (Carpenter et al., '81a; Moon Edley and Graybiel, '83). Available data suggest that descending projections from PPN are small (Moon Edley and Graybiel, '83). The precise role of PPN in the activities of the globus pallidus, substantia nigra, and the subthalamic nucleus remains undefined, but because this nucleus interrelates nuclei that have either no cortical input (e.g., globus pallidus and substantia nigra) or no reciprocal connections (e.g., substantia nigra and globus pallidus; substantia nigra and subthalamic nucleus), it may serve to integrate the activities of these nuclei.

Pallidosubthalamic Projections. The lateral pallidal segment projects mainly to the subthalamic nucleus and projections are topographically organized (Nauta and Mehler, '66; Carpenter and Strominger, '67; Carpenter et al., '68; '81, '81a). The rostral division of the lateral pallidal segment (LPS) projects to the medial two-thirds of the rostral part of the subthalamic nucleus (STN). Cells in the central division of the LPS (flanking the medial pallidal segment) project to the lateral third of the STN throughout most of its rostrocaudal extent (Figs. 11-23 and 11-26, *A* and *B*).

Physiological studies in the monkey and cat indicate that stimulation of the lateral pallidal segment (LPS), or its equivalent, produces a depression of spontaneous activity in cells of the STN (Tsubokawa and Sutin, '72; Ohye et al., '76). In the decorticated rat pallidal stimulation evoked hyperpolarizing potentials, usually followed by depolarizing potentials, considered to be monosynaptic in nature (Kita et al., '83). GABA has been suggested as the probable neurotransmitter in the pallidosubthalamic projection in the cat and rat, because the fall in GAD activity is proportional to the damage of, or blockade of, the LPS

(Fonnum et al., '78a; Rouzaire-Dubois et al., '80).

Pallidonigral Fibers. Several kinds of evidence indicate that pallidal neurons project to substantia nigra. HRP injections of the pars reticulata (SNR) produce retrograde labeling of medium-sized spiny striate neurons and large pallidal neurons, mainly in the lateral segment (Grofová, '75). Pallidonigral projections in the monkey, demonstrated autoradiogrphically by isotope injections of the medial pallidal segment, terminate mainly in the pars compacta (SNC) (Kim et al., '76). Electron microscopic analysis after intraventricular injections of 6-hydroxydopamine, suggest that pallidonigral fibers terminate preferentially upon dopaminergic neurons, while strionigral fibers synapse upon the dendrites of neurons in the pars reticulata (SNR) (Hattori et al., '75). Projections from both pallidal segments to the substantia nigra are considered to have GABA and substance P as their neurotransmitters (Hattori et al., '73; Fonnum et al., '74, '78; Jessell et al., '78; DiFiglia, '81). These projections are relatively minor compared with the massive strionigral projection. Nearly all strionigral fibers end in the SNR, while pallidal afferents to the nigra have a greater distribution upon dopaminergic neurons in the SNC (Hattori et al., '75; Kanazawa et al., '76; Carter and Fibiger, '78).

SUBSTANTIA NIGRA

The substantia nigra (SN), a large nuclear mass dorsal to the crus cerebri and divided into a pars compacta (SNC) and a pars reticulata (SNR), has important connections with the corpus striatum, the subthalamic nucleus and several brain stem nuclei (Figs. 7-9, 11-21, 11-22, and 11-23). This structure and its connections are considered in Chapter 7. Cells of the pars compacta contain high concentrations of dopamine and are recognized as the principal source of striatal dopamine (Ungerstedt, '71; Moore et al., '71). The substantia nigra also contains the highest concentrations in the nervous system of GAD, the enzyme that synthesizes GABA (Hattori et al., '73; Fahn, '76; Okada, '76). The highest concentrations of GAD are in medial parts of SNR; subcellular fractionation studies indicate that 85% of the GAD is present in particles, probably synaptosomes (Fonnum et al., '74). The substantia nigra also contains enkephalin and substance P conveyed respectively by spiny I and II striatal neurons (DiFiglia et al., '82; Gauchey et al., '79); both neurotransmitters are found in the SNR. In addition the substantia nigra contains serotonin (5-HT) and its synthesizing enzyme which are present within dense core vesicles mainly in the SNR (Reubi and Emson, '78). Most of the serotonergic fibers arise from the dorsal nucleus of the raphe (Dray et al., '78).

The substantia nigra receives afferents from the striatum, the globus pallidus, the subthalamic nucleus, the dorsal nucleus of the raphe, and the pedunculopontine nucleus (Fig. 11-25*D*). In addition the nucleus accumbens projects topographically upon both subdivisions of the substantia nigra (Swanson and Cowan, '75; Nauta et al., '78). Efferent fibers from the substantia nigra fall into two classes: (1) dopaminergic and (2) nondopaminergic. Dopaminergic fibers arise from the SNC and project to all parts of the striatum and the dorsal nucleus of the raphe (Beckstead et al., '79). Virtually all other nigrofugal fibers arise from cells of the pars reticulata. Nondopaminergic nigral efferent fibers, constituting a large part of the output system of the corpus striatum, can be grouped as: (1) nigrothalamic fibers, (2) nigrotectal fibers, and (3) nigrotegmental projections. A considerable number of cells in the SNR (estimated between 30 and 50%) project axon collaterals to both the thalamus and to superior colliculus (Bentivoglio et al., '79; Deniau et al., '78; Anderson and Yoshida, '80).

SUBTHALAMIC REGION

The subthalamic region lies ventral to the thalamus, medial to the internal capsule and lateral and caudal to the hypothalamus (Figs. 9-5, 11-15, and 11-22). Nuclei found within the subthalamic region include the subthalamic nucleus, the zona incerta, and the nuclei of the tegmental fields of Forel. Prominent fiber bundles passing through this region include the ansa lenticularis, the lenticular fasciculus (Forel's field H_2), the thalamic fasciculus

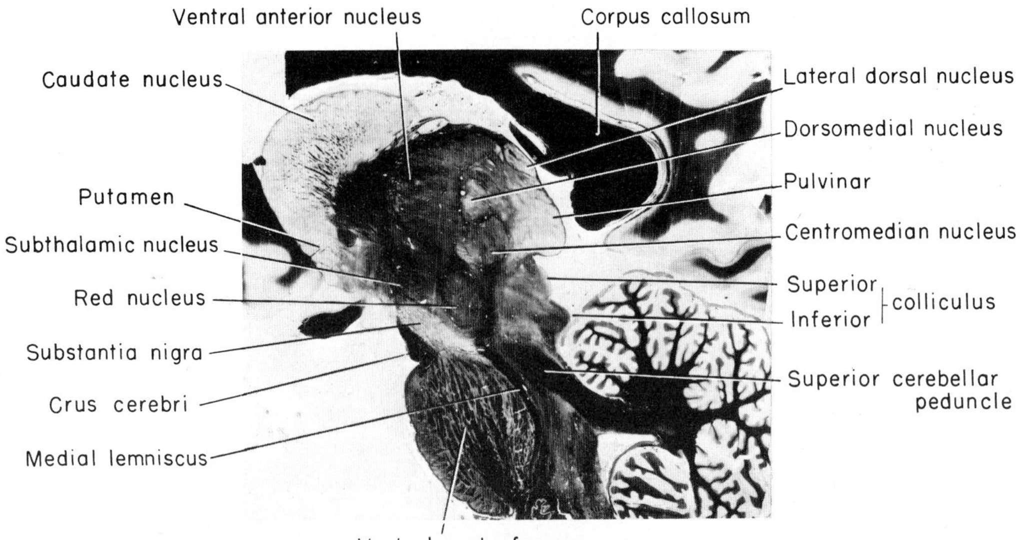

Figure 11.21. Sagittal section through medial regions of the corpus striatum, thalamus and upper brain stem, showing the relationships of caudate nucleus and putamen as well as those of the subthalamic nucleus, the red nucleus and the substantia nigra. (Weigert's myelin stain; photograph). (From Carpenter and Sutin, *Human Neuroanatomy*, 1983; courtesy of Williams & Wilkins.)

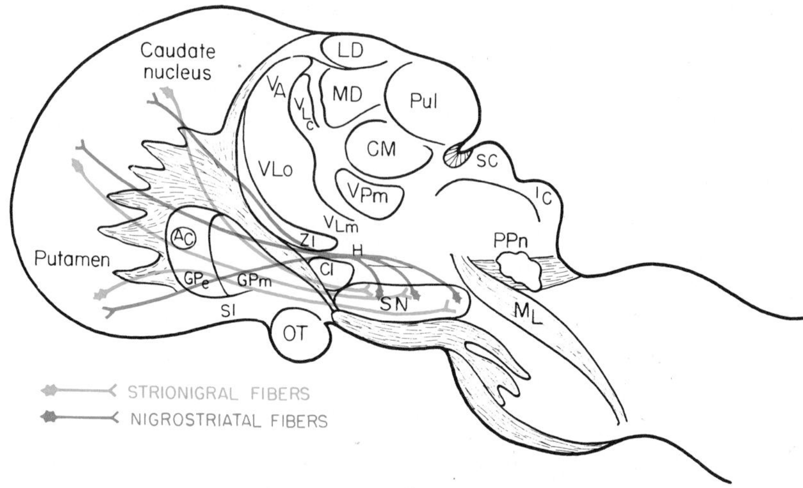

Figure 11.22. Schematic diagram of the strionigral feedback system in a sagittal plane. Strionigral fibers (*blue*) project topographically upon cells of the pars reticulata of the nigra and have GABA as their major neurotransmitter. Cells of the pars compacta of the nigra give rise to reciprocally arranged nigrostriatal fibers (*red*) which convey dopamine to specific loci within the striatum. Abbreviations used: *AC*, anterior commissure; *CM*, centromedian nucleus; *H*, Forel's field H; *IC*, inferior colliculus; *LD*, lateral dorsal nucleus; *LPS*, lateral pallidal segment; *MD*, dorsomedial nucleus; *ML*, medial lemniscus; *MPS*, medial pallidal segment; *OT*, optic tract; *PPn*, pedunculopontine nucleus; *Pul*, pulvinar; *SC*, superior colliculus; *SI*, substantia innominata; *SN*, substantia nigra; *STN*, subthalamic nucleus; *VA*, ventral anterior nucleus; *VLc*, *VLo*, and *VLm*, ventral lateral nucleus, pars caudalis, pars oralis and pars medialis, respectively; *VPm*, ventral posterior medial nucleus; *ZI*, zona incerta. (From Carpenter and Sutin, *Human Neuroanatomy*, 1983; Courtesy of Williams & Wilkins.)

(Forel's field H_1), and the subthalamic fasciculus (Fig. 11-20).

Subthalamic Nucleus. This nucleus, located on the inner surface of the peduncular portion of the internal capsule, has the shape of a thick biconvex lens (Figs. 9-4, 9-5, 11-15, 11-20, and 11-22). Caudally the medial part of the nucleus (STN)

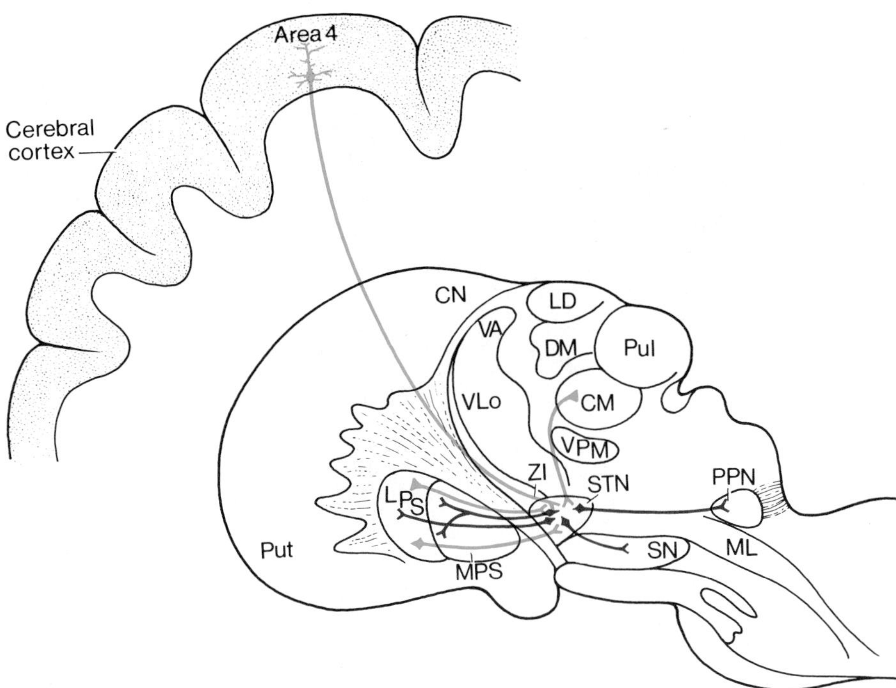

Figure 11.23. Schematic diagram of the connections of the subthalamic nucleus (*STN*) in a sagittal plane. Afferents to STN (*blue*) are derived from the motor cortex, the centromedial nucleus (CM) and the lateral pallidal segment (*LPS*). STN efferents (*red*) project to both pallidal segments, the substantia nigra (*SN*) and the pedunculopontine nucleus (*PPN*). In the rat single STN neurons project to both the pallidum and the SN (van der Kooy and Hattori, '80a). See Figure 11-22 for abbreviations.

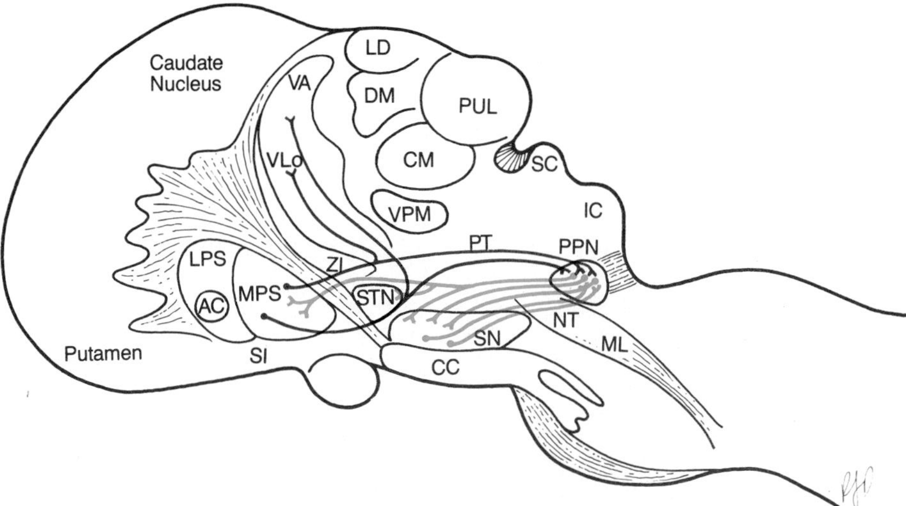

Figure 11.24. Schematic diagram of pallidotegmental (PT) and nigrotectegmental (NT) projections to pedunculopontine nucleus (PPN) in a sagittal plane. Neurons in the medial pallidal segment (MPS) give rise to ascending fibers (*red*) that project to the ventral anterior (VA) and ventral lateral (VLo) thalamic nuclei and descending collaterals (*red*) that end in PPN (Parent and De Bellefeuille, '82). Cells in the pars reticulata of the substantia nigra (SN) (*green*) also project to PPN. Ascending fibers fron PPN (*blue*) project mainly to the pars compacta of SN, although small numbers of fibers project to the MPS and the subthalamic nucleus (STN) (Carpenter et al., '81a). Abbreviations used: *AC*, anterior commissure; *CC*, crus cerebri; *CM*, centromedian nucleus; *DM*, dorsomedial nucleus; *H*, field H of Forel; *LD*, lateral dorsal nucleus; *LPS*, lateral pallidal segment; *ML*, medial lemniscus; *PUL*, pulvinar; *SC*, superior colliculus; *SI*, substantia innominata; *VPM*, ventral posteromedial nucleus; *ZI*, zona incerta.

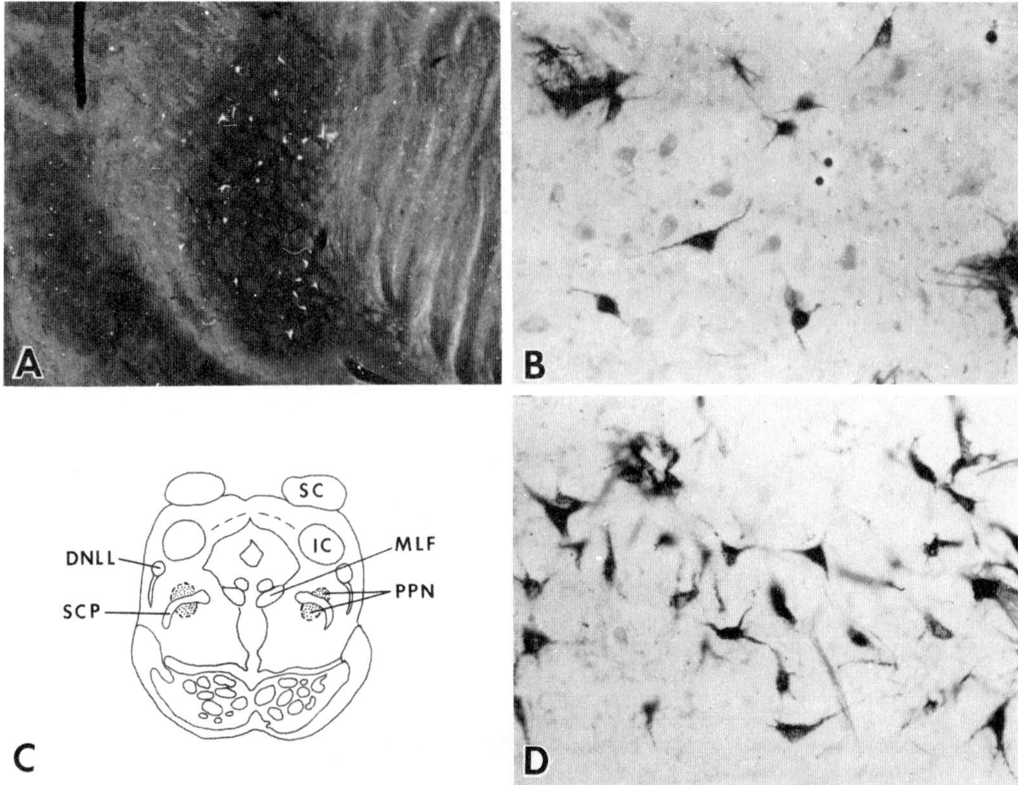

Figure 11.25. Connections of the pedunculopontine nucleus (*PPN*) in the monkey demonstrated by the retrograde transport of horseradish peroxidase (HRP). An injection of HRP into the pedunculopontine nucleus, shown diagrammatically in *C*, retrogradely labeled cells in caudal parts of the medial pallidal segment (*A*) and the pars reticulata of the substantia nigra (*B*). Cells of the pedunculopontine nucleus in *C* lie on both sides of the superior cerebellar peduncle (SCP) at caudal midbrain levels. (*D*) Photomicrograph of retrograde transport of HRP to cells of the pedunculopontine nucleus following an injection of the substantia nigra. Abbreviations used: *DNLL*, dorsal nucleus of lateral lemniscus; *IC*, inferior colliculus; *MLF*, medial longitudinal fasciculus; *SC*, superior colliculus. (*A*, dark-field, ×12; *B*, ×128; *D*, ×128.) (From Carpenter and Sutin, *Human Neuroanatomy*, 1983; courtesy of Williams & Wilkins.)

overlies rostral portions of the substantia nigra. Cells of the subthalamic nucleus are spindle-shaped, pyramidal, or round with branching processes, and their concentration has been described as varying in different parts of the nucleus. Statistical and comparative analyses strongly suggest there is only one variety of Golgi type I neuron in the subthalamic nucleus which is nearly identical in cat, monkey, and man (Yellnik and Percheron, '79). Fluorescent double labeling studies in the rat indicated that virtually all STN neurons (94%) are projection neurons (van der Kooy and Hattori, '80a). Each STN neuron gives rise to 6 or 7 dendritic stems which branch successively into an ellipsoidal domain, usually parallel with the rostrocaudal axis of the nucleus. Dendritic spines are not numerous and most often are located distally. Comparisons of dendritic morphology in the rat and primate indicate: (1) a smaller number of dendritic stems and a larger number of dendritic branching points in the rat, and (2) similar ellipsoidal dendritic arborizations. The dendritic field of a single subthalamic neuron in the rat is calculated to cover the entire nucleus, while in the cat it would cover only half of the nucleus; the dendritic field would cover a fifth of the nucleus in the monkey and a ninth of the nucleus in man (Hammond and Yelnik, '83). Thus, while subthalamic nucleus neurons in rat and primate are similar, their relationships to the nucleus as a whole have evolved to confer upon the primate the potential for a much more specific organization. An important feature disclosed by HRP intracellularly labeled neurons is the presence of axonal collaterals on one group of STN cells (Kita et al., '83a). Neurons in the subthalamic nucleus can be divided into two groups: (1) projection neurons and (2) projection neurons with axonal collaterals distributed within the STN. Although almost all STN neurons project to both the globus pallidus and the substantia nigra, axonal branches projecting to the pallidum are thicker. While subthalamic nucleus is small in the monkey, its relative size is essentially the same as in the human.

Afferents to the Subthalamic Nucleus. Afferent projections to the subthalamic nucleus which have a firm anatomical basis arise from the motor, premotor and prefrontal cortex, the thalamus, the lateral pallidal segment and the pedunculopontine nucleus (PPN). The dominant input to the STN arises from the lateral pallidal segment (Figs. 11-26, *A* and *B*).

Corticosubthalamic Fibers. Although degeneration studies suggested that the STN received very few cortical projections, autoradiographic findings in the monkey have established this afferent connection (Künzle and Akert, '77). A systematic analysis revealed an ipsilateral somatotopically organized projection from the precentral motor cortex to the STN, restricted to the lateral moiety (Fig. 11-23) (Hartmann-von Monakow et al., '78). The somatotopic arrangement demonstrated a face region along the laterodorsal border of the nucleus, a leg region more central, and an arm area between these representations. Area 6 projections, and those from areas 8 and 9, were to more medial and ventral regions of the nucleus. Electron microscopic confirmation of corticosubthalamic fibers indicated terminations by asymmetrical synapses on small distal dendrites and spines (Romansky et al., '79). Physiological data indicate that corticosubthalamic fibers have an excitatory monosynaptic action upon STN neurons (Kitai and Deniau, '81).

Thalamosubthalamic Fibers. A relatively small, but definite, projection from the centromedian-parafascicular nuclear complex (CM-PF) has been established in the rat and the cat by axoplasmic transport studies (Sugimoto et al., '83). Cells in CM-PF giving rise to this projection are scattered throughout the complex and have no unique morphological features; projections of these cells are most concentrated in ventral and ventromedial regions of the rostral third of the STN (Fig. 11-23). Electron microscopic autoradiography indicates that terminal fibers have asymmetrical boutons with round synaptic vesicles (Sugimoto and Hattori, '83). It has been suggested that some cells in CM-PF may project collateral fibers to both the striatum and the STN.

Pallidosubthalamic Projections. The most massive input system to the STN arises from the lateral pallidal segment (Nauta and Mehler, '66; Kim et al., '76; Carpenter et al., '68, '81, '81a). This topographically organized pathway was described earlier in the section concerning pallidal efferent fibers (see p. 310 and Figs. 11-15, 11-20, and 11-26). Data in the monkey show that even though the STN is a small nucleus it appears to have input and output regions (Carpenter et al., '81). The lateral third of the STN receives the bulk of the inputs originating from the lateral pallidal segment (LPS) and the motor cortex, the two largest afferent systems (Fig. 11-26*B*). The rostromedial part of the STN receives inputs from the rostral part of the LPS and from CM-PF (Fig. 11-26*A*). It is significant that cells in the medial and caudal parts of STN project predominantly to the medial pallidal segment and that few, if any, subthalamopallidal fibers arise from the lateral third of the STN.

Tegmentosubthalamic Fibers. The pedunculopontine nucleus (PPN) which receives inputs from the cerebral cortex, the medial pallidal segment and the pars reticulata of the substantia nigra (SNR), is considered to project directly to the subthalamic nucleus. Both anterograde and retrograde transport studies in the cat have demonstrated this projection (Nomura et al., '80; Moon Edley and Graybiel, '83). Autoradiographic data also reveal projections from PPN to the zona incerta, the SNC and the intralaminar thalamic nuclei. The subthalamic nucleus is considered to give rise to a small projection to PPN (Nauta and Cole, '78; Jackson and Crossman, '81; Moon Edley and Graybiel, '83).

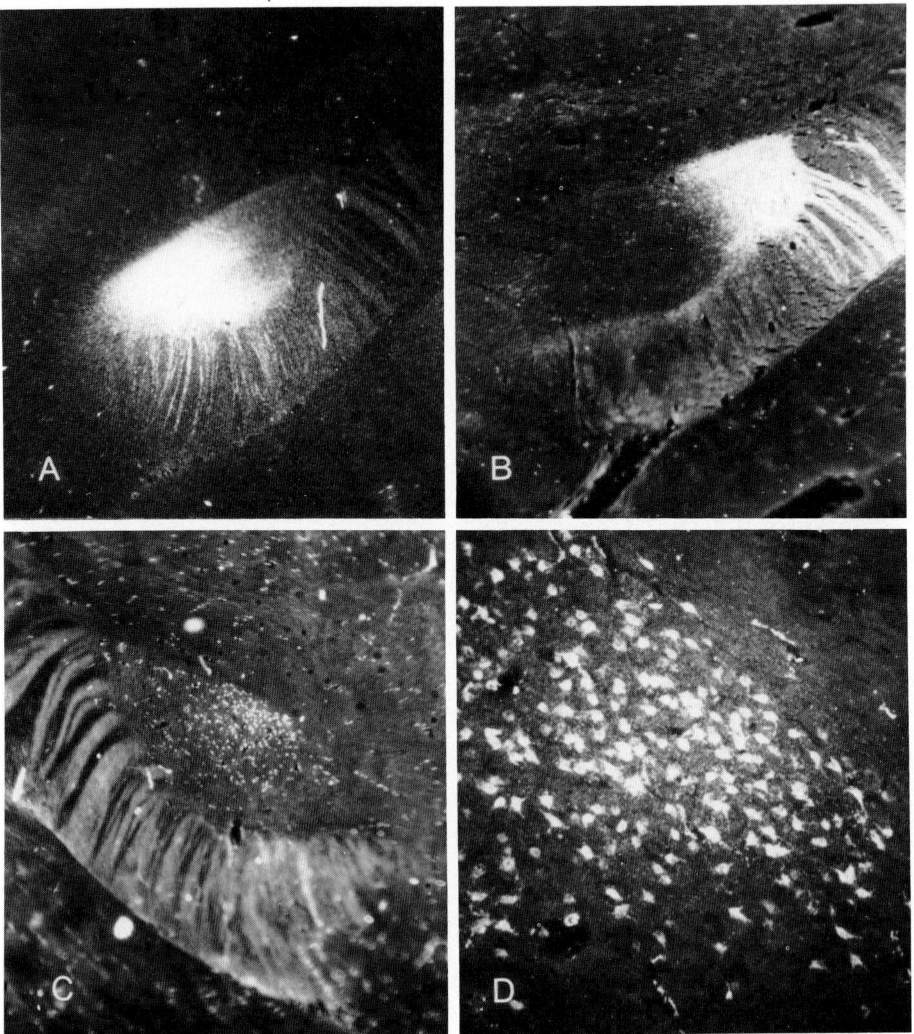

Figure 11.26. Dark-field photomicrographs of the subthalamic nucleus (STN) in the monkey, demonstrating connections with the globus pallidus. *A* and *B* are autoradiographs of [^{3}H]amino acids transported from the lateral pallidal segment (LPS) to the STN. Fibers from the rostral part of the LPS project to medial part of STN rostrally (*A*), while central portions of the LPS flanking the medial pallidal segment project to lateral third of the STN in its central part (*B*) (*C* and *D*) Retrograde transport of horseradish peroxidase (HRP) to cells of the STN following injection of the enzyme into the central part of the lateral pallidal segment. (From Carpenter and Sutin, *Human Neuroanatomy*, 1983; courtesy of Williams & Wilkins.)

Reciprocal connections between PPN and STN appear relatively minor compared with those that interrelate PPN with the substantia nigra and with the medial pallidal segment.

Subthalamic Efferent Projections. The major efferents from the subthalamic nucleus (STN) project to both segments of the globus pallidus and to the substantia nigra (Figs. 11-23 and 11-26, *C* and *D*). Each of these pathways has been discussed separately in relation to pallidal and nigral afferent systems (see pp. 306 and 194).

Considerable evidence suggests that single cells in the STN project fibers to both pallidal segments and to the pars reticulata of the SN (Deniau et al., '78; van der Kooy and Hattori, '80a; Carpenter et al., '81a; Kita et al., '83). Branches of axon collaterals projecting to globus pallidus are thicker than those passing to the SN and have faster rates of conduction (Kita et al.,

'83; '83a). In the rat subthalamopallidal collaterals of branches to the globus pallidal terminate within the entopeduncular nucleus, the equivalent of the primate medial pallidal segment. Stimulation of the STN in the rat produces short latency inhibition in the entopeduncular nucleus (pallidum) and short latency excitation in the substantia nigra (Hammond et al., '78, '83). Dural responses of a different nature are not fully explained, but are presumed to involve local interneurons.

Subthalamic Fasciculus. This bundle consists of fibers from the lateral pallidal segment that project to the STN and fibers from the STN which project to both pallidal segments. These fibers project through peduncular portions of the internal capsule caudal to the lenticular fasciculus (Fig. 11-15).

In man relatively discrete lesions in the STN, usually hemorrhagic, give rise to violent, forceful, and persistent choreoid movements, referred to as *hemiballism.* These unusually violent involuntary movements occur contralateral to the lesion and involve primarily the proximal musculature of the upper and lower extremities, though they may involve the facial and cervical musculature (Whittier, '47).

Zona Incerta. This structure is a strip of gray matter situated between the thalamic and lenticular fasciculi (Figs. 9-5 and 11-15). It is composed of diffuse cell groups which laterally are continuous with the thalamic reticular nucleus. This zone receives corticofugal fibers from the precentral cortex.

Prerubral Field (Forel's Field H). This field contains pallidofugal fibers and scattered cells which constitute the nucleus of the prerubral field (Figs. 9-5, 11-15 and 11-22). The nuclei of the prerubral field, together with similar cells scattered along pallidofugal pathways, have been referred to collectively as the *subthalamic reticular nucleus.*

FUNCTIONAL CONSIDERATIONS

Over 70 years ago Wilson ('12) introduced the term "extrapyramidal" motor system (without definition) in his classic description of hepatolenticular degeneration, a familial disorder of copper metabolism characterized by degeneration of the striatum, cirrhosis of the liver, flapping tremor, muscular rigidity, and a golden-brown pigmentation of the cornea (i.e., the Kayser-Fleischer ring). There seemed to be no question that the corpus striatum formed the centerpiece of this so-called system. Although this term has been defined, debated, and interpreted in innumerable ways, it now appears generally accepted that the corpus striatum has meaningful connections with only a limited array of brain stem nuclei, chief among which are the substantia nigra, the subthalamic nucleus, and portions of the ventral tier thalamic nuclei. Whether the corpus striatum and this limited array of brain stem nuclei form a system hardly needs to be debated. However, the weight of available evidence suggests that the so-called extrapyramidal system is not a complete and independent motor system. The corpus striatum and related nuclei exert their influences upon motor activities by way of thalamic neurons that project upon motor cortical areas. Motor cortical neurons, whose activities are modulated by thalamic neurons, project fibers to, and exert motor control, at all levels of the neuraxis, mainly contralaterally. Neither the corpus striatum nor anatomically related brain stem nuclei project directly to spinal levels.

The corpus striatum, subthalamic nucleus, substantia nigra, and pedunculopontine nucleus are interrelated with each other by an orderly linkage and with specific parts of the neuraxis that can modulate somatic motor activities. The striatum, representing the receptive component of the corpus striatum, receives inputs from broad regions of the cerebral cortex, the intralaminar thalamic nuclei, the substantia nigra, and the midbrain raphe nuclei. Impulses from these sources are mediated by a variety of different neurotransmitters, most of which appear to be excitatory. Striatal output, originating from two types of spiny neurons, projects to both segments of the globus pallidus and the pars reticulata of the substantia nigra. GABA is the principal neurotransmitter in striopallidal and strionigral fiber systems, but some fibers of both projections have enkephalin and substance P as their neurotransmitter.

The output systems of the corpus striatum arise from morphologically similar cells in the medial pallidal segment (MPS) and the pars reticulata of the substantia nigra. Thalamic projections of the medial pallidal segment and the pars reticulata of the substantia nigra (SNR) are distinctive without overlap; nuclear subdivisions of the thalamus receiving these outputs do not exert their major effects upon the primary motor cortex. Thalamic relay nuclei influenced by the output of the MPS appear to project to the premotor and supplementary motor areas. Most physiological data suggest that pallidothalamic and nigrothalamic projections exert primarily inhibitory effects upon thalamic neurons. It seems likely that striatal inhibition of neurons in the MPS and SNR projecting to the thalamus may result in disinhibition of thalamic neurons which act upon the cortical neurons.

The substantia nigra receives inputs from both components of the corpus striatum (i.e., striatum and pallidum) and from all closely related subcortical nuclei (i.e., the subthalamic nucleus, the pedunculopontine nucleus, and the dorsal nucleus of the raphe). The major output of the substantia nigra (pars compacta), exclusive of that to the thalamus and tectum, conveys dopamine to the striatum (Carpenter et al., '76). The subthalamic nucleus in comparison to the substantia nigra receives major inputs from only two sources, the lateral pallidal segment and the motor cortex. A single type of subthalamic nucleus neuron projects collateral branches to the globus pallidus and the pars reticulata of the substantia nigra. The neurotransmitter of subthalamopallidal fibers appears to be GABA; subthalamonigral fibers appear to convey excitatory influences, but the neurotransmitters involved are unknown. Efferents of the subthalamic nucleus appear organized in a manner to modulate the activities of output systems originating from the medial pallidal segment and the pars reticulata of the substantia nigra.

Clinically two basic types of disturbances are associated with diseases of the corpus striatum. These disturbances are: (1) various types of abnormal involuntary movements, referred to as *dyskinesia*, and (2) disturbances of muscle tone. Types of dyskinesia occurring in association with these diseases include *tremor*, *athetosis*, *chorea*, and *ballism*.

Tremor. This, the most common form of dyskinesia, is a rhythmical, alternating, abnormal involuntary activity having a relatively regular frequency and amplitude. A major clinical criterion used to describe and classify different tremors is whether the tremor occurs "at rest" or during voluntary movement. The type of tremor commonly seen in paralysis agitans (parkinsonism), involves primarily the digits, the head and the lips, and occurs during the absence of voluntary movement. During voluntary movement the tremor ceases. Tremor classically associated with cerebellar lesions becomes evident during voluntary and associated movements and ceases when the patient is "at rest." Tremor also is seen in association with weakness (paresis), emotional excitement and as a side effect of a variety of drugs. In general tremor is exaggerated when the patient is anxious, self-conscious, or exposed to cold. Tremor disappears during sleep and under general anesthesia.

Athetosis. This term is used to designate slow, writhing, vermicular involuntary movements, involving particularly the extremities. It may involve also the axial muscle groups and the muscles of the face and neck. The movements blend with each other to give the appearance of a continuous mobile spasm. Athetoid movements involving primarily the axial musculature produce severe torsion of the neck, shoulder girdle, and pelvic girdle. This form of the disturbance, referred to as *torsion spasm* or *torsion dystonia*, is considered as a variant of athetosis; differences between torsion dystonia and athetosis are considered to be due largely to inherent mechanical differences between axial and appendicular musculature.

Chorea. Chorea is a brisk, graceful series of successive involuntary movements of considerable complexity which resemble fragments of purposeful voluntary movements. These movements involve primarily the distal portions of the extremities, the muscles of facial expression, the tongue, and the deglutitional musculature. Most forms of choreoid activity are associated with hypotonus. *Sydenham's chorea* occurs in childhood in association with rheumatic heart disease, and most patients make a complete recovery from this form of chorea. *Huntington's chorea* is a hereditary disorder characterized by choreiform movements and progressive dementia. Although sporadic cases occur, the disorder is inherited as a Mendelian dominant.

Ballism. Ballism, a violent, forceful, flinging movement, involves primarily the proximal appendicular musculature, and muscles about the shoulder and pelvic girdles. It represents the most violent form of dyskinesia known. Ballism is almost invariably associated with discrete lesions in the subthalamic nucleus or its connections. The dyskinesia occurs contralateral to the lesion and is associated with marked hypotonus.

Although athetosis, chorea, and ballism each present distinguishing features, basic resemblances among these forms of dyskinesia probably are greater than their differences (Carpenter, '58). Characteristics common to these dyskinesias include: (1) variable amplitude and frequency, (2) occurrance of movements in immediate and delayed sequence, (3) variations in the duration of single movements, and (4) a highly integrated, complex activity pattern. While each of these types of involuntary motor activity is specialized to a degree, there are indications that athetosis, chorea, and ballism may form a spectrum of choreoid activity in which athetosis and ballism represent extreme forms. Although it is customary to associate increased muscle tonus with most syndromes of the corpus striatum, this is not always found. The initial symptom of paralysis agitans is frequently a *rigidity* of the muscles, which gradually increases over a period of years. The increase in muscle tone is present to a nearly equal degree in antagonistic muscle groups (i.e., in both flexor and extensor muscles). Rigidity in the early stages can be demonstrated by passively flexing or extending the muscles of the extremities, or by attempting to rotate the hand in a circular fashion at the wrist. These movements are interrupted by a series of jerks, referred to as the cogwheel phenomenon. In later stages of the disease rigidity may be so severe as to completely incapacitate the patient.

Athetosis usually is associated with variable degrees of paresis and spasticity. It is suggested that the slow, writhing character of this dyskinesia may be due in part to the associated spasticity. Although muscle tone is increased greatly during athetoid movements and persists after the completion of the movement, muscle tone may thereafter gradually diminish. Chorea and ballism usually are associated with variable degrees of hypotonus.

NEURAL MECHANISMS INVOLVED IN DYSKINESIA

The various types of dyskinesia and excesses of muscle tone associated with diseases of the corpus striatum and related nuclei are regarded as positive disturbances. Such disturbances cannot arise directly from destruction of specific neural structures, but must represent the functional capacity of surviving intact structures. Accordingly positive disturbances, such as tremor, athetosis, chorea, and ballism, are believed to be the result of release phenomena. This theory implies that a lesion in one structure removes the controlling and regulating influences which that structure previously exerted upon another neural mechanism. This concept forms the basis for neurosurgical attempts to alleviate and abolish dyskinesia and increased muscle tone without producing paresis. However, not all disturbances associated with diseases of the corpus striatum can be regarded as positive phenomena. Patients with paralysis agitans also exhibit a mask-like face, infrequent blinking of the eyes, a slow dysparthric speech, a stooped posture, a slow shuffling gait, loss of associated movements (e.g., swinging of the arms while walking), slowness of voluntary movements (bradykinesia), and general poverty of movements. These disturbances can be regarded as negative symptoms. The negative symptoms of parkinsonism largely concern disorders of postural fixation, equilibrium, locomotion, phonation, and articulation, and are considered to be deficits due to destroyed neural structures (Martin and Hurwitz, '62; Martin, '67).

Clinicopathological studies of most forms

of dyskinesia, categorized as extrapyramidal, indicate widespread neuropathological changes. In these disorders the corpora striata suffer severe pathological alterations, but specific brain stem nuclei and parts of the cerebral cortex may be affected also. In parkinsonism (paralysis agitans) pathological changes most consistently affect the substantia nigra. In parkinsonism there is a virtual absence of dopamine in the neostriatum and substantia nigra (Hornykiewicz, '66). This finding suggests that in parkinsonism there exists a decreased ability of the affected brain tissues to form dopamine. Dopamine, formed in the large cells of the pars compacts of the nigra, is conveyed to the neostriatum via nigrostriatal fibers and stored in nerve terminals. Data based upon intracellular recordings suggest that dopamine released by stimulating the substantia nigra is excitatory (Kitai et al., '76; Kitai, '81; Wilson et al., '82). Both striopallidal and strionigral projections have GABA as their principal neurotransmitter (Bak et al., '75; Jessell et al., '78; Ribak, '81). Since GABA is regarded as an inhibitory transmitter, neurons in both the pallidum and the pars reticulata of the substantia nigra may be inhibited by striatal efferents. The above rationale forms the basis for giving L-dihydroxyphenylalanine (L-dopa) in the treatment of parkinsonism. This compound passes the blood-brain barrier and is a precursor of dopamine. The effectiveness of L-dopa can be enhanced by the use of a peripheral decarboxylase inhibitor which prevents systemic decarboxylation of L-dopa to dopamine.

Athetosis most frequently is associated with pathological processes involving the striatum and cerebral cortex, though lesions are sometimes found in the globus pallidus and thalamus (Carpenter, '50). Hemiathetosis may develop after a hemiparesis, or in association with it, as a consequence of a necrotizing cerebrovascular lesion destroying portions of the internal capsule and striatum (Figs. 14-9 and 14-10). Athetoid activity occurs contralateral to the lesion.

With respect to chorea, there is relatively little information available, except concerning chronic progressive chorea, or Huntington's chorea. This hereditary disease is characterized by an insidious onset in adult life. Pathological changes are widespread but have a special predilection for the cerebral cortex and striatum.

In brains of patients dying with Huntington's chorea (Bird and Iversen, '74) it has been demonstrated that striatal neurons have reduced concentrations of glutamic acid decarboxylase (GAD), γ-aminobutyric acid (GABA) and choline acetyltransferase (ChAc). GAD is the enzyme responsible for the biosynthesis of GABA and is localized mainly in inhibitory neurons which release GABA as their transmitter (Iversen, '72). In these same patients concentrations of tyrosine hydroxylase (T-OH) and dopamine were normal in the corpus striatum. The most consistent lesion in Huntington's chorea appears to be a loss of GABA-containing neurons in the corpus striatum. It is well known that L-dopa given in large doses to patients with Parkinson's disease may cause choreiform movements to appear. L-Dopa also tends to exacerbate choreiform activity in patients with Huntington's chorea. The most effective drugs for ameliorating choreiform dyskinesia are those which deplete catecholamines, such as reserpine and dopamine receptor antagonists. The presence of normal dopaminergic systems in association with reduced availability of GABA (and often acetylcholine) may be the key neuropharmacological feature of Huntington's chorea (Bird and Iversen, '74). Clinical attempts to overcome deficiencies of GABA and acetycholine by administering GABA-mimetic drugs or inhibitors of acetylcholine hydrolysis have so far met with limited success. This has been explained by the inability of GABA or the GABA agonist imidazoleacetic acid to cross the blood-brain barrier in sufficient concentrations.

The biochemical changes which characterize Huntington's (chorea) disease in humans can be mimicked in the rat by striatal injections of kainic acid, an analogue of glutamate (Schwarcz and Coyle, '77; Mason and Fibiger, '78). After injections of kainic acid, the activities of GAD and ChAc were reduced 80% whereas the activity of T-OH was increased 80%. The striatal content of dopamine and the synaptosomal uptake of dopamine were unchanged. The neurotoxic effects of kainic acid appear related to the excessive stimulation of glutamate receptors that results in degeneration, first in cell somata and then in dendrites and axons (Schwarcz and Coyle, '77; Hattori and McGeer, '77). The long-term effects of striatal kainic acid lesions and the reduction in activities of GABA-ergic and cholinergic neurons are not as severe as those in Huntington's disease (Zaczek, et al., '78).

Ballism appears to be the only form of dyskinesia resulting from a discrete lesion. The lesion usually is confined to the subthalamic nucleus or its immediate connections (Whittier, '47).

Attempts to produce dyskinesia in experimental animals by creating lesions in parts of the basal ganglia have been notoriously unsuccessful. For reasons not understood, lesions destroying large parts of the substantia nigra do not produce any of the disturbances associated with parkinsonism, although these lesions destroy large parts of the nigrostriatal dopamine system (Carpenter and McMasters, '64).

Recently it has been discovered that a meperidine-analog (1-methyl-4-phenyl-4-1,2,56-tetrahydropyridine, MPTP) appearing in illicit drugs (cocaine-meperidine) in concentrations of 2.5 to 3% was sufficient when given intravenously to produce a chronic form of parkinsonism (Langston et al., '83). This compound was the product of a clandestine laboratory attempting to synthesize 1-methyl-4-phenyl-4-propionoxy-piperdine (MPPP). Individuals taking this drug and hospitalized 2 to 6 weeks after its first use have presented a classic picture of Parkinson's disease. In a patient who died of a drug overdose, moderately severe destruction within the substantia nigra was comparable in severity with that seen in idiopathic parkinsonism. All patients exhibiting this syndrome responded to L-dopa and carbidopa. Using this meperidine-analog, it has been possible to produce in the monkey a model of Parkinson's disease with all the major clinical features (Kolata, '83). This meperidine-analog selectively destroys cells of the substantia nigra that produce dopamine.

The only other form of dyskinesia, aside from cerebellar tremor, produced in an experimental animal is that resulting from discrete lesions in the subthalamic nucleus. This dyskinesia closely resembles that which occurs in man with lesions in the same nucleus. In the monkey, violent choreoid and ballistic activity occurs contralateral to localized lesions in the subthalamic nucleus which: (1) destroy approximately 20% of the nucleus, and (2) preserve the integrity of surrounding pallidofugal fiber systems. This abnormal involuntary activity has been called subthalamic dyskinesia (Whittier and Mettler, '49; Carpenter et al., '50). Subthalamic dyskinesia in the monkey is enduring, associated with distinct hypotonus and can be ameliorated or abolished contralaterally by subsequent stereotaxic lesions in the medial pallidal segment, the ventral lateral nucleus of the thalamic and the motor cortex (Carpenter et al., '50; Carpenter and Mettler, '51; Carpenter, '61). Subthalamic dyskinesia produced in the rhesus monkey by discrete lesions of the subthalamic nucleus (STN) has been considered to be the physiological expression of the removal of inhibitory influences, generated in the STN, which normally act upon the medial segment of the globus pallidus. Lesions destroying up to 20% of the volume of the substantia nigra and producing extensive cell loss in the pars compacta had no effect upon subthalamic dyskinesia (Strominger and Carpenter, '65). Subthalamic dyskinesia has been produced in the monkey by small injections of kainic acid into the STN; dyskinesia appeared on the third postoperative day and was identical to that resulting from electrolytic lesions (Hammond et al., '79). The most illuminating development has been the production of subthalamic dyskinesia in the baboon and monkey by localized injections of GABA antagonists, picrotoxin and bicuculline methiodide, into awake animals via implanted cannulae (Crossman et al., '80; '84). The latency from injection of the GABA antagonist to appearance of unequivocal dyskinesia varied from 5 to 125 minutes and was shortest in well-targeted injections. The duration of the dyskinesia varied from 2 to 4 hours and was followed by an uneventful recovery. These data suggest interruption, or pharmacological blockade, of subthalamopallidal fibers having GABA as their neurotransmitter may be the essential feature in the neural mechanism of subthalamic dyskinesia.

Surgical attempts to ameliorate and abolish various forms of dyskinesia and excesses of muscle tone are based on the thesis that these disturbances are the physiological expression of release phenomena. This implies that disease or pathological alterations of certain neural structures have removed inhibitory influences normally acting upon other intact neural structures, and that this overactivity, or excessive function, is responsible for the dyskinesia. Thus, attention has been focused mainly upon the globus pallidus and the ventral lateral nucleus of the thalamus, since these structures appear to be of greatest importance in the subcortical integration of nonpyramidal motor function. In many instances localized lesions produced by various technics in these structures have abolished, or significantly reduced, many forms of dyskinesia.

The cerebral cortex is acknowledged to play an important role in the neural mechanisms of all forms of dyskinesia. Almost all forms of abnormal involuntary movement cease during sleep and are abolished by general anesthesia. Most forms of dyskinesia are exaggerated in situations where the patient becomes self-conscious, overly anxious, or excited. The fact that ablations of the motor cortex or interruption of the corticospinal tract at various locations abolish dyskinesia suggests that impulses responsible for the dyskinesia probably are transmitted to segmental levels via the corticospinal tract.

CHAPTER 12

Olfactory Pathways, Hippocampal Formation, and the Amygdala

The term rhinencephalon refers to the olfactory brain. Although some authors use this term broadly to include those regions of the brain concerned with both the reception and integration of olfactory information, not all regions of the brain from which potentials can be recorded in response to olfactory stimulation are concerned exclusively with olfactory sense. Some of these regions have lost their original olfactory specificity. A strict definition of the rhinencephalon includes the olfactory bulb, tract, tubercle and striae, the anterior olfactory nucleus, parts of the amygdaloid complex, and parts of the prepyriform cortex. The term rhinencephalon, in this restricted sense, is equivalent to the *paleopallium* or primitive olfactory lobe (Valverde, '65). The *archipallium*, the oldest cortical derivative, is represented by the hippocampal formation, the dentate gyrus, the fasciolar gyrus and the indusium griseum (supracallosal gyrus). The hippocampal formation reaches its greatest development in microsomatic man and is well formed in anosomatic cetaceans, some of which lack olfactory bulbs.

OLFACTORY PATHWAYS

Olfactory Receptors. The olfactory membrane is a yellowish brown patch of specialized epithelium in the upper part of the nasal cavity. Olfactory receptors are located in this membrane (Fig. 12-1). Small sensory cells scattered among supporting cells in the olfactory epithelium have two processes, a coarse peripheral one, passing to the surface, and a fine central one, projecting through the basement membrane. From the coarse peripheral processes a variable number of short olfactory hairs arise. The delicate central processes, which constitute the unmyelinated *olfactoria fila*, converge to form small fascicles and pass from nasal cavity via foramina in the cribriform plate of the ethmoid bone. These exceedingly small fibers, with a very slow conduction rate, enter the ventral surface of the olfactory bulb. The olfactory fila,

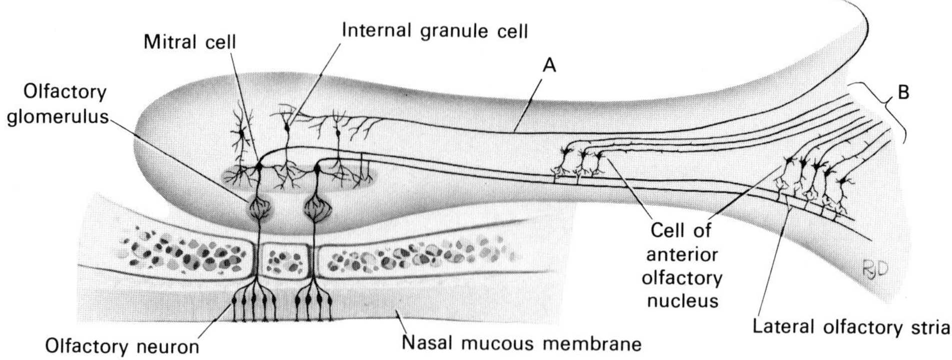

Figure 12-1. Diagram of the olfactory bulb and tract showing relationships of the olfactory receptors and neurons in the nasal mucosa with cells in the olfactory bulb. Cells of the anterior olfactory nucleus form scattered groups caudal to the olfactory bulb. Centrally projecting fibers from the anterior olfactory nucleus are labeled *B*, while a fiber from the contralateral anterior olfactory nucleus is labeled *A* (after Cajal, '11).

representing the central processes of bipolar cells in the olfactory epithelium, collectively constitute the *olfactory nerve* (N. I.). Morphologically the olfactory epithelium represents a primitive type of sensory cell which supports the concept that olfaction is the oldest and most primitive of the special senses. The olfactory receptor is a bipolar neuron with a life span measured in days; new axons are continually growing into the olfactory bulb and form new synapses.

Olfactory Bulb. This flattened ovoid body resting on the cribriform plate of the ethmoid bone is the terminal "nucleus" of the olfactory nerve (Figs. 12-1 and 12-2). Most of the fibers of the olfactory nerve enter the anterior tip of the olfactory bulb. Structurally the olfactory bulb has a laminar organization, but in man this is difficult to demonstrate. Within the gray matter of the olfactory bulb are several types of nerve cells, the most striking of which are the large, triangular *mitral cells,* so named because of their resemblance to a bishop's mitre (Figs. 12-1 and 12-3). Primary olfactory fibers synapse with the brushlike terminals of vertically descending dendrites of the mitral cells to form the *olfactory glomeruli.* Smaller cells of the olfactory bulb, known as *tufted cells,* have a number of dendrites, one of which participates in the formation of the glomerulus. Granule cells of various sizes are found throughout the olfactory bulb but are most dense toward the center of the bulb, forming the granular cell layer (Fig. 12-3; Price and Powell, '70). Granule cells have no axons, and their dendrites have spines, or gemmules, which form dendrodendritic synapses with mitral cells. The morphological features of these junctions suggest dual synapses; one from granule cell to mitral cell, and one from mitral cell to granule cell (Fig. 12-3). This arrangement is called a reciprocal synapse. Granule cells inhibit mitral cells, and the mitral cells appear to excite the granule cells (Getchell and Shepherd, '75). Although afferent fibers in the olfactory bulb do not appear to be localized in any patterned way (Clark and Warwick, '46), a regional organization of olfactory nerve projections to the olfactory bulb has been demonstrated in mammals (Adrian, '42; Clark, '51, '57). Localized lesions in different regions of the olfactory epithelium produce degeneration in specific regions of the glomerular layer (Land, '73). Groupings of glomeruli show marked variations in the intensity of degeneration and some normal glomeruli are present in regions containing degeneration. A selective projection from receptors in small regions of the olfactory epithelium to specific glomeruli, or groups of glomeruli, could provide the anatomical basis for selective responses to odors. Axons of the mitral and tufted cells enter the olfactory tract as *secondary olfactory fibers* (Fig. 12-1).

Caudal to the olfactory bulb are scattered groups of neurons, intermediate in size between mitral and granule cells, that form the *anterior olfactory nucleus* (Fig. 12-4). Some cells of this loosely organized nucleus

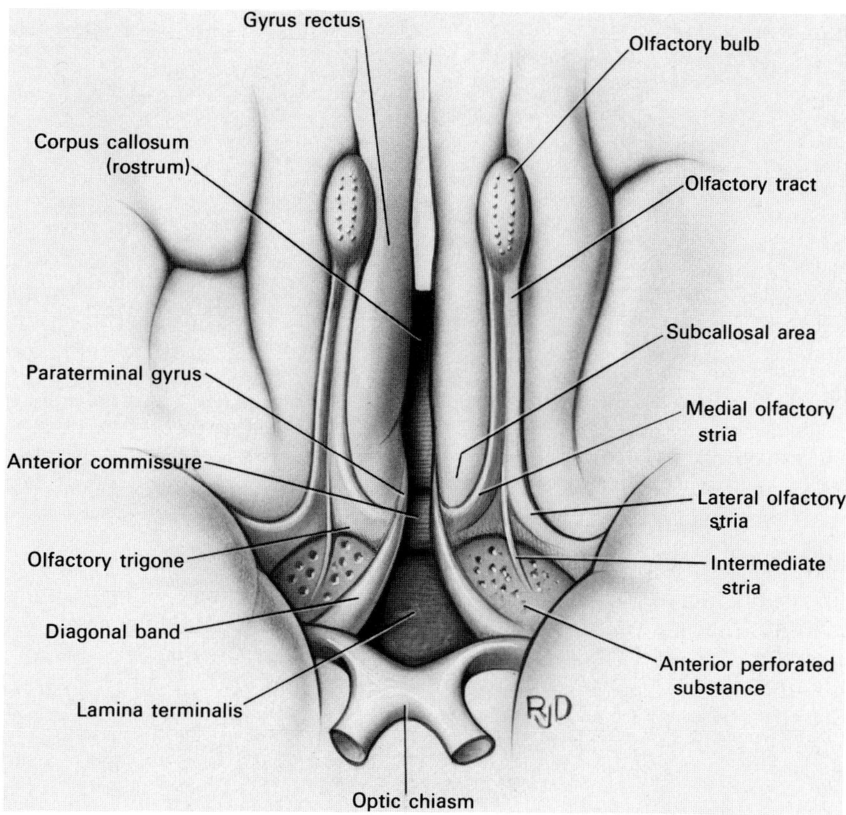

Figure 12-2. Diagram of olfactory structures on the inferior surface of the brain. The optic nerves and chiasm have been retracted caudally to expose the olfactory area.

are found along the olfactory tracts near the base of the hemisphere. Dendrites of these cells pass among the fibers of the olfactory tract, from which they receive impulses. Axons of the cells of the anterior olfactory nucleus pass centrally, cross in the anterior part of the anterior commissure and enter the contralateral anterior olfactory nucleus and olfactory bulb (Powell et al., '65; Valverde, '65; Broadwell, '75; Fig. 12-4).

The olfactory bulb receives a monoaminergic innervation, with serotonin (5-hydroxytryptamine, 5-HT) terminals synapsing upon periglomerular cell dendrites in glomeruli (Fig. 12-3) and norepinephrine varicosities distributed throughout the granular and external plexiform layers (Halász et al., '78). At least 10% of the periglomerular cells, and some tufted cells, show tyrosine hydroxylase immunoreactivity. Several lines of evidence indicate that these cells synthesize dopamine as their transmitter.

Olfactory Tract. This tract passes toward the anterior perforated substance and divides into well-defined *lateral* and *medial olfactory striae.* A thin covering of gray substance over the olfactory striae composes the *lateral* and *medial olfactory gyri* (Figs. 12-2 and 12-4). The lateral olfactory stria and gyrus pass along the lateral margin of the anterior perforated substance to reach the prepyriform region (Figs. 12-5 and 12-6). These fibers terminate in the prepyriform cortex and in the corticomedial part of the amygdaloid nuclear complex (Powell et al., '65).

Olfactory Lobe. This lobe develops as a longitudinal bulge on the basal surface of the hemisphere, where it is separated from the neopallium by the rhinal sulcus (Fig. 2-8). The posterior portion of this lobe differentiates into the olfactory area (anterior

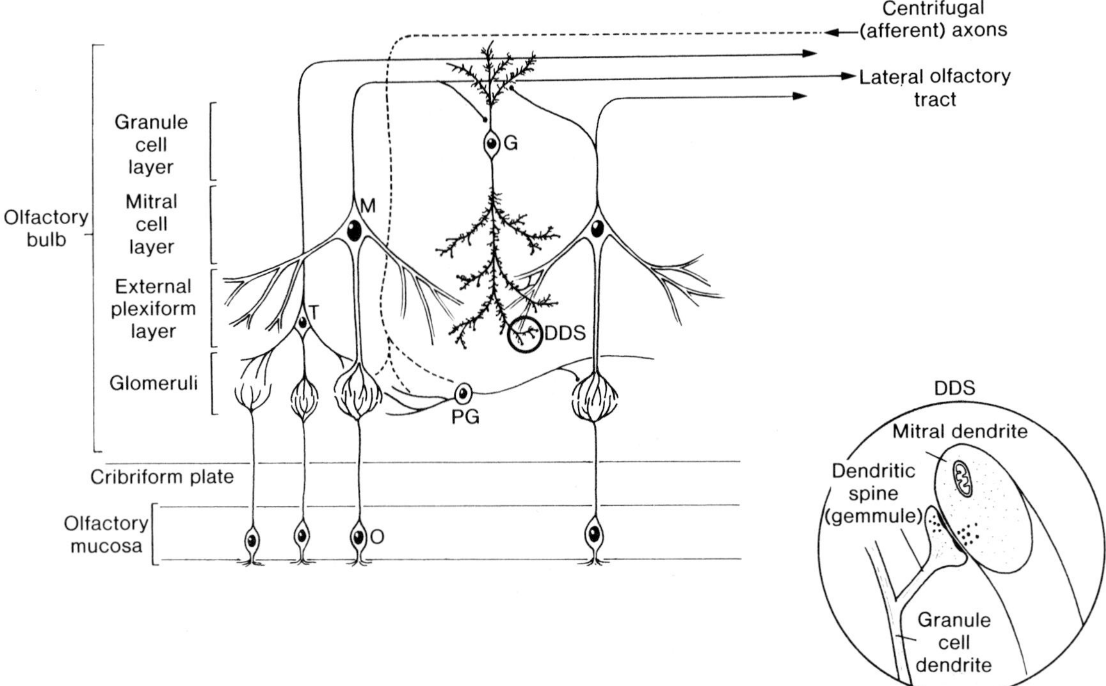

Figure 12-3. A simplified schematic diagram of the major classes of cells in the olfactory bulb. The sensory receptors (*O*) in the olfactory mucosa are illustrated at the bottom of the figure. The central process of the receptor cells enter the olfactory bulb and synapse upon a dendritic tuft of a mitral cell to form a synaptic complex called a glomerulus. Axons of mitral cells (*M*) pass centrally to form the lateral olfactory tract. Mitral axons also have recurrent collaterals which synapse upon granule cells. The granule cells (*G*) have no axons, but dendritic spines on external dendrites form reciprocal dendro-dendritic synapses (DDS and insert) with mitral dendrites. Periglomerular cells (*PG*), represent several morphological types of cells, linking glomeruli. Tufted cells (*T*) are morphologically similar to mitral cells, but their cell bodies are dispersed throughout the external plexiform layer. (From Carpenter and Sutin, *Human Neuroanatomy*, 1983; courtesy of Williams & Wilkins.)

perforated substance) and other olfactory structures on the anteromedial part of the temporal lobe, collectively known as the pyriform lobe.

The *pyriform lobe*, so named because of its pear shape in certain species, is divided into several regions (Fig. 12-5). These include the *prepyriform*, the *periamygdaloid*, and the *entorhinal areas.* The prepyriform area, often referred to as the lateral olfactory gyrus, extends along the lateral olfactory stria to the rostral amygdaloid region (Fig. 12-6). Since its afferent fibers are derived from the lateral olfactory stria, it is regarded as an olfactory relay center. The periamygdaloid area is a small region dorsal and rostral to the amygdaloid nuclear complex; it is intimately related to the prepyriform area. The entorhinal area, the most posterior part of the pyriform lobe, corresponds to area 28 of Brodmann and constitutes a major portion of the anterior parahippocampal gyrus in man (Fig. 12-6). Fibers of the lateral olfactory stria, arising in the olfactory bulb, give collaterals to the anterior olfactory nucleus and the olfactory tubercle and terminate in the prepyriform cortex and in parts of the amygdaloid nuclear complex.

The prepyriform cortex and the periamygdaloid area, which receive fibers from the lateral olfactory stria, constitute the *primary olfactory cortex.* Olfaction appears to be unique among the sensory systems, in that impulses in this system project to the cortex without being relayed by thalamic nuclei.

The prepyriform cortex projects fibers to

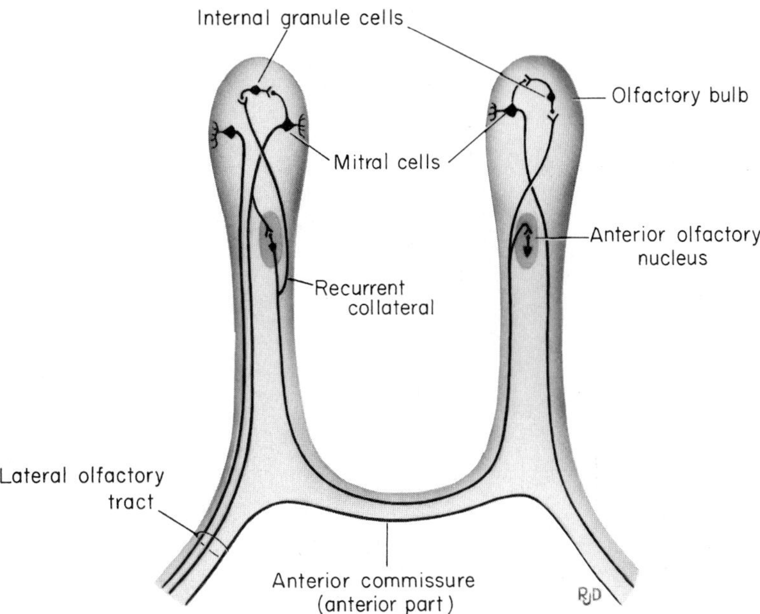

Figure 12-4. Schematic diagram of interconnections of the olfactory bulbs and anterior olfactory nuclei. Collaterals of mitral cell axons synapse upon apical dendrites of pyramidal-shaped cells of the anterior olfactory nucleus. These cells give rise to fibers that cross in the anterior part of the anterior commissure (Fig. 12-9) and synapse upon cells in the contralateral anterior olfactory nucleus and internal granule cells in the olfactory bulb. Recurrent collaterals of axons of the anterior olfactory nuclei project back to the ipsilateral olfactory bulb to terminate upon internal granule cells, which can in turn activate mitral cells. The principal axons of mitral cells enter the lateral olfactory tract (based on Valverde, '65). (From Carpenter and Sutin, *Human Neuroanatomy*, 1983; courtesy of Williams & Wilkins.)

the entorhinal cortex (area 28), the basal and lateral amygdaloid nuclei, the lateral preoptic area, the nucleus of the diagonal band, the medial forebrain bundle, and parts of the dorsomedial nucleus of the thalamus. The entorhinal cortex is regarded as a *secondary olfactory cortical area* (Fig. 13-5), although a projection from the olfactory bulb has been traced to ventral parts of the entorhinal cortex (Broadwell, '75; Kosel et al., '81). Efferent fibers from the entorhinal cortex are projected to the hippocampal formation, and to the anterior insular and frontal cortex via the uncinate fasciculus. No fibers from the prepyriform cortex pass to the hippocampal formation.

The lateroposterior quadrant of the orbitofrontal cortex receives olfactory information via relays in the pyriform and entorhinal cortex (Fig. 12-5). In addition the pyriform cortex projects to the dorsomedial nucleus (DMmc) of the thalamus which in turn projects to the orbitofrontal cortex. Lesions in the lateroposterior quadrant of the orbitofrontal cortex may impair olfactory discrimination in the monkey (Tanabe et al., '75).

Different parts of the amygdaloid nuclear complex receive olfactory inputs. Direct projections from the olfactory bulb pass to the cortical and medial amygdaloid nuclei, while indirect, but substantial, olfactory impulses pass to the basal and lateral amygdaloid nuclei, via relays in the prepyriform cortex. It is of interest that direct and indirect olfactory pathways to the amygdaloid complex terminate in different components and that these two pathways probably influence almost the entire amygdaloid nuclear complex.

Fibers originating from the cells of the anterior olfactory nucleus project: (1) peripherally to internal granule cells of the ipsilateral olfactory bulb, and (2) via the anterior part of the anterior commissure to the contralateral anterior olfactory nucleus

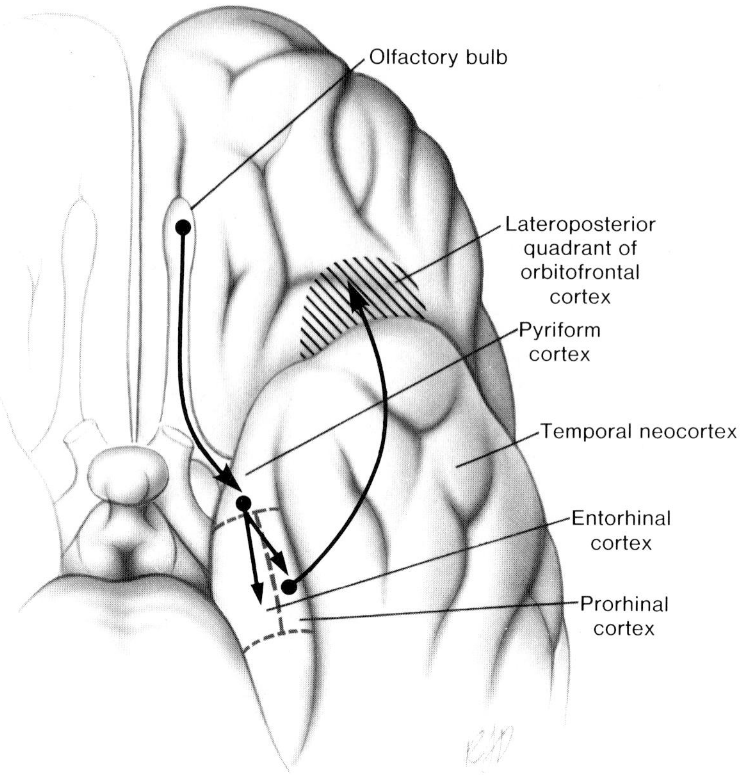

Figure 12-5. Diagram of the inferior surface of the frontal and temporal lobes of a primate brain showing olfactofrontal connections. The lateroposterior quadrant of the orbitofrontal cortex receives olfactory information relayed from the lateral entorhinal area (prorhinal cortex). The lateral entorhinal area also receives olfactory information indirectly from the pyriform cortex (based upon Potter and Nauta, '79). (From Carpenter and Sutin, *Human Neuroanatomy*, 1983; courtesy of Williams & Wilkins.)

and olfactory bulb (Valverde, '65; Powell et al., '65). Impulses from the anterior olfactory nucleus on one side thus reach internal granule cells of the olfactory bulb on both sides, and the contralateral anterior olfactory nucleus. Internal granule cells in the olfactory bulb relay impulses to mitral cells (Fig. 12-4).

The medial olfactory stria and gyrus are less distinct in man and become continuous with the subcallosal area and the paraterminal gyrus (Figs. 12-2 and 12-6). Some of the fibers in this stria may reach the olfactory tubercle and the anterior perforated substance.

The *anterior perforated substance* is a rhomboid-shaped region bounded by the medial and lateral olfactory striae and the optic tract (Figs. 2-8, 12-2, and 12-8). This region is studded with perforations made by penetrating blood vessels (Fig. 14-8). The posterior border of this region is formed by an oblique smooth band, the *diagonal band of Broca* (Fig. 12-2).

The *subcallosal area* and the *paraterminal gyrus* together constitute the septal area. The term *septal area* refers to the cortical part of this region, beneath which are the septal nuclei. The *medial* and *lateral septal nuclei* lie rostral to the anterior commissure and the preoptic area near the base of the septum pellucidum (Figs. 12-6 and 12-7). The medial septal nucleus becomes continuous with the nucleus and tract of the diagonal band and has connections with the amygdaloid nuclear complex. The septal nuclei receive afferents from the hippocampal formation via the fornix; afferents to the medial septal nucleus ascend in the medial forebrain bundle and mammillary peduncle (Fig. 12-7). Efferent fibers from the septal nuclei project via: (1) the stria

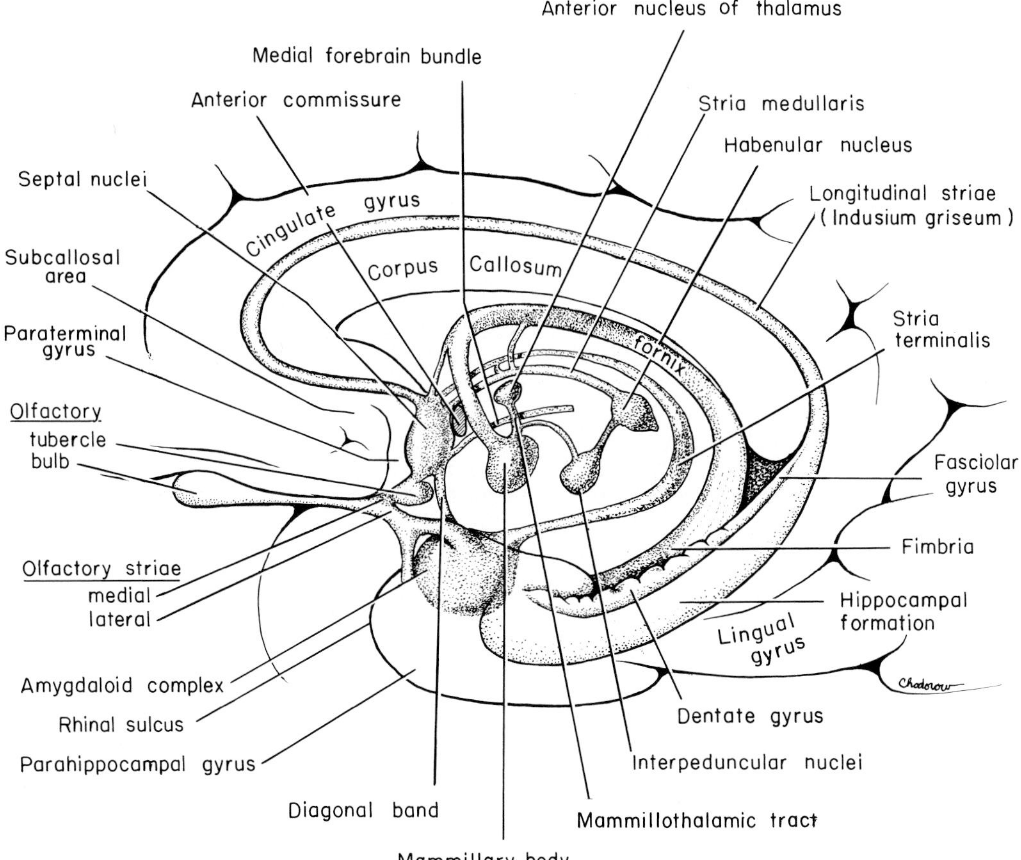

Figure 12-6. Semischematic drawing of rhinencephalic structural relationships as seen in medial view of the right hemisphere. Both deep and superficial structures are indicated. (Modified from a drawing by Krieg, '53.) (From Carpenter and Sutin, *Human Neuroanatomy*, 1983; courtesy of Williams & Wilkins.)

medullaris to the medial habenular nucleus, (2) the medial forebrain bundle to the lateral hypothalamus and midbrain tegmentum, and (3) the fornix to the hippocampal formation (Figs. 10-11 and 12-15).

Clinical Considerations. The ability of the human nose, in concert with the brain, to discriminate thousands of different odor qualities is well known, but the physiological and psychological bases for such discriminations are unknown. Olfactory discrimination does not appear to be based upon morphologically distinct types of receptors, but there is some evidence that certain odors may be distinguished by their relative effectiveness in stimulating particular regions of the olfactory epithelium. Current theories suggest that spatial and temporal factors probably play important roles in the neural coding of olfactory responses (Moulton and Beidler, '67).

Other evidence indicates that the sense of smell is based upon molecular geometry (Amoore et al., '64). Molecules identical in every respect, except that one is the mirror image of the other, may have different odors. Seven primary odors (i.e., camphoraceous, musky, floral, pepperminty, ethereal (ether-like), pungent and putrid) are considered to be equivalent to the three primary colors, because every known odor can be produced by appropriate mixtures of primary odors. Molecules with the same primary odor appear to have particular configurations, and these configurations are thought to fit appropriately shaped receptors in olfactory nerve endings. Certain molecules which may fit more than one

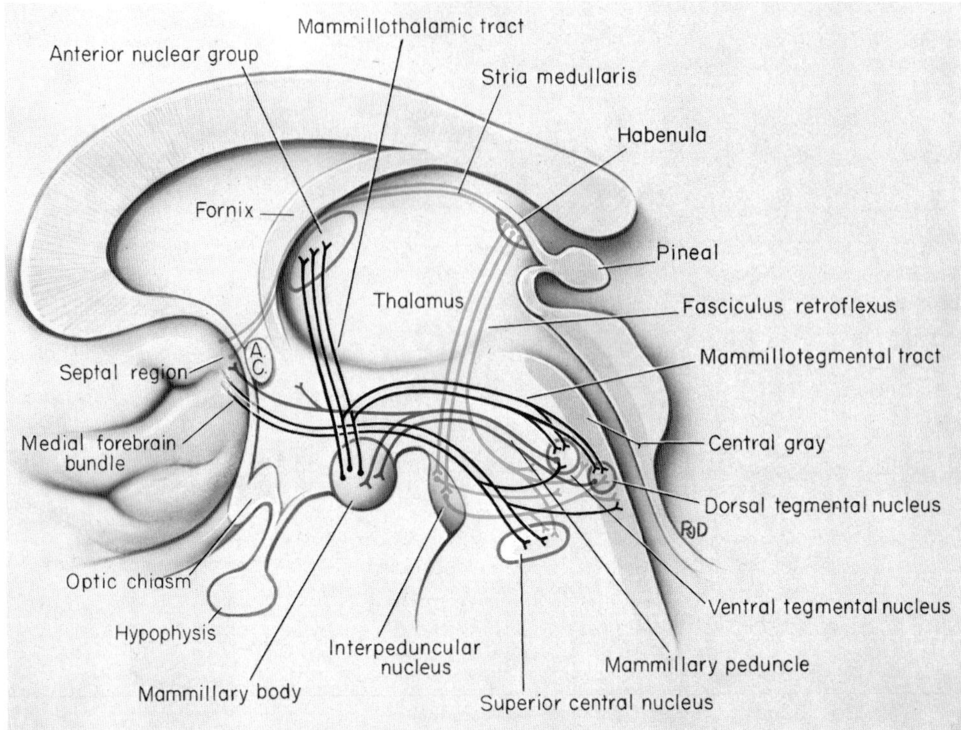

Figure 12-7. Semischematic diagram of limbic pathways interrelating the telencephalon and diencephalon with medial midbrain structures. The medial forebrain bundle and efferent fibers of the mammillary body are shown in *black*. The *medial forebrain bundle* originates from the septal and lateral preoptic regions, traverses the lateral hypothalamic area and projects into the midbrain tegmentum. The mammillary princeps (*black*) divides into two bundles, the *mammillothalamic tract* and the *mammillotegmental tract*. Ascending fibers of the *mammillary peduncle*, arising from the dorsal and ventral tegmental nuclei, are shown in *red*; most of these fibers pass to the mammillary body, but some continue rostrally to the lateral hypothalamus, the preoptic regions and the medial septal nucleus. Fibers arising from the septal nuclei project caudally in the medial part of the *stria medullaris* (*blue*) to terminate in the medial habenular nucleus. Impulses conveyed by this bundle are distributed to midbrain tegmental nuclei via the fasciculus retroflexus (based on Nauta, '58). (From Carpenter and Sutin, *Human Neuroanatomy*, 1983; Williams & Wilkins.)

receptor are considered to signal complex odors.

From a clinical viewpoint the importance of the olfactory system in man is slight, since this special sense plays a less essential role than in lower vertebrates. In certain instances valuable clinical information can be obtained by testing olfactory sense by appropriate methods. Olfaction is tested in each nostril separately by having the patient inhale or sniff nonirritating volatile oils or liquids with characteristic odors. Substances which stimulate gustatory end organs, or peripheral endings of the trigeminal nerve in the nasal mucosa, are not appropriate for testing olfaction. Comparisons between the two sides are of great importance. While the olfactory nerves are rarely the seat of disease, they frequently are involved by disease or injury of adjacent structures. Fractures of the cribriform plate of the ethmoid bone or hemorrhage at the base of the frontal lobes may cause tearing of the olfactory filaments. The olfactory nerves may be involved as a consequence of meningitis or abscess of the frontal lobe.

Unilateral anosmia may be of important diagnostic significance in localizing intracranial neoplasms, especially meningiomas of the sphenoidal ridge or olfactory groove. Hypophysial tumors affect the olfactory bulb and tract only when they extend above the sella turcica. Olfactory "hallucinations" frequently are a consequence of lesions in-

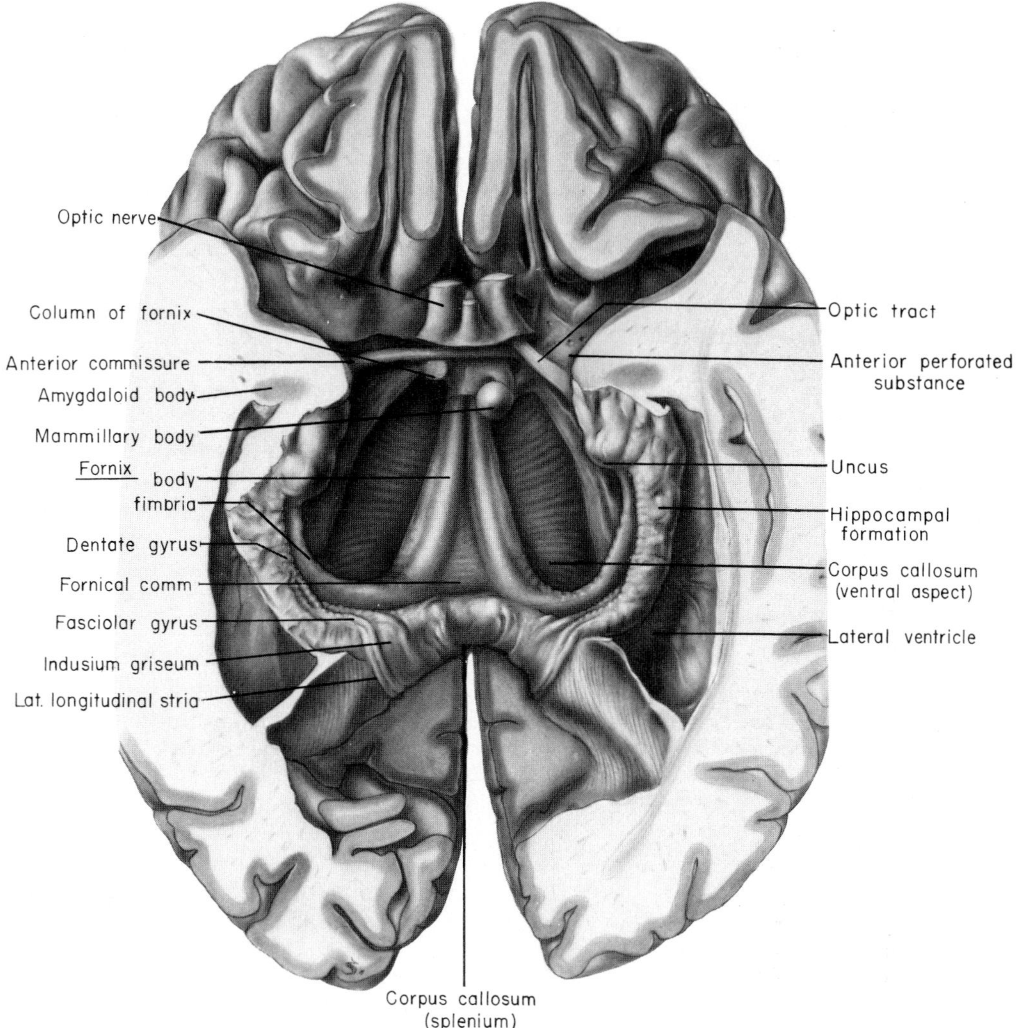

Figure 12-8. Dissection of the inferior surface of the brain showing the configuration of the fornix, the hippocampal formation, the dentate gyrus and related structures. (Reproduced with permission from F. A. Mettler, *Neuroanatomy*, Ed. 2; The C. V. Mosby Company, St. Louis, 1948.) (From Carpenter and Sutin, *Human Neuroanatomy*, 1983; Williams & Wilkins.)

volving or irritating the parahippocampal gyrus, the uncus, or adjoining areas around the amygdaloid nuclear complex. The olfactory sensations which these patients experience usually are described as disagreeable in character and may precede a generalized convulsion. Such seizures are referred to as "uncinate fits."

ANTERIOR COMMISSURE

The anterior commissure crosses the median plane as a compact fiber bundle immediately in front of the anterior columns of the fornix (Figs. 2-6, 2-22, 9-7, 12-8, and 12-9). Proceeding laterally it splits into two portions. The small anterior, or olfactory, portion, greatly reduced in man, loops rostrally and connects the gray substance of the olfactory tract on one side with the olfactory bulb of the opposite side. Fibers in this part of the anterior commissure arise from the anterior olfactory nucleus, cross to the opposite side, and project to the contralateral anterior olfactory nucleus and to granule cells in the olfactory bulb (Fig. 12-4).

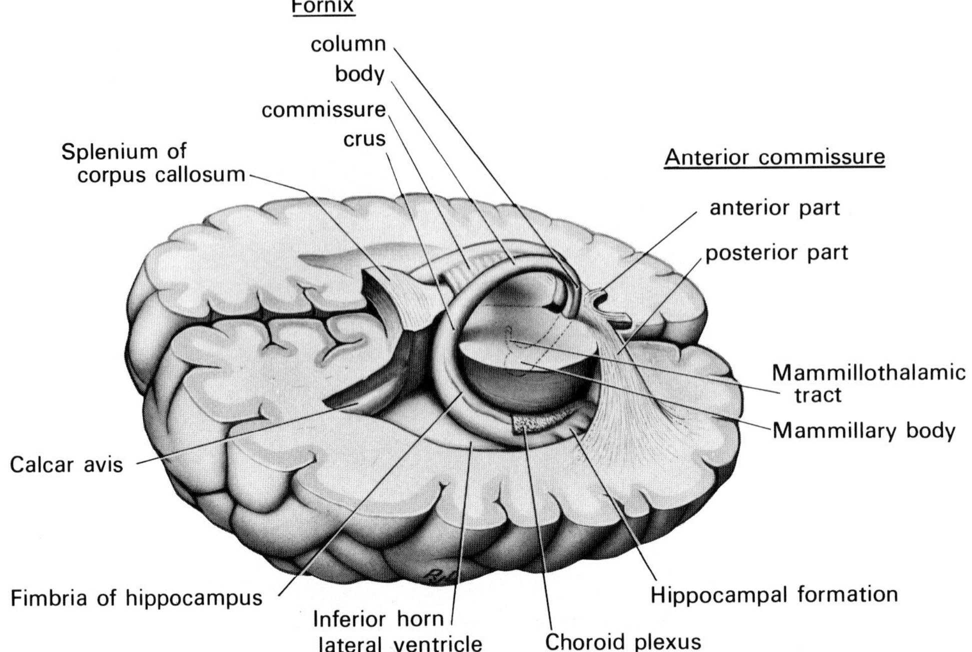

Figure 12-9. Drawing of a brain dissection showing the hippocampal formation, the fornix system and the anterior and posterior parts of the anterior commissure. In this drawing only postcommissural fibers of the fornix are shown projecting to the mammillary body. (From Carpenter and Sutin, *Human Neuroanatomy*, courtesy of Williams & Wilkins.)

The larger posterior portion forms the bulk of the anterior commissure. From its central region fibers of the anterior commissure pass laterally and backward through the most inferior parts of the lateral segments of the globus pallidus and putamen (Figs. 9-7 and 9-8). Further laterally the fibers of the anterior commissure enter the external capsule and come into apposition with the inferior part of the claustrum. Fibers of the posterior portion of the anterior commissure mainly interconnect the middle temporal gyri, although some fibers pass into the inferior temporal gyrus (Fig. 12-9).

HIPPOCAMPAL FORMATION

The hippocampal formation is laid down in the embryo on the medial wall of the hemisphere along the hippocampal fissure. This fissure lies immediately above and parallel to the choroidal fissure, which marks the invagination of the choroid plexus into the ventricle (Fig. 12-10). With the formation of the temporal lobe, both these fissures are carried downward and forward, each forming an arch extending from the region of the interventricular foramen to the tip of the inferior horn of the lateral ventricle. The various parts of the hippocampal arch do not develop to the same extent. The upper portion of the hippocampal fissure is invaded by the crossing fibers of the corpus callosum and ultimately becomes the callosal sulcus (Fig. 2-6) which separates this massive commissure from the overlying pallium. The part of the hippocampal formation which remains above the corpus callosum undergoes little differentiation; in the adult, it forms a thin vestigial convolution, the indusium griseum (Fig. 12-8).

The temporal part of the arch, not affected by the corpus callosum, differentiates into the hippocampal formation. As the hippocampal fissure deepens, the invaginated portion bulges into the inferior horn and becomes the *hippocampus* (Fig. 12-9). The lips of the fissure give rise to the *dentate* and *parahippocampal gyri.* These relationships can be seen in transverse sections (Fig. 12-10). Proceeding from the collateral

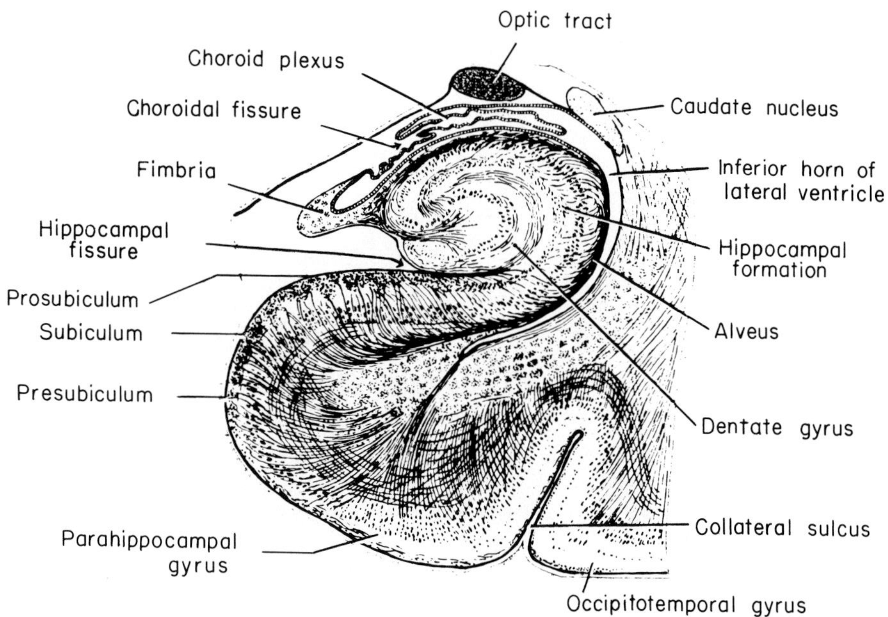

Figure 12-10. Transverse section through the human hippocampal formation and parahippocampal gyrus. The presubiculum, subiculum and prosubiculum represent the region of transition between parahippocampal gyrus and the hippocampus and are archipallial. (From Carpenter and Sutin, *Human Neuroanatomy*, 1983; courtesy of Williams & Wilkins.)

sulcus, the *parahippocampal gyrus* extends to the hippocampal fissure, where it dips into the ventricle to form the *hippocampal formation.* The latter curves dorsally and medially and, on reaching the medial surface, curves inward again to form a semilunar convolution, the *dentate gyrus* or *fascia dentata* (Figs. 12-8 and 12-11). The whole ventricular surface of the hippocampal formation is covered by a white layer, the *alveus*, which is composed of axons from cells of the hippocampus (Fig. 12-10). These fibers converge on the medial surface of the hippocampus to form the *fimbria.* Fibers from the alveus entering the fimbria constitute the beginning of the fornix system (Figs. 12-8 and 12-9). The free thin border of the fimbria is continuous with the epithelium of the choroidal fissure, which lies immediately above it. The choroid plexus, invaginated into the ventricle along this fissure, partly covers the hippocampus (Fig. 12-10).

The superior portion of the parahippocampal gyrus adjoining the hippocampal fissure is known as the *subiculum*, and the area of transition between it and the parahippocampal gyrus, as the *presubiculum* (Fig. 12-10). The presubiculum, subiculum, prosubiculum, hippocampal formation, and dentate gyrus all belong to the archipallium, which has an allocortical structure. The larger inferior portion of the parahippocampal gyrus near the collateral fissure has a six-layered transitional lamination resembling isocortex.

When the hippocampal fissure is opened up, the *dentate gyrus* is seen as a narrow, notched band of cortex between the hippocampal fissure below and the fimbria above (Fig. 12-10). In sagittal sections (Fig. 12-11) the relationships between the hippocampal formation, the dentate gyrus, the amygdaloid nucleus, and the inferior horn of the lateral ventricle can be appreciated. Traced backward, the gyrus accompanies the fimbria almost to the splenium of the corpus callosum. There it separates from the fimbria, loses its notched appearance, and as the delicate *fasciolar gyrus*, passes on to the superior surface of the corpus callosum (Fig. 12-8). It spreads out into a thin gray sheet representing a vestigial convolution, the *indusium griseum* or supracallosal gyrus (Fig. 12-8). Imbedded in the indusium are two slender bands of myelin-

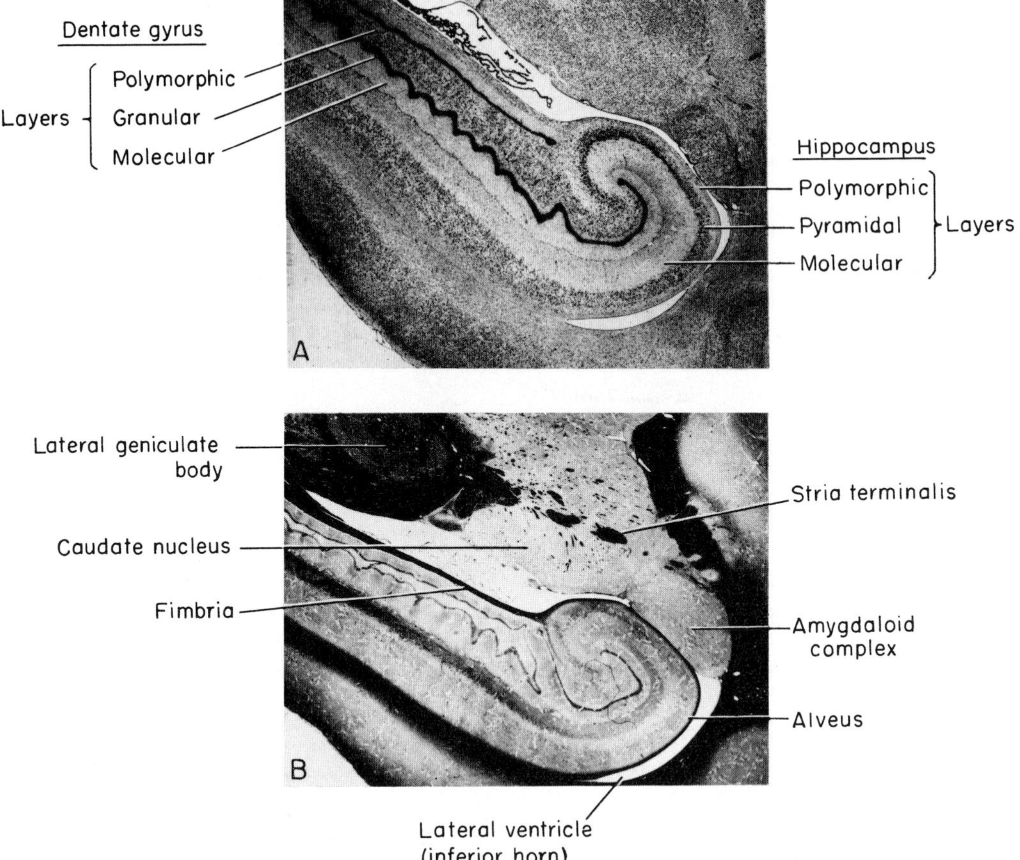

Figure 12-11. Sagittal sections through the hippocampal formation and dentate gyrus in the rhesus monkey demonstrating relationships of these structures to the inferior horn of the lateral ventricle, the tail of the caudate nucleus and the amygdaloid nuclear complex. In *A*, the cellular layers of the hippocampal formation and dentate gyrus are identified. In *B*, the alveus, fimbria, tail of the caudate nucleus, stria terminalis, amygdaloid complex and part of the lateral geniculate body are identified. (*A*, Nissl stain, ×8; *B*, Weil stain, ×9.) (From Carpenter and Sutin, *Human Neuroanatomy*, 1983; courtesy of Williams & Wilkins.)

ated fibers which appear as narrow longitudinal ridges on the superior surface of the corpus callosum. These are the *medial* and *lateral longitudinal striae* (Lancisii), which constitute the white matter of these vestigial convolutions. The indusium griseum and the longitudinal striae extend the length of the corpus callosum, pass over the genu, and become continuous with the paraterminal gyrus and the diagonal band (Figs. 2-9 and 12-2).

The cortical zones from the parahippocampal gyrus through the presubiculum, the subiculum, and the prosubiculum to the hippocampal formation and the dentate gyrus show a gradual transition from a six- to a three-layered cellular organization (Fig. 12-11). Although the entorhinal region (area 28) is six-layered cortex, in more medial regions certain layers drop out and undergo rearrangement. The cortex of the hippocampal formation has three fundamental layers. These are the *polymorphic layer*, the *pyramidal layer* and the *molecular layer* (Fig. 12-11). Several secondary laminae are formed by the arrangement of axons and dendrites of cells within the fundamental layers. Axons of pyramidal cells project into the alveus and the fimbria of the fornix.

The most characteristic layer of the hypocampal formation consists of large and small pyramidal cells, which exhibit many morphological differences, especially in

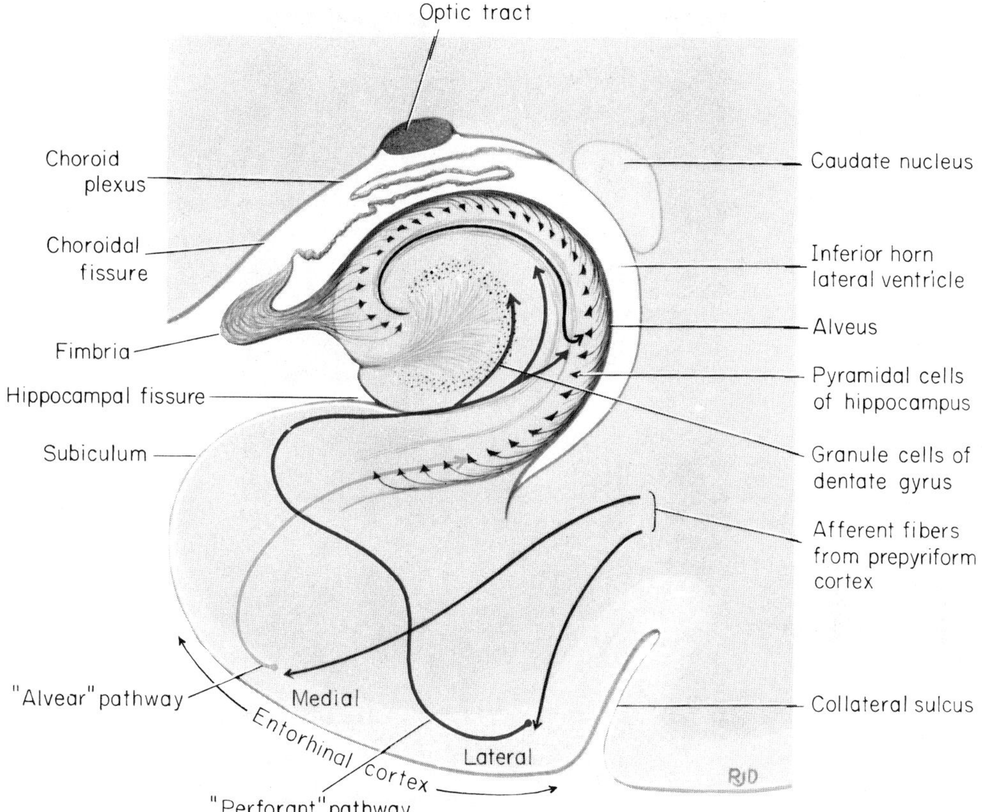

Figure 12-12. Semischematic diagram of the hippocampal formation, dentate gyrus, and entorhinal area. In the dentate gyrus only the granular layer is indicated. In the hippocampal formation only cells and their axons projecting into the alveus are shown. Afferent fibers from prepyriform cortex projecting to the entorhinal cortex are shown in *black*. Projections of the entorhinal cortex to the hippocampal formation follow two pathways: (1) the lateral region gives rise to fibers which follow the so-called "perforant" pathway (*red*), and (2) the medial region gives rise to fibers which follow the so-called "alvear" pathway (*blue*). Axons of pyramidal cells in the hippocampal formation entering the alveus pass to the fimbria of the hippocampus. The dentate gyrus gives rise to fibers that project only to the hippocampal formation. (Based on Lorente de Nó, '34, and a schematic diagram by Peele, '61.) (From Carpenter and Sutin, *Human Neuroanatomy*, 1983; courtesy of Williams & Wilkins.)

dendritic development. Some of the cells, described as double pyramids, have rich dendritic plexuses arising from both poles. Basal and apical dendrites of pyramidal cells enter adjacent layers while their axons enter the alveus (Fig. 12-12). A schematic drawing of a hippocampal pyramidal neuron with sites of synaptic contact of specific afferents is shown in Figure 12-13. *Hippocampal basket cells*, intrinsic neurons, synapse mainly on the somata of pyramidal cells (Shepherd, '79).

Dentate Gyrus. Like the hippocampus, the dentate gyrus consists of three layers: a *molecular layer*, a *granular layer* and a *polymorphic layer* (Fig. 12-11). Layers of the dentate gyrus are arranged in a U- or V-shaped configuration in which the open portion is directed toward the fimbria (Fig. 12-10). The molecular layer of the dentate gyrus is continuous with that of the hippocampus in the depths of the hippocampal fissure. The granular layer, made up of closely arranged spherical or oval neurons, gives rise to axons which pass through the polymorphic layer to terminate upon dendrites of pyramidal cells in the hippocampus. Dendrites of granule cells enter mainly the molecular layer. Cells of the polymorphic layer are of several types, including modified pyramidal cells and so-called basket cells. The dentate gyrus does not give

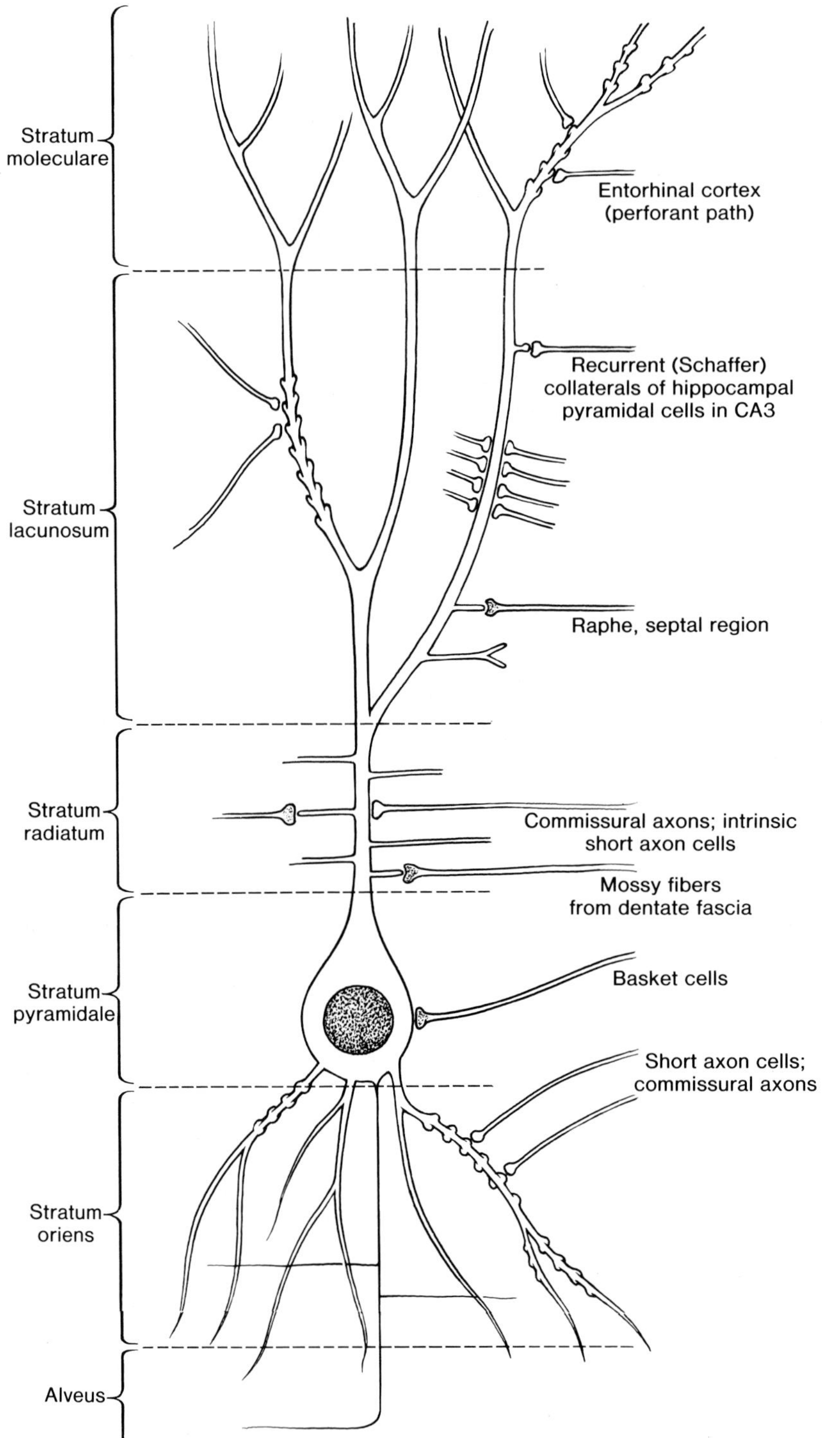

Figure 12-13. A schematic drawing of a CA1 sector hippocampal pyramidal neuron indicating the regions of the cell which receive specific afferent inputs. Specific cell layers of the hippocampal formation can be related to specific parts of the pyramidal cell and to afferent inputs from different sources. Afferent fibers synapse in specific locations upon dendritic shafts, dendritic spines, the cell body and the basal dendrites of the pyramidal cell. (Carpenter and Sutin, *Human Neuroanatomy*, 1983; courtesy of Williams & Wilkins.)

rise to fibers passing beyond the hippocampal formation (Raisman et al., '66).

Histochemical studies provide some clues concerning the operations of the hippocampal formation. Septo-hippocampal projections contain acetylcholinesterase (AChE) terminals (Mellgren et al., '77) and some AChE-containing cell bodies are found within the hilus of the area dentata and scattered throughout the pyramidal cell layer. Noradrenergic innervation of the hippocampal formation arises from cells in the locus ceruleus and projects via the septal region (Lindvall and Björklund, '78). Enkephalin-like immunoreactive axons emerge from the hilar region of the dentate gyrus and terminate as mossy fibers on proximal apical dendrites of hippocampal pyramidal cells (Fig. 12-13). A second group of enkephalin-containing axons follow the "perforant path" from the lateral entorhinal cortex to the hippocampus (Fig. 12-12).

The anatomical connections of the hippocampal formation indicate that it does not receive fibers from the olfactory bulb or the anterior olfactory nucleus, and suggest that it is largely an effector structure. Afferent fibers to this structure arise mainly from the entorhinal area, a portion of the pyriform lobe which does not receive direct olfactory fibers. Fibers from the entorhinal area (area 28) are distributed to the dentate gyrus and hippocampus in their entire posterior portion (Lorente de Nó, '34). Fibers arising from the medial part of the entorhinal area follow the so-called "alvear path" to enter the hippocampus from its ventricular surface (Fig. 12-12). Fibers from the lateral parts of the entorhinal cortex pursue the so-called "perforant path" and traverse the subiculum (Fig. 12-12). These fibers are distributed to all sectors of the hippocampus except the region transitional to the dentate gyrus.

Other afferents to the hippocampal formation project from the medial septal nucleus via the fimbria (Daitz and Powell, '54). Projections from the cingulate cortex reach the presubiculum and entorhinal cortex via the cingulum, but do not enter the hippocampal formation (Raisman et al., '65). Because the entorhinal cortex projects to the hippocampus, impulses from the cingulate cortex can be relayed to the hippocampus (Fig. 12-15).

Fornix. This band of white fibers constitutes the main efferent fiber system of the hippocampal formation. It includes both projection and commissural fibers (Figs. 12-8 and 12-9). It is composed of axons of the large pyramidal cells of the hippocampus and subiculum, which spread over the ventricular surface as the alveus and converge to form the *fimbria* (Swanson and Cowan, '77; Rosene and van Hoesen, '77). Proceeding backward, the fimbriae of the two sides increase in thickness. On reaching the posterior end of the hippocampus, they arch under the splenium of the corpus callosum as the crura of the fornix, at the same time converging toward each other. In this region a number of fibers pass to the opposite side, forming a thin sheet of crossing fibers, the *fornical commissure* (hippocampal commissure, or psalterium), a structure rather poorly developed in man (Figs. 12-8 and 12-9). The two crura then join to form the *body of the fornix,* which runs forward under the corpus callosum to the rostral margin of the thalamus. Here the bundles separate again, and as the *anterior columns of the fornix,* arch ventrally in front of the interventricular foramina and caudal to the anterior commissure (Figs. 10-6 and 10-7). The fimbriae, thin bands of fibers situated laterally, accompany the fornices throughout most of their extent, but rostrally they become incorporated within the main bundles as the latter form the anterior columns of the fornix. Approximately half of the fibers descend caudal to the anterior commissure as the *postcommissural fornix.* Remaining fibers of the fornix pass rostral to the anterior commissure as the *precommissural fornix.*

Postcommissural fornix fibers traverse the hypothalamus en route to the mammillary body, but in their course give off fibers to the thalamus. Fornix fibers passing directly to the mammillary body terminate mainly in the medial nucleus (Figs. 10-2, 10-7 and 12-15). Fibers leaving the postcommissural fornix in the rostral hypothalamus are distributed mainly to the anterior, and the rostral intralaminar thalamic nuclei (Nauta, '56). According to Powell et al. ('57), the anterior nuclei of the thalamus receive as many direct fibers from the fornix as from the mammillothalamic tract (Figs. 9-7 and 9-11). Some postcommissural fornix fibers descend caudally beyond the mammillary bodies to enter the midbrain tegmentum (Guillery, '56; Nauta, '56, '58). Anterograde tracing studies in the rat show that axons in the postcommissural fornix destined for the hypothalamus originate from cell bodies in the subicular cortex and not from hippocampal pyramidal cells (Meibach and Siegel, '77; Swanson and Cowan, '77).

Precommissural fornix fibers, constituting a less compact bundle than the postcommissural fibers, are distributed to septal areas, the lateral preoptic area, and the anterior part of the hypothalamus.

The above anatomical connections indicate the complex pathways by which impulses from the hippocampal formation can be projected to different parts of the neuraxis. Both direct and indirect pathways connect the hippocampal formation with certain thalamic nuclei (i.e., the anterior and the intralaminar), the hypothalamus, and the midbrain reticular formation (Figs. 12-7 and 12-15).

Functional Considerations. Although the hippocampal formation is a large structure and considerable information is available concerning its anatomical connections, relatively little is known about its function. Anatomical and physiological evidence indicate that the hippocampus has no significant olfactory function (Brodal, '47). Comparative anatomists have long known that development of the hippocampus in mammals does not parallel the development of olfactory sense. The hippocampus and dentate gyrus are well developed in cetaceans that are said to be completely anosmatic, and lack olfactory bulbs and nerves.

Localized lesions in the hippocampus and local stimulation of this structure in conscious cats tend to produce similar phenomena (Green, '60). Behavioral changes observed in these animals resemble those occurring in psychomotor epilepsy, and it seems likely that the abnormal fears, hyperesthesia, and pupillary dilatation seen may represent fragments of a seizure. The behavioral changes noted initially after lesions tend to disappear within several weeks, but recur at a later time. The hippocampus has an exceedingly low threshold for seizure activity.

The hippocampus may be concerned particularly with recent memory (Green, '64). Relatively large bilateral lesions of the hippocampus appear to be associated with profound impairment of memory for recent events and with relatively mild behavioral changes (Victor et al., '61). Memory for remote events usually is unaffected. Although general intellectual functions may remain at a fairly high level, these patients demonstrate an inability to learn new facts and skills. Even though the fornix contains most of the efferent fibers from the hippocampal formation, evidence that interruption of these fibers produces memory loss is meager. The mammillary bodies, like the fornix, would seem to be implicated in memory, but experimental data in the rat do not support this thesis (Moss et al., '81).

Korsakoff's syndrome (amnestic confabulatory syndrome), appearing as a sequel to Wernicke's encephalopathy and probably related to a thiamine deficiency associated with alcoholism, is characterized by severe impairment of memory without clouding of consciousness, confusion and confabulatory tendencies. Lesions in this syndrome almost always involve the mammillary bodies and adjacent areas. Amnesia is said to be present in this syndrome only if there is additional thalamic involvement (Victor, '64).

Particularly prominent among concepts relating the hippocampal formation to emotion is the theory proposed by Papez ('37), which attempted to provide an anatomical basis for emotion. Realizing that the term "emotion" denotes both subjective feelings and the expression of these feelings by appropriate autonomic and somatic responses, Papez concluded that: (1) the cortex is essential for subjective emotional experience, and (2) emotional expression must be dependent upon the integrative actions of the hypothalamus. He expressed the belief that the hippocampal formation and its principal projection system, the fornix, provide one of the main pathways by which impulses from the cortex reach the hypothalamus. Impulses reaching the hypothalamus could be projected caudally through the brain stem to effector structures, as well as rostrally to thalamic, and ultimately, cortical levels. The "central

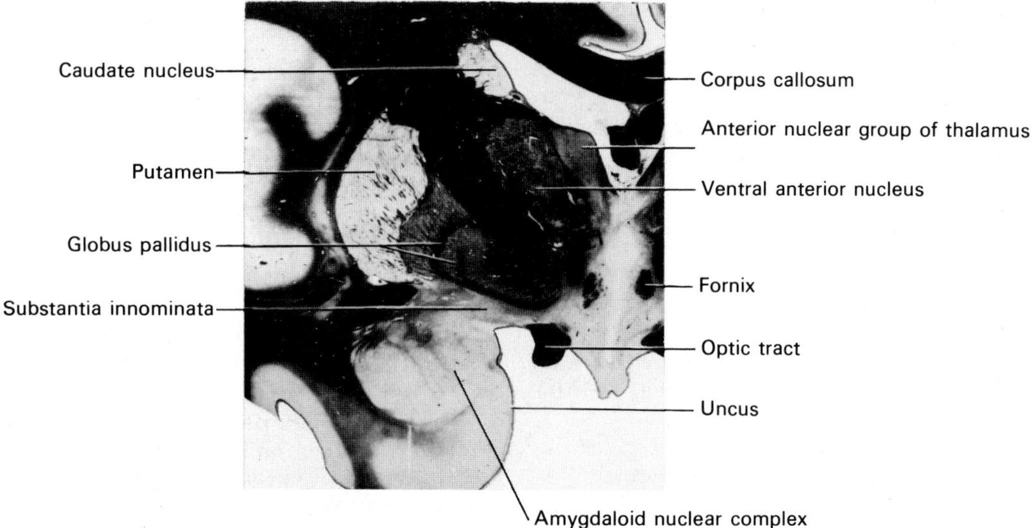

Figure 12-14. Photograph of transverse section through the thalamus, basal ganglia, and amygdaloid nuclear complex. The substantia innominata lies ventral to the globus pallidus and dorsal to the amygdala. (Weil stain.) (From Carpenter and Sutin, *Human Neuroanatomy*, 1983; courtesy of Williams & Wilkins.)

emotive process of cortical origin" was considered to be formed in the hippocampal formation, and transmitted to the mammillary bodies, the anterior nuclei of the thalamus, and the cingulate gyrus. He regarded the cingulate cortex as the receptive region for impulses concerned with emotion, and suggested that radiation of impulses from the cingulate gyrus to other cortical regions added emotional coloring to the psychic process. This circuitous interrelation between cortex and diencephalon was thought to explain how emotional responses could result from either psychic or hypothalamic activity.

AMYGDALOID NUCLEAR COMPLEX

The amygdaloid nuclear complex is a gray mass situated in the dorsomedial portion of the temporal lobe rostral and dorsal to the tip of the inferior horn of the lateral ventricle (Figs. 2-8, 11-2, 12-6, 12-8, and 12-14). It is covered by a rudimentary cortex and caudally is continuous with the uncus of the parahippocampal gyrus.

The amygdaloid complex is divided into two main nuclear masses: (1) a corticomedial nuclear group and (2) a basolateral nuclear group. A central nucleus frequently is included as part of the corticomedial nuclear group. In man the *corticomedial nuclear group* constitutes a dorsal or dorsomedial part of the complex due to a medial rotation of the temporal lobe. Nuclear subdivisions of the corticomedial group include: (1) the anterior amygdaloid area, (2) the nucleus of the lateral olfactory tract, (3) the medial amygdaloid nucleus, and (4) the cortical amygdaloid nucleus. The nucleus of the lateral olfactory tract is the least developed of the amygdaloid nuclei in man. The anterior amygdaloid area, representing the most rostral part of the amygdaloid complex, is rather poorly differentiated. The corticomedial amygdaloid nuclear group lies closest to the putamen and tail of the caudate nucleus.

The largest and best differentiated part of the amygdaloid complex in man is the *basolateral nuclear group*. Subdivisions of this nuclear group are: (1) the lateral amygdaloid nucleus, (2) the basal amygdaloid nucleus, and (3) an accessory basal amygdaloid nucleus. The amygdaloid complex is related medially to the area olfactoria and laterally to the claustrum, while dorsally it is hidden partially by the lentiform nucleus. Caudally the amygdaloid complex is in contact with the tail of the caudate nucleus, which sweeps anteriorly in the roof of the inferior horn of the lateral ventricle (Figs. 11-3, 12-11, and 12-14).

Among the afferent connections of the amygdaloid complex, olfactory fibers are the best established (Fig. 12-6). Fibers originating in the olfactory bulb project via the lateral olfactory tract to terminate in the corticomedial nuclear group. No fibers from the lateral olfactory tract appear to enter the basolateral nuclear group. The basolateral amygdaloid nuclei receive an indirect olfactory input via relays in the prepyriform cortex. Thus nearly all parts of the amygdaloid nuclear complex receive either direct or indirect olfactory pathways.

Important diencephalic projections to the amygdala follow pathways which parallel efferent systems. Fibers arising in the rostral half of the hypothalamus pass via the stria terminalis and ventral to the corpus striatum (ventral amygdalopetal) to all amygdaloid nuclei except the central nucleus (Cowan et al., '65; Szentágothai et al., '68). Retrograde transport studies indicate that hypothalamic afferents to the amygdala arise chiefly from middle and posterior portions of the ipsilateral lateral hypothalamic area (Fig. 10-11); the ventromedial hypothalamic nucleus projects mainly to medial regions of the amygdala (Mehler, '80). This diencephalic input to the amygdaloid nuclear complex passes to all nuclei which receive direct or indirect olfactory afferents (Fig. 10-11). The amygdala receives ipsilateral projections from midline paraventricular thalamic nuclei and from the nucleus subparafascicularis (Mehler, '80). The lateral parabrachial nuclei, which receive ipsilateral afferents from caudal parts of the nucleus solitarius, project ipsilaterally to the central nucleus of the amygdala (Mehler, '80; Beckstead et al., '80).

Opinions differ concerning neocortical projections to the amygdala. Projections from the temporal lobe and cingulate gyrus to the basolateral and lateral nuclei of the amygdala have been described in the monkey (Whitlock and Nauta, '56; Herzog and Van Hoesen, '76; Pandya et al., '73). The orbitofrontal cortex also has been described as a source of amygdaloid afferent fibers (Valverde, '65), and a limited number of afferents arising from parietal and occipital cortex project to the lateral amygdala.

Anatomical evidence concerning nonolfactory sensory afferents to the amygdaloid complex is meager, though electrophysiological studies suggest such connections. Potentials can be evoked in the amygdaloid complex in response to stimulation of nearly all sensory receptors (Gerard et al., '36; Machne and Segundo, '56). Impulses originating from different parts of the body, as well as impulses concerned with different sensory modalities, converge upon the same cells (Gloor, '60).

The amygdala receives noradrenergic afferents from the locus ceruleus and dopaminergic afferents from the region of the ventral tegmental area and substantia nigra in the midbrain (Ungerstedt, '71; Lindvall and Björklund, '78). Dopamine-containing terminals are densest in the central nucleus, but also innervate the lateral and basolateral nuclei. Noradrenergic varicosities are distributed in a similar manner. Axons utilizing each of these neurotransmitters reach the amygdala via both the stria terminalis and ventral pathways. Acetylcholinesterase and choline acetyltransferase are found in highest concentrations in the posterior lateral and basolateral nuclei and in the nucleus of the lateral olfactory tract (Ben-Ari et al., '77a). Enkephalin, substance P and somatostatin are localized mainly in the central and medial nuclei (Ben-Ari et al., '77; Epelbaum et al., '79). In the monkey opiate receptors are distributed throughout the amygdala except for the lateral nucleus (Atweh and Kuhar, '77; La Motte et al., '78).

Stria Terminalis. The most prominent and best established pathway from the amygdaloid nuclear complex is the stria terminalis (Figs. 2-20, 2-24, 9-3, 9-5, 11-4, and 12-6). Most, but not all, of the fibers in this bundle originate from the corticomedial part of the amygdaloid complex (Hall, '63; Cowan et al., '65; Valverde, '65; Raisman, '66; Lammers, '72; De Olmos, '72). Fibers of the stria terminalis arch along the entire medial border of the caudate nucleus near its junction with the thalamus (Fig. 9-6). Rostrally these fibers pass into and terminate in the nuclei of the stria terminalis located lateral to the columns of the fornix and dorsal to the anterior commissure (Heimer and Nauta, '69; De Olmos, '72). This is the most massive termination

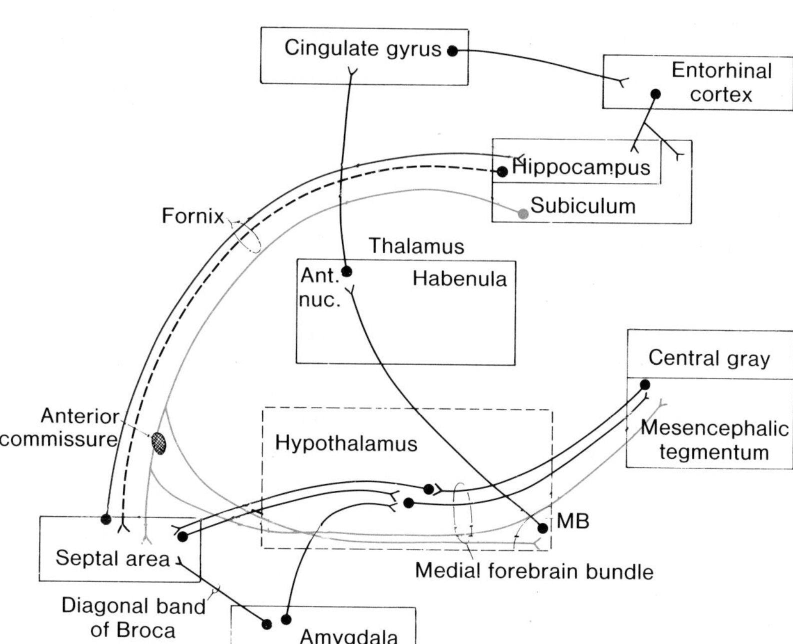

Figure 12-15. Schematic diagram of the major interconnections of structures composing the "limbic system." Fibers arising from the subiculum (*blue*) project via the fornix to the septal area, hypothalamus and mesencephalic tegmentum. Projection fibers from the hippocampal formation in the fornix are represented by *black-dashed* lines. Fibers from the septal area passing to the hippocampus via the fornix are indicated in *red. MB* indicates the mammillary body. (From Carpenter and Sutin, *Human Neuroanatomy*, 1983; courtesy of Williams & Wilkins.)

of the stria terminalis. Part of these fibers, which belong to the postcommissural part of the stria terminalis, also end in the anterior hypothalamic nucleus, and some of the fibers may join the medial forebrain bundle. Fibers of the precommissural part of the stria terminalis terminate in the medial preoptic area and continue caudally to end in a cell-poor zone surrounding the ventromedial hypothalamic nucleus (Fig. 10-4) (Hall, '63; Heimer and Nauta, '67, '69; Dreifuss et al., '68; De Olmos, '72; McBride and Sutin, '77).

Ventral Amygdalofugal Projection. This projection, considered to arise from both the basolateral amygdaloid nuclei and pyriform cortex, emerges from the dorsomedial part of the amygdala and spreads medially and rostrally beneath the lentiform nucleus (Gloor, '55; Nauta, '61; Cowan et al., '65). These fibers pass through the substantia innominata (Figs. 11-13, 12-14 and 12-16) and enter the lateral preoptic and hypothalamic areas, the septal region, and the nucleus of the diagonal band (Broca) (Fig. 12-15). Evidence in the rat suggests that fibers in the projection arise mainly from the periamygdaloid cortex (Valverde, '65; Leonard and Scott, '71); some evidence suggests that ventral amygdaloid fibers are unique to higher mammals.

Amygdalofugal fibers, bypassing the preoptic region and hypothalamus, enter the inferior thalamic peduncle (Fig. 9-8) and project to the midline periventricular nuclei of the thalamus (Mehler, '80). It has been suggested that these fibers arise from the basolateral amygdaloid nuclei, but Valverde ('65) reports they arise chiefly from the anterior amygdaloid area. There is conflicting evidence concerning reciprocal connections between the dorsomedial nucleus of the thalamus and the amygdala (Nauta, '61; Krettek and Price, '74; Mehler, '80). The basolateral amygdaloid nucleus also projects fibers directly to two contiguous areas of neocortex on the medial aspect of the hemisphere rostral and ventral to the genu of the corpus callosum (Krettek and Price, '74). These cortical areas receive inputs from both the dorsomedial nucleus of the thalamus and the amygdala. Additional studies indicate that portions of the amygdala project to the cortex bordering the rhinal sulcus, the entorhinal cortex and the ventral part of the subiculum (Krettek and Price, '74a).

Amygdalostriate Projections. Although degeneration and axoplasmic transport studies have indicated a modest projection from the amygdala to the ventrolateral striatum (Nauta, '61; Krettek and Price, '78; Royce, '78a), recent data suggest a widespread amygdalostriate projection (Kelley et al., '82). This connection arises mainly from the basal lateral amygdaloid nucleus and passes via the longitudinal association bundle and the stria terminalis. Rostrally this projection is dense only in ventromedial regions, while caudally (caudal to the anterior commissure) it encompasses much larger parts of the striatum. No fibers project to the rostro-dorsolateral region of the striatum. Most amygdalostriate fibers are ipsilateral, but a modest symmetrical contralateral distribution (10–15%) is conveyed by the anterior commissure. Amygdalostriate projections appear to overlap the striatal projections from the ventral tegmental area and the raphe nuclei. These observations suggest a division of the striatum into "limbic" and "nonlimbic" parts (Kelley et al., '82). Corticostriate projections from the sensorimotor cortex are mainly to rostro-dorsolateral, "nonlimbic" regions, but there is considerable overlap. It seems likely that the amygdalostriate projection may provide an access route by which the amygdala could influence somatic motor behavior.

Functional Considerations. Even though the amygdaloid complex receives an olfactory input, the importance of this complex for olfactory sense is uncertain. Most evidence suggests that the amygdaloid complex cannot be closely related to olfactory sense since it is well developed in anosmatic aquatic mammals, and bilateral destruction of this complex does not impair olfactory discrimination (Swann, '34; Allen, '41).

Electrical stimulation and ablation of the amygdaloid nuclear complex in animals produces a wide variety of behavioral, visceral, somatic, and endocrine changes (MacLean and Delgado, '53; Shealy and Peele, '57; Gloor, '60; Kaada, '51, '72). Pronounced behavioral changes are elicited by stimulation of the nuclear complex in unanesthetized animals. The most common response to amygdaloid stimulation under such conditions is an "arrest" reaction in which all spontaneous ongoing activities cease as the animal assumes an attitude of aroused attention. This response is indistinguishable from the arousal reaction obtained from brain stem reticular activation and is associated with cortical desynchronization. The "arrest" reaction appears as the initial phase of flight or defense reactions obtained by amygdaloid stimulation. Flight (fear) and defensive (rage and aggression) reactions, termed agonistic behavior, have been elicited from different regions of the amygdaloid complex (Ursin and Kaada, '60). In the amygdaloid complex the intensity of the electrical current determines the intensity of the response, but unlike similar hypothalamic stimulation, the response builds gradually and outlasts the period of stimulation (Zbrożyna, '72). The intense reactions of fear and rage are associated with pupillary dilatation, piloerection, growling, hissing, unmistakable signs of emotional involvement, and participation of the autonomic nervous system. Electrical stimulation of the stria terminalis, or of the ventral amygdalofugal fibers, produces components of the defense reaction, but lesions of the stria terminalis do not alter the responses obtained by stimulating the amygdala (Hilton and Zbrożyna, '63). After lesions completely interrupting the ventral amygdalofugal projections, defense reactions can no longer be obtained by stimulating the amygdaloid complex (Zbrożyna, '72). These findings suggest that the basolateral part of the amygdaloid complex may play an important role in defense reactions. Stimulation of the amygdaloid region in man produces feelings of fear, confusional states, disturbances of awareness and amnesia for events taking place during the stimulation (Feindel and Penfield, '54; Mullan and Penfield, '59; Gloor, '72). Although rage is the most common behavioral response to amygdaloid stimulation in animals, it rarely is associated with temporal lobe seizures, or deep stimulation of the temporal lobe in man (Gloor, '72).

Visceral and autonomic responses include alterations of respiratory rate, rhythm, and amplitude, as well as inhibition of respiration. The most common response of amygdaloid stimulation in unanesthetized animals is an acceleration of the respiratory rate associated with a reduction in amplitude (Kaada, '72). Cardiovascular responses involve both increases and decreases in arterial blood pressure and alterations in heart rate. Pressor responses appear to predominate following amygdaloid stimulation in the unanesthetized animal (Reis and Oliphant, '64). Gastrointestinal motility and secretion may be inhibited or activated, and both defecation and micturition may be induced. Piloerection, salivation, pupillary changes, and alterations of body temperature can occur. These responses are both sympathetic and parasympathetic in nature.

Somatic responses obtained by stimulation of the amygdaloid complex include turning of the head and eyes to the opposite side, and complex rhythmic movements related to chewing, licking and swallowing. The varied somatic and autonomic effects of electrical stimulation of the amygdaloid complex constitute an insignificant part of the syndrome produced by lesions in this complex.

Endocrine responses to stimulation of the amygdaloid nuclear complex include the release of ACTH and gonadotrophic hormone, and lactogenic responses. Stimulation of the amygdaloid areas that produce arousal and emotional responses also produce increased adrenocortical output (Kaada, '72; Zolovick, '72). Bilateral lesions in the medial amygdaloid nuclei produce an elevation of serum levels of ACTH, presumably due to release of an inhibitory influence upon the secretion of ACTH (Bovard and Gloor, '61; Eleftheriou et al., '66). Extensive damage to the amygdala or its hypothalamic projections may attenuate corticosteroid responses (Zolovick, '72). Stimulation of the corticomedial division of the amygdala may induce ovulation, but this response is abolished by transection of the stria terminalis (Shealy and Peele, '57; Everett, '59; Velasco and Taleisnik, '69). The corticomedial amygdaloid nuclei in the female appear to have estrogen concentrating neurons which are part of a system of similar cells extending into hypothalamic and limbic structures (Pfaff and Keiner, '73). The amygdala also is concerned with the luteinizing (LH) and follicle-stimulating (FSH) hormones (Kaada, '72). It is quite clear that the amygdala participates with the hypothalamus in the control and regulation of hypophysial secretions.

Bilateral lesions of the amygdaloid complex in animals consistently produce disturbances of emotional behavior. Animals become placid and display no reactions of fear, rage, or aggression. Previously dominant and abusive animals became tame and did not retaliate to the threats or molestations of other animals. Hypersexuality has been noted as a prominent feature in some experimental studies (Schreiner and Kling, '54; Green et al., '57), but not in all. Hypersexual behavior may occur only when the lesions concomitantly involve the pyriform cortex, since amygdaloid lesions sparing this region do not alter sexual behavior. In most instances hypersexual behavior following bilateral lesions develops after a latent period of several weeks.

In a number of studies in cats removal of the amygdala has led to increased aggressiveness (Bard and Rioch, '37; Bard and Mountcastle, '48; Green et al., '57). Cats displaying postoperative rage frequently developed seizures which were considered to play a role in the savage behavior. Theoretically, the savage behavior is caused by removal of structures exerting inhibitory influences.

Observations in man concerning the effects of bilateral lesions in the amygdaloid complex indicate that these lesions cause a decrease of aggressive and assaultive behavior (Green et al., '51; Pool, '54; Scoville, '54). Stereotaxic lesions in the amygdaloid complex in man (Narabayashi et al., '63; Narabayashi, '72) produce a marked reduction in emotional excitability and tend to normalize social behavior in individuals with severe behavior disturbances. Unilateral lesions in some cases proved sufficient to bring about improvement. Bilateral lesions did not produce the signs and symptoms suggestive of the Klüver-Bucy syndrome. The *Klüver-Bucy syndrome* is characterized by conversion of wild intractable animals (monkeys) to docile beasts which show no evidence of fear, rage or aggression (Klüver and Bucy, '39). These animals display apparent "psychic blindness," a compulsion to examine objects visually, tactually and orally, bizarre sexual behavior and certain changes in dietary habits. Almost all objects are examined, smelled, and mouthed; if the object is not edible, it is discarded. Hypersexuality is characterized by the indiscriminate partnerships sought with both male and female animals. The Klüver-Bucy syndrome has been described in man following large bilateral removal of portions of the temporal lobe (Terzian and Ore, '55; Terzian, '58).

The amygdaloid complex also plays an important role in food and water intake. Bilateral ablations of the amygdala may result in striking hyperphagia, or in hypophagia. Lesions of the basolateral nucleus of the amygdala result in hyperphagia (Fonberg, '68), while stimulation of this part of the amygdala produces an arrest of feeding behavior (Fonberg and Delgado, '61). It has been postulated that this part of the amygdaloid complex inhibits the lateral hypothalamic area, which is regarded as the feeding center of the hypothalamus (Oomura et al., '70; Kaada, '72).

The corticomedial part of the amygdaloid complex is a facilitatory area concerned with food intake. Stimulation of this region produces increases in food intake, as does stimulation of the stria terminalis (Robinson and Mishkin, '62, '68). The amygdala appears to exert its influence upon feeding by modulating the activity of hypothalamic mechanisms. As might be expected the effects of amygdaloid lesions are less severe than those involving the hypothalamus.

SUBSTANTIA INNOMINATA

A heterogeneous group of telencephalic structures on the medial and ventral aspect of the cerebral hemispheres collectively are referred to as the basal forebrain. Despite the location of these structures on the surface of the brain, they lack a cortical organization, but have been described as having a "corticoid" architecture (Mesulam et al., '83). The basal forebrain extends from the olfactory tubercle anteriorly to the hypothalamic region posteriorly and overlaps the area known as the anterior perforated substance (Fig. 12-2). Although the precise boundaries of the basal forebrain are not clearly defined, it appears generally agreed to include the septal area, the olfactory tubercle, parts of the amygdala and the area under the anterior commissure (i.e., the subcommissural region), known as the *substantia innominata* (Figs. 11-13, 12-14, and 12-16). The subcommissural region contains a number of cell groups in contact with fiber bundles traversing the region, which include the diagonal band (Broca), the anterior commissure, the medial forebrain bundle, the ansa lenticularis, the ansa peduncularis and the inferior thalamic peduncle (Fig. 9-8). In the subcommissural region the most conspicuous cells are a group of magnocellular hyperchromic neurons, known as *nucleus basalis* (Meynert, 1872). The term substantia innominata is used inconsistently and frequently as a synonym for the nucleus basalis (Figs. 11-13, 12-14 and 12-16). Large basophilic neurons with similar morphological characteristics are present in the medial septum, dorsal and ventral parts of the nucleus of the diagonal band, and in largest numbers along the ventral and lateral margins of the lateral pallidal segment (Hedreen et al., '84). In the nucleus basalis about 90% of the neurons are cholinergic and have widespread projections to the cerebral cortex (Mesulam et al., '83). These authors suggest that the nucleus basalis may be the single major source of cholinergic innervation of the entire cerebral cortex. In this sense, the basal nucleus appears analogous to the raphe nuclei and the locus ceruleus which constitute the major sources of serotonergic and noradrenergic innervation, respectively, to widespread regions of the cerebral cortex.

The recent interest in the basal nucleus (substantia innominata) is related to the discovery that neurons in this nucleus selectively degenerate in Alzheimer's disease and its variant, senile dementia of the Alzheimer's type, the most common dementia occurring in middle and late life (Katzman, '76; Wang, '77; Whitehouse et al., '81). The loss of cholinergic input from neurons in

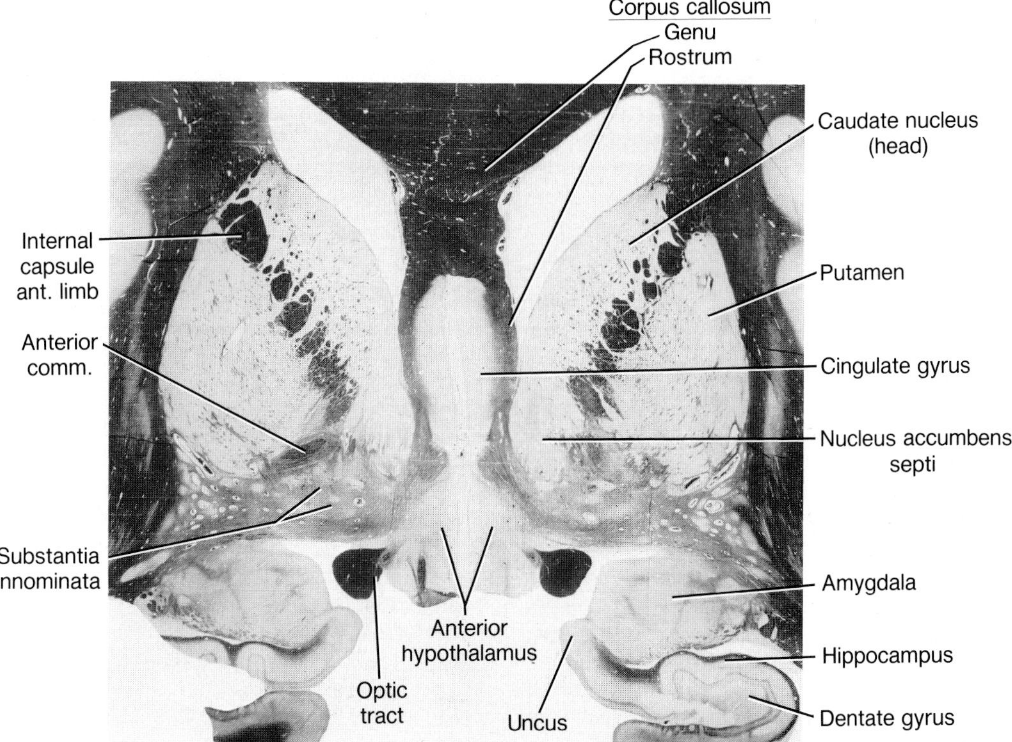

Figure 12-16. Section cut parallel to longitudinal axis of the brain stem through the genu and rostrum of the corpus callosum, the head of the caudate nucleus, the putamen, the substantia innominata, the amygdala and the hippocampal formation. This section reveals the nucleus accumbens septi, ventromedial to the head of the caudate nucleus. The *substantia innominata* lies in the subcommissural region, ventral to the corpus striatum and contains the large hyperchromic neurons known as the *basal nucleus of Meynert.* Cells of the basal nucleus are a major source of cholinergic innervation of the entire cerebral cortex. (Human brain, Weigert's myelin stain.)

the nucleus basalis appears to be a highly significant factor in the well-documented cortical cholinergic deficiency which occurs in these patients (Bowen et al., '76; Davies and Maloney, '76). Alzheimer's disease usually develops between the ages of 40 and 60, is characterized by progressive dementia with apraxia and speech disturbances. There is loss of memory, slurred speech and disorientation. The pathological picture is associated with diffuse degeneration of the cerebral cortex involving all layers, senile plaques in the cortex, intraneuronal fibrillary tangles and selective degeneration of the cells in the nucleus basalis.

LIMBIC SYSTEM

On the medial surface of the cerebral hemisphere, a large arcuate convolution, formed primarily by the cingulate and parahippocampal gyri, surrounds the rostral brain stem and interhemispheric commissures. These gyri, which encircle the upper brain stem, constitute what Broca referred to as the "grand lobe limbique" (Fig. 12-17).

Limbic Lobe. The limbic lobe includes the subcallosal, cingulate, and parahippocampal gyri, as well as the underlying hippocampal formation and dentate gyrus (Fig. 12-17). From a phylogenetic and cytoarchitectural point of view, the limbic lobe consists of *archicortex* (hippocampal formation and dentate gyrus), *paleocortex* (pyriform cortex of the anterior parahippocampal gyrus) and *juxtallocortex* or *mesocortex* (cingulate gyrus). The striking feature of the limbic lobe is that it appears early in phylogenesis and possesses a certain constancy in gross and microscopic structure. The extent to which these var-

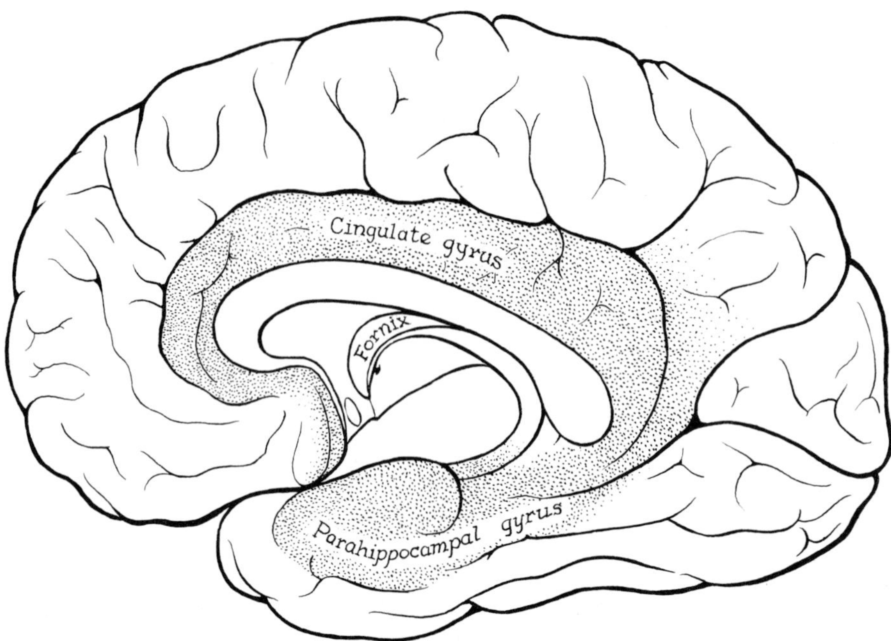

Figure 12-17. Drawing of the medial surface of the hemisphere. *Shading* indicates the limbic lobe which encircles the upper brain stem. This cortex lies on the most medial margin of the hemisphere (i.e., the limbus) and includes archicortex, paleocortex and juxtallocortex. (From Carpenter and Sutin, *Human Neuroanatomy*, 1983; courtesy of Williams & Wilkins.)

ious cortical areas form a functional unit is not understood.

Limbic System. An even more extensive and inclusive designation is the *limbic system.* This term is used to include all of the limbic lobe (Fig. 12-17) as well as associated subcortical nuclei (Fig. 12-6), such as the amygdaloid complex, septal nuclei, hypothalamus, epithalamus, and various thalamic nuclei. The medial tegmental region of the midbrain also is regarded as a part of the limbic system since this region contains both ascending and descending pathways which directly or indirectly are related to the hippocampal formation and the amygdaloid nuclear complex (Figs. 12-7 and 12-15). Despite the heterogeneity and diffuse nature of the so-called limbic system, there are compelling observations that structures comprising this system are involved in neural circuitry that gives rise to a subcortical continuum that begins in the septal area and extends in a paramedian zone through the preoptic region and hypothalamus into the rostral mesencephalon. In this view the hypothalamus is regarded as the central part of this system which suggests the term "septo-hypothalamo-mesencephalic continuum" (Nauta, '72).

The role of the cerebral cortex in the subjective aspects of emotion has been emphasized repeatedly, yet the neocortex appears to have relatively few hypothalamic connections and comparatively little autonomic representation. The intimate relationship of the limbic lobe with the hypothalamus, and the inclusion of these neural structures within the limbic system, have caused many authors to refer to the limbic system as the "visceral brain." Papez's proposed mechanism of emotion, which implicated structures of the limbic system, received experimental support from the studies on monkeys deprived of parts of both temporal lobes (Klüver and Bucy, '39; Klüver, '52).

Various visceral, somatic, and behavioral responses also are obtained by electrical stimulation of the anterior cingulate cortex and the orbital-insular-temporal cortex. Elevation, as well as depression, of arterial blood pressure results from electrical stimulation of these regions in experimental animals (Kaada, '60). Points from which pressor and depressor effects can be obtained frequently are only a few millimeters apart; most authors report that declines in blood pressure are more frequent and of greater magnitude. Effects upon arterial pressure do not appear to be secondary to respiratory changes. Other autonomic responses obtained in experimental animals include inhibition of peristalsis, pupillary dilatation, salivation, and bladder contraction. Perhaps the most striking effect of stimulating these regions is profound inhibition of respiratory movements which involves mainly the inspiratory phase, occurs almost instantaneously, and cannot be held in abeyance for longer than 35 seconds. Acceleration of respiratory movements can be elicited by stimulating portions of the cingulate gyrus posterior to the zone yielding maximum inhibitory effects (Kaada, '60).

Somatic effects obtained by stimulating the anterior cingulate and the orbital-insular-temporal cortex include: (1) inhibition of spontaneous movements, (2) inhibition and facilitation of cortically induced and reflex movements, and (3) chewing, licking and swallowing movements.

The behavioral changes observed in unanesthetized animals with stimulation of the cingulate gyrus are referred to as an "arrest reaction." This reaction consists of an immediate cessation of other activities, an expression of attention or surprise, and movements of the head and eyes to the opposite side (Kaada, '60). Animals remain alert during stimulations and respond to external stimuli. Stimulation of posterior cingulate areas may induce sexual reactions, enhanced grooming, and seemingly pleasurable reactions (MacLean, '58). Neither unilateral nor bilateral ablations of the cingulate cortex, or of the cortex of the orbital-insular-temporal polar region, appear to disturb basic somatomotor or autonomic functions to any marked degree.

Experiments have shown that electrical stimulation of certain subcortical structures via implanted electrodes in unanesthetized rats, cats, and monkeys produce a patterned self-stimulation behavior (Olds and Milner, '54; Brady, '60). In these studies the experimental arrangement is such that the animals can deliver an electrical stimulus to localized areas of their own brains by pressing a pedal or bar. Self-stimulations of the septal region, the anterior preoptic area, and the posterior hypothalamus by bar pressing may be at rates as high as 5,000 per hour in the rat (Olds, '60). The compulsive behavior seen in these situations, where the only reward is an electric shock to a localized region of the brain, suggests that the stimulus may provide a primary reinforcement for drives related to food or sex. Repeated self-stimulation may occur in the monkey from electrodes implanted in a variety of subcortical sites, such as the head of the caudate nucleus, the amygdaloid complex, the medial forebrain bundle, and the midbrain reticular formation (Brady, '60). Self-stimulation of certain regions of the thalamus and hypothalamus may produce unpleasant or avoidance reactions, but these regions appear relatively small in number compared to those from which some gratification appears to result.

The limbic lobe and system occupy central positions in the neural mechanisms that govern behavior and emotion. The components of the limbic system appear to have their main afferent and efferent relationships with two great functional realms, the neocortex and the viscero-endocrine periphery. Among the most prominent neocortical connections are the fibers of the cingulum which arise from the cingulate cortex (Figs. 2-9 and 2-15) and project to the entorhinal cortex along with fibers from other neocortical areas. The entorhinal cortex is a major site of convergence of cortical inputs to the hippocampal formation (Fig. 12-12). Broadly and simply stated, impulses generated in sensory systems, the cerebral cortex and still undetermined neural structures appear to activate triggering mechanisms that in turn excite visceral and somatic systems whose activities in concert provide the physiological expression of behavior and emotion.

CHAPTER 13

The Cerebral Cortex

The cerebral cortex has an area of approximately 2.5 square feet, but only a third of this is found on the free surface; the remainder is hidden in the depths of the sulci. The thickness of the cortex varies from about 4.5 mm in the percentral gyrus to about 1.5 mm in the depths of the calcarine sulcus. The cortex is thickest over the crest of a convolution, thinnest in the depth of a sulcus, and contains an estimated 14 billion neurons.

The cerebral cortex develops from the telencephalon, which in early stages of histogenesis resembles other parts of the embryonic neural tube. The suprastriatal portion of the early telencephalic vesicle is composed of three concentric zones: (1) a *germinal zone* surrounding the lateral ventricle, (2) the *intermediate zone* which becomes the white matter of the cerebral hemispheres, and (3) a *marginal zone* which becomes the cortical zone or plate. The original columnar epithelial cells extend through all zones (Sidman, '70). Near the end of the 2nd month cells migrate from the intermediate zone into the marginal zone, where they form the superficial layer, the *cerebral cortex.* Gradually the cerebral cortex thickens by the addition and differentiation of migrating cells. Cells become organized into horizontal layers between the 6th and 8th months; six such layers are distinguished in the neocortex. Cells formed at the same time tend to remain in the same layer, while newly formed cells migrate through these layers to more superficial locations (Angevine and Sidman, '61). This "inside-out" sequence of neuronal migration applies to the majority of cortical cells. This six-layer cellular arrangement is characteristic of the entire neopallium, which is referred to as the *neocortex,* isocortex, or homogenetic cortex.

The *paleopallium* (olfactory cortex) and the *archipallium* (hippocampal formation and dentate gyrus) have three basic layers, and collectively constitute the *allocortex* or *heterogenetic cortex.*

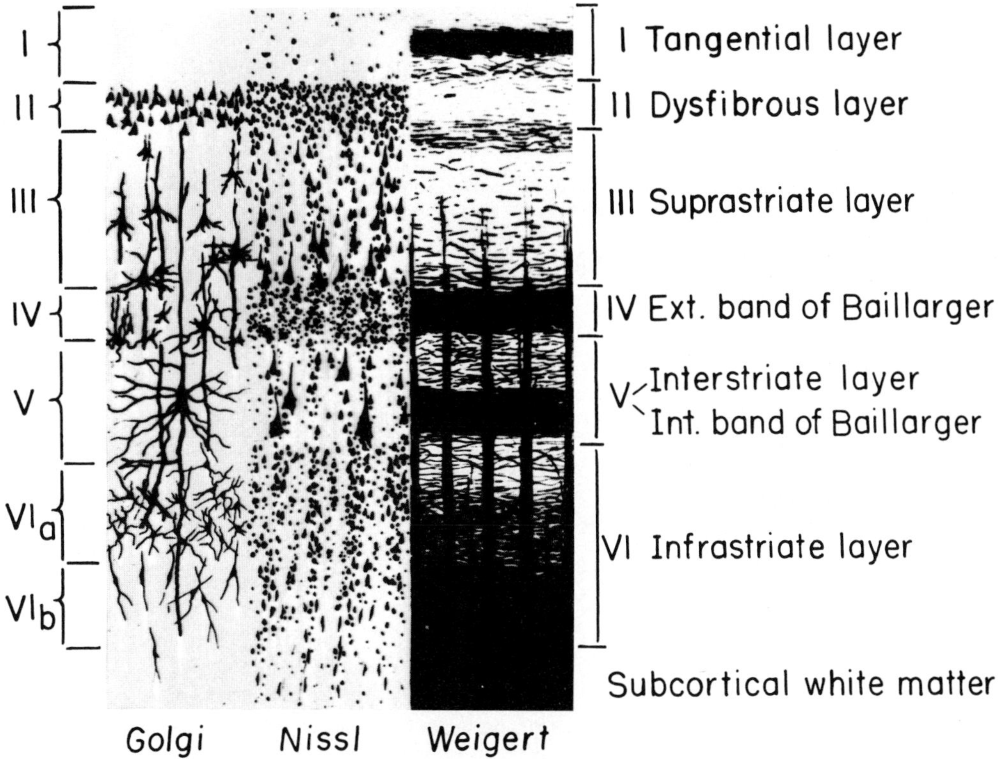

Figure 13-1. The cell layers and fiber arrangement of the human cerebral cortex. Semischemic (after Brodmann, '09). (From Carpenter and Sutin, *Human Neuroanatomy*, 1983; courtesy of Williams & Wilkins.)

CORTICAL CELLS AND FIBERS

The principal types of cells found in the cortex are pyramidal, stellate, and fusiform neurons (Fig. 13-1).

The *pyramidal cells*, which are most characteristic of the cortex, have the form of a pyramid. An *apical dendrite* extends upward toward the pial surface and numerous basal dendrites project horizontally from the cell body. The axon emerges from the base of the cell and enters the white matter. Pyramidal cells have prominent Nissl granules and the cell bodies vary in height from 10 to 50 μm. The giant pyramidal cells, found in the percentral gyrus, may be more than 100 μm in height.

Stellate, or *granule cells* have a polygonal shape, scant cytoplasm, and range in size from 4 to 8 μm. These cells have numerous dendrites, which pass in all directions, and a short axon. Stellate cells are found in all layers of the cortex but are most numerous in layer IV (Figs. 13-1, 13-2, and 13-3).

The *fusiform* or *spindle cells* are found mainly in the deepest cortical layers, with their long axis vertical to the surface. The two poles of the cell are continued into dendrites; the lower dendrites arborize within the layer, while the upper ones ascend toward the surface. The axon arises from the lower part of the cell body, and enters the white matter (Fig. 13-1).

Other cell types found in the cortex are the *horizontal cells of Cajal*, and the cells with ascending axons, known as the *cells of Martinotti.* The former are small fusiform cells found in the most superficial layer. Martinotti cells, present in all layers, are small triangular cells whose axons extend variable distances toward the surface.

Fibers in the cerebral cortex are disposed both radially and tangentially. The former are arranged in delicate, radiating bundles running vertically from the medullary substance toward the cortical surface (Fig. 13-1). They include axons of pyramidal, fusiform, and stellate cells which leave the

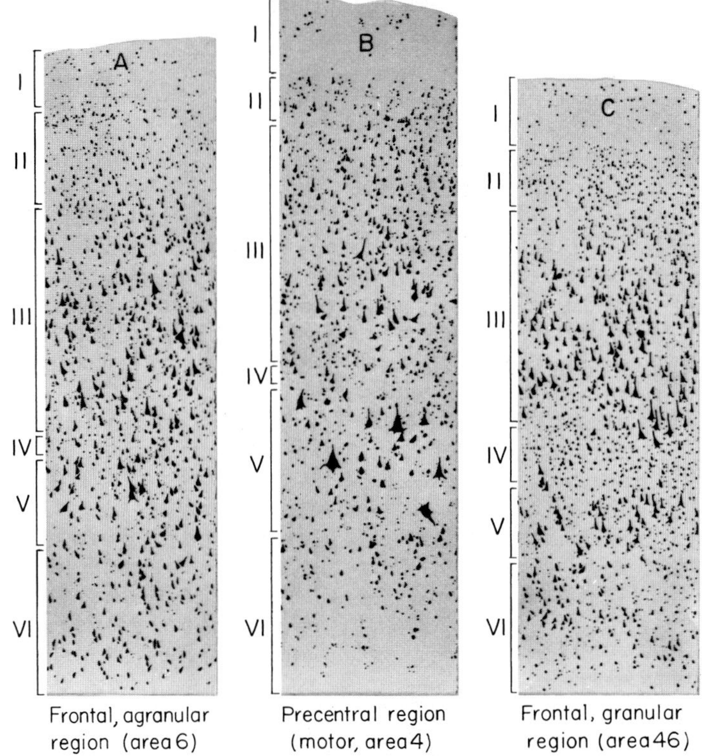

Figure 13-2. Cytoarchitectural pictures of several representative cortical areas (after Campbell, '05). (From Carpenter and Sutin, *Human Neuroanatomy*, 1983; courtesy of Williams & Wilkins.)

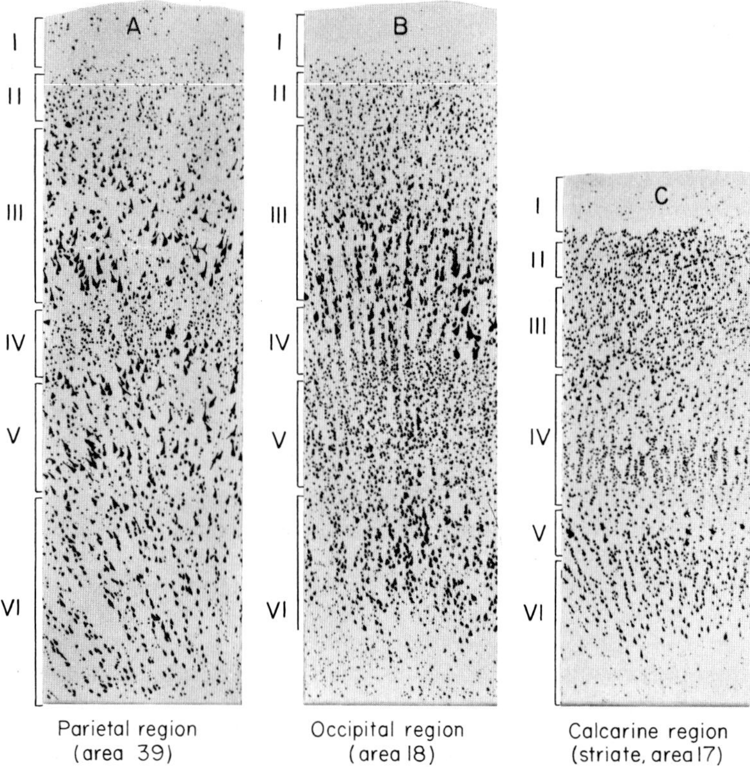

Figure 13-3. Cytoarchitectural pictures of several cortical areas (after Campbell, '05). (From Carpenter and Sutin, *Human Neuroanatomy*, 1983; courtesy of Williams & Wilkins.)

cortex as projection or association fibers, and the entering afferent projection and association fibers, which terminate within the cortex. Tangential fibers run parallel to the cortical surface. These fiber bundles are composed of the terminal branches of afferent projection and association fibers, axons of horizontal and granule cells, and collateral branches of pyramidal and fusiform cells. Horizontal fibers in large part represent terminal portions of radial fibers. Tangential fibers are not distributed evenly throughout the cortex but are concentrated at varying depths into horizontal bands. The two most prominent bands are known as the *bands of Baillarger*, which are visible to the naked eye as delicate white stripes in sections of the fresh cortex (Figs. 13-1 and 13-9).

CORTICAL LAYERS

The most striking anatomical feature of cortical organization is its cellular lamination. In Nissl-stained sections the cell bodies are arranged in superimposed horizontal layers. Layers are distinguished by the types, density, and arrangement of their cells. The lamination seen in myelin-sheath-stained sections is determined primarily by the disposition of horizontal fibers which vary in quantity and density in different layers (Figs. 13-1, 13-2, and 13-3). The *neopallium* (neocortex or isocortex), which forms 90% of the hemispheric surface, has six fundamental layers.

In the neocortex the following layers are distinguished in passing from the pial surface to the underlying white matter. I, molecular; II, external granular; III, external pyramidal; IV, internal granular; V, internal pyramidal; and VI, multiform (Figs. 13-1, 13-2, 13-3, and 13-4).

I. The *molecular layer* contains cells with horizontal axons and Golgi type II cells, as well as the terminal dendrites of cells in lower layers. Dendrites and axonal branches form a tangential fiber plexus.

II. The *external granular* layer consists of closely packed granule cells whose dendrites terminate in the molecular layer and whose axons enter deeper layers.

III. The *external pyramidal layer* is composed of two sublayers of pyramidal neurons of different sizes. Apical dendrites of these cells project to the molecular layer, while axons enter the white matter as association or commissural fibers (Jones and Wise, '77; Szentágothai, '78).

IV. The *internal granular layer* is composed of closely packed stellate cells, many of which have short axons ramifying within the layer. Some larger stellate cells project axons to deeper layers. Myelinated fibers of the external band of Baillarger form a prominent horizontal plexus in this layer (Fig. 13-1).

V. The *internal pyramidal layer* consists mainly of medium and large-size pyramidal neurons. Apical dendrites of large pyramidal cells ascend to the molecular layer; dendrites of smaller pyramids ascend to layer IV. Axons of pyramidal cells leave the cortex chiefly as projection fibers. Horizontal fibers in deeper portions of this layer form the internal band of Baillarger (Fig. 13-1).

VI. The *multiform layer* contains predominantly spindle-shaped cells whose long axis is perpendicular to the cortical surface. Spindle cells vary in size; larger cells send dendrites to the molecular layer while those of smaller cells ascend to layer IV. Axons of these cells enter the white matter as projection and association fibers. The layer is pervaded by fiber bundles which enter and leave the white matter (Fig. 13-1).

Besides the horizontal cellular lamination, the cortex also exhibits a vertical or radical arrangement of the cells, which gives the appearance of slender vertical cells columns passing through the whole thickness of the cortex (Fig. 13-3). This vertical lamination, quite distinct in the parietal, occipital, and temporal lobes, is practically absent in the frontal lobe (Fig. 13-2). The columnar arrangement of cells in the cerebral cortex is determined largely by the mode of termination of corticocortical afferents (Szentágothai, '78). Corticocortical afferents are distributed throughout all layers of the cortex in columnar modules 200 to 300 μm in diameter, while terminals of specific sensory afferents usually are restricted to layer IV. Columnar units of corticocortical afferent fibers are all nearly the same size and have dimensions similar to physiological identified columnar units in the sensory cortex (Mountcastle, '57; Hubel and Wiesel, '59; Goldman

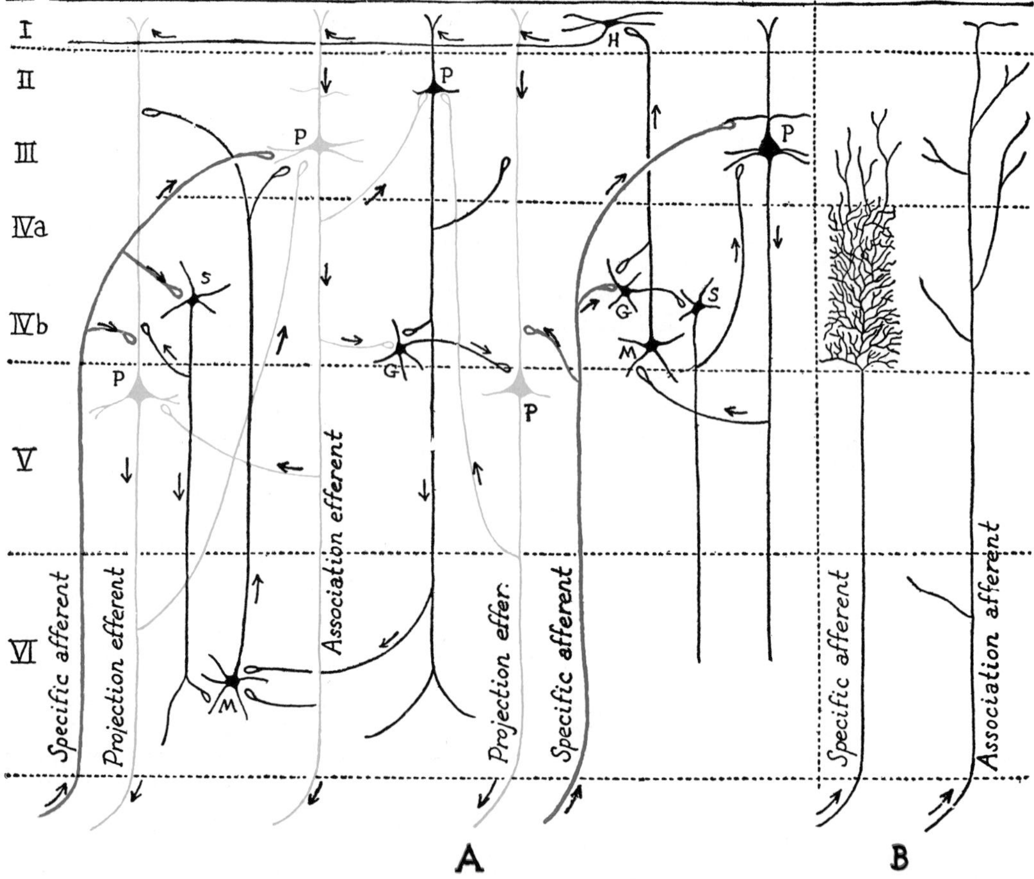

Figure 13-4. (*A*) Diagram showing some of the intracortical circuits. Synaptic junctions are indicated by *loops*. *Red*, afferent thalamocortical fibers; *blue*, efferent cortical neurons; *black*, intracortical neurons; *G*, granule cell; *H*, horizontal cell; *M*, Martinotti cell; *P*, pyramidal cell; *S*, stellate cells. (*B*) Mode of termination of afferent cortical fibers. Based on data by Lorente de Nó ('49). (From Carpenter and Sutin, *Human Neuroanatomy*, 1983; courtesy of Williams & Wilkins.)

and Nauta, '77; Szentágothai, '78). Horizontal lamination in the cerebral cortex is largely determined by the distribution of tangential fibers.

INTERRELATION OF CORTICAL NEURONS

The structure of the cerebral cortex as seen in Nissl or myelin sheath-stained sections is incomplete, for these sections show only the type and arrangement of cell bodies, or the course and distribution of myelinated fibers. An understanding of the neuronal relationships and of the intracortical circuits, can be obtained only by impregnation methods which give a total picture of the cell body and all its processes (i.e., the Golgi method). According to Lorente de Nó ('49), the arrangement of the axonal and dendritic branchings forms the most constant feature of cortical structure (Fig. 13-4).

The afferent fibers of the cortex include projection fibers from the thalamus, association fibers from other cortical areas and commissural fibers from the opposite side. The thalamocortical fibers, especially the specific afferents from the ventral tier thalamic nuclei and the geniculate bodies, pass unbranched to layer IV (Figs. 4-1, 4-3, 4-4, and 9-11). Fibers of the so-called nonspecific thalamocortical system project directly to the cortex from parts of the rostral intralaminar thalamic nuclei (Steriade and Glenn, '82) and via collaterals of thalamostriate fibers arising from the centromedian-parafascicular nuclear complex (Jones and Leavitt, '74). The synaptic termination of nonspecific fibers in the cortex is chiefly axodendritic and widely distributed in all layers, but the principal physiological effects appear to be within the superficial layers (Jasper, '60). The recruiting responses recorded from the cerebral cortex, following stimulation of midline and intralaminar thalamic nuclei, are graded responses thought to represent dendritic hyperpolarization and depolarization.

The cortical neurons may be grouped into cells with descending, ascending, horizontal, and short axons. The last three types serve wholly for intracortical connections. The cells with descending axons (pyramidal, fusiform, and larger stellate cells) furnish all the efferent projection and association fibers, but their axonal collaterals form an extensive intracortical system.

Commissural fibers arise from cells in all cortical regions and interconnect homologous cortical areas. The majority of these fibers pass in the corpus callosum, although some are found in the anterior commissure and the hippocampal commissure. Exceptions to this generalization are found in the regions of the primary motor (area 4) and somesthetic cortex (S I) that represent the hand and foot (Karol and Pandya, '71; Jones and Wise, '77; Jones and Hendry, '80); in the visual cortex, area 17 (Hubel and Wiesel, '67; Zeki, '71; Wong-Riley, '74, '79); and in parts of the auditory cortex (Diamond et al., '68). Commissural cells retrogradely labeled by horseradish peroxidase (HRP) are large pyramidal cells in deep parts of layer III (Jones and Wise, '77). Cortical afferents from commissural neurons extend throughout all cortical layers and fill a column about 200 to 300 μm in diameter (Szentágothai, '78). Similar studies of association fibers in the same hemisphere indicate that most of these fibers arise from the supragranular layers (Jones and Wise, '77). Ipsilateral corticocortical fibers arise from cells in more superficial parts of layer III and from parts of layer II. Terminal branches of association fibers are distributed mainly to layers III and IV (Jones and Powell, '68).

The pyramidal and fusiform cells of layers V and VI have a very characteristic pattern of dendritic and axonal branchings. All the pyramidal cells of layer V give off basilar dendrites to their own layer and an apical dendrite which, in most cases, extends to the molecular layer. The spindle cells of layer VI have similar branches; ascending dendritic shafts terminate respectively in layers I and IV, while other dendrites arborize in layer VI. The axons of pyramidal and spindle neurons are continued as projection fibers. All of these axons send horizontal collaterals to layers V and VI where they contribute to the horizontal plexuses. In addition, many cells have one or more recurrent collaterals which ascend unbranched through layer IV and arborize in layers II and III.

The horizontal laminar arrangement of the cells in the cerebral cortex has served as a major criteria to map the distinctive cytoarchitectonic areas. This lamination also serves to segregate different efferent projections from the cortex. Each of the major efferent pathways emanating from sensory-motor cortex has a specific laminar or sublaminar origin (Jones and Wise, '77). The somata of the majority of cells whose axons are distributed intracortically (both ipsilaterally and contralaterally) lie in the supragranular layers (layers II and III). Cortical neurons whose axons project to subcortical structures are located in the infragranular layers, particularly layer V. In the supragranular layers (i.e., above layer IV), cells whose axons are distributed ipsilaterally as corticocortical fibers lie superficial to cells projecting axons to the cortex of the opposite hemisphere, and cells with shorter axons tend to lie superficial to those with longer axons. In the infragranular layers (i.e., below layer IV) the somata of corticostriate neurons lie in the most superficial part of layer V while somata giving rise to corticospinal and corticotectal fibers are in the deepest part of the same layer. Somata of neurons giving rise to corticorubral, corticopontine, and corticobulbar fibers lie in intermediate regions of layer V, between corticostriate and corticospinal neurons. Layer VI of the cortex contains the somata of cells that give rise to corticothalamic projections. Cells giving rise to a particular set of efferent connections are of nearly the same size and do not vary in their laminar distribution. Only neurons giving rise to corticospinal fibers show great variation in cell size. Cells of particular efferent systems occur in single or multiple strips oriented mediolaterally across the cortex.

Functional Columnar Organization. Physiological studies of the somatic sensory and visual cortex provide ample evidence that a vertical column of cells, extending across all cellular layers, constitutes the elementary functional cortical unit (Mountcastle, '57; Powell and Mountcastle, '59a; Hubel and Wiesel, '62, '63a). This conclusion is supported by the following: (1) neurons of a particular vertical column are all related to the same, or nearly the same, peripheral receptive field, (2) neurons of the same vertical column are activated by the same kind of peripheral stimulus, and (3) all cells of a vertical column discharge at more or less the same latency following a brief peripheral stimulus. The topographic pattern present on the cortical surface extends throughout its depth. Studies of the visual (striate) cortex demonstrate similar discrete functional columns extending from the pial surface to the white matter that are responsive to a specific kind of retinal stimulation in the form of long narrow rectangles of light ("slits"), dark bars against a light background, or straight-line borders, all of which must have a particular axis of orientation (Hubel and Wiesel, '62, '63a). Microelectrode recordings indicate that functional columns of cells are arranged radially, perpendicular to the cortical layers. Columns display variations in size and cross-sectional area, and the receptive field axis of orientation varies in a continuous manner as the surface of the cortex is traversed. Anatomically an elementary functional unit of the cortex, represented by a column of cells, must contain the afferent, efferent and internuncial fiber systems necessary for the formation of a complete cortical circuit. In the basic columnar units the internal circuitry must vary with differences in cytoarchitecture (Fig. 13-3). The convergence of specific afferents upon cells in the columnar unit appears to imprint a specific sensory feature which is relayed by intracortical connections to other cells in the column. The complex axonal branching suggests that intracortical circuits involve cells in all parts of the column. These vertical circuits are interconnected by short neuronal links, represented primarily by the short axons granule cells. Through these short links, cortical excitation may spread horizontally and involve a progressively larger number of vertical units (Fig. 13-4). Thus a specific afferent fiber may not only fire vertical columns of cells in its immediate vicinity, but may reach more distant units through Golgi type II cell relays.

The cerebral cortex has been envisaged as a mosaic of columnar units of remarkably similar internal structure (Szentágothai, '78). In addition to the functional columnar arrangement described in the sensory cortical areas, there are corticocortical columns delineated primarily by the pattern of termination of association and commissural fibers. The columnar units of corticocortical projections are of the same general size as the functional columns of the sensory cortex. In the corticocortical columns there is a convergence of afferent fibers from multiple modular units that create a vast mosaic of cortical connections. Excitatory inputs from the thalamus and other cortical areas are considered to be processed through a column-oriented circuitry composed of both excitatory and inhibitory neurons. Most interneurons in the cerebral cortex are highly specific with respect to: (1) the neurons from which they receive inputs, (2) the arborization pattern of their axons, and (3) the sites at which they establish synapses on other neurons. The vast majority of stellate, or granular, cells belong to the heterogeneous group, referred to as Golgi type II cells, which do not project fibers beyond the cerebral cortex. Electron microscopic evidence, based upon the types of synaptic contact, suggests that the majority of cortical interneurons are excitatory (asymmetrical synapses with spherical synaptic vesicles). Cortical interneurons identified as putative inhibitory cells constitute a minority of the known interneurons. Both excitatory and inhibitory influences within the cerebral cortex are exerted upon pyramidal cells that represent the principal cortical output neurons.

CORTICAL AREAS

The cerebral cortex does not have a uniform structure. It has been mapped and

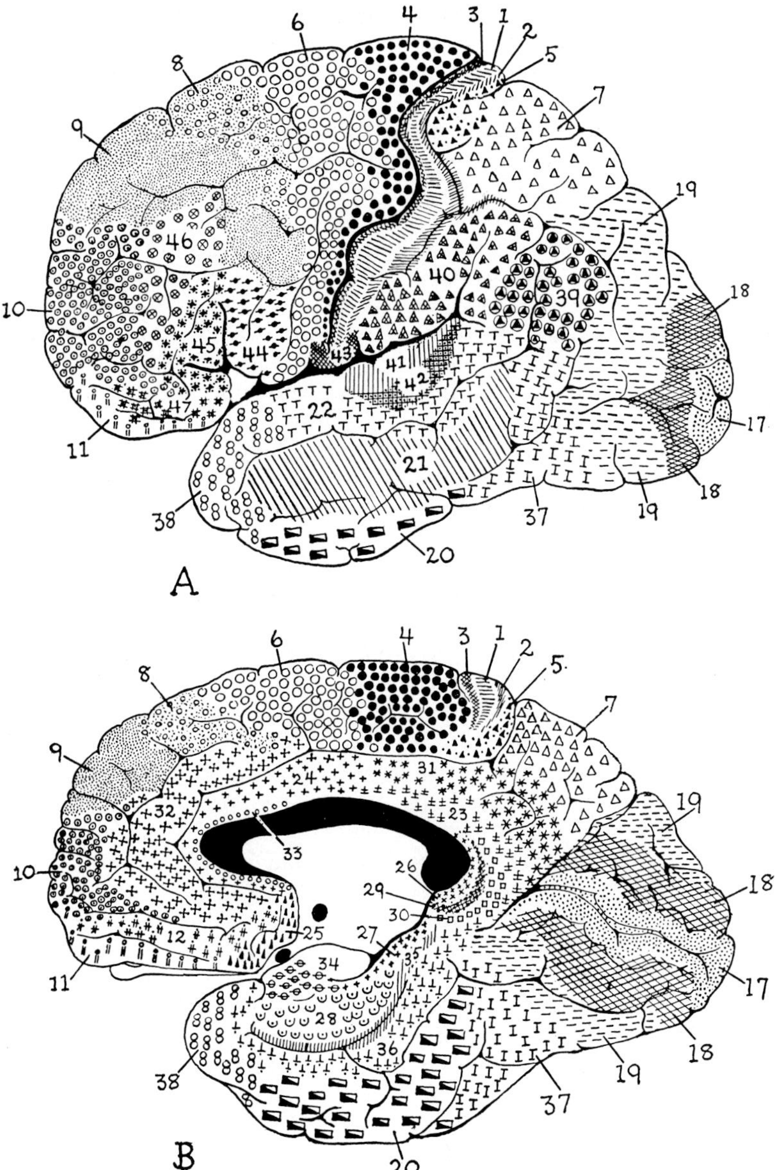

Figure 13-5. Cytoarchitectural map of the human cerebral cortex. (*A*) Convex surface; (*B*) medial surface (after Brodmann, '09). (From Carpenter and Sutin, *Human Neuroanatomy*, 1983; courtesy of Williams & Wilkins.)

divided into a number of distinctive areas that differ from each other in total thickness, in the thickness and density of individual layers, and in the arrangement and number of cells and fibers. In certain areas the structural variations are so extreme that the basic six-layered pattern is practically obscured. Such areas are termed *heterotypical*, as opposed to *homotypical*, which describes cortex in which all six layers are easily distinguished (Brodmann, '09).

Differences in the arrangements and types of cells, as well as the patterns of myelinated fibers, have been used to construct several fundamentally similar maps of the cortex composed of distinctive cytological areas (Fig. 13-5). Campbell ('05) described some 20 cortical areas; Brodmann

('09) increased the number to 47, and Economo ('29) to 109; the Vogts ('19) parcelled the human cerebral cortex into more than 200 areas. The Brodmann map of the cerebral cortex has been used widely for reference (Fig. 13-5).

Virtually all parts of the cerebral cortex are connected with subcortical centers by afferent and efferent projections. In a strict sense there are no circumscribed cortical areas which are purely projective or associative in character. However, there are regions from which the more important descending tracts arise; fibers descending from these areas directly and indirectly influence the activity of lower motor neurons and provide control for both somatic and visceral functions. Motor areas from which muscle movements can be elicited by electrical stimulation lie chiefly in the precentral and premotor regions. Cortical regions which receive direct thalamocortical sensory projections from the ventral tier thalamic nuclei and the geniculate bodies represent the primary sensory areas. The remaining cortical area, not directly related to motor or sensory functions, constitutes the largest part of the cerebral cortex in man; this cortex is referred to as the "association cortex." Afferent fibers to the association cortex are derived from the association nuclei of the thalamus and from the primary sensory areas of the cortex. Although the primary sensory and motor areas are predominant in lower mammals, in that they constitute an unusually large part of the neocortex, there is considerable intermingling of functions. In higher mammals, the primary sensory and motor areas become more specific, and there is an absolute increase in the association cortex (Woolsey, '58).

SENSORY AREAS OF THE CEREBRAL CORTEX

Primary Sensory Areas. The localized cortical regions to which impulses concerned with specific sensory modalities are projected constitute the primary sensory areas of the cerebral cortex. Although certain aspects of the sensation probably enter consciousness at thalamic levels, the primary sensory areas are concerned especially with integration of sensory experience and with the discriminative qualities of sensation. With the exception of olfaction, impulses involved in all forms of sensation reach localized areas of the cerebral cortex via thalamocortical projection systems. The organization of the thalamus is such that all of the specific sensory relay nuclei are located caudally in the ventral tier (Figs. 9-11 and 9-12). The cortical projections of the specific sensory thalamic relay nuclei are to localized areas in the parietal, occipital, and temporal lobes.

Established primary sensory areas in the cerebral cortex are: (1) the *somesthetic area*, consisting of the postcentral gyrus and its medial extension in the paracentral lobule (areas 3, 1, and 2); (2) the *visual* or *striate area*, located along the lips of the calcarine sulcus (area 17); and (3) the *auditory area*, located on the two transvese gyri (Heschl; areas 41 and 42; see Figs. 2-4, 2-9, 6-10, 13-5, 13-6, 13-7, and 13-8). The *gustatory area* is localized to the most ventral part (opercular) of the postcentral gyrus (area 43). The primary olfactory area, consisting of the allocortex of the prepyriform and periamygdaloid regions, has not been assigned numbers under the Brodmann paracellation. Although the *primary vestibular area* in the human cerebral cortex has not been established, studies in the primate indicate it may lie in portions of the postcentral gyrus (Deecke et al., '73, '74; Fredrickson et al., '74).

The primary sensory areas of the cerebral cortex receive the projections of the specific sensory relay nuclei of the thalamus, and are focal regions in the cerebral cortex, where specific sensory modalities are most extensively and critically represented. Evidence suggests that near each primary receptive area there are other cortical zones which also receive sensory inputs.

Secondary Sensory Areas. Near each primary receptive area there are cortical zones which also receive sensory inputs directly from the thalamus, from the primary sensory area, or from both (Friedman et al, '80; Hubel and Wiesel, '65). These cortical zones, adjacent to the primary sensory areas are referred to as *secondary sensory areas*. Secondary sensory areas have been defined primarily in experimental animals by recording evoked potentials in response to peripheral stimuli

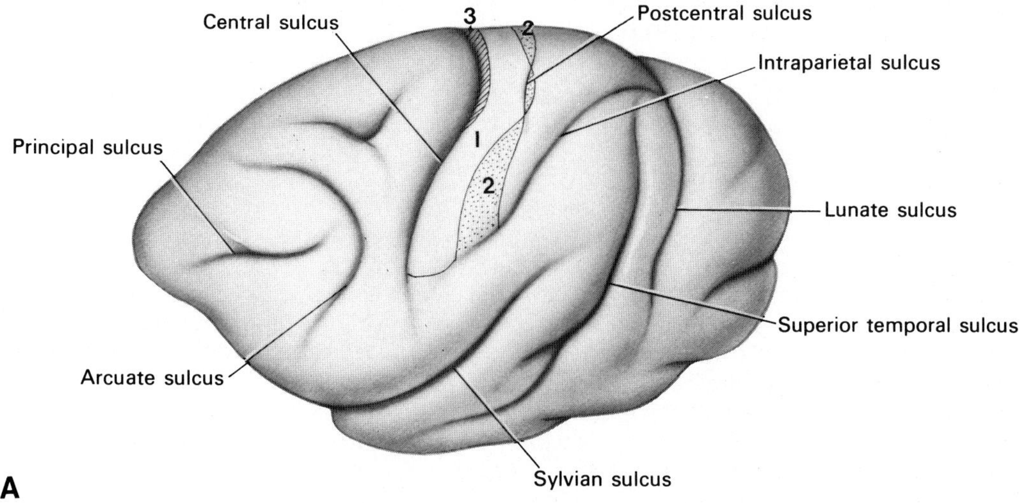

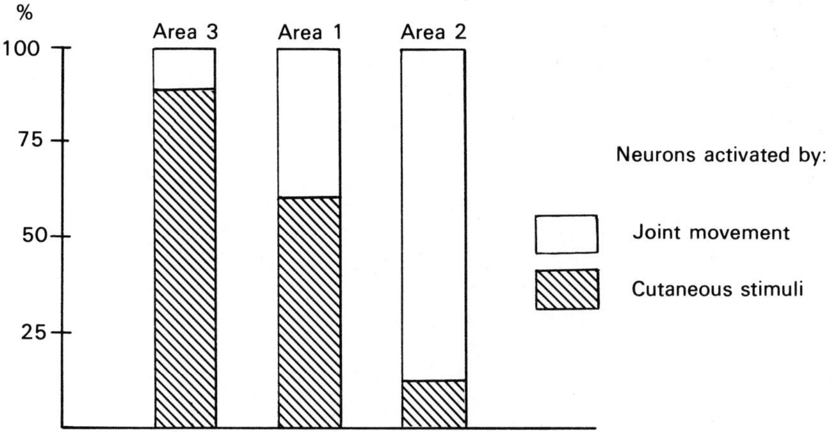

Figure 13-6. (*A*) Diagram of the lateral surface of the monkey cerebral hemisphere showing the extent of the three areas which compose the primary somesthetic cortex. Area *3*, which forms the posterior wall of the central sulcus, is hidden, except for a small dorsomedial region indicated in the diagram. Areas *1* and *2* form the crown and posterior wall of the postcentral gyrus. (*B*) Bar graph indicating the relative prevalence in each cytoarchitectural area of the postcentral gyrus of neuron columns activated by cutaneous stimuli and joint movement (based upon Powell and Mountcastle, '59; and Mountcastle and Powell, '59). (From Carpenter and Sutin, *Human Neuroanatomy*, 1983; courtesy of Williams & Wilkins.)

(Adrian, '40, '41; Woolsey, '58; Rose and Woolsey, '58; Poggio and Mountcastle, '60; Werner and Whitsel, '73). Usually secondary sensory areas are smaller than the primary sensory areas, and the sequence of representation is the reverse, or different than that found in the primary area. Ablations of the secondary sensory areas produce only minor sensory disturbances compared with those resulting from ablations of the primary sensory areas.

Secondary sensory areas, defined primarily in experimental animals, include: (1) a *second somatic sensory area* (somatic sen-

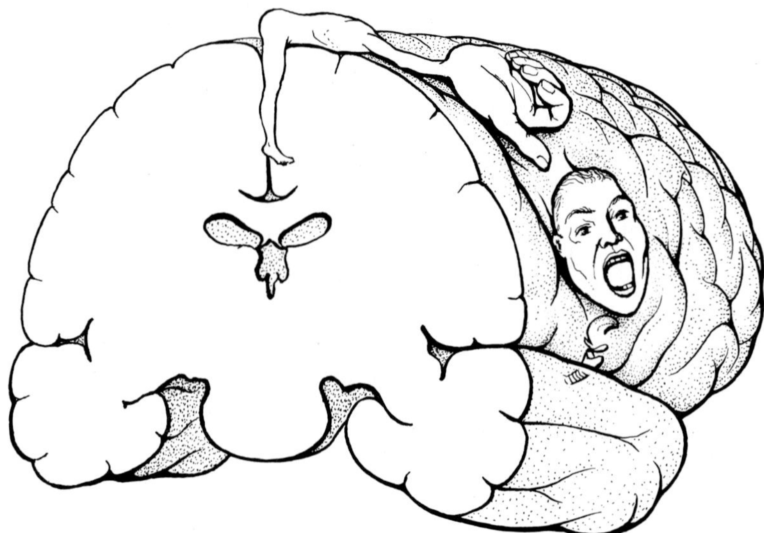

Figure 13-7. Schematic representation of somatotopic localization of the body in the motor cortex. Parts of the body are drawn in proportion to the extent of their cortical representation. The resulting disproportionate figure is called the motor "homunculus." A similar pattern of localization with respect to somesthetic sense is found in the postcentral gyrus (after Penfield and Rasmussen, '50). (From Carpenter and Sutin, *Human Neuroanatomy*, 1983; courtesy of Williams & Wilkins.)

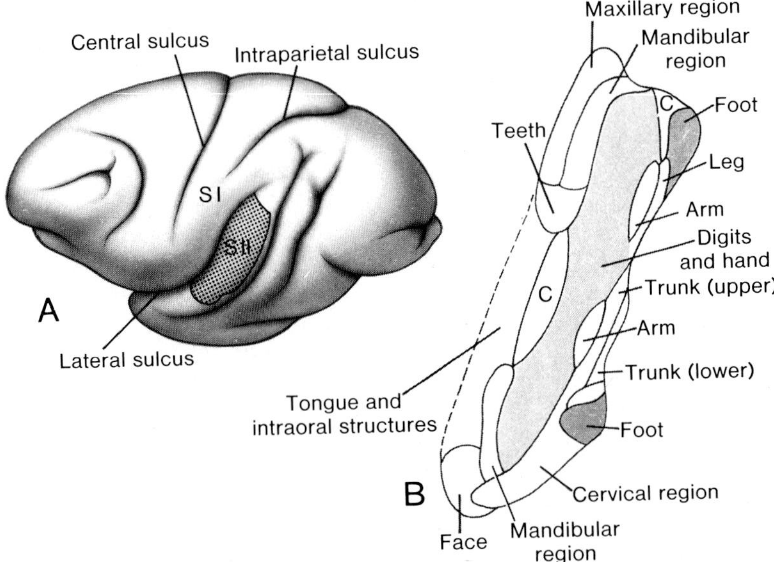

Figure 13-8. Diagrams of the position and somatotopic organication of the second somatic area (SS II) in *Macacus cynomologus*. Most of SS II lies buried in the depths of the lateral sulcus and has been identified on the basis of its cytoarchitecture and connections with the ventrobasal complex and projections from the primary somesthetic cortex (S I). In (*A*), SS II is shown in a flattened view on the cortical surface. In (*B*), the body representation in SS II is outlined as determined from recordings in awake monkeys. Different regions of the body are represented by a series of oblique strips parallel to the lateral sulcus, with the face and intraoral structure most rostral. The area in *blue* represents the digits and hand, while the areas in *red* represents the foot. Areas designated *C* are regions with poorly defined receptive fields (based on Robinson and Burton, '80). (From Carpenter and Sutin, *Human Neuroanatomy*, 1983; courtesy of Williams & Wilkins.)

sory area II, SS II), located ventral to the primary sensory and motor areas along the superior lip of the lateral sulcus (Fig. 13-8), (2) a *secondary auditory area* (auditory area II), surrounding the primary auditory area (auditory area I) (Figs. 13-17 and 13-18), and (3) a *secondary visual area* (visual area II), described in the rabbit, cat and monkey, which is coextensive with the area defined anatomically as area 18. A second somatic sensory area (SS II) has been demonstrated in man (Penfield and Rasmussen, '50), stimulation of which produces various sensations in the upper and lower extremities. Representation of the extremities is chiefly contralateral, though ipsilateral representation also is present. In man no discrete cortical representation has been identified for the face, tongue, mouth or throat in SS II. Because of close functional interrelationships, primary and secondary sensory areas will be discussed together.

Primary Somesthetic Area (S I). The cortical area subserving general somatic sensibility, superficial as well as deep, is located in the postcentral gyrus and in the posterior part of the paracentral lobule. Histologically the gyrus is composed of three narrow strips of cortex (areas 3, 1, 2) which differ in their architectural structure (Fig. 13-5). The anterior part, area 3, is clearly distinguishable from the posterior part; areas 1 and 2 show a more gradual morphological change. Cortical area 3 is characterized by its thinness and lies along the posterior wall of the central sulcus. Areas 1 and 2 form respectively the crown and posterior wall of the postcentral gyrus (Fig. 13-6).

The postcentral gyrus receives the thalamic projections from the ventral posterior nuclei (VPLc and VPM), which relay impulses from the medial lemniscus, the spinothalamic tracts, and ascending gustatory pathways. The majority of the cells of the ventral posterolateral (VPLc) and ventral posteromedial (VPM) thalamic nuclei project to area 3. Area 1, however, receives the exclusive projections of about 30% of the cells in these nuclei, but it also receives collaterals of fibers passing to area 3. Most of the fibers projecting to area 2 appear to be collaterals of fibers passing primarily to areas 3 and 1. Although most of the information concerning thalamocortical projections is based upon retrograde cellular degeneration, studies of discrete lesions in the ventral posterior thalamic nuclei reveal that coarse fibers project profusely to area 3 while fibers projecting to areas 1 and 2 are fine and distribute terminals sparsely throughout these two areas (Jones and Powell, '70, '73). Autoradiographic studies of the projections of the ventral posterior thalamic nuclei confirm the substantial projection to area 3, but do not resolve the question concerning collateral projections to areas 1 and 2 (Jones, '75). Because neurons in area 3 respond preferentially to light tactile stimuli and cells in areas 1 and 2 are excited mainly by deep stimuli and joint movement, it would be expected that different populations of thalamic neurons might project to areas 3, 1 and 2 (Powell and Mountcastle, '59; Werner and Whitsel, '68). In the somatosensory cortex most of the thalamic afferents terminate in layer IV.

The various regions of the body are represented in specific portions of the postcentral gyrus, the pattern corresponding to that of the motor area (Fig. 13-7). Thus the face area lies in the most ventral part, while above it are the sensory areas for the hand, arm, trunk, leg and foot in the order named; the lower extremity is represented in the paracentral lobule (Fig. 2-6). The cortical areas representing the hand, face, and mouth regions are disproportionally large. The digits of the hand, particularly the thumb and index finger, are well represented. The cortical area related to sensations from the face occupies almost the entire lower half of the postcentral gyrus; the upper part of the face is represented above, while the lips and mouth are represented below. The tongue and pharyngeal region are localized in more ventral areas. In attempts to present a readily apparent visual pattern of the sequence of sensory representation in the cerebral cortex, Penfield has drawn a "sensory homunculus" relating different parts of the body to appropriate areas of the cortex. The "sensory homunculus" corresponds to the "motor homunculus" (Fig. 13-7). The distorted representation of the body surface in the primary sensory area has been said to reflect the peripheral innervation density. Those regions of the body with higher densities of receptor elements have more extensive cortical representation, while those regions with relatively few receptors have a minimal representation.

Physiological studies (Powell and Mountcastle, '59a; Mountcastle and Powell, '59) in the monkey indicate that the majority of neurons in the postcentral gyrus are activated by mechanical stimulation and are selectively excited by stimulation of receptors within either skin or deep tissues, but not by stimulation of both (Fig. 13-6). Over 90% of the neurons in area 2 are related to receptors in deep tissues of the body, while the majority of neurons in area 3 are activated only by cutaneous stimuli; different columns of neurons in area 1 are related to either cutaneous or deep receptors. This differential representation of sensory modalities is closely correlated with the gradient of morphological change that characterizes these three cytoarchitectural areas. Afferent impulses from receptors in joint capsules and pericapsular tissues, stimulated by joint movement, are conveyed by the posterior columns, the medial lemnicus, and thalamic relay neurons to particular cell columns in the postcentral gyrus. Impulses conveyed by this system subserve position sense and kinesthesis. Cell columns of the postcentral gyrus responsive to cutaneous stimuli (Mountcastle and Powell, '59a) indicate that receptive fields on the body surface are constant. There is no evidence that the position of the stimulus within the receptive field is coded in terms of the temporal characteristics of the response. The majority of cortical neurons driven by cutaneous stimuli adapt quickly to steady stimuli. The above observations pertain only to the somatic afferent system composed of primary dorsal root afferents in the posterior columns, lemniscal fibers arising from the posterior column nuclei, and thalamocortical fibers arising from the ventral posterolateral nucleus. This is a system of great synaptic security, poised for action at high frequency levels, and possessing the neural attributes required for discriminatory functions.

Stretch receptors in muscle and tendons probably do not provide information useful in perception of joint position. Although most of the afferent impulses from stretch receptors project to the cerebellum (Oscarsson, '65; Rosén and Sjölund, '73), the rostral margin of the primary somesthetic area, designated as area 3a, receives impulses from Ia muscle afferents via the ventrobasal complex (Oscarsson and Rosén, '66; Jones and Powell, '69, '70). It is not clear whether area 3a is a distinct cortical area, a component of the sensory or motor cortex, or a transitional zone (Jones and Porter, '80). The medullary relay centers for group I muscle afferents are in the rostral part of the nuclei gracilis and cuneatus; autoradiographic data indicate that these nuclei project only to VPLc (Tracey et al., '80). The above findings suggest that VPLc may project to the posterior part of so-called area 3a. This region is considered a part of the somesthetic cortex, but unresolved questions remain concerning how impulses from stretch receptors may be utilized for conscious perception of limb positions and movement.

Although fibers of the spinothalamic tract project to the ventral posterolateral nucleus (VPLc) of the thalamus, fibers of this system also project bilaterally upon portions of the intralaminar and posterior thalamic nuclei (Mehler et al., '60; Boivie, '70, '79; Jones and Burton, '74; Burton and Jones, '76). Thus impulses conducted in the anterolateral part of the spinal cord terminate upon multiple thalamic nuclei. Cells of the ventral posterior nucleus project to areas 3, 1, and 2 (S I), as well as to the second somatic area (SS II) (Figs. 13-6, 13-7, and 13-8), a sensory area located along the superior bank of the lateral sulcus (Jones and Powell, '69, '69a, '70, '73). Both of these cortical projections are topographically organized. Early evidence suggested that cells of the posterior thalamic nucleus projected most of their fibers to the second somatic area (SS II) and that this area might be concerned with perception of pain (Knighton, '50; Poggio and Mountcastle, '60; Mehler, '66a; Whitsel et al., '69). Autoradiographic studies indicate that the medial part of the posterior thalamic nucleus which receives most of the somatic afferents projects to a retroinsular cortical area caudal to SS II (Burton and Jones,

'76). Physiological studies of the response properties of SS II in the monkey that are in good agreement with the anatomical definition of this area indicate that neurons in this area respond to somatic stimuli similar to those recorded in S I (Robinson and Burton, '80).

Studies in the monkey disclose that the primary somesthetic area and somatic sensory area II (SS II) are reciprocally and topographically connected with each other and with the motor cortex (area 4) within the same hemisphere (Jones and Powell, '69). Each of these sensory areas also sends an organized projection to the supplementary motor area. The most remarkable feature of these somatic sensory areas is the interlocking of topographic subdivisions. Parts of the primary somesthetic area, the somatic sensory area II and the motor cortex, related to the same portion of the periphery, are interconnected. Commissural connections also exist for the somatic sensory cortex. The primary somesthetic area has connections with its counterpart, and with somatic sensory area II on the opposite side; somatic sensory area II projects to its counterpart on the opposite side but only to regions of the primary somesthetic cortex which represent perioral regions (Jones and Powell, '69a).

Stimulation of the postcentral gyrus in man produces sensations described by the patient as numbness, tingling, or a feeling of electricity. Occasionally the patient may report a sensation of movement in a particular part of the body, though no actual movement is observed. A sensation of pain is rarely produced by these stimulations. Sensations are referred to contralateral parts of the body, except in response to stimulations of the face area. Evidence suggests that the face and tongue are represented bilaterally. Position sense and kinesthetics are represented only contralaterally in the cerebral cortex. Whether the discriminative aspects of tactile sensibility are represented bilaterally in the human cortex is not known. Clinically the sensory deficits caused by lesions in the postcentral gyrus are detectable only on the opposite side.

Microelectrode multinuit mapping of the primary somatosensory cortex in the monkey suggests that the representation of the body surface may be far more complex than indicated by most earlier studies (Merzenich et al., '78). This study suggests two large systematic representations of the body surface, each of which is activated by low threshold stimuli. One representation of the body surface is coextensive with area 3 and the other with area 1 (Fig. 13-6). Each of these somatotopic transformations of the skin surface has some discontinuities where adjoining skin surfaces are not represented. While the two fields of cutaneous representation are basically similar and are approximate mirror images of each other, they differ in size and in the relative proportion of cortex devoted to the representation of various body parts. Because the proportions in each representation differ, both cannot be simple reflections of peripheral innervation density. Area 2 contains a systematic representation of deep body structures (Fig. 13-6). These observations suggest that each of the three distinctive cytoarchitectonic areas that compose the postcentral gyrus may represent different aspects of somatic sensation.

The sensory cortex is not concerned primarily with the recognition of crude sensory modalities, such as pain, thermal sense or mere tactile sense. These crude sensibilities remain after complete destruction of the primary sensory area. "The sensory activity of the cortex . . . endows sensation with three discriminative faculties. These are: (1) recognition of spatial relations, (2) a graduated response to stimuli of different intensity, and (3) appreciation of similarity and difference in external objects brought into contact with the surface of the body" (Head, '20).

Somatic Sensory Area II (SS II). This area lies along the superior bank of the lateral sulcus and extends posteriorly into the parietal lobe (Fig. 13-8). In the monkey the greater part of SS II lies buried in the lateral sulcus (Jones and Powell, '69, '69a, '70). Representation of the various parts of the body has been depicted in reverse sequence to that found in the primary somesthetic area, and the two face areas are adjacent. Parts of the body are described as being represented bilaterally in the secondary somatic sensory area, although contralateral representation predominates.

There have been discrepancies concerning the boundaries, the somatotopic representation, and the modality representation in SS II in different animals, suggesting that this area is not easily defined physiologically (Woolsey, '58; Whitsel et al., '69; Robinson and Burton, '80, '80a, '80b). In the strict anatomical sense SS II is the area on the superior bank of the lateral sulcus (or buried in it) that receives afferents from: (1) the ventral posterior nucleus (VP) of the thalamus (Jones and Powell, '70, '73; Burton and Jones, '76) and (2) both the ipsilateral and contralateral primary somesthetic cortex (S I) (Jones and Powell, '69, '69a; Friedman et al., '80). The somatotopic organization of SS II in the monkey (Fig. 13-8) suggests that the different body regions are represented in successive, obliquely oriented cortical strips parallel with the lateral sulcus (Friedman et al., '80; Robinson and Burton, '80). Neurons with trigeminal receptive fields are found rostrally in SS II and respond to bilateral stimuli (Fig. 13-8). Regions representing the hand are posterior to the face area and form the largest component; regions related to the arm, trunk and hind limbs follow in a rostrocaudal sequence. These cortical strips representing various parts of the body in SS II do not form a topological map of the body surface as depicted in the figurines for S I and SS II. Most of the neurons in SS II respond to cutaneous stimuli in a manner similar to that reported for S I (Robinson and Burton, '80a, '80b). A number of small areas surrounding SS II also respond to cutaneous stimulation, including the retroinsular area which receives projections from the medial part of the posterior thalamic nucleus (Burton and Jones, '76). These carefully controlled studies cast doubt upon the concept that impulses concerned with painful and noxious stimuli are relayed to SS II or the retroinsular cortex via the posterior thalamic nucleus. The efferent cortical connections of SS II are with the primary somesthetic cortex (S I) and with the motor and supplementary motor areas within the same hemisphere (Jones and Powell, '68, '69).

Primary Visual Area. Area 17 is located in the walls of the calcarine sulcus. It occasionally extends around the occipital pole onto the lateral surface of the hemisphere (Figs. 9-23 and 13-5). The exeedingly thin cortex of this area is the most striking example of the heterotypical granulous cortex. Layers II and III are narrow and contain numerous small pyramidal cells (Fig. 13-3). Layer IV, which is very thick, is subdivided by a light band into three sublayers. The upper and lower sublayers are packed with small granule cells. In the middle, lighter layer, fewer small cells are scattered between the large stellate cells. This light layer is occupied by the greatly thickened outer band of Baillarger, here known as the band of Gennari. This band, visible to the naked eye in sections of the fresh cortex, has given this region its name—area striata (Fig. 13-9).

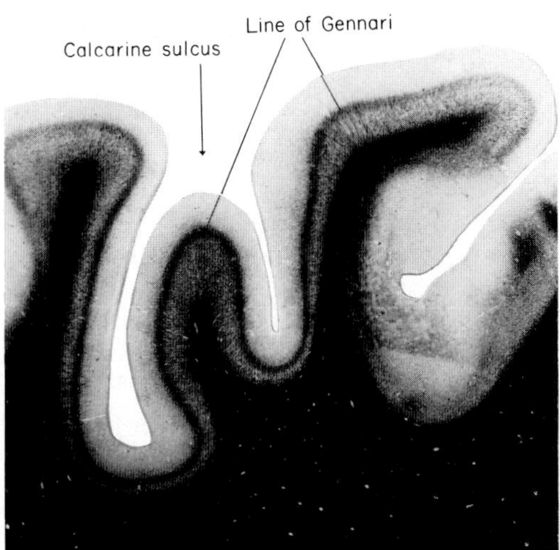

Figure 13-9. Frontal section through calcarine cortex (area striata) showing the line of Gennari. (Weigert's myelin stain; photograph.) (From Carpenter and Sutin, *Human Neuroanatomy*, 1983; courtesy of Williams & Wilkins.)

The visual cortex receives the geniculocalcarine tract, whose course and projection have been discussed (Fig. 9-23; see p. 258). Geniculocalcarine fibers pass in the *external sagittal stratum*, which is separated from the wall of the inferior and posterior horns of the lateral ventricle by the *internal sagittal stratum*, and by fibers of the corpus callosum designated as the *tapetum* (Fig. 2-9). Fibers of the internal sagittal stratum are corticofugal fibers passing from the occipital lobe to the superior colliculus and the lateral geniculate body (Garey et al., '68; Höllander, '74; Kawamura et al., '74).

The macular fibers terminate in the caudal third of the calcarine area, and those from the paracentral and peripheral retinal areas end in respectively more rostral portions (Fig. 9-23). The representation of the macular area in the occipital cortex appears relatively large compared with the macular area of the lateral geniculate body (Fig. 9-20).

Because some unilateral lesions of the visual cortex result in a sparing of macular vision, it has been suggested that the macula may be represented bilaterally. Anatomical evidence supports the thesis that parts of each macular area are represented only in the visual cortex of one hemisphere. Clinically, sparing of macular vision associated with vascular lesions involving the occipital cortex usually is attributed to collateral circulation provided by branches of the middle cerebral artery (Fig. 14-6). Following occlusion of the posterior cerebral artery, these collateral vessels may be sufficient to preserve some macular vision. Similar collateral circulation is not present in the cortical area representing paracentral and peripheral parts of the retina.

Complete unilateral destruction of the visual cortex in man produces a contralateral homonymous hemianopsia in which there is blindness in the ipsilateral nasal field and the contralateral temporal field. Thus a lesion in the right visual cortex produces a left homonymous hemianopsia (Fig. 9-25). Lesions involving portions of the visual cortex, such as the inferior calcarine cortex, produce an *homonymous quadrantanopsia*, in which blindness results in the superior half of the visual field contralaterally. Homonymous hemianopsia can result from lesions involving all fibers of either the optic tract or the optic radiation (Fig. 9-25), but lesions in these locations tend to be incomplete and the visual defects in the two eyes are rarely identical. Frequently patients are unaware of an existing homonyomous hemianopsia and complain primarily of bumping into people and objects on the side of the visual field defect.

An image falling upon the retina initiates a tremendously complex process that results in vision. The transformation of a retinal image into a perceptual image occurs partly in the retina, but mostly in the brain. An impressive series of experimental studies by Hubel and Wiesel in the cat and monkey have provided real insight into the functional organization of the visual cortex.

The receptive field of a cell in the visual system is defined as the region of the retina (or visual field) over which one can influence the firing of that cell. In the retina the receptive field comprises those receptor sets (i.e., rods and cones) and other retinal neurons which influence the firing of one retinal ganglion cell. Receptive fields of retinal ganglion cells are circular, vary somewhat in size, and are of two types: (1) those with an "on" (excitatory) center and an "off" (inhibitory) surround, and (2) those with an "off" (inhibitory) center and an "on" (excitatory) surround (Kuffler, '53). It is well known that retinal ganglion cells fire at a fairly steady rate even in the absence of stimulation. An "on" response is characterized by an increased firing rate of the cell to a light stimulus; in an "off" response the cell's firing rate diminishes when the light stimulus decreases. The physiological basis for the "on" and "off" retinal responses are the concentric receptive fields with either an "on" and "off" center and the reverse type of surround (Fig. 13-10). Lighting up the entire retina diffusely does not affect retinal ganglion cells as strongly as a small circular spot that covers the excitatory region of the receptive field center.

Cells of the lateral geniculate body are of two types and have physiological characteristics similar to retinal ganglion cells, in that: (1) each cell is driven from a circumscribed retinal region (the receptive field), and (2) each receptive field has either an "on," or "off," center with an opposing surround (Hubel and Wiesel, '61). Lateral geniculate neurons are more specialized than retinal ganglion cells in that they are more sensitive to the differences in retinal illumination than to the illumination itself (Fig. 13-10). Cells in different laminae of the lateral geniculate body are driven from receptive fields in one eye, either ipsilaterally or contralaterally, depending upon the uncrossed or crossed connections. In the lateral geniculate body few, if any, cells are influenced binocularly (Hubel and Wiesel,

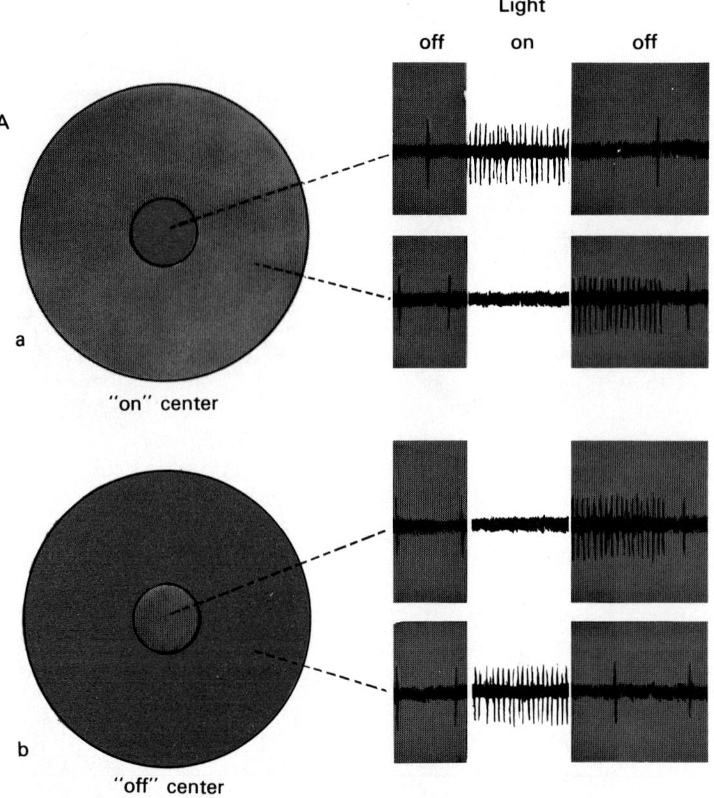

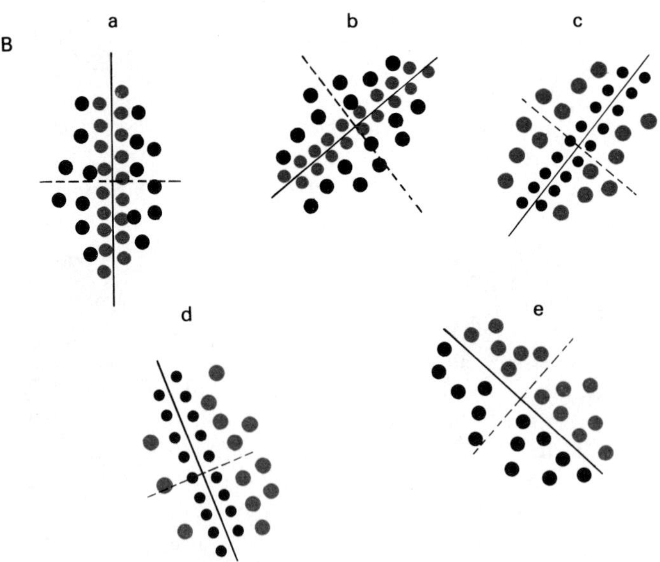

Figure 13-10. (*A*) Receptive fields of retinal ganglion cells and lateral genicular neurons are concentric with either an "on" (excitatory) center and an "off" (inhibitory) surround, or the reverse. In *a*, a spot of light (*red*) filling the "on" center causes the cell to fire vigorously. If the spot of light strikes the surrounding "off" zone, firing of the neuron is suppressed until the light is turned off. In *b*, the responses of a cell with an "off" center and an "on" surround are the reverse. (*B*) Simple cells of striate cortex receive their input from sets of lateral geniculate neurons whose "on" or "off" centers are arranged in straight lines. The receptive field axis of orientation varies for simple cells, as in *a*, *b* and *c*, with excitatory areas represented by *red* dots and inhibitory areas by *black* dots. Although simple cells always have excitatory and inhibitory areas parallel and in a straight line, these areas may be asymmetrical as in *d* and *e* (based on Hubel and Wiesel, '62). (From Carpenter and Sutin, *Human Neuroanatomy*, 1983; courtesy of Williams & Wilkins.)

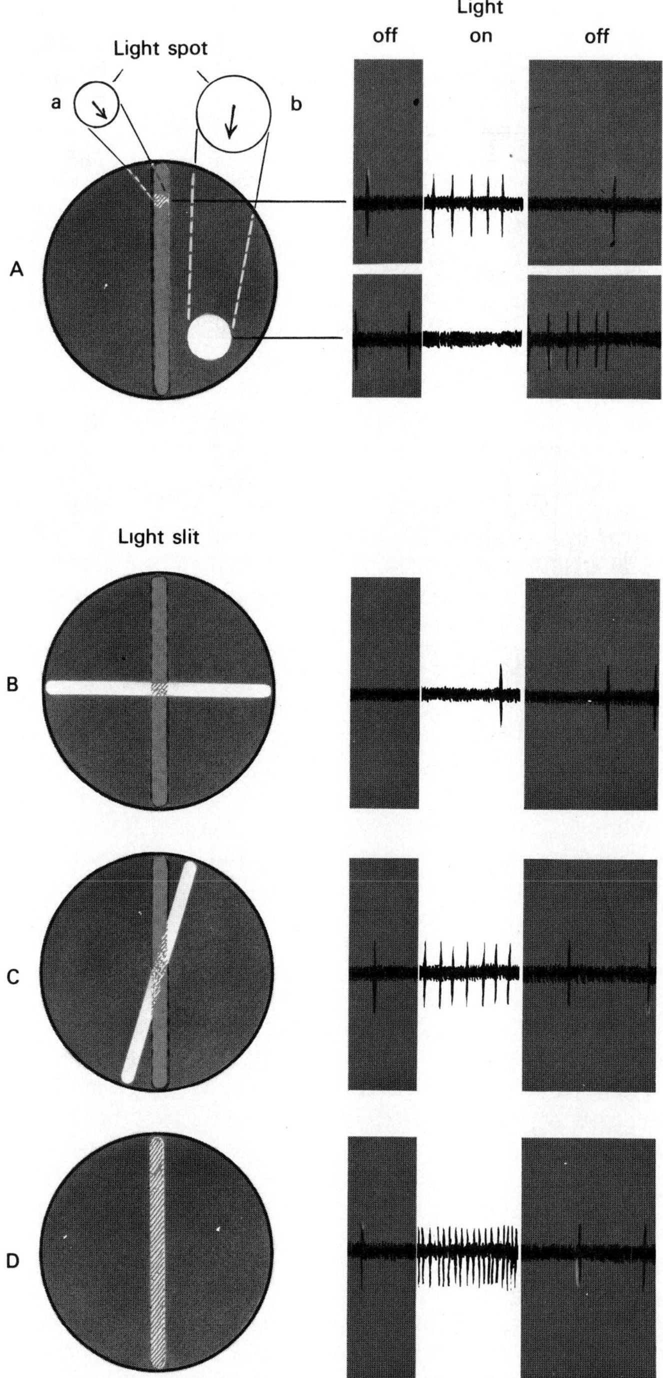

Figure 13-11. Schematic diagram of the functional characteristics of "simple" cells in the striate cortex. In *A*, a small circular spot of light (*a*) shone on the excitatory part of the receptive field (*red*) of a simple cortical cell produces a weak response. A larger spot of light (*b*) shone on the inhibitory surround produces no response. Small spots of light (*a*) produce vigorous responses in retinal ganglion cells and lateral geniculate neurons. The receptive field of the simple cell (*red*) shown above is similar to *a* in Fig. 13-10B. A narrow split of light shone perpendicular to the receptive field axis of orientation (*red*) in *B*, produces virtually no response. Tilting the slit of light as in *C* produces a weak response, while a vertical slit of light, as in *D* which corresponds to receptive field axis of the simple striate cell, produces a vigorous response (after Hubel, '63). (From Carpenter and Sutin, *Human Neuroanatomy*, 1983; courtesy of Williams & Wilkins.)

'62). Visual processing by the brain begins in the lateral geniculate body.

The striate cortex, anatomically far more complex than either the retina or lateral geniculate body, does not have cells with concentric receptive fields. Cells of the striate cortex show a marked specificity in their responses to restricted retinal stimulation (Hubel and Wiesel, '59, '62, '63a, '68). The most effective stimulus shapes are long narrow rectangles of light ("slits"), dark bars against a light background ("dark bars"), and straight-line borders separating areas of different brightness ("edges"). A given cell responds vigorously when an appropriate stimulus is shone on its receptive field, or moves across it, provided the stimulus is presented in a specific orientation (Fig. 13-11). This orientation is referred to as the "*receptive-field axis of orientation*" and it is critical and constant for any particular cell, but it differs for cells in other locations. Cells with the same receptive field axis of orientation are arranged in columns extending from the cortical surface to the white matter (Fig. 13-12).

The cortical columns of the striate cortex may be looked upon as the structural expression of the necessity to encode more than two variables. The two surface coordinates (eccentricity from fovea and distance above or below the horizontal meridian) are used for topographical representation of the visual fields. Engrafted upon this representation are two more variables in columnar form concerned with receptive-field orientation and ocular dominance (Fig. 13-12). The topographical representation of the retinae upon the striate cortex is primary and for each position in the visual field there is neuronal machinery for each orientation and for each eye (Hubel and Wiesel, '74). In the monkey striate cortex there exist two independent and overlapping systems of columns referred to as orientation columns and ocular dominance columns (Hubel and Wiesel, '68). Ocular dominance columns are parallel sheets or slabs arranged perpendicular to the cortical surface which are subdivided into a mosaic of alternating left eye and right eye stripes 250 to 500 μm in width (Hubel and Wiesel, '72). Orientation columns are an order of magnitude smaller than the ocular dominance columns (Fig. 13-12). The horizontal distance corresponding to a complete cycle of orientation columns, representing a rotation through 180°, appears to be roughly equal to a set of left plus right ocular dominance columns with a thickness of 0.5 to 1 mm (Hubel and Wiesel, '74a).

Orientation Columns. The visual cortex is subdivided into discrete columns extending from the surface to the white matter; all cells within each column have the same receptive-field axis orientation. The many varieties of cells in the striate cortex have been grouped into two main functional types, but other subtypes also exist. The main functional cell types are referred to as "*simple*" and "*complex.*"

"Simple" type cells respond to slits of light having the proper receptive-field axis of orientation. A slit of light, oriented vertically in the visual field, may activate a given "simple" cell, whereas the same cell will not respond, though other cells will respond, if the orientation of the slit of light is moved out of the vertical position. The retinal region over which a "simple" type cell can be influenced, is, like the receptive fields of retinal and geniculate cells, divided into "on" and "off" areas (Fig. 13-10). In "simple" cells these "on" areas are narrow rectangles, adjoined on each side by larger rectangular "off" regions. The magnitude of the "on" response depends upon how much of the "on" region is covered by the stimulating light. A narrow slit of light that just fills the elongated "on" region produces a powerful "on" response; stimulation with a slit of light having a different orientation produces a weaker response, because it includes part of the adjacent antagonistic "off" regions (Fig. 13-11). A slit of light at right angles to the optimum orientation for a particular cell, usually produces no response. Thus a large spot of light covering the whole retina evokes no response in "simple" cortical cells, because "on" and "off" effects apparently balance. A particular cortical cell's optimum receptive-field axis of orientation appears to be a property built into the cell by its anatomical connections. The receptive-field axis of orientation differs from one cell column to the next, and may be

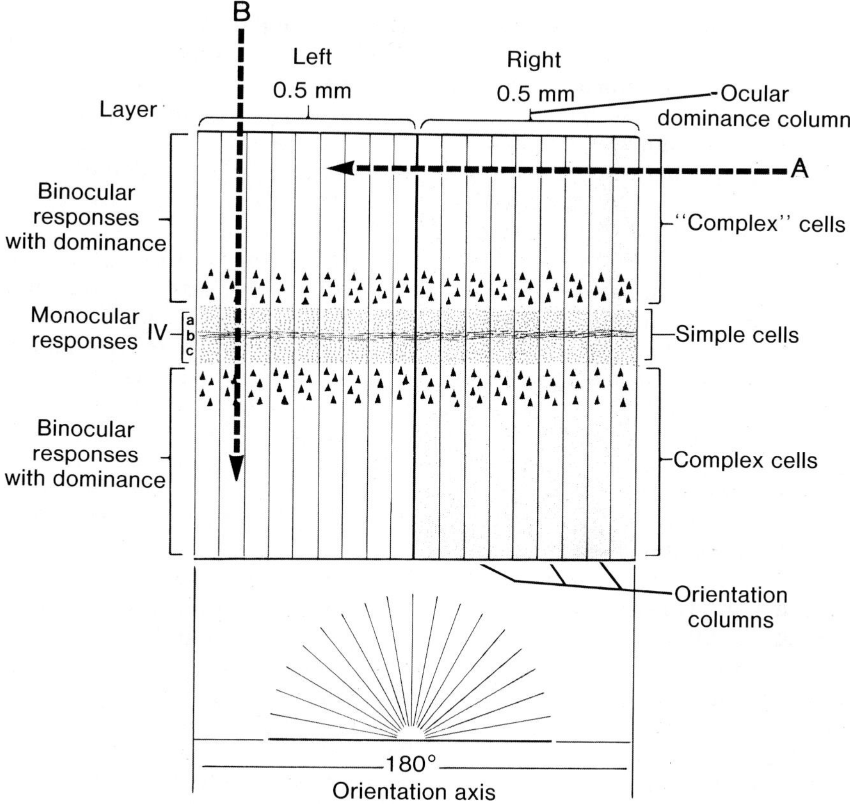

Figure 13-12. Schematic representation of the organization of ocular dominnce and orientation columns in the striate cortex. Ocular dominance columns (0.25 to 0.5 mm) are an order of magnitude larger than orientation columns and a pair of left-right ocular dominance columns (0.5 to 1 mm) are roughly equal to a set of orientation columns representing a complete cycle of orientations through 180°. Input from the lateral geniculate to layer IV is strictly monocular and consists of a series of parallel and alternating stripes—one for the left eye and one for the right eye. Most of the cells in layer IV (*blue*) are "simple" cells. Binocularly influenced cells are predominantly "complex" cells in layers above and below layer IV. A recording electrode inserted tangential to the pial surface, as in arrow *A*, will detect responses to successive stimuli with different orientations, first with right eye dominance and then with left eye dominance. A recording electrode inserted vertically, as in *B*, will indicate responses only to stimuli presented in one axis of orientation. About 50% of the cell above and below layer IV (*blue*) will respond to binocular stimuli, but with consistent left ocular dominance. When the electrode is in layer IV, monocular responses will be recorded (based on Hubel and Wiesel, '74; Hubel et al., '77).

vertical, horizontal or oblique. No one orientation is more common than any other.

"Simple" cells receive their impulses directly from the lateral geniculate body. Presumably a typical "simple" cell receives an input from a large number of lateral geniculate neurons whose "on" centers are arranged in a straight line which corresponds to the receptive field orientation of the simple cell (Fig. 13-10*B*). Thus, for each area of the retina stimulated, each line, and each orientation of the stimulus, there is a particular set of "simple" striate cortical cells that respond. Changing any of the stimulus arrangements will cause an entirely new and different population of "simple" striate cells to respond.

"Complex" type cells, like "simple" cells, respond best to "slits," "bars" or "edges," provided the orientation is suitable. Unlike "simple" cells, these cells respond with sustained firing as the slits of light are moved across the retina, preserving the same receptive field axis of orientation (Hubel and Wiesel, '62). These cells have peculiar characteristics in that a slit of light with the appropriate receptive-field axis of orientation can cause cells to fire vigorously as it moves across the retina in one direction, but reversing the direction of movement of the light stimulus may produce a diminished, or different, response.

Although "complex" cells in the striate cortex have some characteristics similar to those of simple cells, their receptive-fields cannot be mapped into antagonistic "on" and "off" regions. A "complex" cell receives its input from a large number of "simple" cells—all of which have the same receptive-field axis of orientation. Most simple cells in the striate cortex are stellate cells located in layer IV (Fig. 13-12); the majority of complex and hypercomplex cells are pyramidal neurons lying in layers superficial or deep to layer IV (Hubel and Wiesel, '68; Kelly and van Essen, '74). Hypercomplex cells have the properties of two or more complex cells from which they are believed to receive their input. Most cells in layer IV are driven by only one eye while cells in other layers are driven binocularly (Hubel and Wiesel, '68). There are a few cells in layer III of the striate cortex that have a center-surround field organization, but their behavior is much more complex than that of cells in the lateral geniculate body. These findings imply that a vast network of intracortical connections relate "simple" and "complex" cells in the striate cortex in a very specific fashion. They also imply that similar arrangements must exist for all receptive-field axes of orientation.

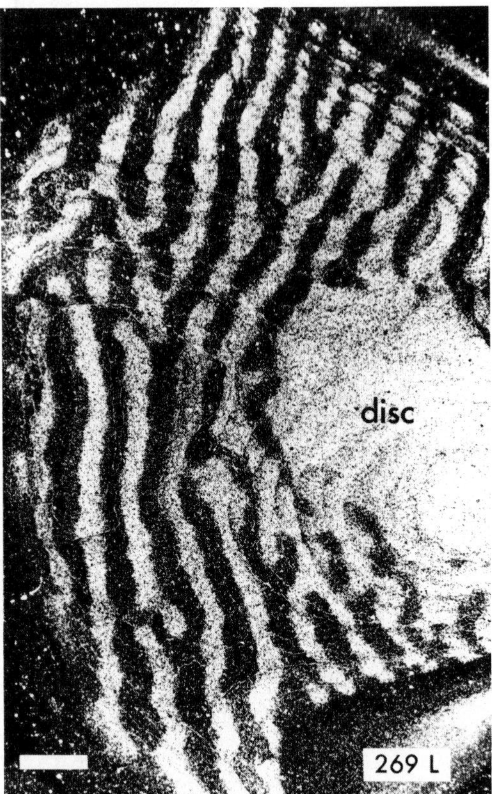

Figure 13-13. Autoradiographic montage of tangential sections of area 17 on the left in a monkey (269 L) whose right eye was removed as an adult. The left eye was injected 4 months later with [^{3}H]proline. The montage shows the normal mosaic pattern of ocular dominance columns with uniformly labeled bands alternating with unlabeled bands. The uniformly labeled area (*disc*) represents the monocular area which covers the blind spot (optic disc) of the enuculated right eye. (From LeVay et al., '80, courtesy of Dr. David Hubel and Allan R. Liss, Inc., New York.) Bar equals 1 mm. (From Carpenter and Sutin, *Human Neuroanatomy*, 1983; courtesy of Williams & Wilkins.)

Attempts have been made to determine the geometry and sequence of the orientation columns in the monkey striate cortex (Hubel and Wiesel, '74). Orientation columns appear to have the form of narrow slabs, as do ocular dominance columns. The arrangement of the columns is highly ordered and recordings made along a tangential microelectrode penetration show that the preferred orientations of cells change in a systematic fashion, in either a clockwise or counterclockwise direction with advancement of the electrode (Fig. 13-12). There is a continuous variation in the preferred orientation with horizontal distance along the cortex. When the electrode crosses from a left-eye region to a right-eye region, there is no noticeable disturbance in the sequence of orientation columns (Fig. 13-12). The horizontal distance along the cortex corresponding to a complete cycle of orientation columns, representing rotations through 180°, is said to be of the same size as a set of left and right ocular dominance columns (0.5 to 1 mm). The principal finding is that orientation columns are arranged with great regularity so that a probe moving along the cortex horizontally generally can be expected to encounter all values of orientation in a regular sequence before any one value is repeated (Hubel and Wiesel, '74a).

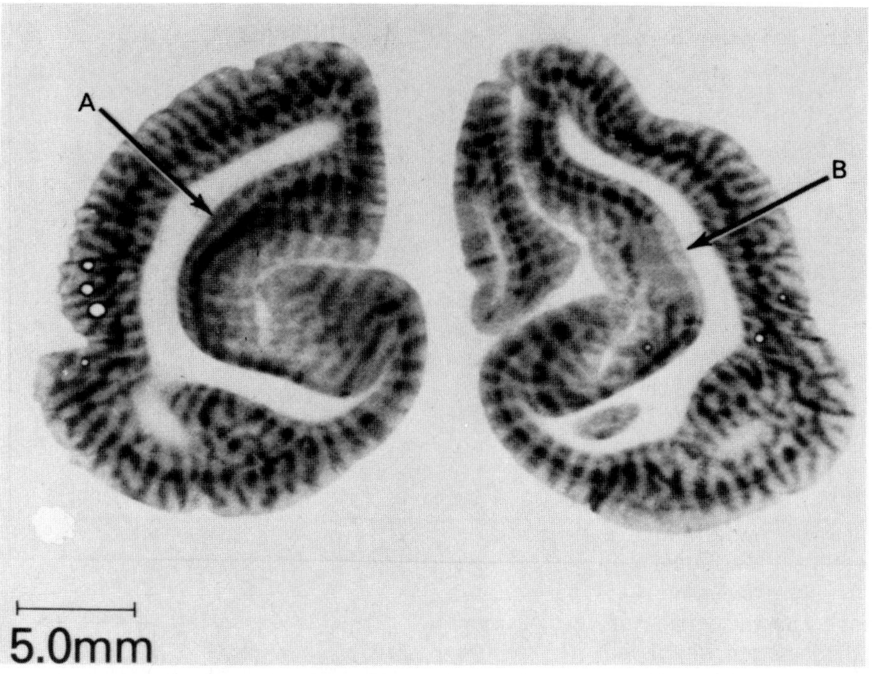

Figure 13-14. Autoradiographic mapping of the visual system in the monkey using 2-[^{14}C]deoxyglucose. Coronal sections of the striate cortex in a monkey with the right eye occluded. The alternate dark and light striations, each 0.3 to 0.4 mm in width, represent ocular dominance columns. These columns are darkest in a band which corresponds to layer IV, but they extend the entire thickness of the cortex. Arrows *A* and *B* point to regions without ocular dominance columns; these regions receive only monocular input. The region indicated by *arrow A* is contralateral to the occluded eye (Fig. 13-13). The region indicated by *arrow B* is ipsilateral to the occluded eye and shows no evidence of radioactivity. Both arrows indicate loci believed to be the cortical representation of the blind spots (Kennedy et al., '76; courtesy of Dr. Louis Sokoloff, Laboratory of Cerebral Metabolism, National Institute of Mental Health, Bethesda, Md.)

Ocular Dominance Columns. Recording from single cells at various levels of the visual system offers a direct means of determining the site of convergence of impulses from the two eyes. In the lateral geniculate body, the first point at which convergence is possible, binocularly influenced cells have not been observed (Hubel and Wiesel, '61). Anatomical findings have provided no evidence that crossed and uncrossed optic tract fibers terminate in an overlapping manner in layers of the lateral geniculate body (Hayhow, '58; Garey and Powell, '68; Hickey and Guillery, '74). It has long been recognized that the primary visual cortex receives projections from both eyes. The receptive fields of all binocularly influenced cortical cells occupy corresponding sites in the two retinas (Hubel and Wiesel, '62). About 80% of the cells in the striate cortex are influenced independently by the two eyes. In a binocularly influenced cell the two receptive fields have the same organization, the same axis of orientation, and a summation occurs when corresponding parts of the two retinas are stimulated simultaneously.

In the monkey, binocular convergence in area 17 is delayed beyond the first and second synaptic stages (Hubel and Wiesel, '68; Hubel et al., '77). Projections of the lateral geniculate body terminate in deep parts of layer IV where they are segregated into a series of parallel alternating stripes, one set connected with the left eye and the other to the right eye. Although input to deep parts of layer IV is essentially monocular, ocular dominance columns extend vertically from the pial surface to the white matter, and show alternate preference for left and right eyes (Figs. 13-12, 13-13, and 13-14). This columnar arrangement is demonstrated by vertical electrode penetrations of the striate cortex in which there is no

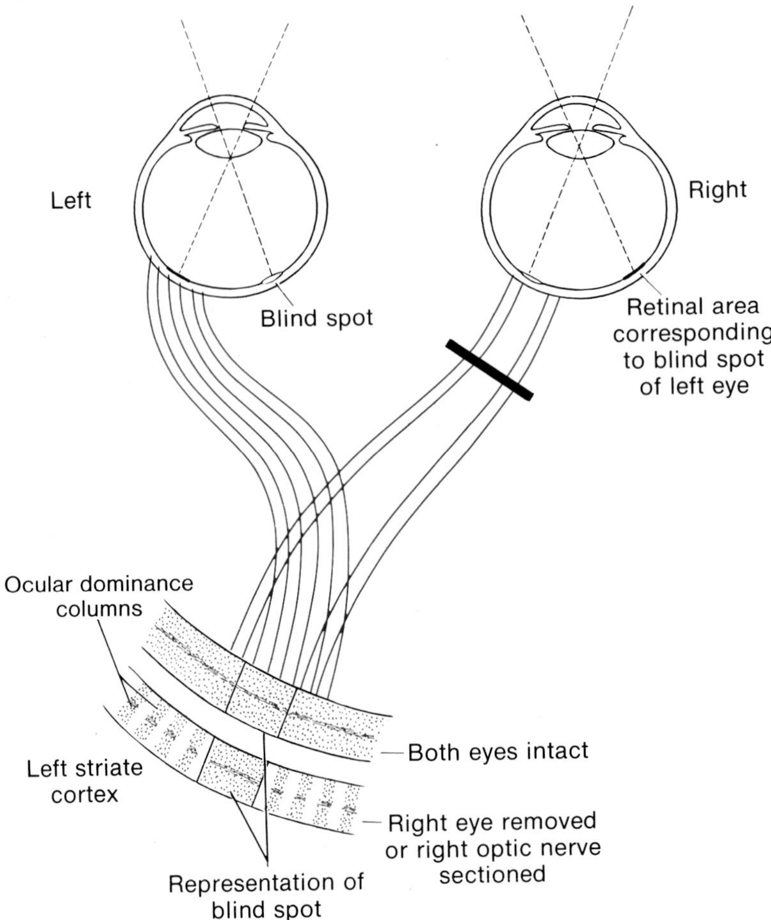

Figures 13-15 and 13-16. Schematic diagrams demonstrating the ocular dominance columns and the blind spot in the striate cortex with the 2-[^{14}C]deoxyglucose metabolic mapping technic in the monkey. In an animal with an intact visual system silver grains are distributed throughout the striate cortex with greatest concentrations in layer IV; neither the blind spot or ocular dominance columns can be demonstrated. Following removal of the right eye, or section of the right optic nerve (*heavy black line*), silver grains are distributed evenly in the representation of the blind spot on the left (Fig. 13-15), but no isotope is evident in the blind spot on the right (Fig. 13-16). Other regions of the striate cortex demonstrated ocular dominance columns on both sides. Fibers from the ipsilateral temporal retina normally cover the blind spot of the opposite eye. The autoradiographs in Fig. 13-14 represent the striate cortex of the right and left hemispheres which are here depicted diagrammatically. (Courtesy of Dr. Louis Sokoloff, National Institute of Mental Health, Bethesda, Md.)

change in eye preference. In tangential penetrations of the striate cortex, the electrode moves from a region in which one eye gives the best response to an adjacent region where the other eye dominates (Hubel et al., '77). In layer IV the responses are monocular, while cells in other layers respond binocularly, but with definite dominance by one eye. The widths of the ocular dominance columns innervated by the ipsilateral or contralateral eye are the same; a set of right and left ocular dominance columns range from 0.5 to 1 mm (Hubel and Wiesel, '74a). Ocular dominance columns are larger than orientation columns and a set of right-left ocular dominance columns corresponds to a complete cycle of orientation columns representing a rotation of receptive field axes through 180° (Fig. 13-12).

The striate cortex is organized into both vertical and horizontal systems. The vertical or columnar system is concerned with retinal position, line orientation, ocular dominance, and perhaps detection of direction of movement; these functional features are mapped in sets of superimposed, but

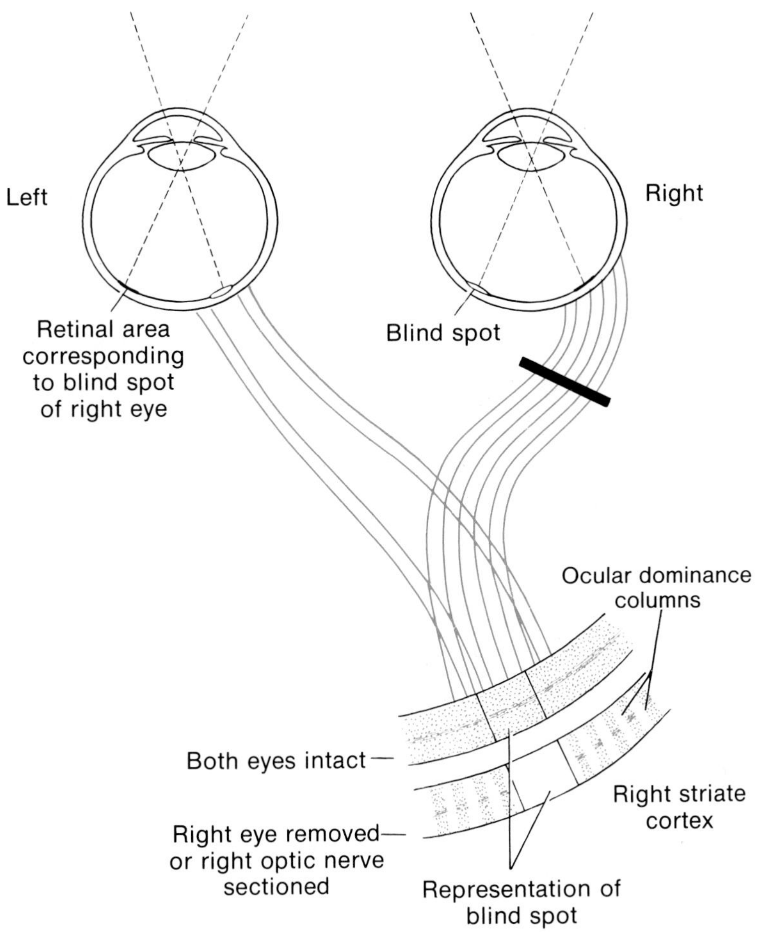

independent, mosaics (Figs. 13-13 and 13-14). The horizontal system segregates cells of different orders of complexity. Cells of the lowest order (simple cells), located in layer IV, are driven monocularly, while those of higher orders (complex and hypercomplex), located in the other layers, are driven by impulses from both eyes (Fig. 13-12).

Ocular dominance columns in the striate cortex have been demonstrated by a variety of neuroanatomical technics. Discrete lesions in a single layer of the lateral geniculate body, produce bands of degenerated fibers in layer IV (250 to 500 μm) of the striate cortex separated by interbands of the same extent free of degeneration (Hubel and Wiesel, '72). The boundaries of ocular dominance columns correspond with a mosaic pattern of dark bands seen in tangential sections of the striate cortex (LeVay et al., '75). Autoradiographic methods, using the principal of transneuronal transport or 2-[^{14}C]deoxyglucose as a metabolic marker to measure glucose utilization, also reveal the characteristic pattern of ocular dominance columns (Wiesel et al., '74; Kennedy et al., '76). Based upon physiological evidence two regions of the striate cortex should not contain ocular dominance columns: (1) the region representing the blind spot of the retina and (2) the cortical region representing the monocular temporal crescent of the visual field. These regions of striate cortex, receiving only monocular visual inputs, have been identified (Figs. 13-13, 13-14, 13-15, and 13-16). The area of the optic disc in the nasal half of each retina transmits no visual impulses to the contralateral striate cortex; this region of striate cortex receives its sole input from the temporal half of the ipsilateral retina.

When an animal is deprived of vision in the right eye and the 2-[^{14}C]deoxyglucose method is employed as a metabolic marker: (1) the left striate cortex shows the striped pattern of ocular dominance columns, except in the representation of the blind spot where metabolic activity is evidenced by a continuous band of isotope uptake, and (2) the right striate cortex shows a similar pattern of striped columns but no evidence of metabolic activity or isotope in the cortical areas representing the blind spot (Figs. 13-14, 13-15, and 13-16). The cortical area representing the monocular crescent of the right visual field, which lies in the left striate cortex, would not contain isotope because all of its input is crossed.

Visual Deprivation. Physiological studies in very young, visually inexperienced, kittens and monkeys, deprived of all vision from birth by visual occluders, have shown that responses in the striate cortex are similar to those of the adult animal with respect to receptive field organization and functional architecture (Hubel and Wiesel, '63; Wiesel and Hubel, '74). In the visually naive young monkey, orientation columns are as highly ordered as in the adult. These observations suggest that the connections responsible for the highly organized behavior of cells in the visual cortex must be present at birth and develop even in the absence of patterned visual experience. Thus the development of orientation specificity in the striate cortex in these two species appears to be genetically determined. The surprising finding in young monkeys deprived of binocular vision for a few weeks after birth was the marked reduction in number of cells in the striate cortex that could be influenced by both eyes. This finding suggested that deprivation of binocular vision for a few weeks after birth may result in deterioration of innate cortical connections subserving binocular vision.

Ocular dominance columns in the monkey are only partially formed at birth and undergo rapid development during the first 6 weeks of life (Hubel et al, '77; LeVay et al, '80). Monocular visual deprivation during the first 6 postnatal weeks causes ocular dominance columns in the deep parts of layer IV related to the open eye to be expanded, while dominance columns related to the closed eye appear shrunken. The number of cells in the striate cortex in layers superficial and deep to layer IV responding to binocular stimuli is greatly reduced (Wiesel and Hubel, '74). These studies indicate that normal binocular visual experience, in the first 6 weeks of life, is necessary for the development of cortical connections that subserve binocular vision.

Secondary Visual Areas. A second visual area (visual area II) has been mapped in the rabbit, cat, and monkey (Thompson et al., '50). Visual area II is a smaller mirror image representation of the primary visual area, located anterolaterally, which anatomically is identical to area 18 in the cat (Fig. 13-5). Lateral to visual area I and II is a third systematic projection of the contralateral visual field (visual area III) which in the cat is identical with area 19 (Hubel and Wiesel, '65).

Area 18 is six-layered granular cortex which lacks the band of Gennari and rostrally merges with area 19 without distinct demarcation. Large pyramidal cells in the third layer of area 18 are useful in establishing its medial and lateral borders (Hubel and Wiesel, '65). Area 18 interrelates areas 17 and 19 of the same and opposite hemispheres by association and commissural fibers. The retinotopic organization of area 18 indicates that the border between areas 17 and 18 corresponds to the representation of the vertical meridian of the visual hemifield (contralateral half of the visual field). Thus as successive recordings are made moving from area 17 to area 18 there is a reversal of the receptive fields (i.e., from peripheral to central followed by a central to peripheral sequence) about the vertical meridian. The isoelevation lines running through both areas 17 and 18 are perpendicular to the representation of the vertical meridian (Tusa et al., '79; Hubel and Wiesel, '65). Visual area II (area 18) represents roughly the central 50° of the visual hemifield which corresponds to the binocular overlap zone in the cat. In area 19 (visual area III) the visual hemifield is represented basically as a mirror image of area 18 and the vertical meridian for area 19 lies on its lateral border. If a recording electrode were moved lateral from the border of area 17 and 18 successive lateral positions in area 18 would represent more peripheral regions of the visual field; when the medial border of area 19 is reached the visual receptive fields would begin to move centrally toward the vertical meridian (Allman and Kass, '74).

Cells of the dorsal division of the lateral geniculate nucleus (LGB) project mainly upon area 17 but some fibers also reach areas 18 and 19 (Edwards et al., '74; Gilbert and Kelly, '75; Wong-Riley, '76; Holländer and Vanegas, '77). Larger cells in the dorsal nucleus of the LGB project to area 18 while cells of all sizes project to area 17 (Gilbert and Kelly, '75; Holländer and Vanegas, '77); some of the larger cells may project collaterals to both areas 17 and 18. The inferior pulvinar and the adjacent part of the lateral pulvinar each contains a representation of the contralateral visual hemifield and project retinotopically upon areas 18 and 19, where fibers end upon cortical layers IV, III, and I, and upon the striate cortex (area 17), where fibers end upon the supragranular layers (Benevento and Rezak, '76; Rezak and Benevento, '79; Rosenquist et al., '74). Fibers projecting to areas 18 and 19 from these parts of the pulvinar constitute important links in the extrageniculate visual projection. In addition area 17 has been demonstrated to project association fibers to area 18 and 19 (Hubel and Wiesel, '65; Martinez-Millán and Holländer, '75). Although there are few commisural connections between area 17 in the two hemispheres, commissural fibers interconnect the junctional region near the border between areas 17 and 18 (Hubel and Wiesel, '67; Zeki, '71; Wong-Riley, '74, '79; Martinez-Millán and Holländer, '75). These fibers arise mainly from the cells in layer III. In both the cat and monkey, cells near the boundary between areas 17 and 18 functionally represent the vertical meridian of the visual hemifield. Thus the vertical meridian of the visual field is bilaterally represented in the visual cortex because of commissural connections. This bilateral representation ensures a uniform visual field free of interruptions along the vertical midline (Hubel and Wiesel, '67; Wong-Riley, '74).

Cells in visual areas II and III respond best to slits of light, dark bars, and edges which have a specific receptive-field axis of orientation. The majority of cells in visual area II are "complex"; in visual area III about half of the cells are complex. Other cells in these areas are referred to as "hypercomplex" cells because of more elaborate properties. Hypercomplex cells have been divided into two types: (1) lower order hypercomplex cells which behave as though their input was derived from two sets of complex cells, one excitatory and one inhibitory, and (2) higher order hypercomplex cells which behave as though they received their input from a large number of lower order hypercomplex cells.

A separate representation of the contralateral visual hemifield (visual area II) adjacent to the primary visual (striate) cortex with a common vertical meridian has been found in all mammalian species studied (Tusa et al., '79). In contrast visual area II (area 19) has not been found in all species and its organization varies. Area 18 (visual area II) largely contains binocular representation of the contralateral visual hemifield and is considered to process visual information related to stereoscopic depth perception (Hubel and Wiesel, '70; Tusa et al., '79).

Primary Auditory Area. In man this area (areas 41 and 42) is located on the two transverse gyri (Heschl) which lie on the dorsomedial surface of the superior temporal convolution, and are buried in the floor of the lateral sulcus (Figs. 2-9, 6-10, 9-12, and 13-5). The middle part of the anterior transverse gyrus and a portion of the posterior gyrus constitute the principal auditory receptive areas (area 41). Remaining parts of the posterior transverse gyrus and adjacent portions of the superior temporal gyrus compose area 42, which is largely an auditory association area. In order to visualize these gyri in an intact brain, it is necessary to separate widely the banks of the lateral sulcus (Figs. 2-4 and 2-9). These two cortical areas are cytoarchitecturally distinct. Area 41 is typical koniocortex, resembling that of areas 3 and 17.

The cortical auditory area receives geniculotemporal fibers (auditory radiation) from the medial geniculate body. The auditory radiation reaches its cortical projection site by passing through the sublenticular portion of the internal capsule (Figs. 6-10 and 9-21). The greater part of the auditory radiation projects to area 41.

Figure 13-17. Schematic diagram of the auditory areas in the cat. The primary auditory area A I has a tonotopic organization with high frequencies (*H*) represented rostrally and low frequencies (*L*) caudally. The dashed vertical lines represent isofrequency bands. The primary auditory area is surrounded by a belt of secondary auditory areas designated as *SF*, suprasylvian fringe, partially in the depth of the suprasylvian sulcus, *EP*, the posterior ectosylvian area, A II, the secondary auditory area, SS II, the second somatic area, *I*, the insular area and *T*, the temporal area (based upon Woolsey, '60; Merzenich et al., '75). (From Carpenter and Sutin, *Human Neuroanatomy*, 1983; courtesy of Williams & Wilkins.)

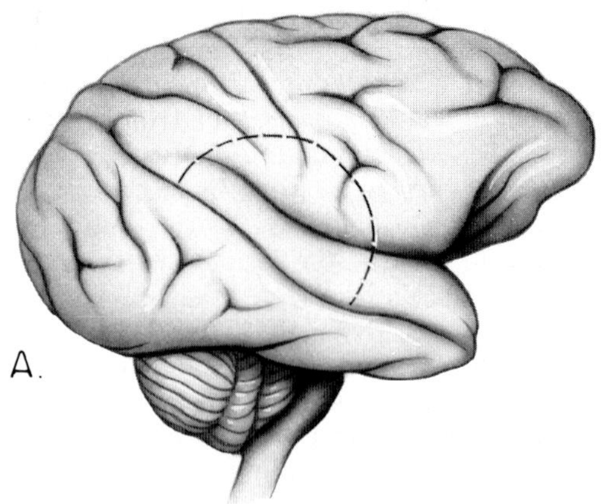

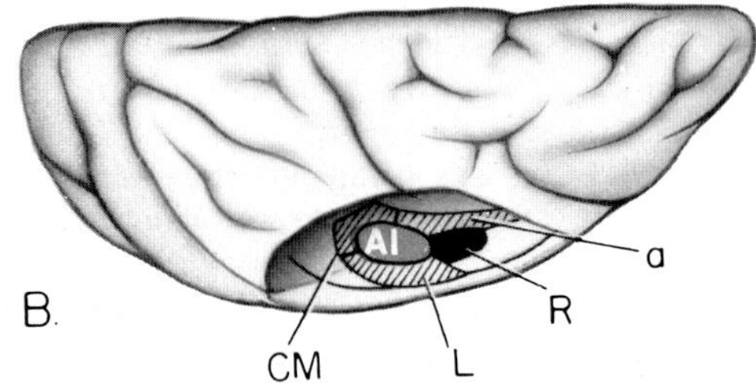

Figure 13-18. (*A*) Drawing of the lateral aspect of the rhesus monkey brain with dashed line indicating region excised to expose the superior temporal plane. (*B*) Dorsal view of the right hemisphere exposing the auditory region in the superior temporal plane. In the primary auditory area, A I (*blue*) low frequencies are represented rostrally and laterally and high frequencies are represented caudally and medially. The area designated *R* (*black*) has a cytoarchitecture similar to A I, an order representation of the auditory spectrum and responds vigorously to auditory stimuli. Auditory area A I and R are surrounded by a belt of secondary auditory cortex (shaded) designated as *a*, *L*, and *CM* (based on Merzenich and Brugge, '73; Imig et al., '77). (From Carpenter and Sutin, *Human Neuroanatomy*, 1983; courtesy of Williams & Wilkins.)

One of the characteristic features of the auditory system is its tonotopic localization. The tonotopic localization present in the cochlea is preserved in auditory relay nuclei of the hindbrain, the inferior colliculus, the medial geniculate body and the cerebral cortex.

The ventral laminated part of the medial geniculate body (MGB), which receives the principal projection from the central nucleus of the inferior colliculus, has a tonotopic organization in which high frequencies are represented medially and low frequencies laterally (Galambos and Rose, '52; Aitkin and Webster, '72; Gross et al., '74). The auditory radiation arises from the ventral laminated part of the MGB (Fig. 9-16) and projects to the primary auditory cortex where there is a spatial representation of tonal frequencies (Casseday et al., '76; Raczkowski et al., '76; Winer et al., '77; Oliver and Hall, '78a; Niimi and Matsuoka, '79). These fibers passing to the primary auditory cortex constitute the *core projection* (Figs. 13-17 and 13-18).

The medial geniculate body also has two other divisions which are not laminated and receive inputs from the lateral tegmental area, the inferior colliculus and several diverse structures (Kudo and Niimi, '78; Oliver and Hall, '78; Moore and Goldberg, '63; Jones and Powell, '71; Casseday et al., '76). These divisions of the MGB, referred to as dorsal and medial (magnocellular) (Morest, '64), project ipsilaterally via the auditory radiation to cytoarchitectonic areas forming a cortical belt around the primary auditory area (Figs. 13-17 and 13-18) (Raczkowski et al., '76; Winer et al., '77; Oliver and Hall, '78a; Niimi and Matsuoka, '79). Fibers arising from the nonlaminated part of the medial geniculate body passing to the secondary auditory areas constitute the *belt projection* (Raczkowski et al., '76; Winer et al., '77; Brodal, '81). There appears to be very little overlap of the auditory projections to the belt area surrounding the primary auditory cortex except for the projection arising from the caudal part of the medial division of the MGB (Oliver and Hall, '78a). The medial magnocellular division appears to project to the entire cortical area receiving fibers from the medial geniculate body, although the laminar distribution of fibers in the cortex is different. The caudal part of the medial nucleus projects primarily upon layer VI, while other subdivisions of the MGB project primarily upon cells in layer IV and parts of layer III.

In the cat, two auditory areas were defined originally on the lateral aspect of the hemisphere below the suprasylvian sulcus by recording evoked potentials from auditory stimuli (Woolsey and Walzl, '42). These auditory areas, designated auditory area I (A I) and auditory area II (A II) were both considered to be tonotopically organized (Fig. 13-17). In the more dorsal auditory area (A I) responses from the basal turn of the cochlea (high frequencies) were represented rostrally while responses from stimulating apical regions of the cochlea (low frequencies) were recorded from caudal regions. In the secondary auditory area (A II), situated ventral to A I, the order of cochlear representation was considered to be the reverse (Fig. 13-17). An additional auditory area in the posterior ectosylvian (EP) region was described subsequently which included parts of A II (Ades, '59). The pattern of tonotopic localization in these and surrounding areas has been found to be much more complex than the initial concept of dual cortical auditory areas (Woolsey, '60).

Microelectrode studies of the frequency representation in auditory area I (A I), indicate a series of isofrequency strips oriented vertically in which high frequencies are represented rostrally and low frequencies caudally (Merzenich et al., '73, '75). In A I there is an orderly representation of frequencies and of cochlear place, in which the basal coils of the cochlea are represented rostrally and the apical region caudally. On an axis perpendicular to the vertical strips (i.e., longitudinal axis of the hemisphere) best-frequencies change as a simple function of cortical location. Isofrequency strips across the cortex are of nearly constant width, but a disproportionally large cortical surface is devoted to higher octaves (Fig. 13-17). This larger representation of high octaves has been considered to be related to greater innervation densities in the basal coils of the cochlea (Spoendlin, '72). On the basis of response characteristics and cytoarchitecture there appear to be at least five secondary auditory fields bordering A I (Fig. 13-17). These areas in the cat have been designated as: (1) the suprasylvian fringe (SF), (2) the posterior ectosylvian area (EP), (3) auditory area II (A II), (4) the insulotemporal area, and (5) parts of the second somatic area SS II (Merzenich et al., '75; Niimi and Matsuoka, '79). In A II no clear tonotopic representation has been established because of the broad tuning curves of its neurons. The tonotopic representation in SF and in EP appears the reverse of that seen in A I (Woolsey, '60, '71). Neurons in the field rostral to A I appear sharply tuned and there is a reversal of frequency progression in passing from A I into this region (Merzenich et al., '75). A I receives its input from the ventral laminated part of the MGB, while A II receives most of its fibers from the medial magnocellular nucleus (Niimi and Matsuoka, '79). The other secondary auditory areas receive their inputs via the belt projection from nonlaminated parts of the MGB (Raczkowski et al., '76; Winer et al., '77; Niimi and Matsuoka, '79).

Since studies of the somesthetic and visual cortex have produced compelling evidence that a vertical column of cells constitutes the elementary functional unit, a similar arrangement might be expected in the auditory cortex. The functional architecture of the auditory cortex appears similar to that of the visual and somesthetic cortex in that cells in the same cell column share the same functional properties. The functional columns in the auditory cortex appear less discrete, do not have such sharp boundaries, and are considered to be much smaller units than in other sensory areas. The isofrequency strips oriented across the primary auditory cortex probably represent, or are composed of, isofrequency cell columns (Merzenich et al., '75). In these columns units throughout the depth of the cortex respond to the same frequency. Both binaural and monaural cell columns have been described (Imig and Adrián, '77). With the exception of some neurons responding only to binaural stimulation, monaural responses were classified as contralateral dominant, ipsilateral dominant, or equidominant. Most neurons in the same perpendicular column display the same aural dominance and binaural interaction.

Studies of the auditory cortex in the monkey have revealed a rather precise tonotopic organization (Merzenich and Brugge, '73; Imig et al., '77). The primary auditory area in the monkey lies caudally on the superior surface of the superior temporal gyrus and can be exposed best by resection of the overlying parietal cortex (Fig. 13-18). Best frequencies in the full auditory range for the monkey were represented in an orderly fashion in the primary auditory area. This is a cytoarchitectonic field coextensive with the koniocortex. Lowest frequencies were represented rostrally and laterally whereas highest frequencies were found caudally and medially (Fig. 13-18). A cortical region immediately rostral to the primary auditory area (A I) has a cytoarchitecture similar to that of A I and appears to respond as vigorously to acoustic stimulation (Imig et al., '77). This rostral field is smaller than A I but contains a complete and orderly representation of the audible frequency spectrum with lower frequencies represented rostral and higher frequencies represented in progressively more caudal and medial regions (Fig. 13-18). The primary auditory area (A I) and the field rostral to it, designated R, appear to constitute the central core of the auditory cortex in the monkey. The primary auditory cortex in the monkey is surrounded by a belt of auditory cortex which is not cytoarchitectonically uniform. This cortical belt, which represents the secondary auditory cortex in the monkey, has been divided into three, or more, auditory fields (Fig. 13-18). In the fields which form this cortical belt, units are less responsive to acoustic stimulation and the frequency organization is more complex than in A I or R. The organization and tonotopic localization in the primary auditory area (A I) appears to be very similar in monkeys, apes, and man.

One of the distinctive features of the auditory system, in contrast to other sensory systems, is the large number of sites at which impulses from one side can be transmitted to contralateral relay nuclei. The largest and most important fiber crossing is in the trapezoid body (Fig. 6-10), but others also are present, including fibers from auditory cortical areas that cross in the corpus callosum. The commissural connections of the auditory cortex in the cat project to homologous areas in the opposite hemisphere (Diamond et al., '68). Auditory area I (A I) projects contralaterally to A I and A II, while A II sends fibers only to A II. Within each subdivision of the auditory cortex there are some areas which receive only small numbers of terminal fibers; the region of A I representing the low frequency range is a clear example. Auditory commissural connections differ greatly from those of the visual cortex (area 17) which are absent except near the common border of areas 17 and 18. Association fibers in the auditory cortex of the cat reciprocally interconnect primary and secondary areas with each other (Diamond et al., '68a).

Physiological studies (Woolsey and Walzl, '42; Rosenzweig, '54) indicate that each cochlea is represented bilaterally in the auditory cortex, although slight differences exist between the two sides. Rosenzweig ('54) has demonstrated that although the cortical effects of stimulating each ear separately are nearly the same, significant differences occur when the position of the stimulus is varied with respect to both ears. When the sound is presented at one side, the cortical response is greatest in the contralateral hemisphere. If the sound is presented in a median plane, the cortical activity in the two hemispheres is equal. These studies suggest a correlation between auditory localization and differential responses in the auditory cortex.

Because audition is represented bilaterally at a cortical level, unilateral lesions of the auditory cortex cause only a partial deafness. The deficits, however, are bilateral, and the greatest loss is contralateral. Removal of one temporal lobe impairs sound localization on the opposite side, especially judgment of the distance of sounds. Clinically, unilateral lesions of the auditory cortex are difficult to recognize.

Electrical stimulation of cortical areas in the temporal lobe near the primary auditory area (i.e., areas 42 and 22) in man produces perceptions described as the noise of a cricket, a bell or a whistle. These sounds may be of high or low pitch, continuous or interrupted, but they do not have changing qualities. These sensations are referred to the contralateral ear. Lesions in Brodmann's area 22 in the dominant hemisphere produce word deafness or sensory aphasia. Although hearing is unimpaired by such lesions, patients cannot interpret the meaning of the sounds.

Gustatory Area. Clinical and experimental evidence suggest that taste sensibility is represented in the parietal operculum (area 43) and in the adjacent parainsular cortex (Börnstein, '40, '40a; Penfield and Rasmussen, '50; Bagshaw and Pribram, '53). Ablations of the precentral and postcentral opercula in the monkey and chimpanzee reportedly cause a loss of taste.

Physiological studies in the rat, cat and monkey indicate that taste impulses conveyed centrally by the chorda tympani and glossopharyngeal nerves are relayed rostrally in the brain stem to the most medial and caudal parts of the ventral posteromedial (VPMpc) nucleus of the thalamus (Blomquist et al., '62; Emmers et al., '62; Emmers, '64).In the cat and monkey the ascending taste pathway is ipsilateral (Figs. 5-21 and 9-14). Rostral regions of the nucleus of the solitary fasciculus project fibers ipsilaterally to VPMpc, while cells in more caudal regions project ascending fibers to both the parabrachial nuclei and VPMpc (Beckstead et al., '80). Thalamic cell groups subserving taste are located medially in VPMpc and are distinct from neurons related to other sensory modalities of the tongue (Blomquist et al., '62; Emmers, '66; Norgren and Wolf, '75). Lesions destroying VPMpc produce gustatory loss in the monkey (Blum et al., '43; Patton et al., '44). In a detailed study of thalamic projections to the insular and opercular cortex in the monkey VPMpc was shown to project to both cortical areas (Roberts and Akert, '63). Gustatory representation in the cerebral cortex is adjacent to the somesthetic area for the tongue, but is separated from the nongustatory lingual area (Norgren and Wolf, '75).

Vestibular Representation. In the cerebral cortex vestibular sense is poorly defined in comparison with other sensory modalities. In man, electrical stimulation of portions of the superior temporal gyrus, particularly regions rostral to the auditory area, provoke sensations of turning movements, referred to as *vertigo*. These sensations are mild compared with the violent vertigo produced by direct stimulation of the labyrinth. Less distinct illusions of body movement have been reported following stimulation of parietal cortex.

Physiological studies in the monkey indicate that vestibular nerve stimulation or angular acceleration of the head about a vertical axis evokes short latency responses in thalamic nuclei. With direct stimulation of the vestibular nerve, responses are recorded contralaterally in the ventral posterior inferior (VPI) and the ventral posterolateral (pars oralis, VPLo) thalamic nuclei (Liedgren et al., '76; Deecke et al., '77). Angular acceleration of the head activates neurons in these thalamic nuclei ipsilaterally and contralaterally, depending upon the direction of rotation (Büttner et al., '77; Magnin and Fuchs, '77). Thalamic units responding to angular acceleration were not numerous and were intermingled with cells activated by touch and pressure. Autoradiographic data reveal that vestibulothalamic projections in the monkey are bilateral and terminate in VPLo, VPI, and VLc (Lang et al., '79). The vestibular projection to the thalamus is small and occurs in patches throughout these nuclear subdivisions of the thalamus. Because thalamic neurons responding to vestibular inputs are few in number, scattered over several subdivisions of the thalamus and intermingled with cells activated by somatosensory input (i.e., kinesthetic sense and pressure), evidence for a specific vestibular relay nucleus in the thalamus is not strong.

The primary cortical projection area of the vestibular nerve in the monkey was found to be in the postcentral gyrus near the lower part of the intraparietal sulcus. This projection area, near the face region of S I, has a cytoarchitecture different than area 2 and is designated as area 2v (Fredrickson et al., '74). Many neurons in cortical area 2v show bimodal inputs, in that they receive both vestibular and deep somatic afferents (Schwarz and Fredrickson, '71). It has been suggested that vestibular and somatosensory afferents that subserve conscious orientation in space converge in this area. Experimental studies indicate that vestibular representation in the human cerebral cortex may be located near the anterior part of the intraparietal sulcus, a region that corresponds to area 2v in the monkey (Fredrickson et al., '74). Vestibular representation in the cerebral cortex is bilateral and lacks the modality specificity which characterizes other primary sensory areas.

CORTICAL AREAS CONCERNED WITH MOTOR ACTIVITY

Corticofugal fibers arise from all regions of the cerebral cortex. These projection fibers convey impulses concerned with motor function, modification of muscle tone and reflex activity, modulation of sensory impulses, and the alteration of the sense of awareness. Corticofugal fibers originate mainly from the deeper cortical layers and project to spinal levels, a variety of brain stem nuclei at all levels, and to all parts of the neostriatum.

The somata of the cells of origin of particular corticofugal fiber systems have a specific laminar or sublaminar distribution (Jones and Wise, '77). Corticospinal neurons lie in the deepest part of layer V, occur in definite clusters, and show great variation in cell size, particularly in area 4. Corticostriate fibers arise from the smallest pyramidal cells in layer V which are concentrated in the superficial part of this layer. Corticopontine, corticobulbar, and corticorubral neurons lie in middle regions of layer V. The majority of corticothalamic cells are found in layer VI but some of these neurons are located in deep parts of layer V. The somata of cortical association and commissural neurons lie in the supragranular layers of the cortex. Cells contributing to distinctive projection systems occur in single or multiple strips 0.5 to 1 mm wide, oriented mediolaterally across the cortex.

Primary Motor Area (M I). Area 4 of Brodmann, commonly designated as the primary motor area M I, is located on the anterior wall of the central sulcus and adjacent portions of the precentral gyrus (Fig. 13-5). This area is broad at the superior margin of the hemisphere, but at the level of the inferior frontal gyrus, it is practically limited to the anterior wall of the central sulcus. On the medial surface of the hemisphere it comprises the anterior portion of the paracentral lobule. The unusually thick cortex of the motor area is agranular in structure, and its ganglionic layer contains the giant pyramidal cells of Betz (Fig. 13-2). These cells are largest in the paracentral lobule, and smallest in the inferior opercular region. The density of Betz cells also varies in different parts of area 4. According to Lassek ('40), 34,000 giant pyramidal cells with cross-sectional areas between 900 and 4,100 μm^2 have been counted in area 4 in the human brain. Cytoarchitecturally area 4 represents a modification of the typical six-layered isocortex in which the pyramidal cells in layers III and V are increased in number and the internal granular layer is obscured. For this reason the cortex is called agranular.

The corticospinal tract, considered to transmit impulses for highly skilled volitional movements to lower motor neurons, arises in large part from area 4. The larger corticospinal fibers are considered to be the axons of giant pyramidal cells. Since the number of fibers in the human corticospinal tract at the level of the pyramid is approximately one million, axons of the giant cells of Betz could account for only a little over 3% of these fibers.

Approximately 90% of the fibers of the corticospinal tract range from 1 to 4 μm in diameter. Of the total number of fibers in the tract, about 40% are poorly myelinated. Small fibers of the corticospinal tract are considered to arise from smaller cells in this and other cortical regions.

Data concerning the cortical areas which contribute fibers to the corticospinal tract and the extent of their individual contributions are incomplete. According to Russell and DeMyer ('61) virtually all fibers of the corticospinal tract arise from area 4, area 6, and parts of the parietal lobe. Approximate percentages of corticospinal fibers arising from these areas were as follows: (1) area 4, 31%, (2) area 6, 29%, and (3) parietal lobe, 40% (Fig. 4-7). Complete decortication, or hemispherectomy, causes all fibers of the corticospinal tract to degenerate.

Retrograde HRP studies in the monkey indicate that corticospinal fibers arise from cells widely distributed in the sensorimotor cortex, all of which are located in the V layer (Coulter et al., '76; Jones and Wise, '77). Labeled corticospinal neurons in the deep parts of layer V are found in areas 6, 4, 3a, 3, 1, 2, 5, and in SS II. Although these neurons show great variation in size, all are pyramidal cells. The largest cells are seen in area 4, while smaller cells, more nearly the same size, are evident in other areas. Cells giving rise to corticospinal projections occur in clusters aligned to form strips oriented mediolaterally across the cortex. Autoradiographic data suggest that major differences exist in the pattern of terminal labeling in the spinal gray following injections of different cytoarchitectonic areas (Coulter and Jones, '77). Isotope injected into cortical areas 3, 1, 2, and 5 label terminals in parts of the posterior horn which correspond to Rexed's laminae III and IV, while injections into areas 4 and 3a label terminals largely in Rexed's lamina VII, but with extensions into regions of spinal motor neurons. No corticospinal neruons project into Rexed's laminae I and II. Some corticospinal neurons end directly upon anterior horn cells in the brachial and lumbosacral enlargements in the monkey (Kuypers, '60; Liu and Chambers, '64); these corticospinal fibers arise from cells in area 4. Branching of corticospinal fibers in the spinal cord indicate that some axons innervate more than one spinal segment. Axons supplying motor neuronal pools innervating distal limb muscles have few collaterals (Shinoda et al., '79). This arrangement is considered to be related to discrete contractions of individual distal limb muscles.

Electrical stimlulation of the primary motor area (M I) evokes discrete isolated movements on the opposite side of the body. Usually the contractions involve the functional muscle groups concerned with specific movements, but individual muscles may be contracted separately. While the pattern of excitable foci is the same for all mammals, the number of such foci, and hence the number of discrete movements, is increased greatly in man. Thus flexion or extension at a single finger joint, twitchings at the corners of the mouth, elevation of the palate, protrusion of the tongue, and even vocalization, all may be evoked by careful stimulation of the proper areas. Charts of motor representation have been furnished by a number of investigators (Figs. 13-7 and 13-19). These data concerning the human brain were collected during neurosurgical procedures in which patients were operated upon under local anesthesia. The location of centers for specific movements may vary from individual to individual, but the sequence of motor representation appears constant. Ipsilateral movements have not been observed in man, but bilateral responses occur in the extraocular muscles and muscles of the face, tongue, jaw, larynx, and pharynx. According to Penfield and Boldrey ('37), the center for the pharynx (swallowing) lies in the most inferior opercular portion of the precentral gyrus; it is followed, from below upward, by centers for the tongue, jaw, lips, larynx, eyelid, and brow, in the order named. Next come the extensive areas for finger movements, the thumb being lowest and the little finger highest; these are followed by areas for the hand, wrist, elbow, and shoulder. Finally in the most superior part are

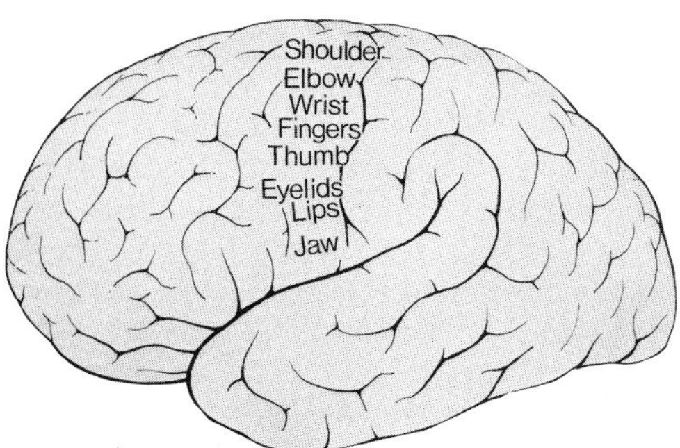

Figure 13-19. Representation of parts of the body in the motor area on the lateral surface of the hemisphere. According to Scarff ('40), the leg usually is represented only in the anterior part of the paracentral lobule. (From Carpenter and Sutin, *Human Neuroanatomy*, 1983; courtesy of Williams & Wilkins.)

the centers for the hip, knee, ankle, and toes. The last named are situated at the medial border of the hemisphere and extend into the paracentral lobule, which also contains the centers for the anal and vesicle sphincters (Fig. 2-6).

The movements elicited by electrical stimulation of the motor cortex probably are not equivalent to voluntary movements, although they are interpreted as "volitional" by the patient. These movements are never skilled movements, comparable to those of complex acquired movements, but consist largely of either simply flexions or extensions at one or more joints. The threshold in different topographical parts of area 4 varies. The region representing the thumb appears to have the lowest threshold, while the face area has the highest threshold. Excessive stimulation of area 4 produces either a focal seizure, or one resembling a Jacksonian convulsion.

The classical view of the somatotopic organization in the motor cortex is a single continuous, distorted representation of the body parts within the primary motor area. This pattern of organization, represented by the motor homunculus or its equivalent, has been extrapolated from studies in which movements have been produced by surface stimulation in a variety of animals and in man. The summation of cortical representation depicted in a single line drawing is regarded as an oversimplification because it rarely takes into account the extent of overlap of various body regions which is a characteristic feature of the motor cortex (Woolsey et al., '51). Studies indicating a double representation of the body surface within areas 3 and 1 in the monkey (Merzenich et al., '78) have raised questions concerning multiple representations of body parts in the primary motor cortex (Strick and Preston, '78). The possibility of multiple representations of the body in motor cortex has been explored in the squirrel monkey in which none of the primary motor area is buried in the central sulcus (Strick and Preston, '78). Microstimulation within layer V revealed a discrete double representation of the hand and wrist with the second hand zone located rostrally. Although all regions of the motor cortex have not been explored in detail, the possibility of dual representation of motor function appears to have some foundation, although it seems unlikely that these systems could be entirely independent. There is at this time no evidence that cells in the motor cortex are organized into functional cell columns as in the somesthetic and visual cortex (Jones, '81).

Ablations of the motor cortex in mammals produce increasingly greater neurological deficits at progressively higher levels of the phylogenetic scale. In the cat even hemidecortication does not impair the animal's ability to walk upon recovery from anesthesia. Ablations of area 4 in the monkey produce a contralateral flaccid paralysis, marked hypotonia, and areflexia. Within a relatively short time myotatic reflexes reappear, along with withdrawal responses to nociceptive stimuli. There is recovery of some motor function in both proximal and distal musculature, but skilled movements are performed slowly with deliberation. No significant spasticity develops in these animals.

Lesions of the motor cortex in man produce neurological deficits similar to those described in the primate, though anatomical details are not so precise. The most reliable data are limited to instances in which all, or parts, of the precentral gyrus have been removed surgically. Ablations limited to the "arm" or "leg" area of the precentral gyrus result in a paralysis of a single limb. The ultimate loss of movement is always greatest in the distal muscle groups, but motor recovery in the affected limb usually is more complete than that associated with nearly total lesions of the motor area (Bucy, '49). Immediately after complete or partial lesions of the precentral gyrus, there is a flaccid paralysis of the contralateral limbs or limb, marked hypotonia, and loss of superficial and myotatic reflexes. Within a relatively short time the Babinski sign can be elicited. The myotatic reflexes generally return early in an exaggerated form.

Premotor Area. This area (area 6) lies immediately rostral to the motor area. It likewise runs dorsoventrally along the whole lateral aspect of the frontal lobe and is continued on the medial surface to the sulcus cinguli (Fig. 13-5). Near the superior

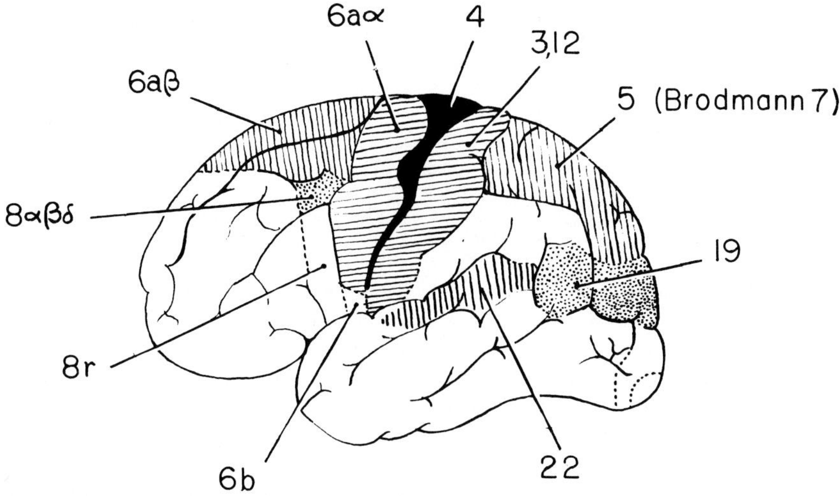

Figure 13-20. The areas of electrically excitable cortex on the lateral surface of the human brain. The motor area is shown in *black*, and the so-called "extrapyramidal areas" are *hatched* except for the eye fields, which are *stippled* (after Foerster, '36). (From Carpenter and Sutin, *Human Neuroanatomy*, 1983; courtesy of Williams & Wilkins.)

border it is quite broad and includes the caudal portion of the superior frontal gyrus. Inferiorly the premotor area narrows, and at the operculum it is limited to the precentral gyrus. Its histological structure resembles that of the motor area, but there are no giant cells of Betz (Fig. 13-2). The presence of pyramidal cells in layers III and V and the narrowness of layer IV make it difficult to distinguish an internal granular layer. For this reason area 6, like area 4, is referred to as agranular frontal cortex. Area 6 has been subdivided into various portions, as shown in Figure 13-20. Electrical stimulation of area 6aα in man produces responses similar to those obtained from area 4. It is probable that this part of area 6 discharges via the corticospinal tract. Unilateral ablations of area 6, not involving the primary or supplementary motor areas, do not produce paresis, grasp reflexes or hypertonia.

Supplementary Motor Area (M II). Observations by early investigators indicated that motor responses in different parts of the body could be elicited by electrical stimulation of the medial surface of the frontal lobe above the cingulate gyrus and rostral to the primary motor area. This motor area, identified in the human brain, has been designated as the supplementary motor area (M II) (Penfield and Rasmussen, '50). The supplementary motor area in man and monkey occupies the medial surface of the superior frontal gyrus rostral to area 4. Detailed descriptions of somatotopic representation within the supplementary motor area of the monkey have been provided by Woolsey et al. ('51). The sequential representation of body parts in this area is shown in Figure 13-21).

The threshold for stimulation of the supplementary motor area (M II) in man and monkey is slightly higher than for the precentral region. Motor responses obtained from the supplementary motor area are not due to spread of excitation to the primary motor area, because they are not significantly altered by: (1) ablation of area 4, or (2) section of the corticospinal tract (Penfield and Jasper, '54; Woolsey, '75). Movements provoked by stimulation of the supplementary motor area have been divided into three types: (1) assumption of postures, (2) maneuvers consisting of complex patterned movements, and (3) infrequent rapid incoordinate movements. The whole pattern of movement seems to be bilateral and synergistic, but most movements are described as tonic contractions of the postural type. Unilateral ablations of the supplementary motor area in man produce no

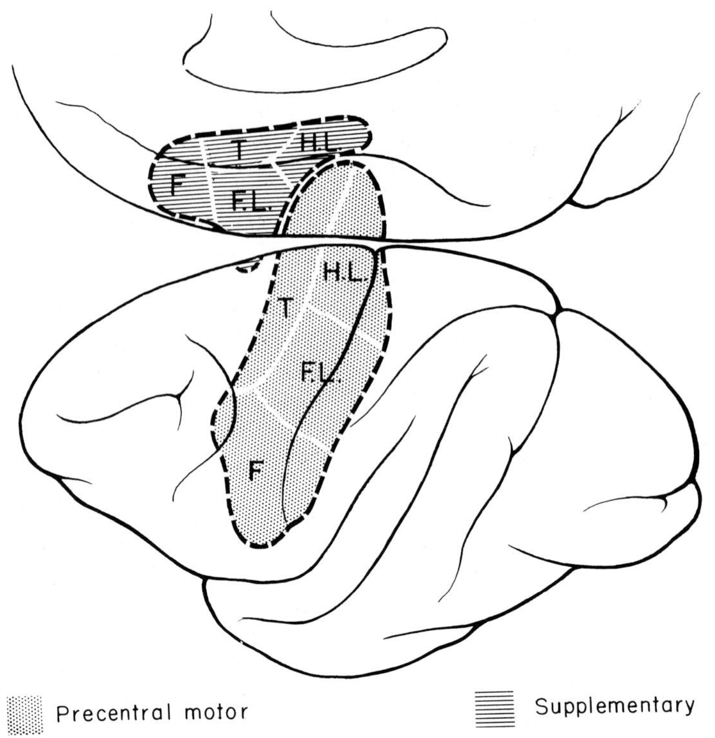

Figure 13-21. Diagram of the precentral and supplementary motor areas in the monkey. The somatotopical representation of different parts of the body are shown: *F*, face area; *T*, trunk; *FL*, forelimb; *HL*, hindlimb. The precentral motor area on the lateral convexity extends over onto the medial aspect of the hemisphere; the *outlined area* shown posterior to the central sulcus represents cortex hidden in the depths of the central sulcus. The supplementary motor area, largely on the medial aspect of the hemisphere, is shown *above* (after Travis, '55a). (From Carpenter and Sutin, *Human Neuronatomy*, 1983; courtesy of Williams & Wilkins.)

permanent deficit in the maintenance of posture or the capacity for movement (Penfield and Rasmussen, '50).

Systematic studies in the monkey of removals of the supplementary motor area alone, and in combination with the precentral motor area, have produced conflicting results. According to Travis ('55, '55a), unilateral ablations of the supplementary motor area in the monkey produce weak transient grasp reflexes in the contralateral limbs, and moderate bilateral hypertonia of the shoulder muscles, but no paresis. Bilateral simultaneous ablations of this area result in disturbances of posture and tonus but produce no paresis. Gradually increasing hypertonia is said to develop during an interval of 2 to 4 weeks. The hypertonia is described mainly in flexor muscles. Myotatic reflexes are hyperactive, and clonus can be demonstrated. The resulting spasticity demonstrates a topographical localization according to the portions of the supplementary motor area removed. These observations were not confirmed in a similar study (Coxe and Landau, '65). Although the ablation method has not yielded specific information concerning the role of the supplementary motor area in motor control, there appears to be some agreement that combined lesions of the supplementary and precentral motor areas on the same side may result in a spastic, rather than a flaccid, paresis (Denny-Brown and Botterell, '48; Travis, '55, '55a; Travis and Woolsey, '56; Brinkman and Kuypers, '73).

Although relatively little is known concerning the functional attributes of the supplementary motor area, the mammalian cerebral cortex seems to possess at least two separate motor areas (Wise and Tanji, '81). The respective roles of these motor areas in control of movement are quite different. It has been suggested that the supplementary motor area may serve mainly to control posture (Wisendanger et al., '74). Studies in conscious, behaving monkeys indicate that neurons in the supplementary motor area are related to movements on both sides of the body and involve distal and proximal musculature equally (Brinkman and Porter, '79). Most of the neurons in the supplementary motor area increase their activity before the onset of movement and large numbers of neurons in this area discharge during movement of either arm. Only a small number of cells in this area respond to peripheral stimuli and the responses are weaker than in the primary motor area (Brinkman and Porter, '79; Wise and Tanji, '81).

The supplementary motor area, as described in man and monkeys, has no clear-cut cytoarchitectonic borders and its neural connections are poorly understood. Corticocortical (association) connections include afferents from the ipsilateral primary sensory area (areas 3, 1, and 2) and from the second somatic area (SS II) (Jones and Powell, '69; Jones et al., '78). Reciprocal connections also exist with the ipsilateral primary motor area (area 4), area 3a, area 5, and the superior part of area 6 on the lateral convexity of the hemisphere (Vogt and Pandya, '78; Pandya and Vignolo, '71). Less well established subcortical projections to the supplementary motor area are derived from the ventral anterior (VA), ventral lateral (VLo), and the paracentral (PCN) thalamic nuclei (Kalil, '75; Kievit and Kuypers, '77; Brinkman and Porter, '79). On the basis of its cortical connections, the supplementary motor area (M II) has been regarded as an area in which sensory impulses converge (Jones, '69; Jones and Powell, '70a). The efferent connections of the supplementary motor area suggest that it plays a direct role in motor control. Cortical efferents project to the primary motor area (area 4) and to lateral portions of area 6 (DeVito and Smith, '59; Jones and Powell, '70a). In addition the supplementary motor area has bilateral projections to the striatum (Kemp and Powell, '70; Jones et al., '77) and ipsilateral projections to thalamic nuclei (VA, VLo, VLc, VPLo) (DeVito and Smith, '59; Wiesendanger et al., '74), the red nucleus and the pontine nuclei. A direct corticospinal projection from the supplementary motor area has been disputed but recent anatomical and physiological studies support the existence of this pathway (Bertrand, '56; Murray and Coulter, '76, '77; Brinkman and Porter, '79). It has been estimated that 5% of cells in the supplementary motor area project axons into the corticospinal tract. In summary, present data support the concept that the supplementary motor area is a separate cortical motor region with striking bilateral motor influences upon both proximal and distal musculature.

Inputs to the Motor Cortical Areas. Although impulses generated in neurons in the primary motor area (M I), the premotor area and in the supplementary motor area (M II) are responsible for movement, motor control, changes in muscle tone, and maintenance of posture, these motor activities are initiated by inputs that arise from the thalamus, other cortical regions, and peripheral receptors. Particularly potent drives upon the motor cortical areas are derived from all divisions of the ventral lateral, and the ventral posterolateral, pars oralis (VPLo) thalamic nuclei (Rispal-Padel et al., '73; Dekker et al, '75; Strick, '76; '76a; Tracey et al., '80; Asanuma et al., '83, '83a, '83b). Crossed projections from the deep cerebellar nuclei terminate in VPLo and in the cell-sparse region of the ventral lateral thalamic nuclear complex, which includes VLc and area x (Olszewski, '52; Percheron, '77; Thach and Jones, '79; Tracey et al., '80; Asanuma et al., '83; Schnell and Strick, '84). The cortical projection area of VPLo and the cell-sparse region of VL has been identified as corresponding to area 4, the primary motor area (M I) (Jones et al, '79; Tracey et al., '80; Asanuma et al., '83; Schell and Strick, '84). These studies indicate that the principal subcortical input to the primary motor cortex is derived from thalamic nuclear subdivisions that receive fibers from the contralateral deep cerebellar nuclei. The uncrossed pallidothalamic fibers, originating from the medial pallidal segment, project to the ventral anterior (VApc), ventral lateral (VLo and VLm), and the centromedian (CM) thalamic nuclei (Nauta and Mehler, '66; Kuo and Carpenter, '73; Kim et al., '76; DeVito and

Anderson, '82). Pallidal inputs to the rostral ventral tier thalamic nuclei do not appear to overlap cerebellothalamic terminations. The cortical projections of VLo are not yet clearly defined, but most evidence suggests this nucleus projects to the premotor area (area 6) (Jones et al., '79; Tracey et al., '80; Asanuma et al., '83). According to Schell and Strick ('84) the thalamic input to the supplementary motor area (M II) originates largely from VLo. The thalamic terminations of projections from the substantia nigra are distinct from those arising from the deep cerebellar nuclei and the globus pallidus. The cortical projections of the magnocellular division of the ventral anterior nucleus (VAmc) and the medial part of the ventral lateral nucleus (VLm) which receive nigral terminations are poorly defined, but appear to exclude area 4, and probably project to areas outside of area 6 (Asanuma et al., '83a).

Neurons of the ventral lateral nucleus show increased activity prior to any movement. This finding suggests that these neurons may play a role in initiating activity in muscles that effect discrete movements and control posture (Strick, '76a). Thalamic neurons which project to the primary motor and premotor cortex are distinct and separate from those that terminate in somatic sensory areas (Jones and Powell, '70; Strick, '76; Kievit and Kuypers, '77). Electron microscopic evidence in the cat indicates that fibers from VL projecting to the motor cortex make synaptic terminations largely in three cortical layers: (1) upper third of layer I (18%), (2) layer III (66%), and (3) layer VI (13%) (Strick and Sterling, '74). Fibers terminating directly in layer V were relatively sparse (3%). The majority of fibers from VL neurons synapse upon dendrite spines and in layer III this input synapses upon the apical dendrites of motor neurons (Betz cells of layer V) and upon interneurons in layer III. Autoradiographic data in the monkey also demonstrated that the largest number of efferents from VL terminate in layer III of area 4 (Jones, '75).

The primary motor area also receives inputs from the primary somesthetic area (S I), the second somatic area (SS II), and the supplementary motor area (Jones and Powell, '68, '69, '73). These cortical inputs to the motor area are of an interlocking nature in that somatotopical subdivisions are connected with each other. Detailed studies suggest that only area 2 of S I projects directly to area 4 (Vogt and Pandya, '78; Jones et al., '78). Area 2 which receives an input from deep somatic receptors also has connections with area 5 via intracortical fibers in layers III and IV. Area 5, difficult to distinguish from area 2, has been shown to project to area 4 and parts of area 6 (Jones et al., '78; Strick and Kim, '78; Zarzecki et al., '78). These data suggest that area 5 has important influences upon the motor cortex and raise questions concerning the nature of this input. About two-thirds of the neurons in area 5 are activated by passive joint rotation. It has been postulated that area 5 contains the "command apparatus" for limb and hand movements in immediate extrapersonal space (Mountcastle et al., '75). Neurons in area 5 have been observed to discharge only when an animal moves its arm towards a desired object or manipulates an object with its hand. The "command" hypothesis suggests that the cortical pathway from area 5 to area 4 is involved in initiating limb and hand movements.

Physiological studies indicate that the motor cortex receives inputs from cutaneous and deep receptors (Rosén and Asanuma, '72; Wiesendanger, '73). Impulses from group I muscle afferent have been recorded in cortical area 3a, but it is not known how these impulses influence the motor cortex, because there is no projection from area 3a to area 4 (Phillips et al., '71; Jones et al., '78). Impulses from joint receptors projecting to area 2 appear to have access to the motor cortex directly and via area 5. Impulses from cutaneous receptors probably reach the motor cortex via relays in the postcentral gyrus. Inputs from cutaneous receptors may be involved in instinctive grasping as well as in the startle reaction (Wisendanger, '73).

Cortical Eye Fields. Rostral to the premotor area is a cortical region particularly concerned with voluntary eye movements. The *frontal eye field* in man occupies principally the caudal part of the middle frontal gyrus (corresponding to parts of area 8, shown in Fig. 13-20), and extends into contiguous portions of the inferior frontal gyrus. The entire frontal eye field does not lie within a single cytoarchitectonic area. Electrical stimulation of the frontal eye field in man causes strong conjugate deviation of the eyes, usually to the opposite side. This cortical field is believed to be a center for voluntary movements of the eyes, which are independent of visual stimuli. These conjugate eye movements are called "movements of command," since they can be elicited by instructing the patient to look to the right or left.

The concept of an *occipital eye center* for conjugate eye movements is based upon the fact that stimulation of occipital cortex produces conjugate eye movements to the opposite side, and lesions in this area are associated with transient deviation of the eyes to the side of the lesion. Unlike the frontal eye field, the occipital eye center is not localized to a small area. Eye responses can be obtained from a wide region of the occipital lobe in the monkey, but the lowest threshold is found in area 17 (Walker and Weaver, '40). The occipital eye centers subserve movements of the eyes induced by visual stimuli, such as following moving objects. These pursuit movements of the eyes are largely involuntary, though they are not present in young infants. The occipital eye centers, unlike the frontal eye fields, are interconnected by fibers passing in the splenium of the corpus callosum. The threshold for excitation in the occipital eye center is higher than in the frontal eye fields; the latency of responses is longer, and eye movements tend to be smoother and less brisk. With a lesion of the occipital eye field, the patient may have difficulty following a slow moving object, but on command can direct the eyes to a particular location. Eye movements on command are impaired by lesions in the frontal eye field, particularly in the dominant hemisphere.

The pathways by which responses from the frontal and occipital eye fields are mediated are thought to involve projections to the superior colliculus. Fibers from area 8 project profusely to the stratum zonale, the stratum opticum, and the intermediate gray stratum (Künzle et al., '76; Künzle and Akert, '77). These corticofugal fibers terminate in the same layers of the superior colliculus that receive fibers from the retina and striate cortex (Hubel et al., '75). None of the corticofugal fibers from the frontal eye field project to the oculomotor nucleus, the accessory oculomotor nuclei, or the paramedian pontine reticular formation. The most massive projection of area 8 is to the paralaminar part of the dorsomedial nucleus with which it has reciprocal connections. The most substantial and highly organized projection to the superior colliculus arises from the visual cortex (Garey et al., '68; Wilson and Toyne, '70; Cynader and Berman , '72).

NONPYRAMIDAL CORTICOFUGAL FIBERS

These cortical projections consist largely of corticoreticular, corticopontine, corticothalamic and corticonuclear fibers.

Corticoreticular Fibers. These fibers arise from all parts of the cerebral cortex, but the largest number arise from the motor and premotor areas. Corticoreticular fibers descend in association with the corticospinal tract but leave this bundle to enter specific areas of the brain stem reticular formation. The majority of these fibers terminate in two fairly well circumscribed areas in the medulla and pons (Fig. 4-14). Some corticoreticular fibers also project to reticular cerebellar relay nuclei. Corticoreticular fibers are distributed bilaterally and nearly symmetrically in these regions of the reticular formation.

Corticopontine Fibers. These fibers arise from extensive regions of the frontal, temporal, parietal and occipital regions of the cerebral cortex (Fig. 7-1). The largest number of corticopontine fibers in the monkey arise from areas 4, 3, 1, 2, 5, and parts of the visual cortex (Jones and Wise, '77; Brodal, '78, '78a). These fibers arise from pyramidal cells in layer V, superficial to the giant pyramidal cells, and are larger than those of other efferent systems except for corticospinal neurons. Corticopontine fibers arising from the visual cortex are from regions representing the peripheral visual field. Contributions to this system from temporal and prefrontal cortex are relatively modest; most of the fibers from the prefrontal areas arise from areas 9 and 8 (Brodal, '68; Astruc, '71).

Corticopontine fibers from the "motor"

and "sensory" areas project somatotopically upon two longitudinally oriented cell columns in the pontine nuclei (Brodal, '68). One cell column is medial and one is lateral. Thus fibers from a particular region of the cerebral cortex end within columnar zones of pontine nuclei which are separated from each other. Most corticopontine fibers end only upon dendrites of pontine neurons and exert a monosynaptic excitatory action (Allen et al., '75; Cooper and Beal, '78). The massive synaptic linkage of corticopontine and pontocerebellar fibers conveys impulses from the cerebral cortex to broad regions of the contralateral neocerebellum.

Corticothalamic Fibers. This large and impressive group of corticofugal fibers arise from specific regions of the cortex and project upon particular thalamic nuclei. In general, cortical areas receiving projections from particular thalamic nuclei give rise to reciprocal fibers which pass back to the same nuclei (Figs. 9-11 and 9-12). The granular frontal cortex projects primarily to the dorsomedial nucleus (DM) of the thalamus. Corticothalamic fibers from the precentral area project upon the ventral lateral nucleus (VL). These projections are more widespread than previously thought in that they pass to VLo, VLm, VLc, and VPLo, as well as to portions of the intralaminar thalamic nuclei (CM, PF, PCN, and CL) (Olszewski, '52; Künzle, '76; Akert and Hartmann-von Monakow, '80). Cortical projections from area 4 to parts of VL and VPLo are reciprocal and topographically arranged. The projections from area 4 to VLc are not as impressive as those from area 6 (Künzle, '78). These data indicate that corticofugal fibers from the precentral gyrus project to thalamic nuclei which receive selective inputs from the deep cerebellar nuclei, the globus pallidus, and the substantia nigra. Area 6 projects fibers to VA, VLc, "area x," VPLo, and the parafascicular nucleus of the thalamus (Künzle, '78). In addition the premotor area has a projection to DMpl. In general, the premotor area shows a thalamic projection pattern in different regions related to either the precentral or prefrontal cortex.

Both the precentral and premotor cortex project upon portions of the intralaminar thalamic nuclei; the largest number of these fibers terminate in the centromedian-parafascicular nuclear complex (CM-PF) (Auer, '56; Niimi et al., '60; Petras, '69; Rinvik, '68; Künzle, '76, '78; Akert and Hartmann-von Monakow, '80). The precentral motor cortex sends fibers ipsilaterally primarily to CM (Künzle, '76). Fibers from the premotor cortex project largely to PF. The intralaminar thalamic nuclei, particular CM-PF, receive substantial projections from the precentral and premotor cortex, but these nuclei project diffusely via collateral branches, upon broad regions of the cortex in a fashion that cannot be regarded as reciprocal (Jones and Leavitt, '74; Kievit and Kuypers, '77).

Efferent fibers from the parietal cortex pass via the sensory radiations of the thalamus to the ventral posterolateral (VPLc) and posteromedial (VPM) thalamic nuclei. Corticothalamic projections from areas 3, 1, and 2 are confined to the ventrobasal complex, except from small projections to the reticular and central lateral thalamic nuclei (Jones et al., '79). No labeled terminals from these areas project to VPLo, the ventral posterior inferior (VPI), the lateral posterior (LP) or the posterior thalamic nuclei.

Parts of the auditory cortex project to the medial geniculate body (MGB) via the sublenticular part of the internal capsule (Fig. 9-21). The cortical projections from the primary and secondary auditory areas are back to the subdivisions of the geniculate body (MGB) (Fig. 9-16) from which they receive inputs (Casseday et al., '76; Oliver and Hall, '78a). The medial geniculate body does not give rise to descending auditory pathways that influence auditory relay nuclei at lower levels of the brain stem, but projections from the auditory cortex to the inferior colliculus (pericentral nucleus; Fig. 7-4) are involved in this activity (Rockel and Jones , '73a; Casseday et al., '76; Oliver and Hall, '78a).

The striate cortex (area 17) sends fibers to the lateral geniculate body (LGB), the superior colliculus, the pretectum, and the inferior pulvinar (Höllander, '74; Lund et al., '75; Gilbert and Kelly, '75). Fibers from area 17, projecting retinotopically to all layers of the lateral geniculate body, arise from cells in layer VI (Höllander, '74; Lund et al., '75). Cells in the V layer of the striate cortex project to the superior colliculus and the inferior pulvinar. Although corticogeniculate and geniculocortical fibers are topographically organized, they are not reciprocal in the true sense, since they arise from and terminate in different layers of the striate cortex.

While reciprocal relationships exist between the principal thalamic nuclei and their cortical projection sites, a different relationship pertains to the reticular and intralaminar thalamic nuclei (Fig. 9-11). The reticular nucleus of the thalamus receives afferents from almost all cortical areas, but there is no evidence that this nucleus projects to the cerebral cortex (Carman et al., '64; Scheibel and Scheibel, '66). However, collaterals of thalamocortical fibers terminate in particular parts of the reticular nucleus (Jones, '75). Also corticothalamic fibers give collaterals to the same portion of the reticular nucleus as the thalamic nucleus which receives the main cortical projection. Thus, the reticular nucleus of the thalamus is strategically situated to sample activities passing in both directions between cerebral cortex and thalamic relay nuclei. The intralaminar thalamic nuclei receive corticofugal fibers; the prefrontal cortex projects upon the rostral intralaminar nuclei, while the premotor and motor cortex send fibers to the CM-PF nuclear complex; parietal and occipital cortex do not project fibers to the intralaminar thalamic nuclei (Powell and Cowan, '67). It has been suggested that the posterior thalamic nuclei may constitute the caudal extension of the intralaminar thalamic nuclei, since they are related primarily to cortex on the lateral surface of the hemisphere caudal to area 4 (Jones and Powell, '71). Most areas of the neocortex project fibers to a particular nucleus of the dorsal thalamus and to either part of the intralaminar or posterior thalamic nuclei. The striate cortex is unique in that it does not project, or receive fibers from, either the intralaminar or posterior thalamic nuclei. The principal projections of the intralaminar nuclei are to the striatum, but an extensive collateral system projects diffusely upon broad regions of the cerebral cortex (Jones and Leavitt, '74). Corticothalamic fibers projecting to the intralaminar thalamic nuclei and the collateral system from these nuclei passing to the cortex are not reciprocal (Kievit and Kuypers, '77; Akert and Hartmann-von Monakow, '80).

CEREBRAL DOMINANCE

Although the two cerebral hemispheres appear as mirror images duplicates of each other, many functions are not represented equally at cortical levels. This appears true even though: (1) impulses from receptors on each side of the body seem to project nearly equally, though largely contralaterally, to symmetrical cortical areas, and (2) certain information received in the cortex of one hemisphere can be transferred to the other via interhemispheric commissures (Meyers, '56).

In certain higher functions, believed to be cortical in nature, one hemisphere appears to be the "leading" one and, in this sense, is referred to as the *dominant hemisphere*. With respect to most of the higher functions, cerebral dominance appears to be one of degree (Zangwill, '60). Cerebral dominance probably is most complete in relation to the complex and highly evolved aspects of language. Handedness also is related to cerebral dominance, though its relationship is less clear-cut than has been assumed. It seems likely that handedness is a graded characteristic. Left-handedness, in particular, is less definite than right-handedness, and less regularly associated with dominance in either hemisphere. There also appears to be a group of disturbances related to language that are said to be commonly associated with imperfectly developed cerebral dominance. These include the improper development of reading, writing, and drawing abilities, poor spatial judgment, and imperfect directional control (Zangwill, '60). In true right-handed individuals it is nearly always the left hemisphere which is dominant and governs language and related processes; but the converse of this is not necessarily true. The degree of cerebral dominance appears to vary widely, not only among individuals, but with respect to different functions. Although a degree of "cerebral ambilaterality" would appear to be a distinct advantage with respect to recovery of speech following a unilateral cerebral injury, it carries the risk, or possibility, of difficulty in learning to read, spell and draw. The relationship between handedness and speech is perhaps a more natural one than is commonly realized, since some gesturing often accompanies speech and in certain situations may substitute for it. Most clinicians relate handedness and speech to the dominant hemisphere.

The dominant hemisphere, usually the left, is primarily concerned with processing language, arithmetic, and analytic functions, while the nondominant hemisphere is concerned with spatial concepts, recognition of faces, and some elements of music (Sperry, '74). Ideographic (pictographic) language may be processed by the nondominant hemisphere because of its spatial and pictorial capabilities, while grammatical language using script depends upon analytic functions of the dominant hemisphere. The visual sign language used by deaf persons appears to be processed primarily in the left hemisphere.

Cerebral dominance is considered to have a genetic basis, but its hereditary determination probably is not absolute. Pathological and psychological factors also influence handedness, and many determining factors remain unknown.

Many cortical functions are concerned only with contralateral regions of the body, and unilateral lesions affecting these functions produce a disturbance contralaterally, regardless of cerebral dominance. This appears particularly true of the primary motor and sensory areas. It also is the case with lesions of the parietal cortex which result in *asterognosis*, or inability to recognize form, size, texture, and identity of an object by touch alone. In certain parietal lobe lesions particular deficits occur more commonly in the nondominant hemisphere. One such syndrome is characterized by a disorder of the body image in which the patient: (1) fails to recognize parts of his own body, (2) fails to appreciate the existence of hemiparesis, and (3) neglects the part of his body which he denies.

SLEEP

Sleep has been considered a unique passive state, interpreted physiologically as the expression of functional deafferentation of the ascending reticular activating system. The awake state was explained in terms of increased activity in this ascending system, while sleep was correlated with passive dampening of this system. Recent advances indicate that sleep is an active, complex neural phenomenon initiated by sleep-inducing structures and mediated by biochemical transmitters. Sleep is not a single phenomenon, but a series of successive functionally related states, which depend upon different active mechanisms, some of which can be selectively modified, or suppressed (Lindsley, '60; Kleitman, '63; Jouvet, '67, '69). In mammals, two recurring, distinctive and related sleep states can be readily recognized. These are referred to as slow wave sleep and paradoxical sleep.

Slow wave sleep is characterized in the EEG by synchronized cortical activity consisting of spindles (11 to 16 cycles/sec) and/or by high voltage slow waves. During slow wave sleep, tone remains in the neck muscles, spinal reflex activity is present and changes in autonomic activity are minimal. After a time this state is succeeded by a totally different sleep state, known as paradoxical sleep.

Paradoxical sleep is characterized by an EEG pattern with low voltage fast activity which resembles that of the alert, waking state. This sleep state occurs intermittently after variable periods of slow wave sleep and has precise behavioral criteria: (1) abolition of antigravity muscle tone, especially in the cervical region; (2) depression of spinal reflex activity; (3) reduction in blood pressure, bradycardia, and irregular respiration; and (4) bursts of rapid eye movements (REM). The EEG pattern in this sleep state is similar to that which characterizes the awake state and for this reason it is called paradoxical sleep.

In paradoxical sleep rapid eye movements (REM) of 50 to 60 per minute occur in a stereotyped pattern different from that seen in the waking state. REM are associated with subcortical and cortical activities, which have been termed *pontogeniculo-occipital* (PGO) *activity*. Phasic activities of high voltage can be recorded from the pontine reticular formation, the lateral geniculate body and the occipital cortex.

PGO activity occurs transiently during slow sleep, and always precedes paradoxical sleep. During paradoxical sleep, PGO waves are fairly constant, and it is likely that the same electrical events are triggering both these activities and the REM (Jouvet, '69). Bursts of ascending impulses from the medial and inferior vestibular nuclei have been implicated in the REM (Pompeiano and Morrison, '65; Pompeiano, '67). Lesions in the medial and inferior vestibular nuclei abolish the bursts of REM, but paradoxical sleep maintains its low voltage, fast activity in the EEG.

Information concerning the biogenic amines has provided some understanding of their role in sleep states (Jouvet, '67, '69). In the cat, reserpine, which depletes both serotonin and norepinephrine, produces a tranquil state and suppresses both slow wave and paradoxical sleep. Most monoamine oxidase (MAO) inhibitors have a suppressive effect upon paradoxical sleep and increase slow wave sleep. Histofluorescence techniques have demonstrated that most serotonin-containing neurons are located in the raphe system (Ungerstedt, '71; Felten et al., '74), and central norepinephrine-containing neurons are located principally in the locus ceruleus (Ungerstedt, '71; Dahlström and Fuxe, '64). Inhibition of serotonin synthesis leads to insomnia which is reversible; injections of the immediate precursor of serotonin (5-hydroxytryptamine) causes a return to normal sleep. Nearly total destruction of serotonin-containing neurons in the raphe also produces insomnia. It has been suggested that serotonin may be most intimately associated with slow wave sleep, but many intricate facets of the sleep process remain poorly defined.

The relationship between slow wave sleep and paradoxical sleep is not simple, but evidence suggests that serotonergic neurons, involved in slow wave sleep, also may act as part of the triggering mechanism for paradoxical sleep (Jouvet, '69). Serotonergic neurons triggering paradoxical sleep are located in caudal regions of the pontine raphe; lesions at this level depress paradoxical sleep relative to slow sleep. The structures responsible for paradoxical sleep are thought to lie outside of the raphe system, and include the locus ceruleus, a cell group containing norepinephrine and monoamine oxidase. Monoamine oxidase inhibitors and bilateral lesions of the locus ceruleus have been described as selectively suppressing paradoxical sleep. Some doubt has been cast upon the thesis that the locus ceruleus triggers paradoxical sleep by other studies in which bilateral lesions of this structure have failed to suppress paradoxical sleep even though norepinephrine has been greatly diminished in the cerebral cortex (B. E. Jones, et al., '77). Certain cholinergic mechanisms also have been implicated in the mechanism of paradoxical sleep, in that atropine suppresses this form of sleep, while direct injections of acetylcholine in the locus ceruleus produce paradoxical sleep. Thus, the complex neuropharmacological events which underlie paradoxical sleep involve a number of different neurotransmitters, not all of which are known.

INTEGRATED CORTICAL FUNCTIONS

One of the striking features of the human brain is its elaborate neural mechanisms for complex correlations, sensory discriminations and the utilization of former experiences and reactions. These mechanisms involve *associative memory* and *mnemonic reactions.* The ability to retain, modify and reuse neuronal chains probably provides the basis of conscious and unconscious memory.

In a general way, the central sulcus divides the cerebral cortex into a posterior receptive portion and an anterior part related to motor functions. The posterior portion contains all the primary receptive areas which receive specific sensory impulses from lower centers in the brain stem. Regions in immediate contact with the receptive centers, known as *parasensory areas,* serve for the combination and elaboration of primary impulses into more complex sensory perceptions. In more distant *association areas* impulses conveyed from various sensory regions may overlap (e.g., the inferior parietal lobule) and form the basis for multisensory perceptions. The interaction of different sensory impulses initiated by "feeling" and "seeing" an object or person excite memory constellations which lead to recognition. The arousal of associative mnemonic complexes has been termed "gnosis," and it forms the basis of understanding and knowledge. Disorders of these mechanisms caused by lesions in association areas of the cerebral cortex are known as gnostic disturbances, or *agnosias*. In these conditions tactile, visual or auditory stimuli may no longer evoke appropriate memory constellations. When these gnostic disturbances involve the associative mechanisms underlying the comprehension of language, they form part of the complex known as the *aphasias*.

Closely related to both agnosia and aphasia is another group of disorders characterized by difficulty in performing skilled, learned movements even though no paralysis or sensory loss is present. These disorders which affect the motor side of higher sensory-motor integration, are referred to as the *apraxias*. There are only two ways a patient can show that he recognizes an object: (1) by naming or describing the object, or (2) by demonstrating its use. If the patient can demonstrate the use of an object, but is unable to name it, he has an aphasia. If he can name the object, or describe it, but does not know how to use it, he has an apraxia. The above example demonstrates that agnosia partially underlies both aphasia and apraxia.

CHAPTER 14

Blood Supply of the Central Nervous System

The central nervous system is metabolically one of the most active systems of the body. Although the brain constitutes only about 2% of the body weight, it requires 17% of the cardiac output and 20% of the oxygen utilized by the body. Estimates of cerebral blood flow based upon the nitrous oxide method of Kety and Schmidt ('48) indicate a normal blood flow of about 50 ml/100 g of brain tissue per minute. Thus, a brain of average weight has a normal blood flow of about 750 ml per minute. The mean oxygen consumption in a normal conscious subject is about 3.3 ml/100 g of brain tissue per minute, or about 46 ml per minute for the entire brain. The brain is not a homogeneous organ and metabolic activity and nutritive requirements in various regions reflect the functional activity of neuronal systems. This differential functional activity in neuronal systems can be demonstrated autoradiographically by injection of 2-[^{14}C]deoxyglucose, a glucose analog, which passes the blood-brain barrier, is partially metabolized by functionally active neurons, and is trapped in the neurons (Kennedy et al., '75, '76; Plum et al., '76). This technic, developed only at the tissue level, reveals surprising details of neuronal activity under controlled conditions (Figs. 13-14, 13-15, and 13-16).

Even brief interference with cerebral circulation can cause neurological or mental disturbances. Neural tissue deprived of an adequate blood supply undergoes necrosis. Impairment of local or regional blood supply constitutes the most common cause of central nervous system lesions. Vascular lesions most commonly result from arteriosclerosis of cerebral and cervical (i.e., internal carotid artery) vessels which reduce blood flow and can lead to thrombosis. Vascular occlusions also may result from emboli (i.e., fragments of blood clots, fat, and

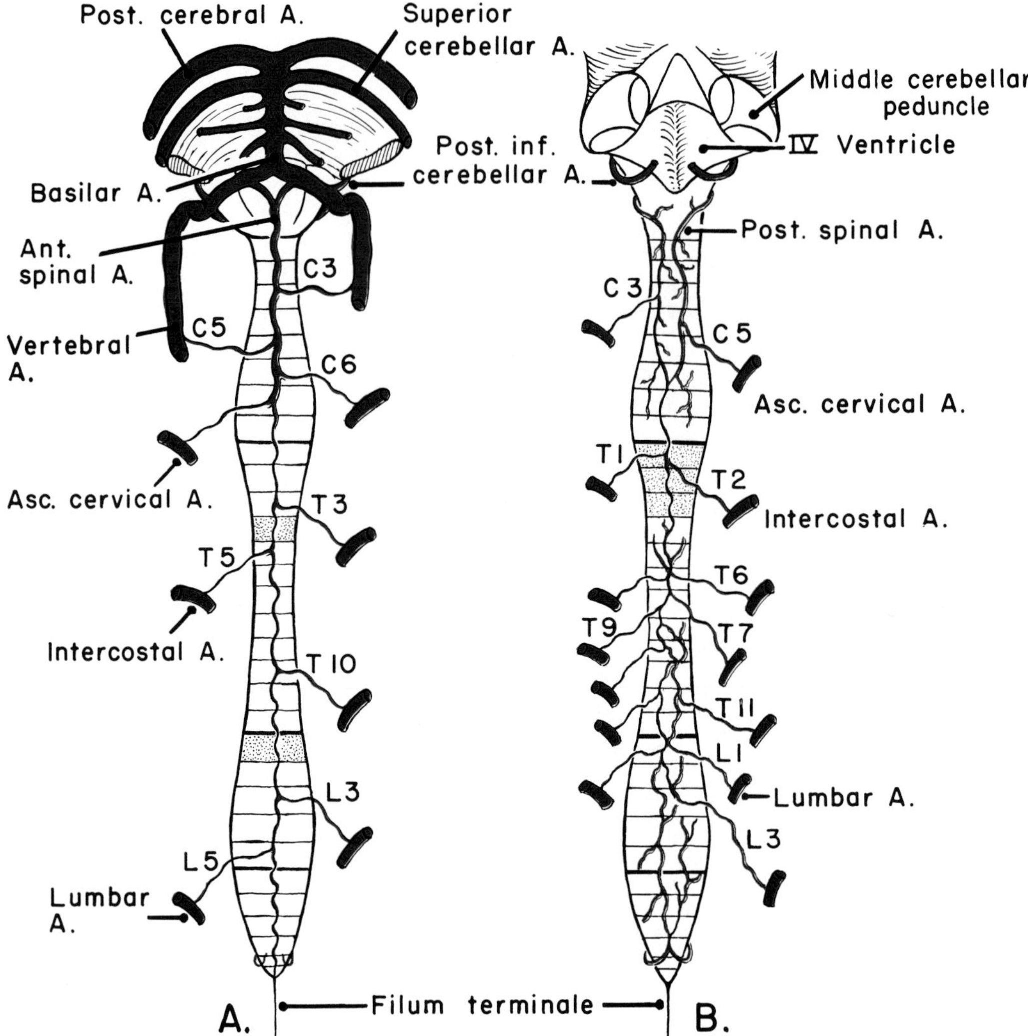

Figure 14-1. Diagram of the arterial supply of the spinal cord. (*A*) Anterior surface and arteries; (*B*) posterior surface and arteries. Vulnerable segments of the spinal cord are *stippled. Letters* and *numbers* indicate the most important radicular arteries (based on Bolton, '39; Suh and Alexander, '39; Zulch, '54). (From Carpenter and Sutin, *Human Neuroanatomy*, 1983; courtesy of Williams & Wilkins.)

tumors or air bubbles). Hemorrhage into brain tissue, the brain ventricles, or the meninges may result from vascular lesions. Probably the most common cause of spontaneous hemorrhage into the brain and subarachnoid space is rupture of cerebral aneurysms (abnormal sacculations), most of which are of congenital origin. Neural lesions resulting from interruptions of the blood supply often can be localized to specific cerebral arteries on the basis of characteristic sensory and motor deficits.

BLOOD SUPPLY OF THE SPINAL CORD

The spinal cord is supplied by: (1) branches of the *vertebral arteries* that descend, and (2) multiple *radicular arteries derived from segmental vessels* (Fig. 14-1). As the vertebral arteries ascend along the anterolateral surfaces of the medulla, each gives rise to two paired descending vessels: (1) the posterior spinal artery, and (2) the anterior spinal artery.

Posterior Spinal Arteries. Paired pos-

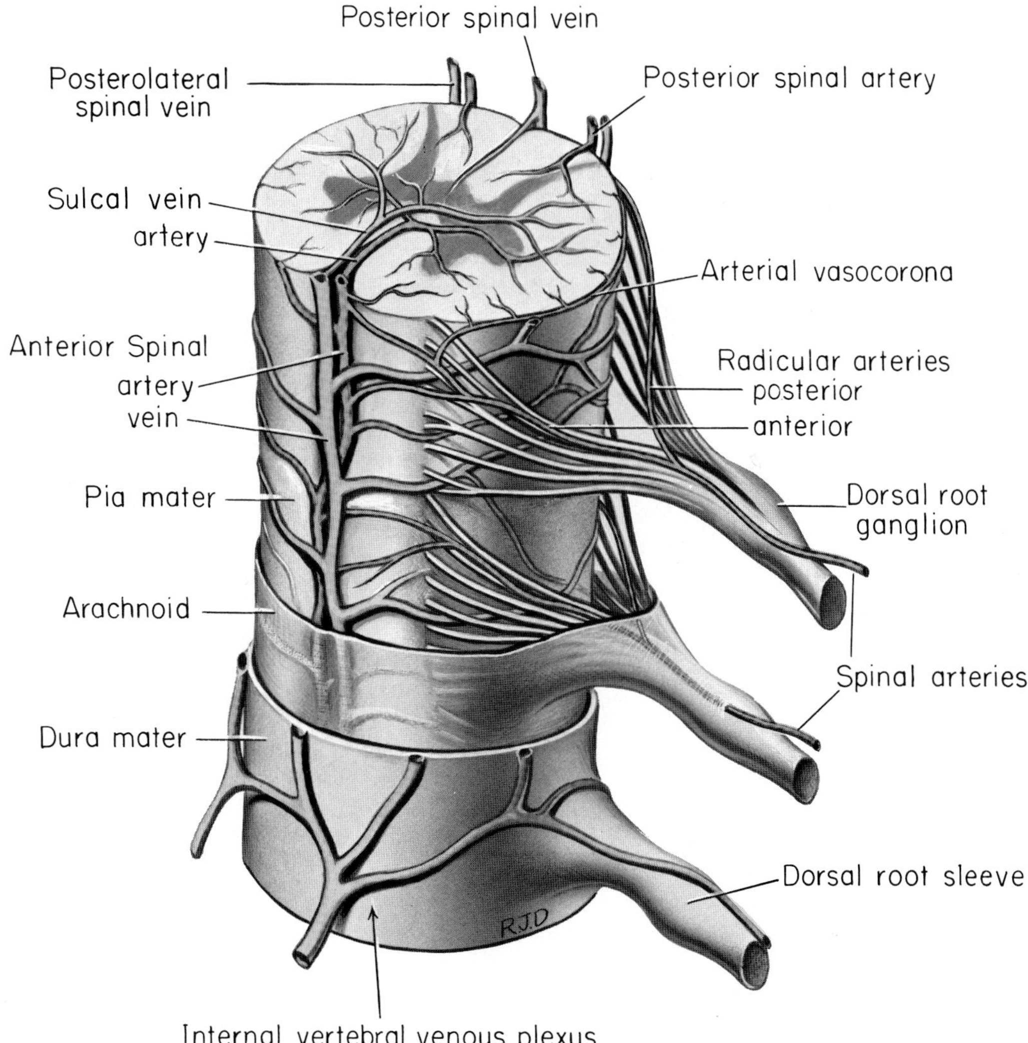

Figure 14-2. Blood supply and venous drainage of the spinal cord shown with respect to the meninges and internal structure. (From Carpenter and Sutin, *Human Neuroanatomy*, 1983; courtesy of Williams & Wilkins.)

terior spinal arteries descend on the posterior surface of the spinal cord, medial to the dorsal roots, receive variable contributions from the posterior radicular arteries, and form two longitudinal plexiform channels near the dorsal root entry zone (Fig. 14-2). At times the posterior spinal arteries become discontinuous, or so small they appear discontinuous. These vessels receive blood from the posterior radicular arteries and distribute it to the posterior third of the spinal cord (Turnbull, '72).

Anterior Spinal Arteries. The paired anterior spinal arteries unite to form a single descending midline vessel that supplies midline rami to the lower medulla and sulcal branches that enter the anterior median fissure of the spinal cord (Fig. 14-1). The continuity of the anterior spinal artery is dependent upon anastomotic branches which it receives from the anterior radicular arteries (Suh and Alexander, '39). Anterior radicular arteries join the anterior spinal artery by branching gently upward or sharply downward. Where two anterior radicular arteries reach the same level of the spinal cord a diamond-shaped arterial configuration results. In the thoracic region the anterior spinal artery may narrow to such an extent that it may not function as an adequate anastomosis, if the anterior radicular arteries, above or below it should be occluded. An arterial ring encircling the conus medullaris communicates with the most caudal part of the anterior spinal artery.

The anterior and posterior spinal arteries are anastomotic channels extending the length of the spinal cord which receive branches from the radicular arteries. Branches of the vertebral arteries provide the principal blood supply of virtually the entire cervical spinal cord.

Radicular Arteries. These arteries are derived from segmental vessels (i.e., ascending cervical, deep cervical, intercostal, lumbar, and sacral arteries), pass through the intervertebral foramina, and divide into *anterior* and *posterior radicular arteries* which provide the principal blood supply of thoracic, lumbar, sacral, and coccygeal spinal segments (Fig. 14-2). Radicular arteries are situated most frequently on the left side in the thoracic and lumbar regions of the spinal cord, while the cervical spinal cord is supplied equally from either side. Radicular arteries course along the ventral surface of the roots they accompany. Where the epineurium blends with the dura mater, the radicular arteries enter the subarachnoid space. A single radicular artery may become either an anterior or posterior radicular artery, or divide to form both (Turnbull, '72). Small twigs leave the arteries to supply the dura mater and the spinal roots they accompany.

Anterior radicular arteries contributing to the anterior spinal artery vary from 2 to 17, but most commonly number between 6 and 10 arteries. The cervical spinal cord receives from 0 to 6 anterior radicular arteries, while the thoracic cord receives 2 to 4 and the lumbar cord has 1 or 2. One anterior radicular artery in the lumbar region, appreciably larger than all others, is known as the *artery of Adamkiewicz* or the artery of the lumbar enlargement (Lazorthes et al., '57). This radicular artery usually travels with a lower thoracic or upper lumbar spinal root most frequently on the left side. The thoracic spinal cord has the greatest length between radicular arteries, which means that occlusion of one of these vessels may seriously compromise its circulation. In addition certain spinal regions which receive their blood supply from more than one source are particularly vulnerable if they are suddenly deprived of blood from one of these sources (Fig. 14-1). The upper thoracic (T1–T4) and first lumbar spinal segments are among the most vulnerable regions of the spinal cord. The intercostal arteries do not interconnect with other arteries in the same extensive fashion as the extraspinal arteries in the cervical and lumbosacral regions. Thus occlusion of one intercostal artery in a vulnerable region can result in a spinal cord infarction. This clinical picture is seen with dissecting aneurysms of the aorta or as a result of surgery on the aorta where more than one intercostal artery may be blocked (Turnbull, '73). Spinal cord segment L1 is another vulnerable region, where the anterior aspect of the cord is susceptible to vascular insult (Fig. 14-1).

The *posterior radicular arteries*, numbering between 10 and 23, divide on the posterolateral surface of the spinal cord and join the paired posterior spinal arteries. Although these vessels are more often on the left side, left predominance is not as evident as with the anterior radicular arteries.

The *anterior spinal artery* gives rise to a number of sulcal branches which enter the anterior median fissure of the spinal cord; these branches pass alternately to the right or left except for an occasional sulcal artery that divides into right and left branches (Fig. 14-2). Central branches arising from the anterior spinal artery are not only more numerous in the cervical and lumbar regions of the spinal cord, but they are of larger caliber than in the thoracic region (Hassler, '66). Sulcal branches of the anterior spinal artery supply the anterior horn, the lateral horn, the central gray, and the basal part of the posterior horn. In addition these branches supply the anterior and lateral funiculi. Peripheral portions of the lateral funiculi receive branches from the *arterial vasocorona*. The *posterior spinal arteries* supply the posterior horns and the posterior funiculus (Fig. 14-2).

Spinal Veins. Veins draining the spinal

cord have a distribution generally similar to that of spinal arteries. Anterior longitudinal venous trunks consist of anteromedian and anterolateral veins (Fig. 14-2). Sulcal veins entering the anteromedian vein drain anteromedial portions of the spinal cord; each sulcal vein drains regions on both sides of the spinal cord. Anterolateral regions of the spinal cord drain into anterolateral veins and into the *venous vasocorona*. The *anteromedian* and *anterolateral spinal veins* are drained by 6 to 11 anterior radicular veins which empty into the epidural venous plexus. One large radicular vein in the lumbar region is referred to as the *vena radicularis magna*; other smaller radicular veins are distributed along the spinal cord.

Posterior longitudinal venous trunks, consisting of a *posteromedian vein* and paired *posterolateral veins*, drain the posterior funiculus, and posterior horns (including their basal regions) and the white matter in the lateral funiculi adjacent to the posterior horn. The posterior longitudinal veins are drained by 5 to 10 posterior radicular veins that enter the epidural venous plexus. The longitudinal veins are connected with each other by coronal veins (venous vasocorona) which encircle the spinal cord.

The *internal vertebral venous plexus* (epidural venous plexus), located between the dura mater and the vertebral periosteum, consists of two or more anterior and posterior longitudinal venous channels which are interconnected at many levels from the clivus to the sacral region (Crock and Yoshizawa, '77). At each intervertebral space there are connections with thoracic, abdominal, and intercostal veins, as well as with the external vertebral venous plexus. Since there are no valves in this spinal venous network, blood flowing through these channels may pass directly into the systemic venous system. When intraabdominal pressure is increased, venous blood from the pelvic plexus passes upward in the internal vertebral venous system. When the jugular veins are obstructed, blood leaves the skull via this plexus. The importance of the continuity of this venous plexus with the prostatic plexus has been cited as a route by which neoplasms may metastasize (Batson, '40). Epidural venograms reveal many details of the internal vertebral venous plexus and usually fill the pediculate veins which outline the superior and inferior margins of the intervertebral foramina (Fig. 14-3).

BLOOD SUPPLY OF THE BRAIN

The entire brain is supplied by two pairs of arterial trunks, the internal carotid arteries and the vertebral arteries.

Internal Carotid Artery. This artery can be divided into four segments: cervical, intrapetrosal, intracavernous, and cerebral (supraclinoid) portions. The intracavernous and cerebral portions of this artery are referred to as the "carotid siphon" by neuroradiologists because of their characteristic configuration. The *intracavernous segment* of the internal carotid artery lies close to the medial wall of the cavernous sinus, courses nearly horizontally and bears important relationships to cranial nerves III, IV, VI, and portions (division I) of nerve V which lie within the sinus. The abducens nerve lies immediately adjacent to the internal carotid artery within the sinus. The *cerebral segment* begins as the artery emerges from the cavernous sinus and passes medial to the anterior clinoid process (Fig. 14-17). This portion of the artery, extending upward and backward, gives rise to all major branches of the internal carotid artery. The *cervical segment* which extends from the bifurcation of the common carotid to the carotid canal in the petrous bone has no branches. The *intrapetrosal segment* of this vessel is surrounded by dense bone. Small branches given off from the intrapetrosal and *intracavernous segments* pass into the tympanic cavity, the cavernous and inferior petrosal sinuses, the trigeminal ganglion and the meninges of the middle fossa.

Major branches of the internal carotid artery are the *ophthalmic*, *posterior communicating*, and *anterior choroidal arteries* (Fig. 14-4). Lateral to the optic chiasm the internal carotid artery divides into a smaller *anterior cerebral artery* and a larger *middle cerebral artery*. The middle cerebral artery is regarded as the direct continuation of the internal carotid artery.

Vertebral Artery. The vertebral artery arises from the first part of the subclavian artery, enters the foramen transversarium

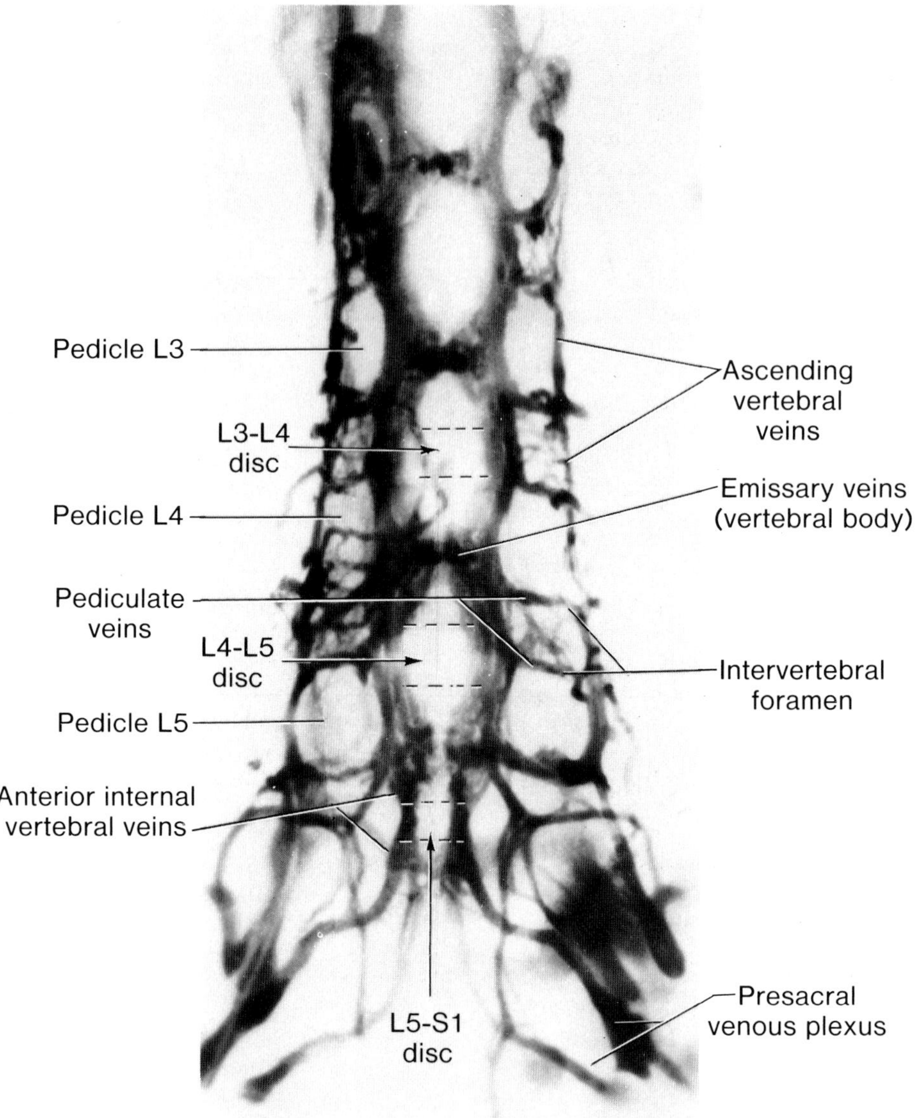

Figure 14-3. Epidural venogram done retrograde from one ascending lumbar vein. Venogram reveals details of the internal vertebral venous plexus including ascending vertebral veins, emissary veins from vertebral body, pediculate veins at the superior and inferior margins of the intervertebral foramina, the anterior internal vertebral veins and the presacral venous plexus. The pedicles of L3, L4, and L5 are well outlined and the approximate position of the intervertebral discs at three levels are indicated by *dashed lines.* (From Carpenter and Sutin, *Human Neuroanatomy*, 1983; courtesy of Williams & Wilkins.)

of the 6th cervical vertebra, and ascends in the foramina transversaria of all higher cervical vertebrae. The artery pierces the posterior altanto-occipital membrane and the dura mater to enter the posterior fossa through the foramen magnum. The vertebral arteries course along the anterolateral surfaces of the medulla and unite at the caudal border of the pons to form the basilar artery (Figs. 14-4, 14-12, and 14-13). Cervical portions of the vertebral artery give rise to spinal (radicular) and muscular branches.

Intracranial branches of the vertebral

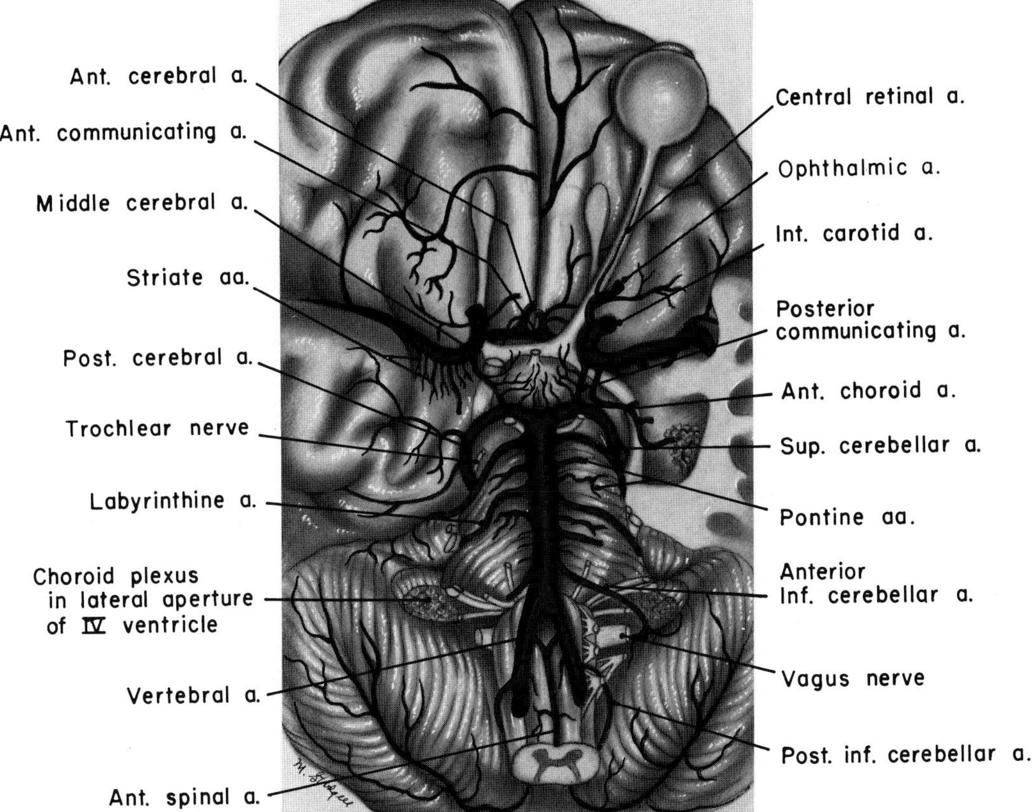

Figure 14-4. Formation and branches of the arterial circle on the inferior surface of the brain. (From Carpenter and Sutin, *Human Neuroanatomy*, 1983; courtesy of Williams & Wilkins.)

and basilar arteries supply the cervical spinal cord (via anterior and posterior spinal arteries), the medulla, pons, midbrain, cerebellum, posterior parts of the diencephalon, and parts of the occipital and temporal lobes of the brain. A labyrinthine branch of the basilar artery supplies the cochlea and vestibular apparatus (Fig. 14-4).

Cerebral Arterial Circle. The cerebral arterial circle (Willis) is an arterial wreath encircling the optic chiasm, the tuber cinereum, and the interpeduncular region formed by anastomotic branches of the internal carotid artery and the most rostral branches of the basilar artery (Figs. 14-4 and 14-8). This arterial circle is formed by the anterior and posterior communicating arteries, and proximal portions of the anterior, middle, and posterior cerebral arteries. The anterior cerebral arteries run medially and rostrally toward the interhemispheric fissure; in front of the optic chiasm these two arteries are joined by a connecting vessel, the *anterior communicating artery*. The *posterior communicating arteries* arise from the internal carotid arteries; run caudomedially, and anastomose with proximal portions of the posterior cerebral arteries. The posterior cerebral arteries are formed by the bifurcation of the basilar artery at the rostral border of the pons. The cerebral arterial circle is said to equalize blood flow to various parts of the brain, but normally there is little exchange of blood between the right and left sides of the arterial circle because of the equality of blood pressure. The arterial circle and its branches on the inferior surface of the brain are shown in Figures 14-4 and 14-8.

From the arterial circle and the principal cerebral arteries two types of branches arise, central and cortical. *Central arteries*, arising from the arterial circle and proximal

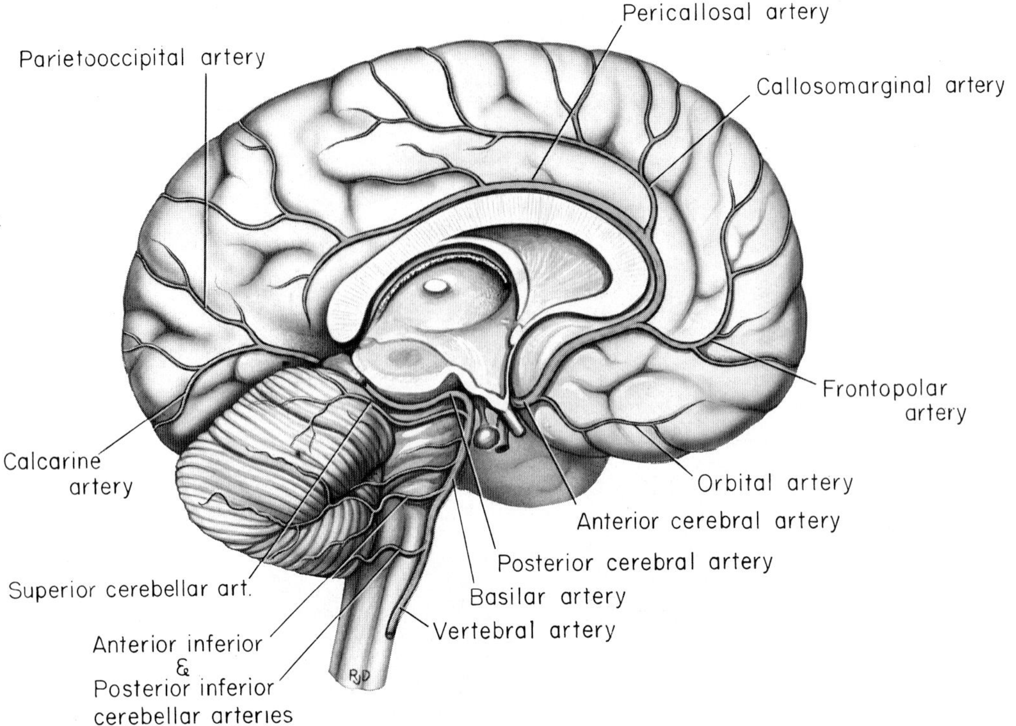

Figure 14-5. Principal arteries on the medial surface of the cerebrum shown together with the arteries of the brain stem and cerebellum. (From Carpenter and Sutin, *Human Neuroanatomy*, 1983; courtesy of Williams & Wilkins.)

portions of the principal cerebral arteries, penetrate the substance of the brain and supply deep structures (Figs. 14-9, 14-10, and 14-11). The anterior and posterior choroidal arteries, respectively, branches of the internal carotid, and the posterior cerebral arteries, may be included in this group. Penetrating vessels, particularly those of central branches, have been referred to as end-arteries, suggesting that they do not anastomose with other arteries. In the human brain there are no end-arteries, but anastomoses between these small branches usually are not sufficient to maintain adequate circulation if a major vessel is occluded suddenly. *Cortical* branches of each major cerebral artery pass in the pia mater to large regions of the cerebral cortex, undergo considerable branching, and form freely anastomosing superficial plexuses (Figs. 14-5, 14-6, and 14-7). Smaller arteries arising from these plexuses penetrate the cortex at nearly right angles and run for variable distances.

CORTICAL BRANCHES

The cortical branches of the cerebral hemisphere are derived from the anterior, middle, and posterior cerebral arteries.

Anterior Cerebral Artery. This artery originates at the bifurcation of the internal carotid artery lateral to the optic chiasm and nerve (Fig. 14-4). The anterior cerebral artery passes rostromedially, dorsal to the optic nerve, and approaches the corresponding artery of the opposite side with which it connects via the anterior communicating artery (Figs. 14-5 and 14-8). The artery enters the interhemispheric fissure, passes upward on the medial surface of the hemisphere, and continues posteriorly on the superior surface of the corpus callosum. The anterior cerebral artery gives rise to: (1) the *medial striate artery*, (2) *orbital branches*, (3) the *frontopolar artery*, (4) the *callosomarginal artery*, and (5) the *pericallosal artery*.

The *medial striate artery* (recurrent ar-

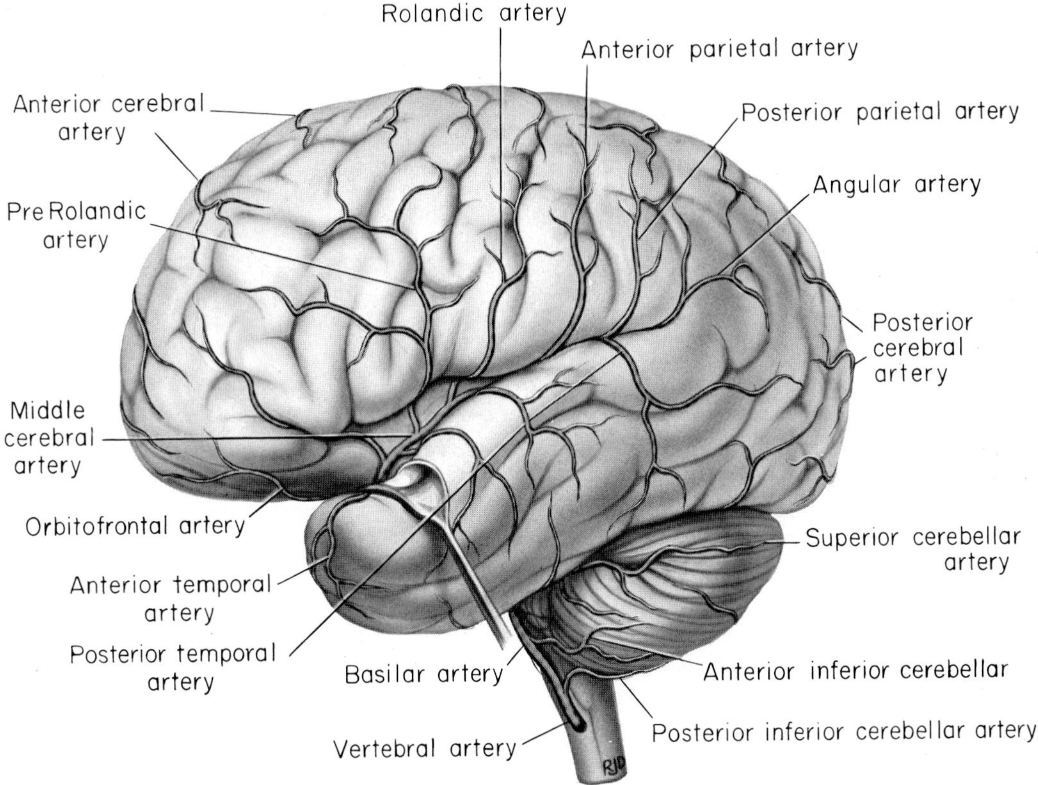

Figure 14-6. Principal arteries on the lateral surface of the cerebrum and cerebellum. (From Carpenter and Sutin, *Human Neuroanatomy*, 1983; courtesy of Williams & Wilkins.)

tery of Heubner), which may arise proximal or distal to the anterior communicating artery, courses caudally and laterally, and enters the anterior perforated space. This vessel supplies the anteromedial part of the head of the caudate nucleus, adjacent parts of the internal capsule and putamen, and parts of the septal nuclei (Figs. 14-8, 14-9, and 14-10). Several small branches of the artery frequently supply the inferior surface of the frontal lobe (Perlmutter and Rhoton, '76).

Orbital branches of the anterior cerebral artery, arising from the ascending part of this artery ventral to the genu of the corpus callosum, extend rostrally to supply the orbital and medial surfaces of the frontal lobe.

A *frontopolar artery* is given off as the anterior cerebral artery curves around the genu of the corpus callosum; branches of this artery supply medial parts of the frontal lobe and extend onto the convexity of the hemisphere.

The *callosomarginal artery*, a major branch of the anterior cerebral artery, arises distal to the frontopolar artery and passes caudally in the callosomarginal sulcus. Branches of this artery supply the paracentral lobule and parts of the cingulate gyrus.

The *pericallosal artery*, regarded as the terminal branch of the anterior cerebral artery, courses caudally along the dorsal surface of the corpus callosum and supplies the medial surface of the parietal lobe, including the precuneus.

Anomalies of the anterior cerebral artery occur in about 25% of brains; these include unpaired arteries and instances where branches are given off to the contralateral hemisphere (Baptista, '63). Occlusion of the trunk of one anterior cerebral artery may produce a contralateral hemiplegia

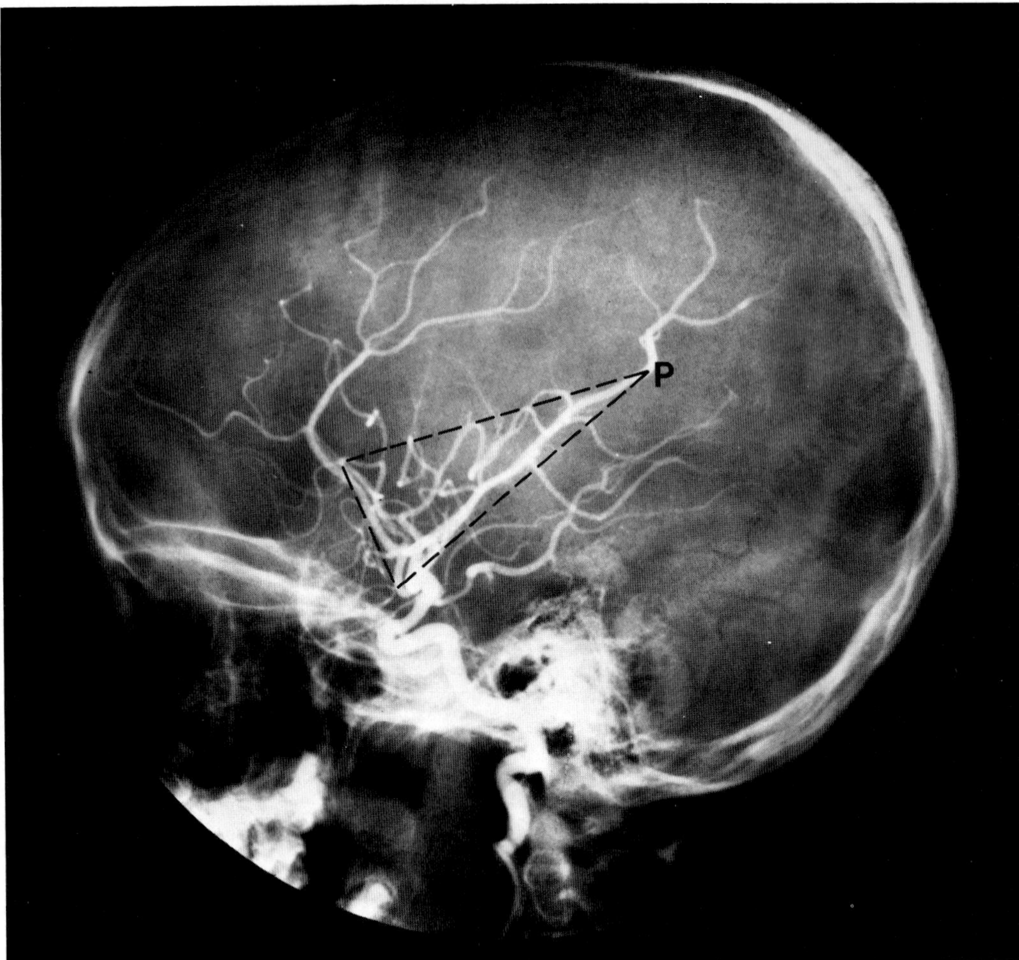

Figure 14-7. Cerebral angiogram demonstrating the Sylvian triangle. There are 5 to 8 branches of the *middle cerebral artery* on the surface of the insula. As they course upward, they reach the deepest portion of the sulcus formed by the junction of the insula and the frontoparietal operculum. Upon reaching this point, the middle cerebral branches change direction and proceed downward a short distance to emerge from the lateral sulcus (Sylvian fissure). The points of reversal can be identified in the angiogram and a line drawn from the most anterior to the most posterior point (*P*) forms the upper margin of the Sylvian triangle. The inferior margin of the triangle is a line from the most posterior point (the angiographic Sylvian point, P) to the anterior extremity of the middle cerebral artery. The anterior border is a line drawn from the rostral extremity of the middle cerebral artery to the first turn of the opercular branch. The triangle contains branches of the middle cerebral vessels as they are disposed on the insula. (Courtesy of the late Dr. Ernest H. Wood, Columbia University, College of Physicians and Surgeons; Taveras and Wood, '76.) (From Carpenter and Sutin, *Human Neuroanatomy*, 1983; courtesy of Williams & Wilkins.)

which is greatest in the lower limb. Obstruction of both anterior cerebral arteries is associated with bilateral paralysis, especially in the lower limbs and impaired sensation that mimics a spinal cord lesion.

Middle Cerebral Artery. The middle cerebral artery, the continuation of the internal carotid artery beyond the origin of the anterior cerebral artery, passes laterally over the anterior perforated substance to enter the lateral cerebral fossa between the temporal lobe and the insula (Figs. 14-4, 14-6, 14-7, and 14-8). This artery, the largest and most complex of the cerebral arteries, divides into a number of large branches which course upward and backward; as

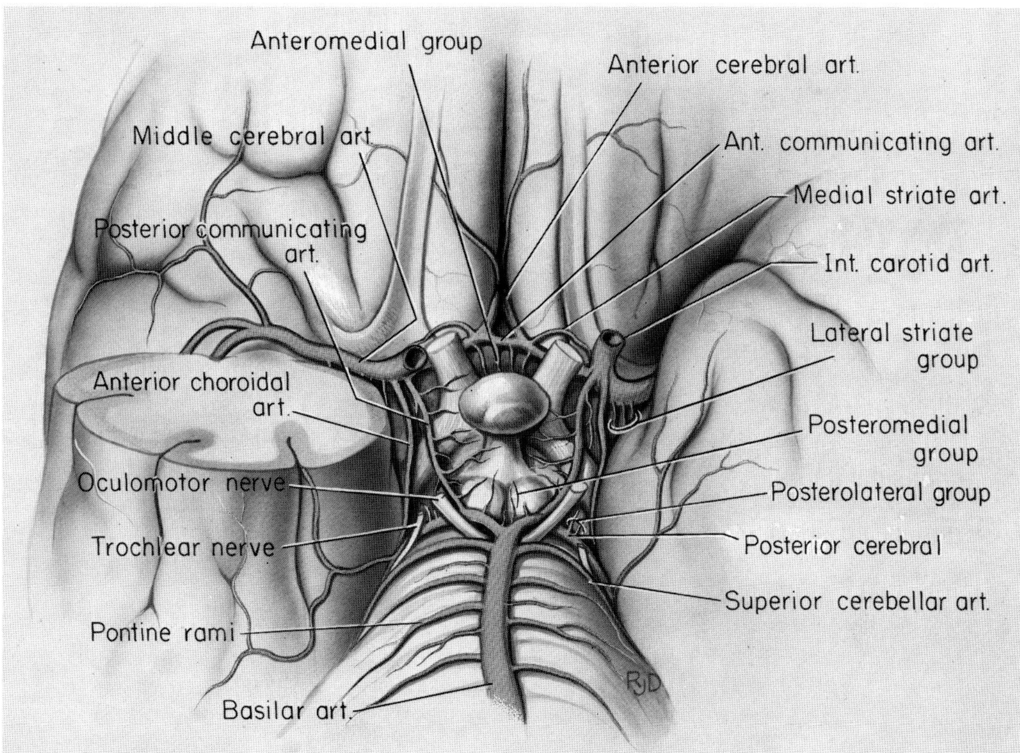

Figure 14-8. The cerebral arterial circle at the base of the brain showing the distribution of the ganglionic branches. These vessels form *anteromedial*, *posteromedial*, *posterolateral*, and *lateral striate* arterial groups. The *medial striate* and *anterior choroidal arteries* also are shown. (From Carpenter and Sutin, *Human Neuroanatomy*, 1983; courtesy of Williams & Wilkins.)

these branches reach the dorsal margin of the insula, they loop abruptly downward toward the lateral sulcus (Gibo et al., '81). The course of the branches of the middle cerebral artery in the insular region is of great importance in the interpretation of cerebral angiograms (Taveras and Wood, '76). In the insular region 5 to 8 branches of the middle cerebral artery lie within what is called the Sylvian triangle (Fig. 14-7). The Sylvian point (or apex) is established angiographically by the most posterior branch of the middle cerebral artery to emerge from the lateral fissure. The inferior margin of the Sylvian triangle is formed by the lower branches of the middle cerebral artery, while the superior margin is formed by looping branches of this artery that are reversing their course. Displacement of branches of the middle cerebral artery in the Sylvian triangle by mass lesions can be detected readily in cerebral angiograms and the direction of displacement provides important information concerning localizing lesions.

Branches of the middle cerebral artery emerge from the lateral sulcus to be distributed in a "fanlike" fashion over the lateral convexity of the hemisphere. These cortical branches supply lateral parts of the orbital gyri, the inferior and middle frontal gyri, most of the precentral and postcentral gyri, the superior and inferior parietal lobules, and the superior and middle temporal gyri, including the temporal pole. The largest cortical branches appear to supply the temporo-occipital and angular areas (Gibo et al., '81). The cortical arteries arise from stem arteries and supply individual cortical regions. In general, one or two cortical arteries pass to each cortical region supplied. The cortical branches to the frontal, anterior temporal and anterior parietal regions are smaller than those to posterior parietal, posterior temporal and temporo-occipital regions, but they are more numerous.

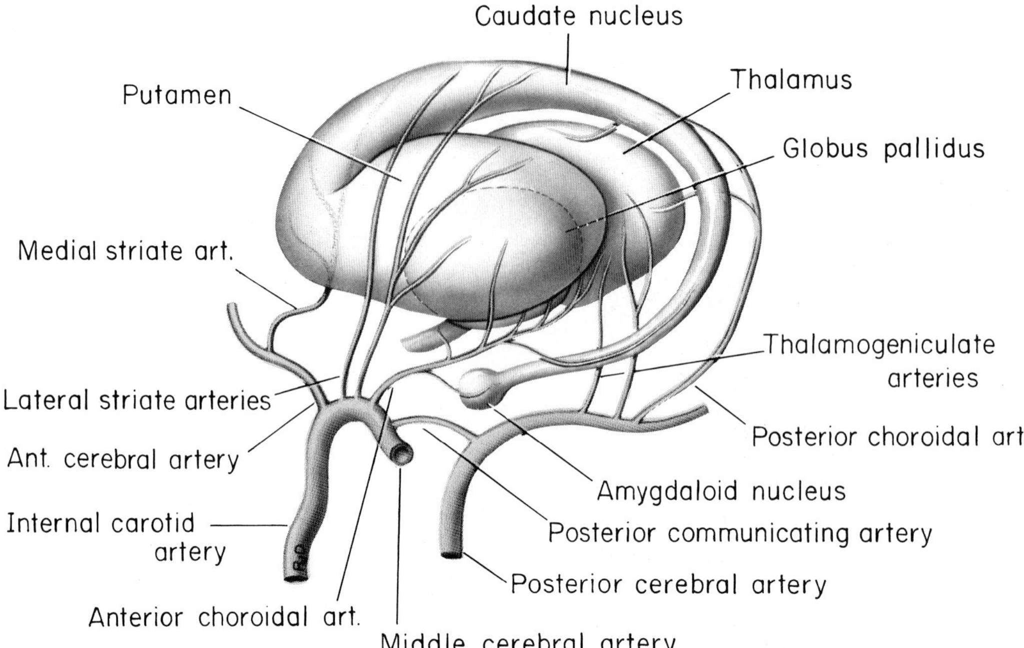

Figure 14-9. Diagrammatic representation of the arterial supply of the corpus striatum and thalamus (modified from Aitken, '09.) (From Carpenter and Sutin, *Human Neuroanatomy*, 1983; courtesy of Williams & Wilkins.)

Branches of the middle cerebral artery include: (1) the *lenticulostriate arteries*, (2) the *anterior temporal artery*, (3) the *orbitofrontal artery*, (4) *pre-Rolandic* and *Rolandic branches*, (5) *anterior* and *posterior parietal branches*, and (6) a *posterior temporal branch* which extends caudally to supply lateral portions of the occipital lobe. Angular branches supplying the angular gyrus constitute the terminal part of the middle cerebral artery.

The extensive and important region nourished by the middle cerebral artery includes the motor and premotor areas, the somesthetic and auditory areas, and large regions of the association cortex concerned with integrative functions. Occlusion of the middle cerebral artery near the origin of its cortical branches may produce: (1) a severe contralateral hemiplegia, most marked in the upper extremity and face; (2) a contralateral sensory loss for position sense and discriminating tactile sense; and (3) severe aphasia, when the dominant hemisphere is involved.

Posterior Cerebral Arteries. These arteries, formed by the bifurcation of the basilar artery, pass laterally around the crus cerebri (Figs. 14-4, 14-5, and 14-8). After receiving anastomoses from the posterior communicating arteries, these arteries continue along the lateral aspect of the midbrain, and then pass above to the tentorium to course on the medial and inferior surfaces of the temporal and occipital lobes. Branches of the posterior cerebral artery extend onto the lateral surfaces of the hemisphere to supply parts of the inferior temporal gyrus, variable portions of the occipital lobe and parts of the superior parietal lobule (Fig. 14-6). Branches of the posterior cerebral artery also are distributed to the brain stem, the choroid plexus of the third and lateral ventricles, and to regions of the cerebral cortex (Zeal and Rhoton, '78).

The posterior cerebral artery divides into two main branches: (1) the *posterior temporal artery* and (2) the *internal occipital artery*.

The *posterior temporal artery* gives off an anterior temporal branch which supplies the inferior surface of the temporal lobe anteriorly and frequently anastomoses with branches of the middle cerebral artery. Pos-

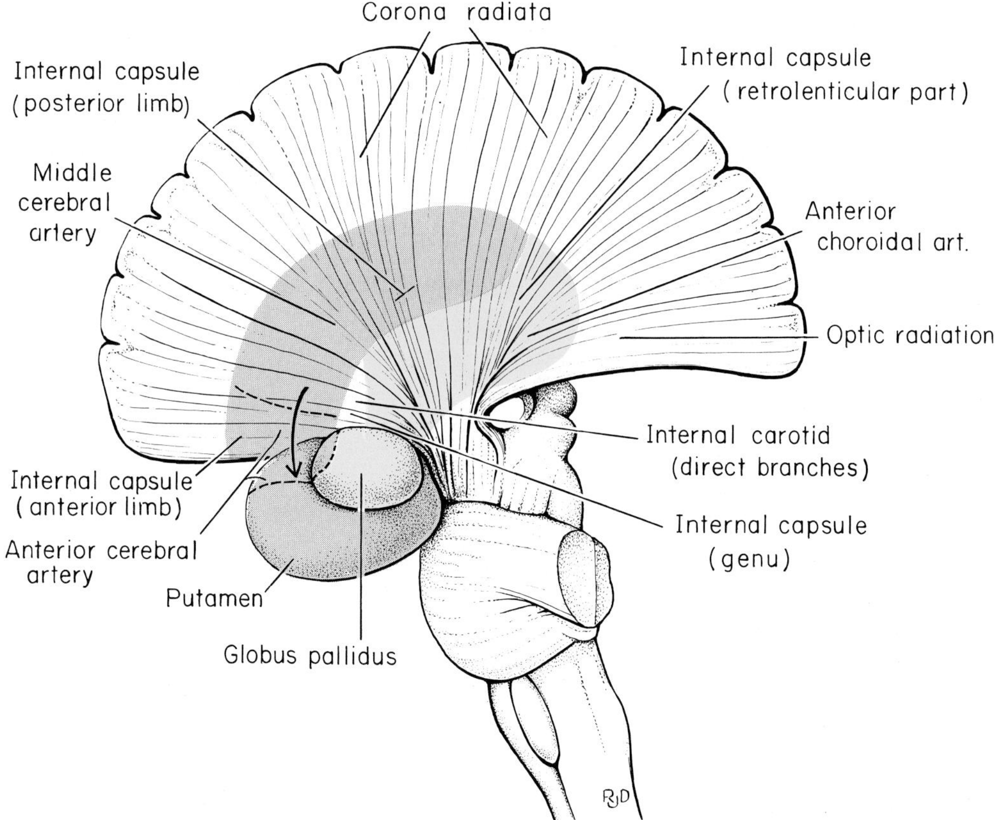

Figure 14-10. Diagram of the blood supply of the internal capsule and corpus striatum. The putamen and globus pallidus are shown rotated ventrally away from the internal capsule. Regions supplied by branches of the *middle* and *anterior cerebral arteries* are shown in *red*; portions of the internal capsule and corpus striatum supplied by the *anterior choroidal artery* are in *yellow.* Direct branches of the *internal carotid artery* supply the genu of the internal capsule (Alexander, '42). (From Carpenter and Sutin, *Human Neuroanatomy*, 1983; courtesy of Williams & Wilkins.)

terior branches of the posterior temporal artery supply the occipitotemporal and lingual gyri (Fig. 2-8).

The *internal occipital artery* divides into the *parieto-occipital* and the *calcarine arteries*, both of which supply different medial regions of the medial aspect of the occipital lobe and portions of the splenium of the corpus callosum (Fig. 14-5). The calcarine artery is of major importance because it supplies the primary visual cortex. Occlusion of the posterior cerebral artery, or the calcarine artery, produces a contralateral homonymous hemianopsia; macular vision often is spared due to anastomoses between branches of the middle and posterior cerebral arteries near the occipital pole.

Cerebral angiography, a technic based upon the injection of radiopaque solutions into cerebral vessels and rapid serial roentgenograms, reveals not only the position and configuration of the cerebral vessels, but it shows the various phases of filling and emptying of vessels by the radiopaque solutions (Taveras and Wood, '76). This radiographic technic is particularly useful in localizing cerebral aneurysms and vascular malformations; in addition it often provides information concerning occlusive vascular disease and space-occupying intracranial masses. While cerebral angiography provides invaluable diagnostic information, it usually is not possible to visualize the small terminal arteries.

CENTRAL ARTERIES

These ganglionic branches arise from proximal portions of the major cerebral and communicating arteries, and supply the diencephalon, basal ganglia, and internal capsule. Penetrating ganglionic arteries are arranged in four groups, designated as anteromedial, anterolateral, posteromedial, and posterolateral (Fig. 14-8).

The *anteromedial arteries* arise from the anterior cerebral and anterior communicating arteries, enter the most medial part of the anterior perforated substance, and are distributed to the anterior hypothalamus, the preoptic area, and the supraoptic region.

The *posteromedial arteries* arise from the whole extent of the posterior communicating artery and the most proximal part of the posterior cerebral artery. Rostral branches of this group supply the hypophysis, infundibulum, and tuberal regions of the hypothalamus; deep penetrating branches, distributed to anterior and medial parts of the thalamus, are referred to as *thalamoperforating arteries* (Fig. 14-12). Caudal branches of this group supply the mammillary bodies and subthalamic region, as well as medial nuclei of the thalamus. The most caudal branches of this group are distributed to medial regions of the midbrain tegmentum and crus cerebri.

The *posterolateral arteries* arise from the posterior cerebral artery, lateral to its anastomosis with the posterior communicating artery (Fig. 14-8). These penetrating branches supply the caudal half of the thalamus (i.e., the geniculate bodies, pulvinar, lateral nuclear group, and large parts of the ventral tier nuclei). These branches of the posterior cerebral artery are referred to as the *thalamogeniculate arteries* (Fig. 14-9).

The *anterolateral group of arteries*, commonly referred to as *striate arteries*, arise primarily from proximal portions of the middle cerebral artery. The medial striate artery (Heubner), derived from the anterior cerebral artery, belongs to this group (Fig. 14-9). These arteries enter the anterior perforated substance and supply portions of the corpus striatum and internal capsule (Figs. 14-9 and 14-10). The medial striate artery supplies the rostroventral part of the head of the caudate nucleus and adjacent portions of the putamen and internal capsule. The lateral striate arteries, derived from the middle cerebral artery, supply remaining portions of the striatum (i.e., caudate nucleus and putamen), except for extreme caudal parts of the putamen and the tail of the caudate nucleus (Fig. 14-11). These arteries also nourish the lateral part of the globus pallidus, the anterior limb of the internal capsule, and dorsal portions of the posterior limb of the internal capsule.

Choroidal Arteries. The anterior and posterior choroidal arteries are distinctive central branches (Figs. 14-4, 14-8, 14-9, and 14-10). The *anterior choroidal artery* usually arises from the internal carotid artery distal to the posterior communicating artery (Carpenter et al., '54). This artery, characterized by its long subarachnoid course and its relatively small caliber, first passes caudally across the optic tract, and then laterally toward the rostromedial surface of the temporal lobe; it enters the inferior horn of the lateral ventricle through the choroidal fissure (Fig. 12-10). Structures supplied by this artery, in addition to the choroid plexus, include the hippocampal formation, portions of both pallidal segments (i.e., lateral parts of the medial segment and medial parts of the lateral segment), a large ventral part of the posterior limb of the internal capsule, and the entire retrolenticular part of the internal capsule (Fig. 14-10). Small branches of this artery supply parts of the optic tract, parts of the amygdaloid complex, ventral parts of the tail of the caudate nucleus, posterior parts of the putamen, and ventrolateral parts of the thalamus.

The *posterior choroidal arteries*, arising from the posterior cerebral artery, consist of one medial and two lateral choroidal arteries (Figs. 14-9 and 14-12). The *medial posterior choroidal artery* curves around the midbrain to reach the region of the pineal body; it gives off branches to the tectum, the choroid plexus of the third ventricle, and the superior and medial surfaces of the thalamus. The *lateral posterior choroidal arteries* partially encircle the brain stem, enter the choroidal fissure and supply more caudal parts of the choroid plexus in the lateral ventricle; some branches of this artery anastomose with branches of the anterior choroidal artery.

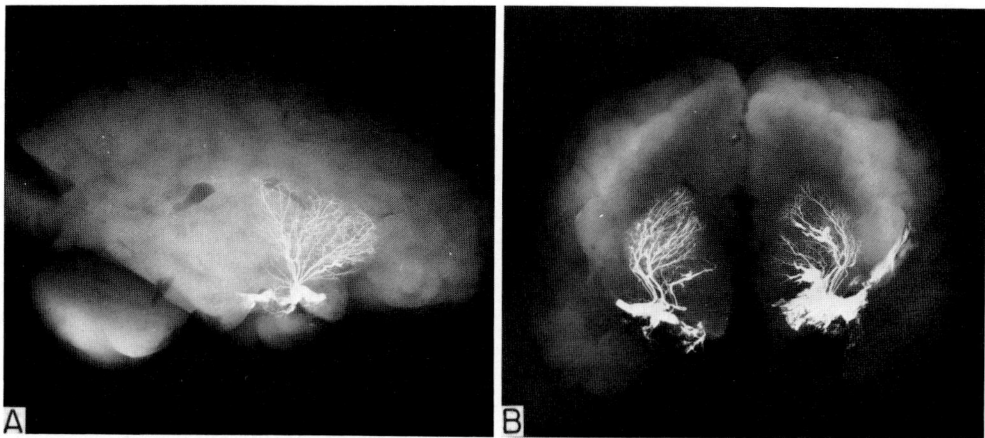

Figure 14-11. Roentgenograms of fresh cadaver brains in which individual arteries have been injected with radiopaque material. (*A*) Lateral and (*B*) frontal views, respectively, of the deep ganglionic branches of the *middle cerebral artery* that penetrate the brain in the anterior perforated substance. (Courtesy of Dr. Harry A. Kaplan.) (From Carpenter and Sutin, *Human Neuroanatomy*, 1983; courtesy of Williams & Wilkins.)

BLOOD SUPPLY OF THE CORPUS STRIATUM, INTERNAL CAPSULE, AND DIENCEPHALON

The *striatum* is nourished mainly by the lateral striate arteries derived from the middle cerebral artery (Figs. 14-9 and 14-10). Rostromedial parts of the head of the caudate nucleus are supplied by the medial striate artery (Heubner) while the tail of the caudate nucleus and the caudal part of the putamen receive branches of the anterior choroidal artery. The lateral segment of the globus pallidus is supplied by branches of both the lateral striate and anterior choroidal arteries (Mettler et al., '56). The lateral part of the medial pallidal segment receives branches from the anterior choroidal artery, while branches of the posterior communicating artery nourish the most medial portions of this pallidal segment.

The *internal capsule*, both anterior and posterior limbs, is supplied primarily by the lateral striate branches of the middle cerebral artery (Figs. 14-10 and 14-11). The medial striate artery supplies a rostromedial part of the anterior limb of the internal capsule. As a rule, the genu of the internal capsule receives some direct branches from the internal carotid artery, while ventral parts of the posterior limb and its entire retrolenticular part are supplied by branches of the anterior choroidal artery (Salamon and Lazorthes, '71).

The *thalamus* is nourished mainly by branches of the posterior cerebral artery (Figs. 14-9 and 14-12). *Thalamoperforating branches*, referred to as the posteromedial arteries, course dorsally and medially to supply chiefly medial and anterior regions of the thalamus (Foix and Hillemand, '25); Salmon and Lazorthes, '71). These arteries, arising from the most medial part of the posterior cerebral artery and from the terminal part of the basilar artery, course dorsally into the diencephalon and nourish paraventricular regions of the hypothalamus and medial regions of the thalamus (Hara and Fujino, '66; George et al., '75). Perforating branches of these arteries, visualized in vertebral angiograms (Fig. 14-12), may be displaced, deformed, or stretched by space-occupying lesions or enlargment of the third ventricle. *Thalamogeniculate branches*, referred to as the posterolateral arteries, supply the pulvinar and the lateral nuclei of the thalamus. These arteries arise from the posterior cerebral artery as it winds around the crus cerebri and from the choroidal arteries (Lazorthes and Salamon, '71; Carpenter et al., '54). The *medial posterior choroidal artery* supplies the choroid plexus of the third ventricle and superior and medial portions of the thalamus. The *inferior thalamic arteries*, arising from the posterior communicating artery and the bifurcation of the basilar artery, course rostrally and dorsally, and enter inferior portions of the thalamus

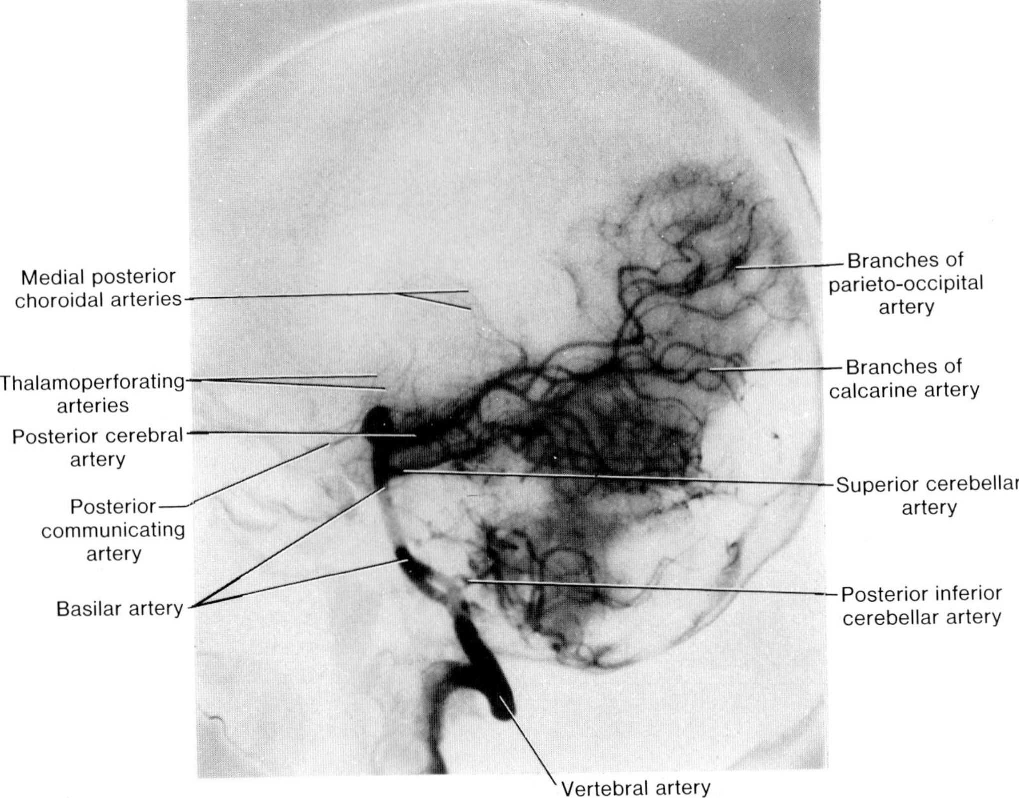

Figure 14-12. Lateral projection of a vertebral angiogram demonstrating major branches of the vertebral basilar system. (Courtesy of Dr. Daniel Hottenstein and Keith Himes, Holy Spirit Hospital, Camp Hill, Pa.) (From Carpenter and Sutin, *Human Neuroanatomy*, 1983; courtesy of Williams & Wilkins.)

(Lazorthes and Salamon, '71). These arteries supply regions of the thalamus rostral to the territory of the thalamoperforating arteries.

The anterior hypothalamus and preoptic region receive their blood supply from the anteromedian ganglionic arteries. More caudal regions of the hypothalamus and the subthalamic region are supplied by branches of the posteromedian group of ganglionic arteries, derived from the posterior cerebral and posterior communicating arteries.

VERTEBRAL BASILAR SYSTEM

The intracranial part of each vertebral artery gives rise to: (1) a *posterior spinal artery*, (2) an *anterior spinal artery*, (3) a *posterior inferior cerebellar artery*, and (4) a *posterior meningeal artery*. The two vertebral arteries unite to form the basilar artery at the lower border of the pons (Figs. 14-1 and 14-4). Branches of the basilar artery include: (1) the *anterior inferior cerebellar arteries*, (2) the *labyrinthine arteries*, (3) numerous *paramedian* and *circumferential pontine rami*, (4) the *superior cerebellar arteries*, and (5) the *posterior cerebral arteries*. The labyrinthine arteries do not supply the brain stem but pass laterally through the internal auditory meati to the inner ear (Fig. 14-4). The posterior cerebral arteries, representing the terminal branches of the basilar artery, furnish branches which supply parts of the midbrain, thalamus, and large regions of the temporal and occipital lobes (Figs. 14-12 and 14-13). With the exception of the most rostral portions of the crus cerebri, the entire blood supply of the medulla, pons, mesencephalon, and cerebellum is derived from the vertebral basilar system. Although many of the branches of the vertebral and

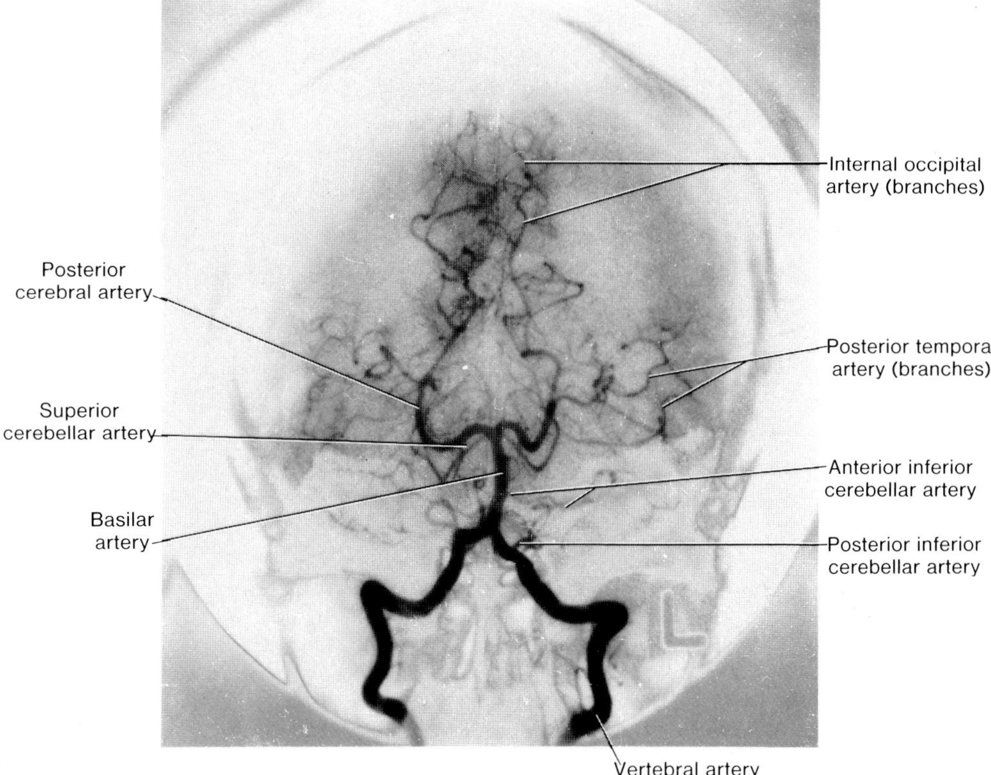

Figure 14-13. Vertebral angiogram as seen in the Towne projection using a substraction technic. (Courtesy of Dr. Daniel Hottenstein and Keith Himes, Holy Spirit Hospital, Camp Hill, Pa.) (From Carpenter and Sutin, *Human Neuroanatomy*, 1983; courtesy of Williams & Wilkins.)

basilar arteries are of small caliber, major branches can be demonstrated in vertebral angiograms (Figs. 14-12 and 14-13). Both posterior cerebral arteries usually are filled by contrast media following injection of one vertebral artery.

Medulla and Pons. These portions of the brain stem are supplied by the anterior and posterior spinal arteries, the posterior inferior cerebellar arteries, and branches of the vertebral and basilar arteries (Figs. 14-1, 14-14, and 14-15). The anterior inferior and superior cerebellar arteries make smaller contributions. There is great variation in the extent of areas supplied by individual vessels and considerable overlap in some regions.

The *posterior spinal artery* supplies the gracile and cuneate fasciculi and their nuclei, and the caudal and dorsal portions of the inferior cerebellar peduncle (Figs. 14-1 and 14-14). When missing, its territory often is taken over by the posterior inferior cerebellar artery.

The *anterior spinal artery* supplies a paramedian region of the medulla which includes the pyramids, the medial lemniscus, medial longitudinal fasciculus, most of the hypoglossal nucleus, caudal parts of the solitary nucleus and dorsal motor nucleus of the vagus, and the medial accessory olive (Fig. 14-14).

Bulbar branches of the vertebral artery supply the pyramids at the lower border of the pons, cephalic parts of the hypoglossal nucleus, and most of the inferior olivary complex. These branches also nourish the reticular formation and parts of the solitary nucleus and the dorsal motor nucleus of the vagus. At caudal medullary levels branches of the vertebral artery are distributed to practically the entire lateral medullary region between the medullary pyramids and the fasciculus cuneatus (Fig. 14-14). Two

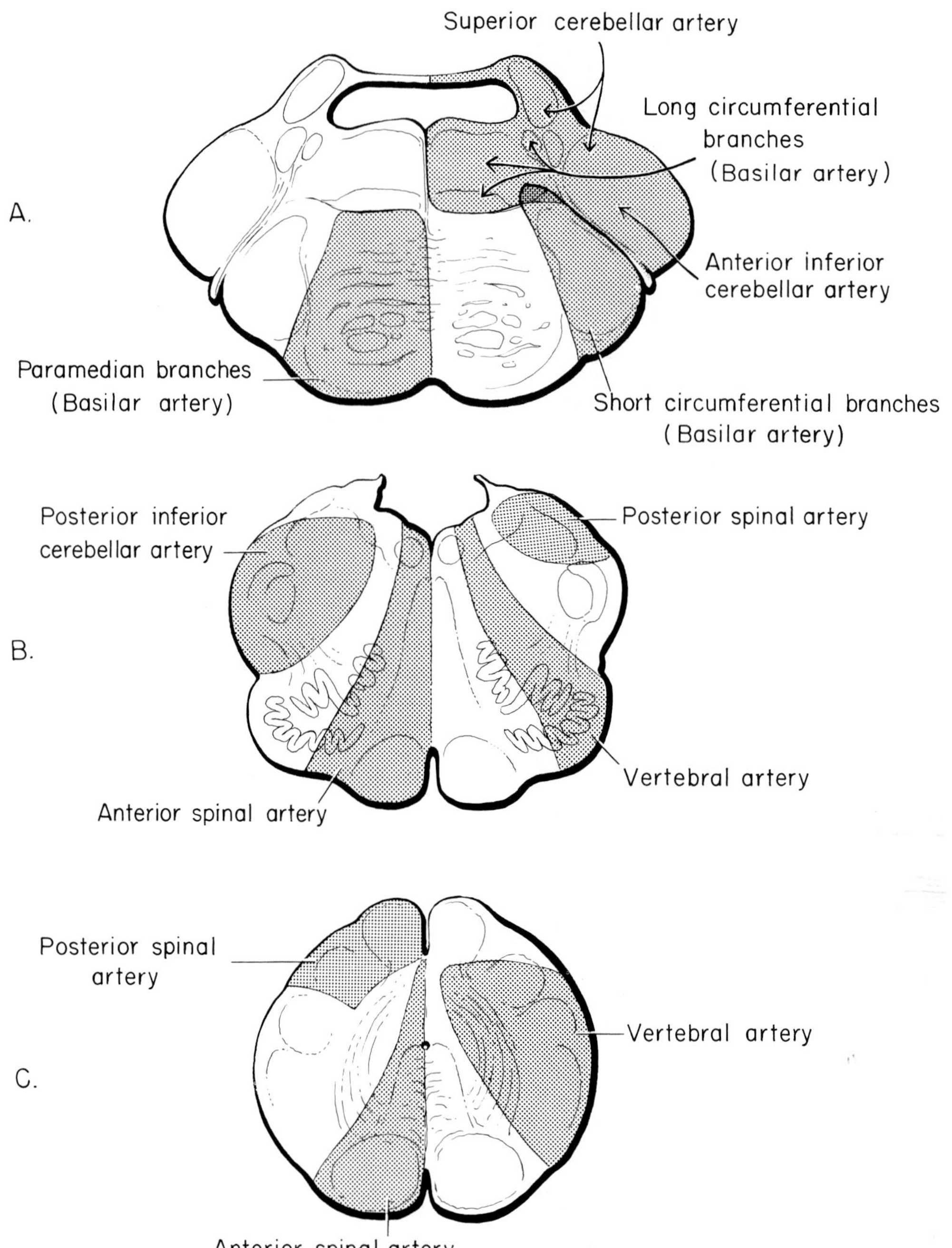

Figure 14-14. Diagrams of the arterial supply of the medulla and pons. Medullary levels shown are through the posterior column nuclei (*C*) and the inferior olivary nuclear complex (*B*) (based on Stopford, '15, '16). The pons (*A*) is supplied by paramedian and circumferential branches of the basilar artery (Frantzen and Olivarius, '57). (From Carpenter and Sutin, *Human Neuroanatomy*, 1983; courtesy of Williams & Wilkins.)

types of arteries enter the medulla. Short arteries supply small branches to the spinal trigeminal, spinothalamic, and spinocerebellar tracts, while long arteries supply deeper regions. Some of the long arteries reach the floor of the fourth ventricle. The medullary region supplied by these branches includes structures involved in the lateral medullary syndrome (Baker, '61; Stephens and Stilwell, '69).

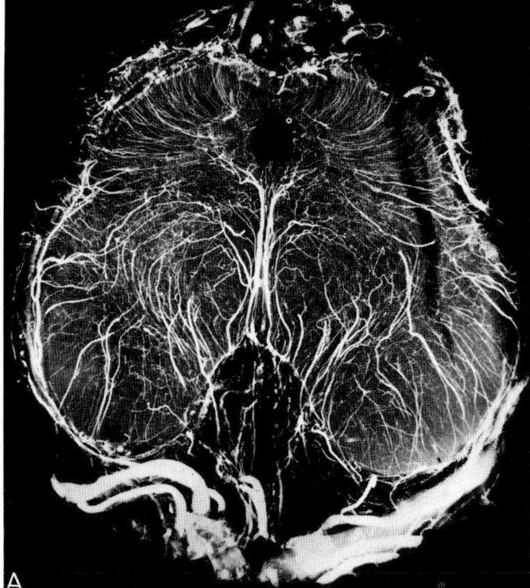

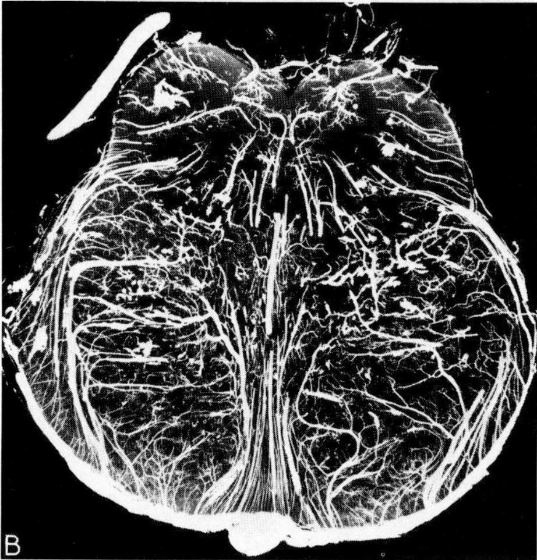

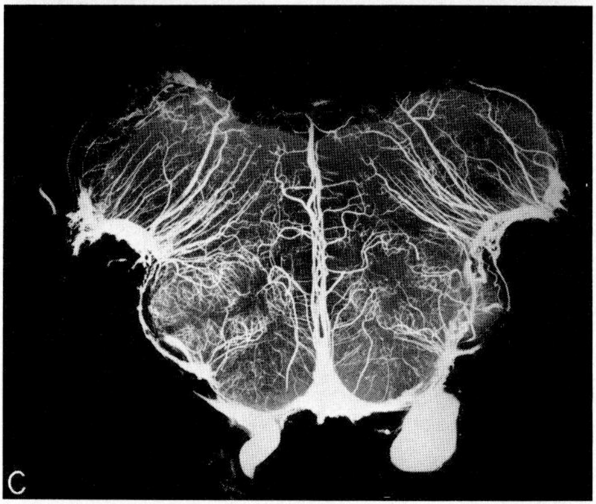

Figure 14-15. Microangiograms of the blood supply of the midbrain, pons and medulla made from 4 mm thick injected specimens. In the midbrain (*A*) the tegmentum is supplied mainly by branches of the *posterior cerebral* and *superior cerebellar arteries*, but it also receives contributions from the paramedian and both long and short circumferential arteries. The upper pons (*B*) receives paramedian and circumferential branches from the *basilar artery*, as well as branches of the *superior cerebellar artery* distributed to dorsal regions. The vascular pattern in the upper medulla (*C*) should be compared with the diagram of Figure 14-14. (Courtesy of Dr. O. Hassler, '67.) (From Carpenter and Sutin, *Human Neuroanatomy*, 1983; courtesy of Williams & Wilkins.)

The *posterior inferior cerebellar artery* supplies the lateral medullary region rostral to that supplied by direct bulbar branches of the vertebral artery (Fig. 20-16). This retro-olivary region of the medulla contains the spinothalamic tracts, the spinal trigeminal nucleus and tract, the nucleus ambiguus, the dorsal motor nucleus of the vagus and the emerging fibers from these nuclei, as well as the ventral part of the inferior cerebellar peduncle (Figs. 14-12, 14-13, 14-14, and 14-15). Descending autonomic fibers also are found within this region of the medulla and pons.

The ventral portion of the pons is supplied by three groups of arteries derived from the basilar artery (Fig. 14-14). These arterial branches are grouped as: (1) paramedian, (2) short circumferential, and (3) long circumferential.

Paramedian branches supply a medial pontine region which includes the pontine nuclei, and the corticospinal, corticopontine, and corticobulbar tracts. These branches give rise to smaller rami which nourish ventromedial parts of the pontine tegmentum.

Short circumferential arteries supply the adjacent anterolateral part of the pons, and variable parts of overlying tegmentum (Fig. 14-14).

Long circumferential arteries course laterally over the anterior surface of the pons and anastomose with smaller branches of the anterior inferior cerebellar arteries. These arteries supply lateral parts of the middle cerebellar peduncle, as well as most of the pontine tegmentum. The caudal pontine tegmentum is supplied by branches of the long circumferential and anterior inferior cerebellar arteries; the rostral pontine tegmentum receives branches of the long circumferential and superior cerebellar arteries (Figs. 14-14 and 14-15). Structures within the distribution of these arterial branches include the reticular formation, the medial lemniscus, the medial longitudinal fasciculus, the spinothalamic and spinocerebellar tracts, the middle and superior cerebellar peduncles, and the cranial nerve nuclei of the pons.

Sudden occlusion of paramedian arteries usually produces a hemiplegia, transitory hemisensory disturbances and variable disturbances of conjugate eye movements. Obstruction of the short circumferential arteries on one side usually results in ipsilateral cerebellar and autonomic disturbances and impairment of contralateral sensation. Occlusion of the long circumferential arteries and other arteries supplying the pontine tegmentum produces cranial nerve disturbances, paresis of conjugate eye movements, contralateral hemianesthesia, ipsilateral cerebellar disturbances, and frequently nystagmus. Complete or partial thrombosis of the basilar artery may produce precipitous loss of muscle tone, dilated or pinpoint pupils that do not react to light, and bilateral Babinski responses. Neurological disturbances usually are bilateral, but may be asymmetrical and exhibit certain fluctuations.

Mesencephalon. Most of the blood supply of the mesencephalon is derived from branches of the basilar artery (Fig. 14-15). Arteries supplying this part of the brain stem include branches of: (1) the *posterior cerebral artery*, (2) the *superior cerebellar artery*, (3) the *posterior communicating artery*, and (4) the *anterior choroidal artery*. Branches of these arteries, like those supplying the pons, can be grouped into paramedian arteries and long and short circumferential arteries.

Paramedian arteries, derived from the posterior communicating artery and proximal portions of the posterior cerebral arteries, form an extensive plexus in the interpeduncular fossa, enter the brain stem in the posterior perforated substance, and supply the rapheal region, the oculomotor complex, the medial longitudinal fasciculus, the red nucleus, and medial parts of the substantia nigra and crus cerebri (Fig. 14-15). Vascular lesions involving paramedian arterial branches at midbrain levels frequently produce a *superior alternating hemiplegia*, characterized by ipsilateral oculomotor disturbances and a contralateral hemiplegia (Weber's syndrome). This syndrome results from lesions involving portions of the crus cerebri and fibers of the oculomotor nerve. A less frequent lesion in the paramedian tegmental zone destroys portions of the red nucleus, the superior cerebellar peduncle, and intraaxial rootlets of the oculomotor nerve (Benedikt's syndrome).

Short circumferential arteries, arising from the interpeduncular plexus and proximal portions of the posterior cerebral and superior cerebellar arteries, supply central and lateral parts of the crus cerebri, the substantia nigra, and lateral portions of the midbrain tegmentum.

Long circumferential arteries arise primarily from the posterior cerebral artery; the most important of these, the *quadrigeminal*, or *collicular artery*, encircles the brain stem and supplies the superior and inferior colliculi. The tectum also is supplied by branches of the medial posterior choroidal artery and the superior cerebellar artery.

Venous Drainage. Although the veins of the hindbrain seldom accompany arterial branches in the same vascular sheath, the intraparenchymatous venous angioarchitecture resembles that of the arteries. Anastomoses between intraparenchymatous veins occur mainly at the capillary level. In the lower medulla posterior veins are larger than anterior veins and penetrate deeper regions. Large veins, draining the choroid plexus of the fourth ventricle, most of the pons and the upper medulla, empty into the sigmoid or the petrosal sinuses (Fig. 14-16). Veins draining the caudal medulla empty into anterior and posterior spinal veins. Paramedian veins which run to the ventral surface of the brain stem are inclined caudally in the upper pons, but are perpendicular to the axis of the brain stem in more caudal regions. At the junction of pons and medulla a large vein consistently drains the floor of the fourth ventricle. Veins from ventral portions of the pons drain into paired longitudinal venous plexuses lateral to the basilar artery. Numerous veins of the mesencaphalon arise from capillaries, run close to the arteries, and form peripheral plexuses in the pia. Blood from these plexuses is collected by basal veins which drain into either the great cerebral vein or the internal cerebral veins (Fig. 14-19).

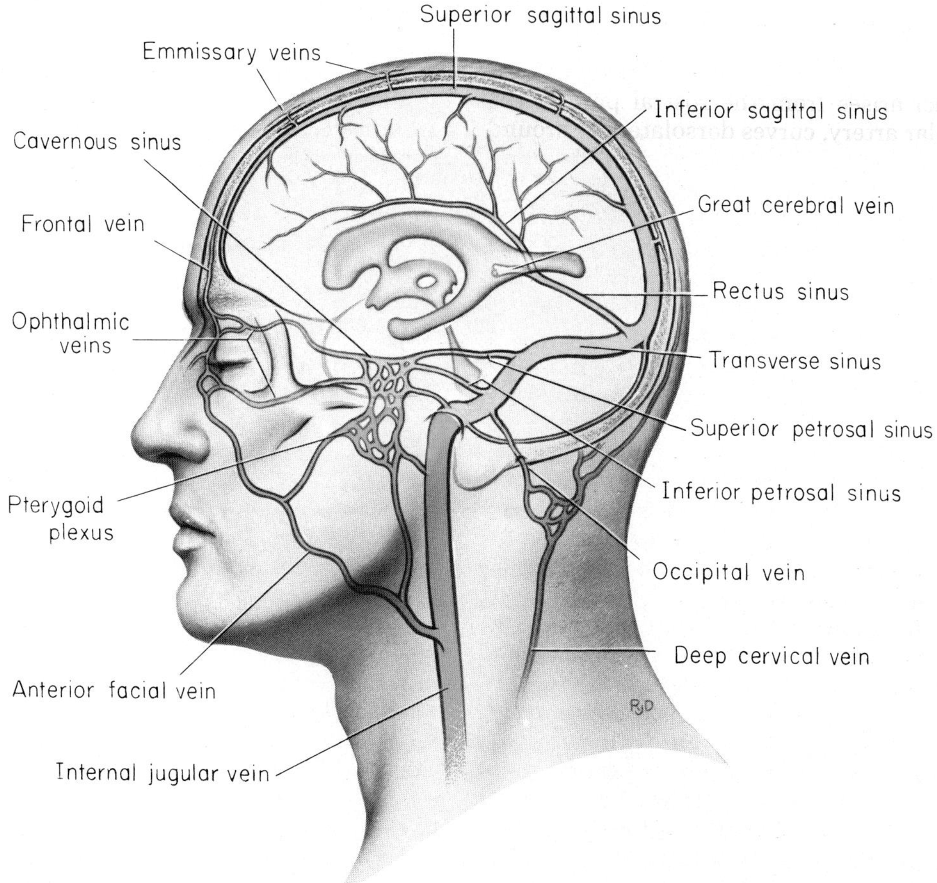

Figure 14-16. The dural sinuses and their principal connections with extracranial veins. Intracranial venous sinuses and veins are *light blue*; extracranial veins are *dark blue.* (From Carpenter and Sutin, *Human Neuroanatomy*, 1983; courtesy of Williams & Wilkins.)

Cerebellum. Each half of the cerebellum is supplied by three arteries: (1) the *superior cerebellar*, (2) the *anterior inferior cerebellar*, and (3) the *posterior inferior cerebellar.* The superior cerebellar artery passes on the superior surface of the cerebellum, while the other arteries run on the inferior cerebellar surface.

Posterior Inferior Cerebellar Artery. This vessel derived from the vertebral artery (Figs. 14-12 and 14-13), courses rostrolaterally along the surface of the medulla where small perforating rami supply the dorsolateral region of the medulla. This artery then curves upward onto the inferior surface of the cerebellum where branches supply the inferior vermis (uvula and nodulus), the cerebellar tonsil, and the inferolateral surface of the cerebellar hemisphere (Figs. 2-29 and 14-5). Medial branches of this artery supply parts of the choroid plexus of the fourth ventricle.

Anterior Inferior Cerebellar Artery. This artery, the most caudal large vessel arising from the basilar artery (Fig. 14-13), supplies caudal parts of the pontine tegmentum, and passes caudally and laterally to reach the inferior surface of the cerebellum (Fig. 14-5). This artery supplies the pyramis, tuber, flocculus, and parts of the inferior surface of the cerebellar hemisphere. Penetrating branches supply portions of the dentate nucleus and the surrounding white matter. Some branches of this artery contribute to choroid plexus of the fourth ventricle.

Superior Cerebellar Artery. This vessel arises from the rostral part of the basilar artery, curves dorsolaterally around the brain stem, and passes onto the superior surface of the cerebellum (Figs. 14-5, 14-12, and 14-13). This artery divides into two main branches: (1) a medial branch supplying the superior cerebellar vermis and adjacent regions, and (2) a lateral branch whose rami convey blood to the superior surface of the cerebellar hemisphere. Perforating arteries from these branches supply the deep cerebellar nuclei, the superior medullary velum, and the corpus medullare; some branches contribute to the choroid plexus of the fourth ventricle.

Cerebellar veins have a course similar to that of the arteries. Superior and inferior median veins drain respective portions of the vermis, paravermal regions, and the deep cerebellar nuclei. The superior vein drains into the great cerebral vein (Fig. 14-19), while the inferior vein empties into the rectus and transverse sinuses (Fig. 14-16). Superior and inferior lateral veins drain respective portions of the cerebellar hemispheres; these veins empty into the superior and inferior petrosal sinuses (Fig. 14-16).

CEREBRAL VEINS AND VENOUS SINUSES

Fine veins emerge from the substance of the brain, form pial venous plexuses, and drain into larger venous channels, the cerebral veins. The cerebral veins pass through the subarachnoid space and empty into the endothelial-lined sinuses of the dura mater. These sinuses lie between the periosteal and meningeal layers of the dura, exhibit great tautness, do not collapse easily and are devoid of valves (Figs. 1-1, 1-2, and 1-3). The dural sinuses, draining superiorly and posteriorly, converge near the internal occipital protruberance to form the *confluens sinuum* (Figs. 1-1 and 14-16). Two *transverse sinuses*, arising from the confluens, convey blood to the internal jugular vein on each side. Superficial veins of the scalp communicate with the dural sinuses via small *emissary veins* which perforate the skull.

The *superior sagittal sinus*, lying along the superior margin of the falx cerebri, extends from the foramen cecum to the confluens (Fig. 14-16). This sinus increases in size as it passes caudally and its central portion contains *venous lacunae* which vary in number and size. These venous lacunae contain arachnoidal protrusions, known as arachnoid villi.

The *inferior sagittal sinus* runs along the inferior margin of the falx cerebri (Fig. 14-16); caudally it is joined by the great cerebral vein, and forms the rectus sinus. The *rectus sinus*, located at the junction of the falx cerebri and tentorium cerebelli, empties into the confluens (Fig. 1-3).

The two *transverse sinuses* arise from the confluens sinuum, pass laterally and forward in a groove in the occipital bone, and at the occipitopetrosal junction each sinus curves downward and backward as the sigmoid sinus (Fig. 1-3). The *sigmoid sinus* is drained by the *internal jugular vein.* The confluens often is asymmetrical; the superior sagittal sinus usually drains into the right transverse sinus, while the rectus sinus drains into the left transverse sinus (Fig. 1-1).

The *cavernous sinus* is a large irregular network of communicating venous channels on each side of the sphenoid sinus, the sella turcica, and the pituitary gland that extends from the superior orbital fissure to the petrous portion of the temporal bone (Harris and Rhoton, '76). This sinus encloses the internal carotid artery; the oculomotor, trochlear, and abducens nerves; and the ophthalmic division of the trigeminal nerve (Fig. 14-17). The cavernous sinus of each side is connected with the other by the *basilar venous plexus* (Fig. 14-17), and by venous channels which pass anterior and posterior to the hypophysis. The opthalmic vein and the sphenoparietal sinus drain into the cavernous sinus. The cavernous sinus drains posteriorly into the superior and inferior petrosal sinuses, which enter respectively the transverse sinus and the bulb of the internal jugular vein. Fine venous nets also connect the cavernous sinus with the pterygoid and pharyngeal venous plexuses.

Cerebral Veins. The cerebral veins consist of deep and superficial groups and, like the dural sinuses, are devoid of valves. Superficial veins draining the cortex and subcortical white matter empty into the superior sagittal or basal sinuses (i.e., cavernous, petrosal and transverse). The deep

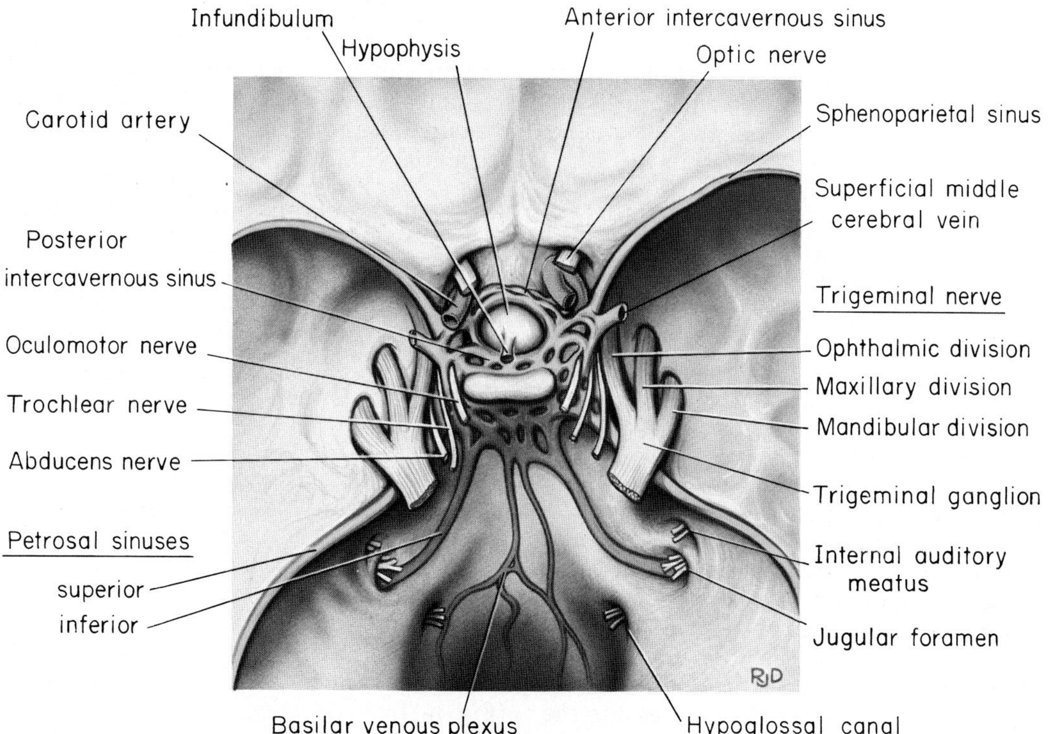

Figure 14-17. The cavernous sinus, its venous connections, and related structures. (From Carpenter and Sutin, *Human Neuroanatomy*, 1983; courtesy of Williams & Wilkins.)

cerebral veins, draining the choroid plexus, periventricular regions, diencephalon, basal ganglia, and deep white matter, empty into the internal cerebral and the great cerebral veins. These two groups of veins are interconnected by numerous anastomotic channels.

Superficial Cerebral Veins. These veins arise from the cortex and subcortical white matter, anastomose freely in the pia, and form larger veins which empty into the dural sinuses (Fig. 14-18). These larger veins include the superior and inferior cerebral veins and the superficial middle cerebral vein.

The *superior cerebral veins*, collecting blood from the convex and medial surfaces of the hemisphere drain into the superior sagittal sinus. These veins, 10 to 15 in number, enter the sinus by coursing obliquely forward; blood flow in these veins, as they enter the sinus, is opposite to that in the sinus. Some veins on the medial surface of the hemispheres drain into the inferior sagittal sinus.

The *inferior cerebral veins* drain the basal hemispheric surface and ventral parts of the lateral surface. Inferior cerebral veins on the basal surface of the hemisphere empty into the basal sinuses. In rostral regions these veins enter the cavernous and sphenoparietal sinuses; caudally these veins empty into the petrosal and transverse sinuses.

The *superficial middle cerebral vein* courses along the lateral sulcus and receives smaller veins on the lateral surface of the hemisphere (Fig. 14-18). This large vein empties into the cavernous sinus (Fig. 14-17). The superficial middle cerebral vein also receives anastomotic branches, the most constant and prominent of which are the *superior anastomotic* (Trolard) and the *inferior anastomotic* (Labbé) *veins.* These anastomotic veins connect the superficial middle cerebral vein respectively with the superior sagittal and transverse sinuses.

Large cortical regions on the inferior and medial surfaces of the hemisphere are drained by a number of veins that empty into the internal cerebral veins or into the great cerebral vein. Anastomotic channels,

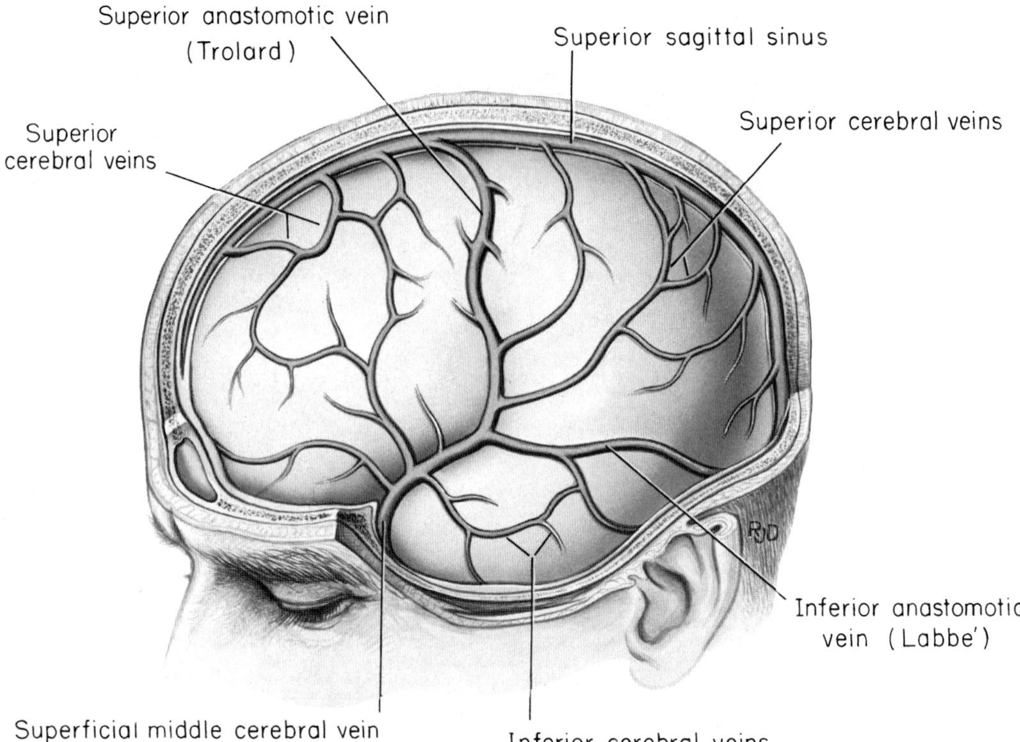

Figure 14-18. The external cerebral veins on the convexity of the hemisphere. (From Carpenter and Sutin, *Human Neuroanatomy*, 1983; courtesy of Williams & Wilkins.)

connecting superficial and deep veins, include the basal vein (Rosenthal), the occipital vein, and the posterior callosal vein. It is best to consider these veins in relation to the deep cerebral veins.

Deep Cerebral Veins. The deep cerebral veins of major importance are: (1) the *internal cerebral veins*, (2) the *basal veins* (Rosenthal), and (3) the *great cerebral vein* (Galen).

The *internal cerebral veins* (paired) are located near the midline in the tela choroidea of the roof of the third ventricle (velum interpositum). These veins extend caudally from the region of the interventricular foramina over the superior and medial surface of the thalamus (Fig. 14-19). In the rostral part of the quadrigeminal cistern these paired veins join to form the great cerebral vein. The internal cerebral vein on each side receives: (1) The *thalamostriate vein*, (2) the *choroidal vein*, (3) the *septal vein*, (4) the *epithalamic vein*, and (5) the *lateral ventricular vein*.

The *thalamostriate vein*, running forward at the junction of the thalamus and caudate nucleus, receives the *anterior terminal vein* and numerous *transverse caudate veins* (Figs. 14-19 and 14-20). Distally, the transverse caudate veins enter the white matter adjacent to the lateral angle of the lateral ventricle; their smaller tributaries in this region form the *longitudinal caudate veins.* The *superior striate veins*, draining superior parts of the striatum and internal capsule, empty into the longitudinal and transverse caudate veins (Fig. 14-20).

The *choroidal vein* extends distally into the inferior horn of the lateral ventricle (Fig. 14-19). The *septal vein* drains the septum pellucidum and portions of the corpus callosum. The *epithalamic vein* drains the dorsal part of the diencephalon. The *lateral ventricular vein* extends over the surface of the thalamus and the tail of the caudate nucleus; it drains the white matter of the parahippocampal gyrus and part of the choroid plexus.

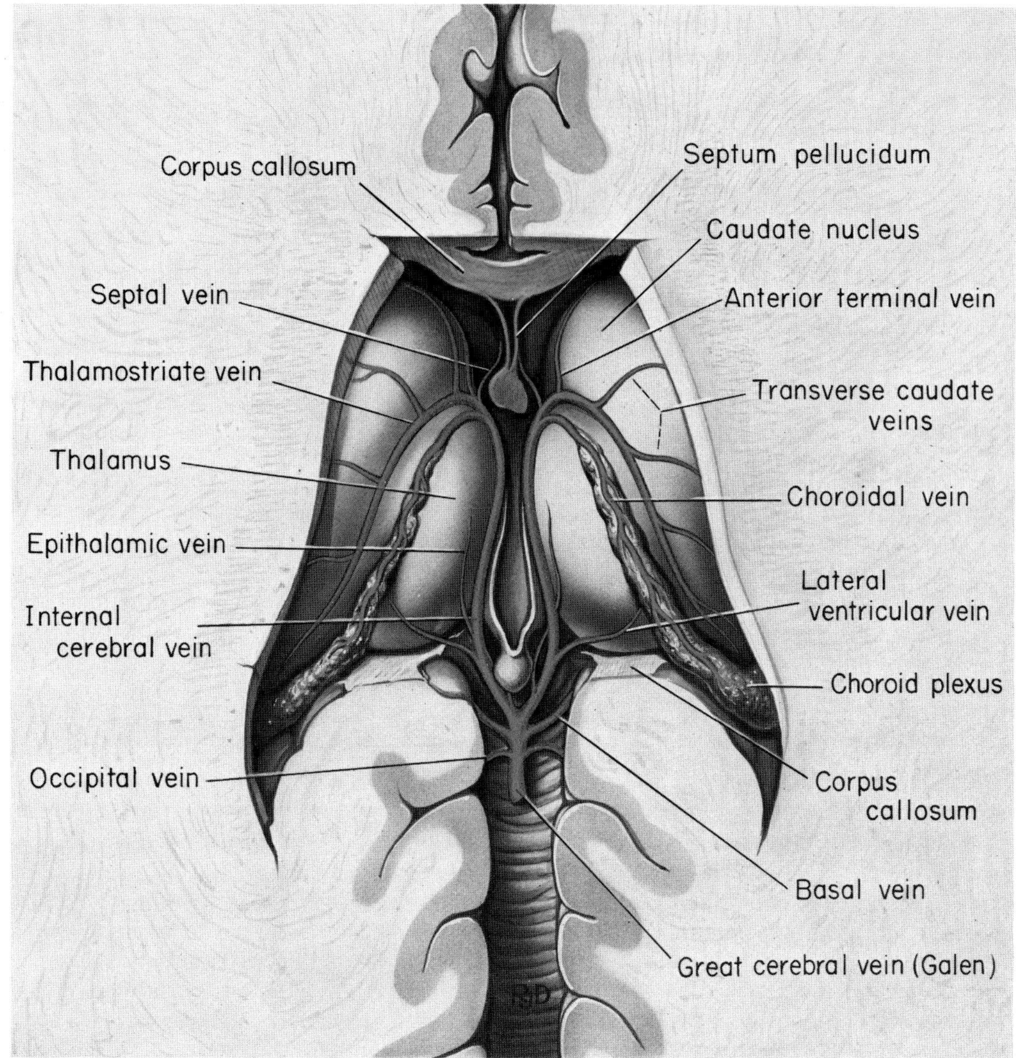

Figure 14-19. The internal cerebral veins and their tributaries (modified from Schwartz and Fink, '26). (From Carpenter and Sutin, *Human Neuroanatomy*, 1983; courtesy of Williams & Wilkins.)

The *basal vein* (Rosenthal) arises near the medial part of the anterior lobe (Figs. 14-19 and 14-20). This vein receives: (1) the *anterior cerebral vein*, (2) the *deep middle cerebral vein*, and (3) the *inferior striate veins*.

The *anterior cerebral vein* accompanies the anterior cerebral artery and drains the orbital surface of the frontal lobe, and rostral portions of both the corpus callosum and cingulate gyrus. The *deep middle cerebral vein*, located in the depths of the lateral sulcus, drains insular and opercular cortex. The *inferior striate veins* drain ventral portions of the striatum, emerge through the anterior perforated substance, and empty into the deep middle cerebral vein.

The *great cerebral vein* (Galen) receives the paired basal internal cerebral veins, the paired internal cerebral veins, the paired basal veins, the paired occipital veins, and the posterior callosal vein (Figs. 14-19 and 14-20). This short vein passes caudally beneath the splenium of the corpus callosum and empties into the rectus sinus. The paired *occipital veins* drain inferior and me-

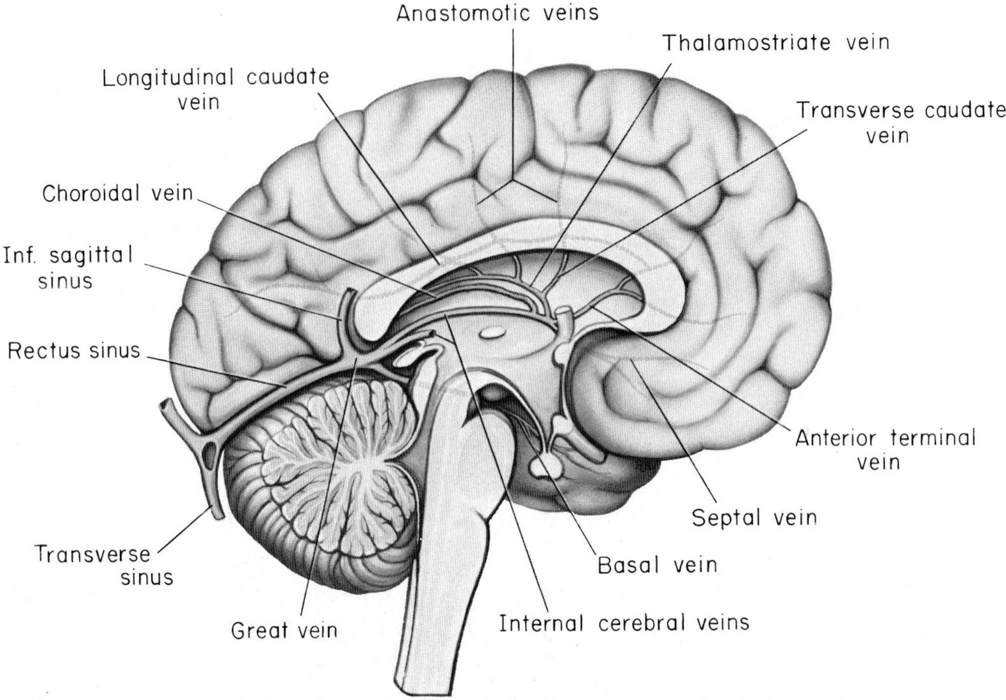

Figure 14-20. Midsagittal view of the internal cerebral veins showing the relationship of the great vein to the rectus sinus (Schlesinger, '39). (From Carpenter and Sutin, *Human Neuroanatomy*, 1983; courtesy of Williams & Wilkins.)

dial surfaces of the occipital lobe and adjacent parietal regions. The *posterior callosal vein* drains the splenium of the corpus callosum and adjacent medial surfaces of the brain.

Angiographic studies also provide information concerning both deep and superficial cerebral veins (Taveras and Wood, '76). In serial roentgenograms the superficial frontal veins fill before the parietal veins. The deep veins are the last to fill and they retain sufficient concentrations of radiopaque material to permit visualization for a longer period of time. Visualization of the deep cerebral veins provides more important diagnostic information than the superficial veins which exhibit variable configurations. The thalamostriate vein and some of its major tributaries can provide information concerning the size and configuration of the lateral ventricle.

References

ADES, H. W. 1959. Central auditory mechanism. In J. FIELD (Editor), *Handbook of Physiology*, Sect. 1, Vol. I. American Physiological Society, Washington, D.C., Ch. 24, pp. 585–613.

ADRIAN, E. D. 1940. Double representation of the feet in the sensory cortex of the cat (abstract). J. Physiol. (Lond.), **98:** 16P–18P.

ADRIAN, E. D. 1941. Afferent discharges to the cerebral cortex from peripheral sense organs. J. Physiol. (Lond.), **100:** 159–191.

ADRIAN, E. D. 1942. Olfactory reactions in the brain of the hedgehog. J. Physiol. (Lond.), **100:** 459–473.

ADRIAN, E. D. 1943. Afferent areas in the cerebellum connected with the limbs. Brain, **66:** 289–315.

AGHAJANIAN, G. K., FOOTE, W. E., AND SHEARD, M. H. 1968. Lysergic acid diethylamide: Sensitive neuronal units in the midbrain raphe. Science, **161:** 706–708.

AGHAJANIAN, G. K., BLOOM, F. E., AND SHEARD, M. H. 1969. Electron microscopy of degeneration within the serotonin pathway of rat brain. Brain Res., **13:** 266–273.

AGHAJANIAN, G. K., HAIGLER, H. J., AND BENNETT, J. L. 1975. Amine receptors in the CNS. III. 5-Hydroxytryptamine in brain. In L. L. IVERSON, S. D. IVERSON, AND S. H. SNYDER (Editors), *Handbook of Psychopharmacology*, Ed. 6. Plenum Press, New York, pp. 63–96.

AITKEN, H. F. 1909. A report on the circulation of the lobar ganglia made to DR. JAMES B. AYER (with a postscript by J. B. AYER, M.D.). Boston Med. Surg. J., **160:** Suppl. 18.

AITKEN, L. M., AND WEBSTER, W. R. 1971. Tonotopic organization in the medial geniculate body of the cat. Brain Res., **26:** 402–405.

AITKEN, L. M., AND WEBSTER, W. R. 1972. Medial geniculate body of the cat: Organization and responses to tonal stimuli of neurons in the ventral division. J. Neurophysiol., **35:** 365–380.

AITKEN, L. M., WEBSTER, W. R., VEALE, J. L., AND CROSBY, D. C. 1975. Inferior colliculus. I. Comparison of response properties of neurons in central, pericentral and external nuclei of adult cat. J. Neurophysiol., **38:** 1196–1207.

AKELAITIS, A. J. 1943. Study of language function (tactile and visual lexia and graphia) unilaterally following section of the corpus callosum. J. Neuropathol. Exp. Neurol., **2:** 226–262.

AKERT, K., AND HARTMANN-VON MONAKOW, K. 1980. Relationships of precentral, premotor and prefrontal cortex to the mediodorsal and intralaminar nuclei of the monkey thalamus. Acta Neurobiol. Exp. (Warsz.), **40:** 7–25.

AKERT, K., POTTER, H. D., AND ANDERSON, J. W. 1961. The subfornical organ in mammals. I. Comparative and topographical anatomy. J. Comp. Neurol., **116:** 1–14.

ALBE-FESSARD, D., AND KRUGER, L. 1962. Duality of unit discharge from cat centrum medianum in response to natural and electrical stimulation. J. Neurophysiol., **25:** 3–20.

ALBE-FESSARD, D., AND ROUGEUL, A. 1958. Activités d'origine somesthésique évoquées sur le cortex non-spécific du chat anesthésié au chloralose: Rôle du centre médian du thalamus. Electroencephalogr. Clin. Neurophysiol., **10:** 131–152.

ALBE-FESSARD, D., LEVANTE, A., AND LAMOUR, Y. 1974. Origin of spinothalamic tract in monkeys. Brain Res., **65:** 503–509.

ALEXANDER, L. 1942. The vascular supply of the striopallidum. Proc. Assoc. Res. Nerv. Ment. Dis., **21:** 77–132.

ALLEN, G. I., KORN, H., OSHIMA, T., AND TOYAMA, K. 1975. The mode of synaptic linkage in the cerebroponto-cerebellar pathway of the cat. II. Responses of single cells in the pontine nuclei. Exp. Brain Res., **24:** 15–36.

ALLEN, W. F. 1941. Effect of ablating the pyriform-amygdaloid areas and hippocampi on positive and negative olfactory conditioned reflexes and on conditioned olfactory differentiation. Am. J. Physiol., **132:** 81–92.

ALLMAN, J. M., AND KAAS, J. H. 1974. The organization of the second visual area (VII) in the owl monkey: A second order transformation of the visual hemifield. Brain Res., **76:** 247–265.

ALTMAN, J., AND CARPENTER, M. B. 1961. Fiber projections of the superior colliculus in the cat. J. Comp. Neurol., **116:** 157–178.

AMOORE, J. E., JOHNSTON, J. W., JR., AND RUBIN, M. 1964. The stereochemical theory of odor. Sci. Am., **210:** 42–49.

ANDÉN, N.-E., CARLSSON, A., DAHLSTRÖM, A., FUXE, K., HILLARP, N.-Å., AND LARSSON, K. 1964. Demonstration and mapping out of nigrostriatal neurons. Life Sci., **3:** 523–530.

ANDÉN, N.-E., DAHLSTRÖM, A., FUXE, K., AND LARSSON, K. 1965. Further evidence for the presence of nigro-striatal dopamine neurons in the rat. Am. J. Anat., **116:** 329–333.

ANDÉN, N.-E., DAHLSTRÖM, A., FUXE, K., LARSSON, K., OLSON, L., AND UNGERSTEDT, U. 1966. Ascending monoamine neurons to the telencephalon and diencephalon. Acta Physiol. Scand., **67:** 313–326.

ANDÉN, N.-E., FUXE, K., HAMBERGER, B., AND HÖKFELT, T. 1966a. A quantitative study on the nigro-neostriatal dopamine neuron system in the rat. Acta Physiol. Scand., **67:** 306–312.

ANDERSON, M. E., AND YOSHIDA, M. 1980. Axonal branching patterns and location of nigrothalamic and nigrocollicular neurons in the cat. J. Neurophysiol., **43:** 883–895.

ANGAUT, P. 1969. The fastigio-tectal projections: An anatomical experimental study. Brain Res., **13:** 186–189.

ANGAUT, P. 1970. The ascending projections of the nucleus interpositus posterior of the cat cerebellum: An experimental anatomical study using silver impregnation methods. Brain Res., **24:** 377–394.

ANGAUT, P., AND BOWSHER, D. 1965. Cerebello-rubral connexions in the cat. Nature, **208:** 1002–1003.

ANGAUT, P., AND BOWSHER, D. 1970. Ascending projections of the medial (fastigial) nucleus: An experimental study in the cat. Brain Res., **24:** 49–68.

ANGAUT, P., AND BRODAL, A. 1967. The projection of the "vestibulocerebellum" onto the vestibular nuclei in the cat. Arch. Ital. Biol., **105:** 441–479.

ANGEVINE, J. B., JR., AND COTMAN, C. W. 1981. *Principles of Neuroanatomy.* Oxford University Press, New York, 393 pp.

ANGEVINE, J. B., JR., AND SIDMAN, R. L. 1961. Autoradiographic study of cell migration during histogenesis of the cerebral cortex in the mouse. Nature, **192:** 766–768.

ANGEVINE, J. B., JR., MANCALL, E. L., AND YAKOVLEV, P. I. 1961. *The Human Cerebellum. An Atlas of Gross Topography in Serial Sections.* Little, Brown, Boston.

APPELBERG, B. 1960. Localization of focal potentials evoked in the red nucleus and ventrolateral nucleus of the thalamus by electrical stimulation of the cerebellar nuclei. Acta Physiol. Scand., **51:** 356–370.

ASANUMA, C., THACH, W. T., AND JONES, E. G. 1983. Cytoarchitectonic delineation of the ventral lateral thalamic region in the monkey. Brain Res. Rev., **5:** 219–235.

ASANUMA, C., THACH, W. T., AND JONES, E. G. 1983a. Distribution of cerebellar terminations and their relation to other afferent terminations in the ventral lateral thalamic region of the monkey. Brain Res. Rev., **5:** 237–265.

ASANUMA, C., THACH, W. T., AND JONES, E. G. 1983b. Anatomical evidence for segregated focal groupings of efferent cells and their terminal ramifications in the cerebellothalamic pathway of the monkey. Brain Res. Rev., **5:** 267–297.

ASTRUC, J. 1971. Corticofugal connections of area 8 (frontal eye field) in *Macaca mulatta.* Brain Res., **33:** 241–256.

ATWEH, S. F., AND KUHAR, M. J. 1977. Autoradiographic localization of opiate receptors in rat brain. III. The telencephalon. Brain Res., **134:** 393–405.

AUER, J. 1956. Terminal degeneration in the diencephalon after ablation of frontal cortex in the cat. J. Anat., **90:** 30–41.

AXELROD, J., WURTMAN, R. J., AND SNYDER, S. H. 1965. Control of hydroxyindole-*o*-methyltransferase activity in the rat pineal gland by environmental lighting. J. Biol. Chem., **240:** 949–955.

BAGSHAW, M. H., AND PRIBRAM, K. H. 1953. Cortical organization in gustation (*Macaca mulatta*). J. Neurophysiol., **16:** 499–508.

BAILEY, P. 1948. *Intracranial Tumors,* Ed. 2. Charles C Thomas, Publisher, Springfield, Ill.

BAK, I. J., CHOI, W. B., HASSLER, R., USUNOFF, K. G., AND WAGNER, A. 1975. Fine structural synaptic organization of the corpus striatum and substantia nigra in rat and cat. In D. CALNE, T. N. CHASE, AND A. BARBEAU (Editors), *Dopaminergic Mechanisms.* Raven Press, New York, pp. 25–41.

BAK, I. J., MARKHAM, C. H., COOK, M. L., AND STEVENS, J. G. 1978. Ultrastructural and immunoperoxidase study of striatonigral neurons by means of retrograde axonal transport of herpes simplex virus. Brain Res., **143:** 361–368.

BAKER, A. B. 1961. Cerebrovascular disease. IX. The medullary blood supply and the lateral medullary syndrome. Neurology (Minneap.), **11:** 852–861.

BAKER, R. 1977. Anatomical and physiological organization of brain stem pathways underlying the control of gaze. In A. BERTHOZ AND R. BAKER (Editors), *Control of Gaze by Brain Stem Neurons (Developments in Neuroscience,* Vol. 1). Elsevier/North-Holland, Amsterdam, pp. 207–222.

BAKER, R., AND BERTHOZ, A. 1975. Is the prepositus hypoglossi nucleus the source of another vestibulo-ocular pathway? Brain Res., **86:** 121–127.

BAKER, R., AND HIGHSTEIN, S. M. 1975. Physiological identification of interneurons and motoneurons in the abducens nucleus. Brain Res., **91:** 292–298.

BAPTISTA, A. P. 1963. Studies on the arteries of the brain. II. The anterior cerebral artery: Some anatomic features and their clinical implication. Neurology, **13:** 825–835.

BÁRÁNY, E. H. 1972. Inhibition by hippurate and probenecid of *in vitro* uptake of iodipamide and *o*-iodohippurate: A composite uptake system for iodipamide in choroid plexus, kidney cortex and anterior uvea of several species. Acta Physiol. Scand., **86:** 12–27.

BARD, P. 1939. Central nervous mechanisms for emotional behavior patterns in animals. Proc. Assoc. Res. Nerv. Ment. Dis., **19:** 190–218.

BARD, P. 1968. Regulation of the systemic circulation. In V. B. MOUNTCASTLE (Editor), *Medical Physiology,* Ed. 12, Vol. I. C. V. Mosby, St. Louis, Ch. 11, pp. 178–208.

BARD, P., AND MOUNTCASTLE, V. B. 1948. Some forebrain mechanisms involved in expression of rage with special reference to suppression of angry behavior. Proc. Assoc. Res. Nerv. Ment. Dis., **27:** 362–404.

BARD, P., AND RIOCH, D. M. 1937. A study of 4 cats deprived of neocortex and additional portions of the forebrain. Bull. Johns Hopkins Hosp., **60:** 73–147.

BARNES, S. 1901. Degeneration in hemiplegia: With special reference to a ventrolateral pyramidal tract, the accessory fillet and Pick's bundle. Brain, **24:** 463–501.

BASBAUM, A. I., AND FIELDS, H. L. 1979. The origin of descending pathways in the dorsolateral funiculus of the spinal cord of the cat and rat: Further studies on the anatomy of pain modulation. J. Comp. Neurol., **187:** 513–532.

BASBAUM, A. I., CLANTON, C. H., AND FIELDS, H. L. 1976. Opiate and stimulus-produced analgesia: Functional anatomy of medullospinal pathways. Proc. Natl. Acad. Sci. U.S.A., **73:** 4685–4688.

BASBAUM, A. I., CLANTON, C. H., AND FIELDS, H. L. 1978. Three bulbospinal pathways from the rostral medulla of the cat: An autoradiographic study of pain modulating systems. J. Comp. Neurol., **178:**

209–224.

Batini, C., Corvisier, J., Destombes, J., Gioanni, H., and Everett, J. 1976. The climbing fibers of the cerebellar cortex, their origin and pathway in cat. Exp. Brain Res., **26:** 407–422.

Batson, O. V. 1940. The function of the vertebral veins and their role in the spread of metastases. Ann. Surg., **112:** 138–149.

Batton, R. R., III, Jayaraman, A., Ruggiero, D., and Carpenter, M. B. 1977. Fastigial efferent projections in the monkey: An autoradiographic study. J. Comp. Neurol., **174:** 281–306.

Beckstead, R. M., Domesick, V. B., and Nauta, W. J. H. 1979. Efferent connections of the substantia nigra and ventral tegmental area in the rat. Brain Res., **175:** 191–217.

Beckstead, R. M., Morse, J. R., and Norgren, R. 1980. The nucleus of the solitary tract in the monkey: Projections to the thalamus and brain stem nuclei. J. Comp. Neurol., **190:** 259–282.

Bédard, P., Larochelle, L., Parent, A., and Poirier, L. J. 1969. The nigrostriated pathway: A correlative study based upon neuroanatomical and neurochemical criteria in the cat and monkey. Exp. Neurol., **25:** 365–377.

Beitz, A. J. 1976. The topographical organization of the olivo-dentate and dentato-olivary pathways in the cat. Brain Res., **115:** 311–317.

Békésy, G. von. 1960. *Experiments in Hearing*. McGraw-Hill, New York.

Ben-Ari, Y., Le Gal La Salle, G., and Kanazawa, I. 1977. Regional distribution of substance P within the amygdaloid complex and bed nucleus of the stria terminalis. Neurosci. Lett., **4:** 299–302.

Ben-Ari, Y., Zigmond, R. E., Shute, C. C. D., and Lewis, P. R. 1977*a*. Regional distribution of choline acetyltransferase and acetylcholinesterase within the amygdaloid complex and stria terminalis system. Brain Res., **120:** 435–445.

Bender, M. B., and Shanzer, S. 1964. Oculomotor pathways defined by electrical stimulation and lesions in the brain stem of the monkey. In M. B. Bender (Editor), *The Oculomotor System*. Harper & Row, New York, pp. 81–140.

Benevento, L. A., and Fallon, J. H. 1975. The ascending projections of the superior colliculus in the rhesus monkey (*Macaca mulatta*). J. Comp. Neurol., **160:** 339–362.

Benevento, L. A., and Rezak, M. 1976. The cortical projections of the inferior and adjacent lateral pulvinar in the rhesus monkey (*Macaca mulatta*): An autoradiographic study. Brain Res., **108:** 1–24.

Benjamin, R. M., and Akert, K. 1959. Cortical and thalamic areas involved in taste discrimination in the albino rat. J. Comp. Neurol., **111:** 231–260.

Bentivoglio, M., Van Der Kooy, D., and Kuypers, H. G. J. M. 1979. The organization of the efferent projections of the substantia nigra in the rat: A retrograde fluorescent double labeling study. Brain Res., **175:** 1–17.

Berger, H. 1929. Ueber das Elektrenkephalogramm des Menschen. Arch. Psychiat. Nervenkr., **87:** 527–570.

Berkley, K. J., and Hand, P. J. 1978. Projections to the inferior olive of the cat. II. Comparisons of input from the gracile, cuneate and the spinal trigeminal nuclei. J. Comp. Neurol., **180:** 253–264.

Berkley, K. J., and Worden, I. G. 1978. Projections to the inferior olive of the cat. I. Comparisons of input from the dorsal column nuclei, the lateral cervical nucleus, the spino-olivary pathways, the cerebral cortex and the cerebellum. J. Comp. Neurol., **180:** 237–252.

Bertrand, G. 1956. Spinal efferent pathways from the supplementary motor area. Brain, **79:** 461–473.

Bertrand, G. L., Blundell, J., and Musella, R. 1965. Electrical exploration of the internal capsule and neighboring structures during stereotaxic procedures. J. Neurosurg., **22:** 333–343.

Biegon, A., Rainbow, T. C., and McEwen, B. S. 1982. Quantitative autoradiography of serotonin receptors in the rat brain. Brain Res., **242:** 197–204.

Bindslev, N., Tormey, J. McD., Pietras, R. J., and Wright, E. M. 1974. Electrically and osmotically induced changes in permeability and structure of toad urinary bladder. Biochim. Biophys. Acta, **332:** 286–297.

Binkley, S. 1979. A timekeeping enzyme in the pineal gland. Science, **240:** 66–71.

Bird, E. D., and Iverson, L. L. 1974. Huntington's chorea: Postmortem measurement of glutamic acid decarboxylase, choline acetyltransferase and dopamine in basal ganglia. Brain, **97:** 457–472.

Bishop, G. A., McCrea, R. A., Lighthall, J. W., and Kitai, S. T. 1979. An HRP and autoradiographic study of the projection from the cerebellar cortex to the nucleus interpositus anterior and nucleus interpositus posterior of the cat. J. Comp. Neurol., **185:** 735–756.

Bishop, P. O., Kozak, W., Levick, W. R., and Vakkur, G. J. 1962. The determination of the projection of the visual field on to the lateral geniculate nucleus in the cat. J. Physiol. (Lond.), **163:** 503–539.

Björklund, A., Owman, C., and West, K. A. 1972. Peripheral sympathetic innervation and serotonin cells in the habenular region of the rat brain. Z. Zellforsch. Mikrosk. Anat., **127:** 570–579.

Blomquist, A. J., Benjamin, R. M., and Emmers, R. 1962. Thalamic localization of afferents from the tongue in squirrel monkey (*Saimiri sciureus*). J. Comp. Neurol., **118:** 77–87.

Bloom, F. E., Hoffer, B. J., and Siggins, G. R. 1971. Studies on norepinephrine containing afferent to Purkinje cells of rat cerebellum. I. Localization of the fibers and their synapses. Brain Res., **25:** 501–521.

Bloom, F. E., Battenberg, E., Rossier, J., Ling, N., and Guillemin, R. 1978. Neurons containing β endorphin in rat brain exist separately from those containing enkephalin: Immunocytochemical studies. Proc. Natl. Acad. Sci. U.S.A., **75:** 1591–1595.

Blum, M., Walker, A. E., and Ruch, T. C. 1943. Localization of taste in the thalamus of *Macaca mulatta*. Yale J. Biol. Med., **16:** 175–192.

Bobillier, P., Petitjean, F., Salvert, D., Ligier, M., and Seguin, S. 1975. Differential projections of the nucleus raphe dorsalis and nucleus raphe centralis as revealed by autoradiography. Brain Res., **85:** 205–210.

Bobillier, P., Sequin, S., Petitjean, F., Salvert, D., Touret, M., and Jouvet, M. 1976. The raphe nuclei of the cat brain stem. A topographical atlas of their projections as revealed by autoradiography. Brain Res., **113:** 449–486.

BOIVIE, J. 1970. Terminations of the cervicothalamic tract in the cat: An experimental study with silver impregnation methods. Brain Res., **19:** 333–360.

BOIVIE, J. 1978. Anatomical observations on the dorsal column nuclei, their thalamic projection and the cytoarchitecture of some somatosensory thalamic nuclei in the monkey. J. Comp. Neurol., **178:** 17–48.

BOIVIE, J. 1979. An anatomical reinvestigation of the termination of the spinothalamic tract in the monkey. J. Comp. Neurol., **186:** 343–370.

BOLTON, B. 1939. The blood supply of the human spinal cord. J. Neurol. Psychiatry, **2:** 137–148.

BORG, E. 1973. On the neuronal organization of the acoustic middle ear reflex. A physiological and anatomical study. Brain Res., **49:** 101–123.

BORISON, H. L., AND WANG, S. C. 1949. Functional localization of central coordinating mechanisms for emesis in cat. J. Neurophysiol., **12:** 305–313.

BORISON, H. L., AND WANG, S. C. 1953. Physiology and pharmacology of vomiting. Pharmacol. Rev., **5:** 193–230.

BÖRNSTEIN, W. S. 1940. Cortical representation of taste in man and monkey. I. Functional and anatomical relations of taste, olfaction and somatic sensibility. Yale J. Biol., **12:** 719–736.

BÖRNSTEIN, W. S. 1940a. Cortical representation of taste in man and monkey. II. Localization of cortical taste area in man and method of measuring impairment of taste in man. Yale J. Biol., **13:** 133–156.

BOS, J., AND BENEVENTO, L. A. 1975. Projections of the medial pulvinar to orbital cortex and frontal eye fields in the rhesus monkey (*Macaca mulatta*). Exp. Neurol., **49:** 487–496.

BOVARD, E. W., AND GLOOR, P. 1961. Effect of amygdaloid lesions on plasma corticosterone response of the albino rat to emotional stress. Experientia, **17:** 521.

BOWEN, D. M., SMITH, C. B., WHITE, P., AND DAVISON, A. N. 1976. Neurotransmitter-related enzymes and indices of hypoxia in senile dementia and other abiotrophies. Brain, **99:** 459–496.

BOYCOTT, B. B., AND WÄSSLE, H. 1974. The morphological types of ganglion cells of the domestic cat's retina. J. Physiol. (Lond.), **240:** 397–419.

BRADY, J. V. 1960. Temporal and emotional effects related to intracranial electrical self-stimulation. In S. R. RAMEY AND D. S. O'DOHERTY (Editors), *Electrical Studies on the Unanesthetized Brain*. Paul B. Hoeber, New York, Ch. 3, pp. 52–77.

BRAND, S., AND RAKIC, P. 1979. Genesis of the primate neostriatum: [^{3}H]thymidine autoradiographic analysis of the time of neuron origin in the rhesus monkey. Neuroscience, **4:** 767–778.

BRAWER, J. R., MOREST, D. K., AND KANE, E. C. 1974. The neuronal architecture of the cochlear nucleus of the cat. J. Comp. Neurol., **155:** 251–300.

BREMER, R. 1937. L'activité cérébrale au cours du sommeil et de la narcose: Contribution à l'étude du mecanisme du sommiel. Bull. Acad. R. Med., Belg., **2:** 68–86.

BRIGHTMAN, M. W. 1965. The distribution within the brain of ferritin injected into cerebrospinal fluid compartments. I. Ependymal distribution. J. Cell Biol., **26:** 99–123.

BRIGHTMAN, M. W., AND REESE, T. S. 1969. Junctions between intimately apposed cell membranes in the vertebrate brain. J. Cell Biol., **40:** 648–677.

BRIGHTMAN, M. W., REESE, T. S., AND FEDER, N. 1970. Assessment with the electronmicroscope of the permeability to peroxidase of cerebral endothelium and epithelium in mice and sharks. In C. CRONE AND N. A. LASSEN (Editors), *Capillary Permeability*. Academic Press, New York, pp. 468–476.

BRINKMAN, C., AND PORTER, R. 1979. Supplementary motor area in the monkey: Activity of neurons during performance of a learned motor task. J. Neurophysiol., **42:** 681–709.

BRINKMAN, J., AND KUYPERS, H. G. J. M. 1973. Cerebral control of contralateral and ipsilateral hand and finger movements in the split-brain rhesus monkey. Brain, **96:** 653–674.

BROADWELL, R. D. 1975. Olfactory relationships of the telencephalon and diencephalon in the rabbit. II. An autoradiographic and horseradish peroxidase study of the efferent connections of the anterior olfactory nucleus. J. Comp. Neurol., **164:** 389–410.

BROADWELL, R. D., AND BRIGHTMAN, M. W. 1976. Entry of peroxidase into neurons of the central and peripheral nervous systems from extracerebral and cerebral blood. J. Comp. Neurol., **166:** 257–284.

BROCA, P. 1878. Anatomie comparée circonvolutions cérébrales: Le grand lobe limbique et la scissure limbique dans la série des mammifères. Rev. Anthropol. Ser. 2, **1:** 384–498.

BRODAL, A. 1940. Experimentelle Untersuchungen über die olivocerebellare Lokalisation. Z. Gesamte Neurol. Psychiatr., **169:** 1–153.

BRODAL, A. 1947. The hippocampus and the sense of smell. Brain, **70:** 179–222.

BRODAL, A. 1957. *The Reticular Formation of the Brain Stem. Anatomical Aspects and Functional Correlations*. Charles C Thomas, Springfield, Ill.

BRODAL, A. 1976. The olivocerebellar projection in the cat as studied with the method of retrograde axonal transport of horseradish peroxidase. II. The projection of the uvula. J. Comp. Neurol., **166:** 417–426.

BRODAL, A. 1981. *Neurological Anatomy in Relation to Clinical Medicine*, Ed. 3. Oxford University Press, New York.

BRODAL, A., AND HODDEVIK, G. H. 1978. The pontocerebellar projection to the uvula in the cat. Exp. Brain Res., **32:** 105–116.

BRODAL, A., AND HØIVIK, B. 1964. Site and mode of termination of primary vestibulo-cerebellar fibres in the cat. Arch. Ital. Biol., **102:** 1–21.

BRODAL, A., AND JANSEN, J. 1946. The ponto-cerebellar projection in the rabbit and cat. J. Comp. Neurol., **84:** 31–118.

BRODAL, A., AND POMPEIANO, O. 1957. The vestibular nuclei in the cat. J. Anat., **91:** 438–454.

BRODAL, A., AND SZIKLA, G. 1972. The termination of the brachium conjunctivum descendens in the nucleus reticularis tegmenti pontis: An experimental study in the cat. Brain Res., **39:** 337–351.

BRODAL, A., TABER, E., AND WALBERG, F. 1960. The raphe nuclei of the brain stem in the cat. II. Efferent connections. J. Comp. Neurol., **114:** 239–259

BRODAL, A., POMPEIANO, O., AND WALBERG, F. 1962. *The Vestibular Nuclei and Their Connections, Anat-*

omy and Functional Correlations. Charles C Thomas, Springfield, Ill.

BRODAL, P. 1968. The corticopontine projection in the cat. I. Demonstration of a somatotopically organized projection from the primary sensorimotor cortex. Exp. Brain Res., **5:** 212–237.

BRODAL, P. 1972. The corticopontine projection from the visual cortex in the cat. I. The total projection and the projection from area 17. Brain Res., **39:** 297–317.

BRODAL, P. 1975. Demonstration of a somatotopically organized projection onto the paramedian lobule and the anterior lobe from the lateral reticular nucleus: An experimental study with the horseradish peroxidase method. Brain Res., **95:** 221–239.

BRODAL, P. 1978. Principles of organization of the monkey corticopontine projection. Brain Res., **148:** 214–218.

BRODAL, P. 1978a. The corticopontine projection in the rhesus monkey: Origin and principles of organization. Brain, **101:** 251–283.

BRODISH, A. 1964. Role of the hypothalamus in the regulation of ACTH release. In E. BAJUSZ AND G. JASMIN (Editors), *Major Problems in Endocrinology.* S. Karger, Basel.

BRODMANN, K. 1909. *Vergleichende Lokalisation lehre der Grosshirnrinde in ihren Prinzipien dargestellt auf Grund des Zellenbaues.* J. A. Barth, Leipzig, 324 pp.

BROUWER, B., AND ZEEMAN, W. P. C. 1926. The projection of the retina in the primary optic neuron in monkeys. Brain, **49:** 1–35.

BROWN-GRANT, K., AND RAISMAN, G. 1972. Reproductive function in the rat following selective destruction of afferent fibres to the hypothalamus from the limbic system. Brain Res., **46:** 23–42.

BROWNSTEIN, M. J., PALKOVITZ, M., SAAVEDRA, J. M., AND KIZER, J. S. 1975. Tryptophan hydroxylase in the rat brain. Brain Res., **97:** 163–166.

BUCY, P. C. 1949. Effects of extirpation in man. In P. C. BUCY (Editor), *The Precentral Motor Cortex*, Ed. 2. University of Illinois Press, Urbana, Ch. 14, pp. 353–394.

BUNNEY, B. S., AND AGHAJANIAN, G. K. 1976. The precise localization of nigral afferents in the rat as determined by a retrograde tracing technique. Brain Res., **117:** 423–435.

BUNT, A. H., HENDRICKSON, A. E., LUND, J. S., LUND, R. D., AND FUCHS, A. F. 1975. Monkey retinal ganglion cells: Morphometric analysis and tracing of axonal projections with a consideration of the peroxidase technique. J. Comp. Neurol., **164:** 265–286.

BURDE, R. M., AND LOEWY, A. D. 1980. Central origin of oculomotor parasympathetic neurons in the monkey. Brain Res., **198:** 434–439.

BURTON, H., AND JONES, E. G. 1976. The posterior thalamic region and its cortical projection in new world and old world monkeys. J. Comp. Neurol., **168:** 249–302.

BURTON, H., AND LOEWY, A. D. 1977. Projections to the spinal cord from medullary somatosensory relay nuclei. J. Comp. Neurol., **173:** 773–792.

BUTLER, R. A., DIAMOND, I. T., AND NEFF, W. D. 1957. Role of auditory cortex in discrimination of changes in frequency. J. Neurophysiol., **20:** 108–120.

BÜTTNER, U., AND HENN, J. 1976. Thalamic unit activity in the alert monkey during natural vestibular stimulation. Brain Res., **103:** 127–132.

BÜTTNER, U., BÜTTNER-ENNEVER, J. A., AND HENN, V. 1977. Vertical eye movement related unit activity in the rostral mesencephalic reticular formation of the alert monkey. Brain Res., **130:** 239–252.

BÜTTNER, U., HENN, V., AND OSWALD, H. P. 1977a. Vestibular-related neuronal activity in the thalamus of the alert monkey during sinusoidal rotation in the dark. Exp. Brain Res., **30:** 435–444.

BÜTTNER-ENNEVER, J. A. 1977. Pathways from the pontine reticular formation to structures controlling horizontal and vertical eye movements in the monkey. In A. BERTHOZ AND R. BAKER (Editors), *Control of Gaze by Brain Stem Neurons* (Developments in Neuroscience, Vol. 1). Elsevier/North-Holland, Amsterdam, pp. 89–98.

BÜTTNER-ENNEVER, J. A., AND AKERT, K. 1981. Medial rectus subgroups of the oculomotor nucleus and their abducens internuclear input in the monkey. J. Comp. Neurol., **197:** 17–27.

BÜTTNER-ENNEVER, J. A., AND BÜTTNER, U. 1978. A cell group associated with vertical eye movements in the rostral mesencephalic reticular formation of the monkey. Brain Res., **151:** 31–47.

BYSTRZYCKA, E. K. 1980. Afferent projections to the dorsal and ventral respiratory nuclei in the medulla oblongata of the cat studied by the horseradish peroxidase technique. Brain Res., **185:** 59–66.

CAJAL, S. RAMÓN Y. 1909, 1911. *Histologie du système nerveux de l'homme et des vertébres.* Norbert Maloine, Paris. 2 vols.

CAMPBELL, A. W. 1905. *Histological Studies on the Localization of Cerebral Function.* Cambridge University Press, New York, 360 pp.

CANNON, W. B., AND ROSENBLUETH, A. 1949. *The Supersensitivity of Denervated Structures.* Macmillan Company, New York.

CAREY, R. G., BEAR, M. F., AND DIAMOND, I. T. 1980. The laminar organization of the reciprocal projections between the claustrum and striate cortex in the tree shrew, *Tupaia glis.* Brain Res., **184:** 193–198.

CARLETON, S. C., AND CARPENTER, M. B. 1983. Afferent and efferent connections of the medial, inferior and lateral vestibular nuclei in the cat and monkey. Brain Res., **278:** 29–51.

CARLETON, S. C., AND CARPENTER, M. B. 1984. Distribution of primary vestibular fibers in the brain stem and cerebellum of the monkey. Brain Res., **294:** 281–298.

CARMAN, J. B., COWAN, W. M., AND POWELL, T. P. S. 1963. The organization of corticostriate connexions in the rabbit. Brain, **86:** 525–562.

CARMAN, J. B., COWAN, W. M., AND POWELL, T. P. S. 1964. Cortical connexions of the thalamic reticular nucleus. J. Anat., **98:** 587–598.

CARMAN, J. B., COWAN, W. M., POWELL, T. P. S., AND WEBSTER, K. E. 1965. A bilateral corticostriate projection. J. Neurol. Neurosurg. Psychiatry, **28:** 71–77.

CARMEL, P. W. 1970. Efferent projections of the ventral anterior nucleus of the thalamus in the monkey.

Am. J. Anat., **128:** 159–184.

Carpenter, M. B. 1950. Athetosis and the basal ganglia. Arch. Neurol. Psychiatry, **63:** 875–901.

Carpenter, M. B. 1958. The neuroanatomical basis of dyskinesia. In W. S. Fields (Editor), *Pathogenesis and Treatment of Parkonsonism.* Charles C Thomas, Springfield, Ill., Ch. 2, pp. 50–85.

Carpenter, M. B. 1959. Lesions of the fastigial nuclei in the rhesus monkey. Am. J. Anat., **104:** 1–34.

Carpenter, M. B. 1961. Brain stem and infratentorial neuraxis in experimental dyskinesia. A.M.A. Arch. Neurol., **5:** 504–524.

Carpenter, M. B. 1971. Upper and lower motor neurons. In J. A. Downey and R. C. Darling (Editors), *Physiological Basis of Rehabilitation Medicine.* W. B. Saunders, Philadelphia, Ch. 1, pp. 3–27.

Carpenter, M. B. 1971a. Central oculomotor pathways. In P. Bach-y-Rita *et al.* (Editors), *The Control of Eye Movements.* Academic Press, New York, Ch. 4, pp. 67–103.

Carpenter, M. B. 1981. Anatomy of the corpus striatum and brain stem integrating systems. In V. Brooks (Editor), *Handbook of Physiology*, Sect. 1, Vol. II. Motor Control. American Physiological Society, Washington, D.C., Ch. 19, pp. 947–995.

Carpenter, M. B., and Batton, R. R. III. 1980. Abducens internuclear neurons and their role in conjugate horizontal gaze. J. Comp. Neurol., **189:** 191–209.

Carpenter, M. B., and Batton, R. R., III. 1982. Connections of the fastigial nucleus in the cat and monkey. Exp. Brain Res. (Suppl. 6), pp. 250–295.

Carpenter, M. B., and Carleton, S. C. 1983. Comparison of vestibular and abducens projections to the medial rectus subdivision of the oculomotor complex in the monkey. Brain Res., **274:** 144–149.

Carpenter, M. B., and McMasters, R. E. 1964. Lesions of the substantia nigra in the rhesus monkey: Efferent fiber degeneration and behavioral observations. Am. J. Anat., **114:** 293–320.

Carpenter, M. B., and Mettler, F. A. 1951. Analysis of subthalamic hyperkinesia in the monkey with special reference to ablations of agranular cortex. J. Comp. Neurol., **95:** 125–158.

Carpenter, M. B., and Nova, H. R. 1960. Descending division of the brachium conjunctivum in the cat: A cerebello-reticular system. J. Comp. Neurol., **114:** 295–305.

Carpenter, M. B., and Peter, P. 1970/71. Accessory oculomotor nuclei in the monkey. J. Hirnforsch., **12:** 405–418.

Carpenter, M. B., and Peter, P. 1972. Nigrostriatal and nigrothalamic fibers in the rhesus monkey. J. Comp. Neurol., **144:** 93–116.

Carpenter, M. B., and Pierson, R. J. 1973. Pretectal region and the pupillary light reflex: An anatomical analysis in the monkey. J. Comp. Neurol., **149:** 271–300.

Carpenter, M. B., and Strominger, N. L. 1965. The medial longitudinal fasciculus and disturbances of conjugate horizontal eye movements in the monkey. J. Comp. Neurol., **125:** 41–66.

Carpenter, M. B., and Strominger, N. L. 1967. Efferent fiber projections of the subthalamic nucleus in the rhesus monkey: A comparison of the efferent projections of the subthalamic nucleus, substantia nigra and globus pallidus. Amer. J. Anat., **121:** 41–72.

Carpenter, M. B., and Sutin, J. 1983. *Human Neuroanatomy*, ed. 8. Williams & Wilkins, Baltimore.

Carpenter, M. B., Whittier, J. R., and Mettler, F. A. 1950. Analysis of choreoid hyperkinesia in the rhesus monkey: Surgical and pharmacological analysis of hyperkinesia resulting from lesions of the subthalamic nucleus of Luys. J. Comp. Neurol., **92:** 293–331.

Carpenter, M. B., Noback, C. R., and Moss, M. L. 1954. The anterior choroidal artery. Its origins, course, distribution and variations. Arch. Neurol. Psychiatry, **71:** 714–722.

Carpenter, M. B., McMasters, R. E., and Hanna, G. R. 1963. Disturbances of conjugate horizontal eye movements in the monkey. I. Physiological effects and anatomical degeneration resulting from lesions of the abducens nucleus and nerve. Arch. Neurol., **8:** 231–247.

Carpenter, M. G., Fraser, R. A. R., and Shriver, J. 1968. The organization of the pallidosubthalamic fibers in the monkey. Brain Res., **11:** 522–559.

Carpenter, M. B., Stein, B. M., and Shriver, J. E. 1968. Central projections of spinal dorsal roots in the monkey. II. Lower thoracic lumbosacral and coccygeal dorsal roots. Am. J. Anat., **123:** 75–118.

Carpenter, M. B., Harbison, J. W., and Peter, P. 1970. Accessory oculomotor nuclei in the monkey: Projections and effects of discrete lesions. J. Comp. Neurol., **140:** 131–154.

Carpenter, M. B., Stein, B. M., and Peter, P. 1972. Primary vestibulocerebellar fibers in the monkey: Distribution of fibers arising from distinctive cell groups of the vestibular ganglia. Am. J. Anat., **135:** 221–250.

Carpenter, M. B., Nakano, K., and Kim, R. 1976. Nigrothalamic projections in the monkey demonstrated by autoradiographic technics. J. Comp. Neurol., **165:** 401–416.

Carpenter, M. B., Batton, R. R., Carleton, S. C., and Keller, J. T. 1981. Interconnections and organization of pallidal and subthalamic nucleus neurons in the monkey. J. Comp. Neurol., **197:** 579–603.

Carpenter, M. B., Carleton, S. C., Keller, J. T., and Conte, P. 1981a. Connections of the subthalamic nucleus in the monkey. Brain Res., **224:** 1–29.

Carter, D. A., and Fibiger, H. C. 1978. The projections of the entopeduncular nucleus and globus pallidus in rat as demonstrated by autoradiography and horseradish peroxidase histochemistry. J. Comp. Neurol., **177:** 113–124.

Casagrande, V. A., Harting, J. K., Hall, W. C., and Diamond, I. T. 1972. Superior colliculus of the tree shrew: A structural and functional subdivision into superficial and deep layers. Science, **177:** 444–447.

Casseday, J. H., Diamond, I. T., and Harting, J. K. 1976. Auditory pathways to the cortex in *Tapaia glis*. J. Comp. Neurol., **166:** 303–340.

Chambers, W. W., and Sprague, J. M. 1955. Functional localization in the cerebellum. I. Organization in longitudinal corticonuclear zones and their contribution to the control of posture, both extrapyramidal and pyramidal. J. Comp. Neurol., **103:** 105–130.

CHAMBERS, W. W., AND SPRAGUE, J. M. 1955a. Functional localization in the cerebellum. II. Somatotopic organization in cortex and nuclei. Arch. Neurol. Psychiatry, **74:** 653–680.

CHAN-PALAY, V. 1976. Serotonin axons in supraependymal and subependymal in leptomeninges: Their roles in local alterations of cerebrospinal fluid and vasomotor activity. Brain Res., **102:** 103–130.

CHAN-PALAY, V. 1977. *Cerebellar Dentate Nucleus: Organization, Cytology and Transmitters*, Springer-Verlag, Berlin.

CHAN-PALAY, V. 1978. Paratrigeminal nucleus. I. Neurons and synaptic organization. J. Neurocytol., **4:** 405–418.

CHAN-PALAY, V., AND PALAY, S. L. 1970. Interrelations of basket cell axons and climbing fibers in the cerebellar cortex of the rat. Z. Anat. Entwickl.-Gesch., **132:** 191–227.

CHANG, H. T., WILSON, C. J., AND KITAI, S. T. 1981. Single neostriatal efferent axons in the globus pallidus: A light and electron microscopic study. Science, **213:** 915–918.

CHANG, M. M., AND LEEMAN, S. E. 1970. The isolation of a sialogogic peptide from bovine hypothalamic tissue and its characterization as substance P. J. Biol. Chem., **245:** 4784–4790.

CHANG, M. M., LEEMAN, S. W., AND NIALL, H. D. 1971. Amino acid sequence of substance P. Nature (Lond.) New Biol., **232:** 86–87.

CHI, C. C., AND FLYNN, J. P. 1971. Neuroanatomical projections related to biting attack elicited from hypothalamus in cats. Brain Res., **35:** 49–66.

CHU, N.-S., AND BLOOM, F. E. 1973. Norepinephrine-containing neurons: Changes in spontaneous discharge patterns during sleeping and waking. Science, **179:** 908–910.

CLARK, W. E. L. 1932. The structure and connections of the thalamus. Brain, **55:** 406–470.

CLARK, W. E. L. 1941. The laminar organization and cell content of the lateral geniculate body in the monkey. J. Anat., **75:** 419–433.

CLARK, W. E. L. 1951. The projection of the olfactory epithelium on the olfactory bulb in the rabbit. J. Neurol. Neurosurg. Psychiatry, **14:** 1–10.

CLARK, W. E. L. 1957. Inquiries into the anatomical basis of olfactory discrimination. Proc. R. Soc. Lond. (Biol.), **146:** 299–319.

CLARK, W. E. L., AND WARWICK, R. T. 1946. The pattern of olfactory innervation. J. Neurol. Neurosurg. Psychiatry, **9:** 101–111.

CLARK, W. E. L., BEATTIE, J., RIDDOCH, G., AND DOTT, N. M. 1938. *The Hypothalamus.* Oliver & Boyd, Edinburgh.

COGAN, D. G. 1956. *Neurology of the Ocular Muscles*, Ed. 2. Charles C Thomas, Springfield, Ill.

CONNOR, J. D. 1970. Caudate nucleus neurones: Correlation of the effects of substantia nigra stimulation with iontophoretic dopamine. J. Physiol. (Lond.), **208:** 691–703.

CONRAD, L. C., LEONARD, C. M., AND PFAFF, D. W. 1974. Connections of the median and dorsal raphe nuclei in the rat. An autoradiographic and degeneration study. J. Comp. Neurol., **156:** 179–206.

COOPER, M. H., AND BEAL, J. A. 1978. The neurons and the synaptic endings in the primate basilar pontine gray. J. Comp. Neurol., **180:** 17–42.

CORNING, H. K. 1922. *Lehrbuch der topographischen Anatomie für Studierende und Ärzte.* J. F. Bergmann, Munich, pp. 609–614.

COULTER, J. D., AND JONES, E. G. 1977. Differential distribution of corticospinal projections from individual cytoarchitectonic fields in the monkey. Brain Res., **129:** 335–340.

COULTER, J. D., EWING, L., AND CARTER, C. 1976. Origin of primary sensorimotor cortical projections to lumbar spinal cord of cat and monkey. Brain Res., **103:** 366–372.

COURVILLE, J. 1966. Somatotopical organization of the projection from the nucleus interpositus anterior of the cerebellum to the red nucleus: An experimental study in the cat with silver impregnation methods. Exp. Brain Res., **2:** 191–215.

COURVILLE, J. 1975. Distribution of olivocerebellar fibers demonstrated by a radioautographic tracing method. Brain Res., **95:** 253–263.

COURVILLE, J., AND BRODAL, A. 1966. Rubrocerebellar connections in the cat: An experimental study with silver impregnation methods. J. Comp. Neurol., **126:** 471–485.

COURVILLE, J., AND COOPER, C. W. 1970. The cerebellar nuclei of *Macaca mulatta*: A morphological study. J. Comp. Neurol., **140:** 241–254.

COURVILLE, J., AND DIAKIW, N. 1976. Cerebellar corticonuclear projection in the cat: The vermis of the anterior and posterior lobes. Brain Res., **110:** 1–20.

COURVILLE, J., AND FARACO-CANTIN, F. 1978. On the origin of the climbing fibers of the cerebellum: An experimental study in the cat with an autoradiographic tracing method. Neuroscience, **3:** 797–809.

COURVILLE, J., AUGUSTINE, J. R., AND MARTEL, P. 1977. Projections from the inferior olive to the cerebellar nuclei in the cat demonstrated by retrograde transport of horseradish peroxidase. Brain Res., **130:** 405–419.

COWAN, W. M., AND CUÉNOD, M. 1975. The use of axonal transport for study of neuronal connections: A retrospective survey. In *The Use of Axonal Transport for Studies of Neuronal Connectivity.* Elsevier, Amsterdam, pp. 2–23.

COWAN, W. M., RAISMAN, G., AND POWELL, T. P. S. 1965. The connexions of the amygdala. J. Neurol. Neurosurg. Psychiatry, **28:** 137–151.

COWAN, W. M., GOTTLIEB, D. I., HENDRICKSON, A. E., PRICE, J. L., AND WOOLSEY, T. A. 1972. The autoradiographic demonstration of axonal connections in the central nervous system. Brain Res., **37:** 21–51.

COXE, W. S., AND LANDAU, W. M. 1965. Observations upon the effect of supplementary motor cortex ablation in the monkey. Brain, **88:** 763–772.

CROCK, H. V., AND YOSHIZAWA, H. 1977. *The Blood Supply of the Vertebral Column and Spinal Cord in Man.* Springer-Verlag, Berlin, 130 pp.

CRONE, C. 1963. The permeability of capillaries in various organs as determined by use of the "indicator diffusion" method. Acta Physiol. Scand., **58:** 292–305.

CROSSMAN, A. R., SAMBROOK, M. A., AND JACKSON, A. 1980. Experimental hemiballismus in the baboon produced by injection of a gamma-aminobutyric acid antagonist into the basal ganglia. Neurosci. Lett., **20:** 369–372.

CROSSMAN, A. R., SAMBROOK, M. A., AND JACKSON, A. 1984. Experimental hemichorea/hemiballismus in the monkey: Studies on the intracerebral site of action in a drug-induced dyskinesia. Brain, **107:** 579–596.

CUELLO, A. C., AND KANAZAWA, I. 1978. The distribution of substance P immunoreactive fibers in the rat central nervous system. J. Comp. Neurol., **178:** 129–156.

CUMMINGS, J. F., AND PETRAS, J. M. 1977. The origin of spinocerebellar pathways. I. The nucleus cervicalis centralis of the cranial cervical spinal cord. J. Comp. Neurol., **173:** 655–692.

CYNADER, M., AND BERMAN, N. 1972. Receptive-field organization of monkey superior colliculus. J. Neurophysiol., **35:** 187–201.

DAHLSTRÖM, A. 1971. Regional distribution of brain catecholamines and serotonin. Neurosci. Res. Program Bull., **9:** 197–205.

DAHLSTRÖM, A., AND FUXE, K. 1964. Evidence for the existence of monoamine-containing neurons in the central nervous system. I. Demonstration of monoamines in the cell bodies of brain stem neurons. Acta Physiol. Scand., **62** (Suppl. 232): 1–55.

DAITZ, H. M., AND POWELL, T. P. S. 1954. Studies of the connections of the fornix system. J. Neurol. Neurosurg. Psychiatry, **17:** 75–82.

DAVIES, J., AND DRAY, A. 1976. Substance P in the substantia nigra. Brain Res., **107:** 623–627.

DAVIES, P., AND MALONEY, A. J. F. 1976. Selective loss of central cholinergic neurons in Alzheimer's disease. Lancet, **2:** 1403.

DAVSON, H. 1967. *Physiology of the Cerebrospinal Fluid.* Little, Brown, Boston.

DEECKE, L., SCHWARZ, D. W. F., AND FREDRICKSON, J. M. 1973. The vestibular thalamus in the rhesus monkey. Adv. Otorhinolaryngol., **19:** 210–219.

DEECKE, L., SCHWARTZ, D. W. F., AND FREDRICKSON, J. M. 1974. Nucleus ventroposterior inferior (VPI) as the vestibular thalamic relay in the rhesus monkey. I. Field potential investigation. Exp. Brain Res., **20:** 88–100.

DEECKE, L., SCHWARZ, D. W. F., AND FREDRICKSON, J. M. 1977. Vestibular responses in the rhesus monkey ventroposterior thalamus. II. Vestibuloproprioceptive convergence at thalamic neurons. Exp. Brain Res., **30:** 219–232.

DE GROOT, J., AND HARRIS, G. W. 1950. Hypothalamic control of the anterior pituitary gland and blood lymphocytes. J. Physiol., **111:** 335–346.

DÉJÉRINE, J. 1901. *Anatomie des centres nerveaux,* Vol. 2. J. Rueff, Paris, 720 pp.

DEKKER, J. J., KIEVIT, J., JACOBSON, S., AND KUYPERS, H. G. J. M. 1975. Retrograde axonal transport of horseradish peroxidase in the forebrain of the rat, cat and rhesus monkey. In M. SANTINI (Editor), *Prospectives in Neurobiology* (Golgi Centennial Symposium). Raven Press, New York, pp. 201–208.

DEMPSEY, E. W., AND MORISON, R. S. 1942. The production of rhythmically recurrent cortical potentials after localized thalamic stimulation. Am. J. Physiol., **135:** 293–300.

DEMPSEY, E. W., AND MORISON, R. S. 1943. The electrical activity of a thalamocortical relay system. Am. J. Physiol., **138:** 283–298.

DENIAU, J. M., HAMMOND, C., CHEVALIER, G., AND FÉGER, J. 1978. Evidence for branched subthalamic nucleus projections to substantia nigra, entopeduncular nucleus and globus pallidus. Neurosci. Lett., **9:** 117–121.

DENIAU, J. M., HAMMOND, C., RIZK, A., AND FÉGER, J. 1978a. Electrophysiological properties of identified output neurons of the rat substantia nigra (pars compacta and pars reticulata): Evidences for the existence of branched neurons. Exp. Brain Res., **32:** 409–422.

DENNY-BROWN, D., AND BOTTERELL, E. H. 1948. The motor functions of the agranular frontal cortex. Proc. Assoc. Res. Nerv. Ment. Dis., **27:** 235–345.

DE OLMOS, J. S. 1972. The amygdaloid projection field in the rat studied with the cupric-silver method. In B. E. ELEFTHERIOU (Editor), *The Neurobiology of the Amygdala.* Plenum Press, New York, pp. 145–204.

DESCARRIES, L., WATKINS, K. C., GARCIA, S., AND BEAUDET, A. 1982. The serotonin neurons in nucleus raphe dorsalis of adult rat: A light and electron microscope radioautographic study. J. Comp. Neurol., **207:** 239–254.

DEVITO, J. L., AND ANDERSON, M. E. 1982. An autoradiographic study of efferent connections of the globus pallidus in *Macaca mulatta.* Exp. Brain Res., **46:** 107–117.

DEVITO, J. L., AND SMITH, O. A., JR. 1959. Projections from the mesial frontal cortex (supplementary motor area) to the cerebral hemispheres and brain stem of the *Macaca mulatta.* J. Comp. Neurol., **111:** 261–277.

DEVITO, J. L., ANDERSON, M. E., AND WALSH, K. E. 1980. A horseradish peroxidase study of afferent connections of the globus pallidus in *Macaca mulatta.* Exp. Brain Res., **38:** 65–73.

DIAMOND, I. T., JONES, E. G., AND POWELL, T. P. S. 1968. Interhemispheric fiber connections of the auditory cortex in the cat. Brain Res., **11:** 177–193.

DIAMOND, I. T., JONES, E. G., AND POWELL, T. P. S. 1968a. The association connections of the auditory cortex of the cat. Brain Res., **11:** 560–579.

DIAMOND, I. T., JONES, E. G., AND POWELL, T. P. S. 1969. The projection of the auditory cortex upon the diencephalon and brain stem in the cat. Brain Res., **15:** 305–340.

DIETRICHS, E., AND WALBERG, F. 1979. The cerebellar projection from the lateral reticular nucleus as studied with retrograde transport of horseradish peroxidase. Anat. Embryol. (Berl.), **155:** 273–290.

DIETRICHS, E., AND WALBERG, F. 1979a. The cerebellar corticonuclear and nucleocortical projections in the cat as studied with anterograde and retrograde transport of horseradish peroxidase. I. The paramedian lobule. Anat. Embryol. (Berl.), **158:** 13–39.

DIFIGLIA, M., PASIK, P., AND PASIK, T. 1976. A Golgi study of neuronal types in the neostriatum of monkeys. Brain Res., **114:** 245–256.

DIFIGLIA, M., ARONIN, N., AND LEEMAN, S. E. 1981. Immunoreactive substance P in the substantia nigra of the monkey: Light and electron microscopic localization. Brain Res., **233:** 381–388.

DIFIGLIA, M., ARONIN, N., AND MARTIN, J. B. 1982. Light and electron microscopic localization of immunoreactive leu-enkephalin in monkey basal ganglia. J. Neurosci., **2:** 303–320.

DIVAC, I., LAVAIL, J. H., RAKIC, P., AND WINSTON, K. R. 1977. Heterogenous afferents to the inferior parietal lobule of the rhesus monkey revealed by the retrograde transport method. Brain Res., **123:** 197–207.

DOW, R. S., AND MORUZZI, G. 1958. *The Physiology and Pathology of the Cerebellum*. University of Minnesota Press, Minneapolis.

DOWLING, J. E., AND BOYCOTT, B. B. 1966. Organization of the primate retina: Electron microscopy. Proc. R. Soc. Lond. (Biol.), **166:** 80–111.

DRAY, A. 1980. The physiology and pharmacology of mammalian basal ganglia. Progress in Neurology, **14:** 221–335.

DRAY, A., GONYE, T. J., OAKLEY, N. R., AND TANNER, T. 1976. Evidence for the existence of a raphe projection to the substantia nigra in rat. Brain Res., **113:** 45–57.

DRAY, A., DAVIES, J., OAKLEY, N. R., TONGROACH, P., AND VELLUCCI, S. 1978. The dorsal and medial raphe projections to the substantia nigra in the rat: Electrophysiological, biochemical and behavioral observations. Brain Res., **151:** 431–442.

DREIFUSS, J. J., MURPHY, J. T., AND GLOOR, P. 1968. Contrasting effects of two identified amygdaloid efferent pathways on single hypothalamic neurons. J. Neurophysiol., **31:** 237–248.

DUFFY, M. J., MULHALL, D., AND POWELL, D. 1975. Subcellular distribution of substance P in bovine hypothalamus and substantia nigra. J. Neurochem., **25:** 305–307.

EAGER, R. P. 1963. Efferent cortico-nuclear pathways in the cerebellum of the cat. J. Comp. Neurol., **120:** 81–103.

EBESSON, S. O. E. 1968. A connection between the dorsal column nuclei and the dorsal accessory olive. Brain Res., **8:** 393–397.

ECCLES, J. C., LLINÁS, R., AND SASAKI, K. 1966. The excitatory synaptic action of climbing fibres on the Purkinje cells of the cerebellum. J. Physiol. (Lond.), **182:** 268–296.

ECCLES, J. C., ITO, M., AND SZENTÁGOTHAI, J. 1967. *The Cerebellum as a Neuronal Machine*. Springer-Verlag, New York.

ECONOMO, C. V. VON. 1929. *The Cytoarchitectonics of the Human Cerebral Cortex*. Oxford Medical Publications, London.

EDWARDS, S. B. 1972. The ascending and descending projections of the red nucleus in the cat: An experimental study using an autoradiographic tracing method. Brain Res., **48:** 45–63.

EDWARDS, S. B., AND HENKEL, C. K. 1978. Superior colliculus connections with the extraocular motor nuclei in the cat. J. Comp. Neurol., **179:** 451–467.

EDWARDS, S. B., ROSENQUIST, A. C., AND PALMER, L. A. 1974. An autoradiographic study of ventral lateral geniculate projections in the cat. Brain Res., **72:** 282–287.

EDWARDS, S. B., GINSBURGH, C. L., HENKEL, C. K., AND STEIN, B. E. 1979. Sources of subcortical projections to the superior colliculus in the cat. J. Comp. Neurol., **184:** 309–330.

EHRLICH, P. 1885. *Das Sauerstoff-Bedürfnis des Organismus. Eine Farbenanalytische Studie*. Herschwald, Berlin, pp. 69–72.

ELDE, R., HOKFELT, T., JOHANSSON, O., AND TERENIUS, L. 1976. Immunohistochemical studies using antibodies to leucine-enkephalin: Initial observations on the nervous systems of the rat. Neuroscience, **1:** 349–351.

ELEFTHERIOU, B. E., ZOLOVICK, A. J., AND PEARSE, R. 1966. Effects of amygdaloid lesions on pituitary-adrenal axis in the deer-mouse. Proc. Soc. Exp. Biol. Med., **122:** 1259.

ELFVIN, L. G. 1958. The ultrastructure of unmyelinated fibers in the splenic nerve of the cat. J. Ultrastruct. Res., **1:** 428–454.

ELLER, T., AND CHAN-PALAY, V. 1976. Afferents to the cerebellar lateral nucleus: Evidence from retrograde transport of horseradish peroxidase after pressure injections through micropipettes. J. Comp. Neurol., **166:** 285–301.

ELLIOTT, K. A. C., AND JASPER, H. 1949. Measurement of experimentally induced brain swelling and shrinkage. Am. J. Physiol., **157:** 122–129.

ELZE, C. 1932. Centrales Nervensystem. In H. BRAUS, *Anatomie des Menschen. Ein Lehrbuch für Studierende und Ärzte*, Vol. III. J. Springer, Berlin, p. 234.

EMMERS, R. 1964. Localization of thalamic projection of afferents from the tongue in the cat. Anat. Rec., **148:** 67–74.

EMMERS, R. 1966. Separate relays of tactile, thermal and gustatory modalities in the cat thalamus. Proc. Soc. Exp. Biol. Med., **121:** 527–531.

EMMERS, R. 1973. Interaction of neural systems which control body water. Brain Res., **48:** 323–347.

EMMERS, R. 1976. Thalamic mechanisms that process a temporal pulse code for pain. Brain Res., **103:** 425–441.

EMMERS, R., BENJAMIN, R. M., AND BLOMQUIST, A. J. 1962. Thalamic localization of afferents from the tongue in the albino rat. J. Comp. Neurol., **118:** 43–48.

EMSON, P. C., ARREGUI, A., CLEMONT-JONES, V., SANDBERG, B. E. B., AND ROSSOR, M. 1980. Regional distribution of methionine-enkephalin and substance P-like immunoreactivity in normal human brain and in Huntington's disease. Brain Res., **199:** 147–160.

ENGLANDER, R. N., NETSKY, M. G., AND ADELMAN, L. S. 1975. Location of human pyramidal tract in the internal capsule—Anatomical evidence. Neurology (Minneap.), **25:** 823–826.

EPELBAUM, J., ARANCIBIA, L. T., KORDON, C., OTTERSEN, O. P., AND BEN-ARI, Y. 1979. Regional distribution of somatostatin within the amygdaloid complex of the rat brain. Brain Res., **174:** 172–174.

EVERETT, J. W. 1959. Neuroendocrine mechanisms in control of the mammalian ovary. In A. GORBMAN (Editor), *Comparative Endocrinology*. John Wiley & Sons, New York, pp. 168–174.

EVERETT, J. W. 1964. Central neural control of reproductive functions of the adenohypophysis. Physiol. Rev., **44:** 373–431.

FAHN, S. 1976. Regional distribution studies of GABA and other putative neurotransmitters and their enzymes. In E. ROBERTS (Editor), *GABA in Nervous System Function*. Raven Press, New York, pp. 169–186.

FÉGER, J., DENIAU, J. M., DE CHAMPLAIN, J., AND

FELTZ, P. 1979. A survey of electrophysiology and pharmacology of neostriated input-output relations. In I. DIVAC AND R. G. E. OBERG (Editors), *The Neostriatum*. Pergamon Press, Oxford, pp. 71–102.

FEINDEL, W., AND PENFIELD, W. 1954. Localization of discharge in temporal lobe automatism. Arch. Neurol. Psychiatry, **72:** 605–630.

FELTEN, D. L., LATIES, A. N., AND CARPENTER, M. B. 1974. Monoamine-containing cell bodies in the squirrel monkey brain. Am. J. Anat. **139:** 153–166.

FENSTERMACHER, J. D., AND RALL, D. P. 1973. Physiology and pharmacology of cerebrospinal fluid. In *Pharmacology of the Cerebral Circulation*. Pergamon Press, Oxford, Vol. 1, pp. 35–79.

FERNÁNDEZ, C., GOLDBERG, J. M., AND ABEND, W. K. 1972. Response to static tilts of peripheral neurons innervating otolith organs of the squirrel monkey. J. Neurophysiol., **35:** 978–997.

FIBIGER, H. C. 1982. The organization and some projections of cholinergic neurons of the mammalian forebrain. Brain Res. Rev., **4:** 327–388.

FIBIGER, H. C., PUDRITZ, R. E., MCGEER, P. L., AND MCGEER, E. G. 1972. Axonal transport in nigrostriatal and nigrothalamic neurons: Effects of medial forebrain bundle lesions and 6-hydroxydopamine. J. Neurochem., **19:** 1697–1708.

FIELDS, H. L. 1981. An endorphin-mediated analgesia system: Experimental and clinical observations. In J. B. MARTIN, S. REICHLIN, AND K. L. BICK (Editors), *Neurosecretion and Brain Peptides*. Raven Press, New York, pp. 199–212.

FIELDS, H. L., BASBAUM, A. I., CLANTON, C. H., AND ANDERSON, S. D. 1977. Nucleus raphe magnus inhibition of spinal cord dorsal horn neurons. Brain Res., **126:** 441–454.

FINK, R. P., AND HEIMER, L. 1967. Two methods for selective silver impregnation of degenerating axons and their synaptic endings in the central nervous system. Brain Res., **4:** 369–374.

FLUMERFELT, B. A., OTABE, S., AND COURVILLE, J. 1973. Distinct projections to the red nucleus from the dentate and interposed nuclei in the monkey. Brain Res., **50:** 408–414.

FOERSTER, O. 1936. Symptomatologie der Erkrankungen des Grosshirns. Motorische Felder und Bahnen. In O. BUMKE AND O. FOERSTER (Editors), *Handbuch der Neurologie*, Vol. 6. Springer, Berlin, pp. 1–357.

FOIX, C., AND HILLEMAND, J. 1925. Les artères de l'axe encéphalique jusqu'au diencéphale inclusivement. Rev. Neurol. (Paris), **44:** 705–739.

FONBERG, E. 1968. The role of the amygdaloid nucleus in animal behavior. Prog. Brain Res., **22:** 273–281.

FONBERG, E., AND DELGADO, J. M. R. 1961. Avoidance and alimentary reactions druing amygdala stimulation. J. Neurophysiol., **24:** 651–664.

FONNUM, F., AND STORM-MATHISEN, J. 1977. High affinity uptake of glutamate in terminals of corticostriate axons. Nature, **266:** 377–378.

FONNUM, F., AND WALBERG, F. 1973. An estimate of the concentration of δ-aminobutyric acid and glutamate decarboxylase in the inhibitory Purkinje axon terminals in the cat. Brain Res., **54:** 115–127.

FONNUM, F., STORM-MATHISEN, J., AND WALBERG, F. 1970. Glutamate decarboxylase in inhibitory neurons: A study of the enzyme in Purkinje cell axons and boutons in the cat. Brain Res., **20:** 259–275.

FONNUM, F., GROFOVÁ, I., RINVIK, E., STORM-MATHISEN, J., AND WALBERG, F. 1974. Origin and distribution of glutamate decarboxylase in substantia nigra of the cat. Brain Res., **71:** 77–92.

FONNUM, F., GOTTESFELD, Z., AND GROFOVA, I. 1978. Distribution of glutamate decarboxylase, choline acetyltransferase and aromatic amino acid decarboxylase in the basal ganglia of normal and operated rats. Evidence for striatopallidal, striatoentopeduncular and striantonigral GABAergic fibers. Brain Res., **143:** 125–138.

FONNUM, F., GROFOVÁ, I., AND RINVIK, E. 1978a. Origin and distribution of glutamate decarboxylase in the nucleus subthalamicus of the cat. Brain Res., **153:** 370–374.

FONNUM, F., STORM-MATHISEN, J., AND DIVAC, I. 1981. Biochemical evidence for glutamate as neurotransmitter in corticostriate and corticothalamic fibers in rat brain. Neuroscience, **6:** 863–873.

FOX, C. A., AND RAFOLS, J. A. 1975. The radial fibers in the globus pallidus. J. Comp. Neurol., **159:** 177–200.

FOX, C. A., HILLMAN, D. E., SIEGESMUND, K. A., AND DUTTA, C. R. 1967. The primate cerebellar cortex. A Golgi and electron microscopic study. In C. A. FOX AND R. S. SNIDER (Editors), *The Cerebellum, Progress in Brain Research*. Elsevier, Amsterdam, Vol. 25, pp. 174–225.

FOX, C. A., ANDRADE, A. N., HILLMAN, D. E., AND SCHWYN, R. C. 1971. The spiny neurons in the primate striatum: A Golgi and electron microscopic study. J. Hirnforsch., **13:** 181–201.

FOX, C. A., ANDRADE, A. N., SCHWYN, R. C., AND RAFOLS, J. A. 1971/72. The aspiny neurons and the glia in the primate striatum. A Golgi and electron microscopic study. J. Hirnforsch., **13:** 341–362.

FOX, C. A., ANDRADE, A. N., LU QUI, I. J., AND RAFOLS, J. A. 1974. The primate globus pallidus: A Golgi and electron microscopic study. J. Hirnforsch., **15:** 75–93.

FOX, C. A., RAFOLS, J. A., AND COWAN, W. M. 1975. Computer measurements of axis cylinder diameters of radial fibers and "comb" bundle fibers. J. Comp. Neurol., **159:** 201–224.

FRANTZEN, E., AND OLIVARIUS, B. I. F. 1957. On thrombosis of the basilar artery. Acta Psychiatr. Neurol. Scand., **32:** 431–439.

FRASCHINI, F., COLLU, R., AND MARTINI, L. 1971. Mechanisms of inhibitory action of pineal principles on gonadotropin secretion. In G. E. W. WOLSTENHOLME AND J. KNIGHT (Editors), *The Pineal Gland*. Churchill Livingstone, Edinburgh, pp. 259–272.

FREDRICKSON, J. M., KORNHUBER, H. H., AND SCHWARZ, D. W. F. 1974. Cortical projections of the vestibular nerve. In H. H. KORNHUBER (Editor), *Handbook of Sensory Physiology*, Vol. 6 (Part I). Springer-Verlag, Berlin, pp. 565–582.

FRIEDMAN, D. P., JONES, E. G., AND BURTON, H. 1980. Representation pattern in the second somatic sensory area of the monkey cerebral cortex. J. Comp. Neurol., **192:** 21–41.

FROHMAN, L. A. 1980. Neurotransmitters as regulators of endocrine function. In D. T. KRIEGER AND J. C. HUGHES (Editors), *Neuroendocrinology*, Sinauer Associates, Sunderland, Mass., pp. 44–57.

FROTSCHER, M., RINNE, U., HASSLER, R., AND WAGNER, A. 1981. Termination of cortical afferents on identified neurons in the caudate nucleus of the cat. Exp. Brain Res., **41:** 329–337.

FRY, W. J., KRUMINS, R., FRY, F. J., THOMAS, G., BORBELY, S., AND ADES, H. 1963. Origins and distribution of some efferent pathways from the mammillary nuclei of the cat. J. Comp. Neurol., **120:** 195–258.

FUCHS, A. 1977. Role of the vestibular and reticular nuclei in the control of gaze: Reticular, prepositus and other internuclear neuronal activity. In R. BAKER AND A. BERTHOZ (Editors), *Control of Gaze by Brain Stem Neurons: Developments in Neuroscience*. Elsevier/North-Holland, Amsterdam, pp.341–348.

FUKUDA, Y., AND STONE, J. 1974. Retinal distribution and central projections of Y, X and W cells of the cat's retina. J. Neurophysiol., **37:** 749–772.

FUKUSHIMA, K., PETERSON, B. W., UCHINO, Y., COULTER, J. D., AND WILSON, V. J. 1977. Direct fastigiospinal fibers in the cat. Brain Res., **126:** 538–542.

FULTON, J. F., AND INGRAHAM, F. D. 1929. Emotional disturbances following experimental lesions of the base of the brain (pre-chiasmal). J. Physiol., **67:** 27–28.

FULWILER, C. E., AND SAPER, C. B. 1984. Subnuclear organization of the efferent connection of the parabrachial nucleus in the rat. Brain Res. Rev., **7:** 239–259.

FUXE, K., AND ANDÉN, N. E. 1966. Studies on the central monoamine neurons with special reference to the nigro-neostriatal dopamine neuron system. In E. COSTA ET AL. (Editors), *Biochemistry and Pharmacology of the Basal Ganglia*. Raven Press, New York, pp. 123–129.

FUXE, K., AND HÖKFELT, T. 1970. Central monoaminergic systems and hypothalamic function. In L. MARTINI, M. MOLTA, AND F. FRASCHINI (Editors), *The Hypothalamus*. Academic Press, New York, pp. 123–138.

GACEK, R. R. 1961. The efferent cochlear bundle in man. Arch. Otolaryng., **74:** 690–694.

GACEK, R. R. 1971. Anatomical demonstration of the vestibulo-ocular projections in the cat. Acta Otolaryn. (Suppl. 293), 1–63.

GACEK, R. R. 1978. Location of commissural neurons in the vestibular nuclei of the cat. Exp. Neurol., **59:** 479–491.

GACEK, R. R., AND LYON, M. 1974. The localization of vestibular efferent neurons in the kitten with horseradish peroxidase. Acta Otolaryngol. (Stockh.), **77:** 92–101.

GADDUM, J. H., AND HAMEED, K. A. 1954. Drugs which antagonize 5-hydroxytryptamine. Br. J. Pharmacol., **9:** 240–248.

GAINER, H. 1981. The biology of neurosecretory neurons. In J. B. MARTIN, S. REICHLIN, AND K. L. BICK (Editors), *Neurosecretion and Brain Peptides*, Raven Press, New York, pp. 5–20.

GALAMBOS, R. 1956. Suppression of auditory nerve activity by stimulation of efferent fibers to cochlea. J. Neurophysiol., **19:** 424–437.

GALAMBOS, R., AND ROSE, J. E. 1952. Microelectrode studies on medial geniculate body of the cat. III. Response to pure tone. J. Neurophysiol., **15:** 381–400.

GALE, K., HONG, J.-S., AND GUIDOTTI, A. 1977. Presence of substance P and GABA in separate strionigral neurons. Brain Res., **36:** 371–375.

GAREY, L. J., AND POWELL, T. P. S. 1968. The projection of the retina in the cat. J. Anat., **102:** 189–222.

GAREY, L. J., JONES, E. G., AND POWELL, T. P. S. 1968. Interrelationships of striate and extrastriate cortex with the primary relay sites of the visual pathway. J. Neurol. Neurosurg. Psychiatry, **31:** 135–157.

GAUCHEY, C., BEAUJOUAN, J. C., BESSON, M. H., KERDEHUE, B., GLOWINSKI, J., AND MICHELOT, R. 1979. Topographic distribution of substance P in the cat substantia nigra. Neurosci. Lett., **12:** 127–131.

GAZZANIGA, M. S., AND SPERRY, R. W. 1967. Language after section of the cerebral commissures. Brain, **90:** 131–148.

GENIEC, P., AND MOREST, D. K. 1971. The neuronal architecture of the human posterior colliculus. Acta Otolaryngol. [Suppl.] (Stockh.), **295:** 1–33.

GEORGE, A. E., SALAMON, G., AND KRICHEFF, I. N. 1975. Pathologic anatomy of the thalamoperforating arteries in lesions of the third ventricle: Part II. A.J.R., **124:** 231–240.

GERARD, R. W., MARSHALL, W. H., AND SAUL, L J. 1936. Electrical activity of the cat's brain. Arch. Neurol. Psychiatry, **36:** 675–738.

GETCHELL, T. V., AND SHEPHERD, G. M. 1975. Short-axon cells in the olfactory bulb: Dendrodendritic synaptic interactions. J. Physiol. (Lond.), **251:** 523–548.

GEYER, M. A., PUERTO, A., DAWSEY, W. J., KNAPP, S., BULLARD, W. P., AND MANDELL, A. J. 1976. Histologic and enzymatic studies of the mesolimbic and mesostriatal serotoninergic pathways. Brain Res., **106:** 241–256.

GIBO, H., CARVER, C. C., RHOTON, A. L., LENKEY, C., AND MITCHELL, R. J. 1981. Microsurgical anatomy of the middle cerebral artery. J. Neurosurg., **54:** 151–169.

GILBERT, C. D., AND KELLY, J. P. 1975. The projection of cells in different layers of the cat's visual cortex. J. Comp. Neurol., **163:** 81–106.

GILLINGHAM, F. J. 1962. Small localized surgical lesions of the internal capsule in the treatment of dyskinesia. Confin. Neurol., **22:** 385–392.

GLENDENNING, K. K., HALL, J. A., DIAMOND, I. T., AND HALL, W. C. 1975. The pulvinar nucleus of *Galago sensgalensis*. J. Comp. Neurol., **161:** 419–458.

GLENN, L. L., AND STERIADE, M. 1982. Discharge rate and excitability of cortically projecting intralaminar thalamic neurons during waking and sleeping states. J. Neurosci., **2:** 1387–1404.

GLOOR, P. 1955. Electrophysiological studies on the connections of the amygdaloid nucleus in the cat. Electroencephalogr. Clin. Neurophysiol., **7:** 243–264.

GLOOR, P. 1960. Amygdala. In J. FIELD (Editor), *Handbook of Physiology*, Sect. 1, Vol. II. American Physiological Society, Washington, D.C., Ch. 57, pp. 1395–1420.

GLOOR, P. 1972. Temporal lobe epilepsy: Its possible contribution to the understanding of the functional significance of the amygdala and of its interaction with neocortical-temporal mechanisms. In B. E. ELEFTHERIOU (Editor). *The Neurobiology of the Amygdala*. Plenum Press, New York, pp. 423–457.

GLUSMAN, M. 1974. The hypothalamic "savage" syndrome. Proc. Assoc. Res. Nerv. Ment. Dis., **52:** 52–92.

GOBEL, S. 1975. Golgi studies of the substantia gelatinosa neurons in the spinal trigeminal nucleus. J. Comp. Neurol., **162:** 397–416.

GOBEL, S. 1978. Golgi studies of the neurons in layer I of the dorsal horn of the medulla (trigeminal nucleus caudalis). J. Comp. Neurol., **180:** 375–394.

GOBEL, S. 1978a. Golgi studies of the neurons in layer II of the dorsal horn of the medulla (trigeminal nucleus caudalis). J. Comp. Neurol., **180:** 395–414.

GOBEL, S., AND PURVIS, M. B. 1972. Anatomical studies of the organization of the spinal V nucleus: The deep bundles and the spinal V tract. Brain Res., **48:** 27–44.

GOLDBERG, J. M., AND FERNÁNDEZ, C. 1980. Efferent vestibular system in the squirrel monkey: Anatomical location and influence on afferent activity. J. Neurophysiol., **43:** 986–1025.

GOLDMAN, P. S., AND NAUTA, W. J. H. 1977. Columnar distribution of cortico-cortical fibres in the frontal association, limbic and motor cortex of the developing rhesus monkey. Brain Res., **122:** 393–413.

GOLDMAN, P. S., AND NAUTA, W. J. H. 1977a. An intricately patterned prefrontocaudate projection in the rhesus monkey. J. Comp. Neurol., **171:** 369–386.

GOMEZ, D. G., CHAMBERS, A. A., DIBENEDETTO, A. T., AND POTTS, D. G. 1974. The spinal cerebrospinal fluid absorptive pathways. Neuroradiology, **8:** 61–66.

GOMEZ, D. G., POTTS, D. G., AND DEONARINE, J. 1974a. Arachnoid granulations of sheep: Structural and ultrastructural changes with varying pressure differences. Arch. Neurol., **30:** 169–175.

GONZALEZ-VEGAS, J. A. 1974. Antagonism of dopamine-mediated inhibition in the nigrostriatal pathway: A mode of action of some catatonia-inducing drugs. Brain Res., **80:** 219–228.

GORDON, B. 1972. The superior colliculus of the brain. Sci. Am., **227:** 72–82.

GORSKI, R. A., HARLAN, R. E., JACOBSON, C. D., SHRYNE, J. E., AND SOUTHAM, A. M. 1980. Evidence for the existence of a sexually dimorphic nucleus in the preoptic area of the rat. J. Comp. Neurol., **193:** 529–539.

GOULD, B. B. 1979. The organization of afferents to the cerebellar cortex in the cat: Projections from the deep cerebellar nuclei. J. Comp. Neurol., **184:** 27–42.

GOULD, B. B. 1980. Organization of afferents from the brain stem nuclei to the cerebellar cortex in the cat. Adv. Anat. Embryol. Cell Biol., **62:** 1–90.

GOULD, B. B., AND GRAYBIEL, A. M. 1976. Afferents to the cerebellar cortex in the cat: Evidence for an intrinsic pathway leading from the deep nuclei to the cortex. Brain Res., **110:** 601–611.

GRAHAM, J. 1977. An autoradiographic study of the efferent connections of the superior colliculus in the cat. J. Comp. Neurol., **173:** 629–654.

GRAHAM, R. C., JR., AND KARNOVSKY, M. J. 1966. The early stages of absorption of injected horseradish peroxidase in the proximal tubules of the mouse kidney: Ultrastructural cytochemistry by a new technique. J. Histochem. Cytochem., **14:** 291–302.

GRANIT, R. 1955. *Receptors and Sensory Perception*. Yale University Press, New Haven, Conn.

GRANT, G. 1962. Spinal course and somatotopically localized termination of the spinocerebellar tracts: An experimental study in the cat. Acta Physiol. Scand., **56** (suppl. 193): 1–45.

GRAY, E. G. 1961. The granule cells, mossy synapses and Purkinje spinal synapses of the cerebellum: Light and electron microscopic observations. J. Anat., **95:** 345–356.

GRAYBIEL, A. M. 1972. Some extrageniculate visual pathways in the cat. Invest. Ophthalmol., **11:** 322–332.

GRAYBIEL, A. M. 1977. Direct and indirect preoculomotor pathways of the brain stem: An autoradiographic study of the pontine reticular formation in the cat. J. Comp. Neurol., **175:** 37–78.

GRAYBIEL, A. M. 1978. A satellite system of the superior colliculus: The parabigeminal nucleus and its projection to the superficial collicular layers. Brain Res., **145:** 365–374.

GRAYBIEL, A. M., AND HARTWIEG, E. A. 1974. Some afferent connections of the oculomotor complex in the cat: An experimental study with tracer techniques. Brain Res., **81:** 543–551.

GRAYBIEL, A. M., AND RAGSDALE, C. W. 1979. Histochemically distinct compartments in the striatum of human, monkey and cat demonstrated by acetylcholinesterase staining. Proc. Natl. Acad. Sci. U.S.A., **75:** 5723–5726.

GRAYBIEL, A. M., AND RAGSDALE, C. W. 1980. Clumping of acetylcholinesterase activity in the developing striatum of the human fetus and young infant. Proc. Natl. Acad. Sci. U.S.A., **77:** 1214–1218.

GRAYBIEL, A. M., AND SCIASCIA, T. R. 1975. Origin and distribution of nigrotectal fibers in the cat. Neurosci. Abstr., **1:** 271.

GRAYBIEL, A. M., RAGSDALE, C. W., AND MOON EDLEY, S. 1979. Compartments in the striatum of the cat observed by retrograde cell labeling. Exp. Brain Res., **34:** 189–195.

GRAYBIEL, A. M., PICKEL, V. M., JOH, T. H., REIS, D. J., AND RAGSDALE, C. W. 1981. Direct demonstration of a correspondence between the dopamine islands and acetylcholinesterase patches in the developing striatum. Proc. Natl. Acad. Sci. U.S.A., **78:** 5871–5875.

GRAYBIEL, A. M., RAGSDALE, C. W., YONEOKA, E. S., AND ELDE, R. P. 1981a. An immunohistochemical study of enkephalins and other neuropeptides in the striatum of the cat with evidence that the opiate peptides are arranged to form mosaic patterns in register with the striosomal compartments visible by acetylcholinesterase staining. Neuroscience, **6:** 377–397.

GREEN, J. D. 1960. The hippocampus. In J. FIELD (Editor), *Handbook of Physiology*, Sect. 1, Vol. II. American Physiological Society, Washington, D.C., Ch. 56, pp. 1373–1389.

GREEN, J. D. 1964. The hippocampus. Physiol. Rev., **44:** 561–608.

GREEN, J. D., AND HARRIS, G. W. 1949. Observation of the hypophysioportal vessels of the living rat. J. Physiol. (Lond.), **108:** 359–361.

GREEN, J. D., CLEMENTE, C. A., AND DE GROOT, J.

1957. Rhinencephalic lesions and behavior in cats. J. Comp. Neurol., **108:** 505–545.

GREEN, J. R., DUISBERG, R. E. H., AND MCGRATH, W. B. 1951. Focal epilepsy of psychomotor type. A preliminary report of observations on effects of surgical therapy. J. Neurosurg., **8:** 157–172.

GREER, M. A., AND ERWIN, H. L. 1956. Evidence of separate hypothalamic centers controlling corticotropin and thyrotropin secretion by the pituitary. Endocrinology, **58:** 665–670.

GROFOVÁ, I. 1975. The identification of striatal and pallidal neurons projecting to substantia nigra: An experimental study by means of retrograde axonal transport of horseradish peroxidase. Brain Res., **91:** 286–291.

GROFOVÁ, I. 1979. Extrinsic connections of the neostriatum. In I. DIVAC AND R. G. D. OBERG (Editors), *The Neostriatum.* Pergamon, Oxford, pp. 37–51.

GROFOVÁ, I., AND RINVIK, E. 1970. An experimental study on the striatonigral projection in the cat. Exp. Brain Res., **11:** 249–262.

GROSS, N. B., LIFSCHITZ, W. S., AND ANDERSON, D. J. 1974. The tonotopic organization of the auditory thalamus of the squirrel monkey (*Saimiri sciureus*). Brain Res., **65:** 323–332.

GROVES, P. M. 1983. A theory of the functional organization of the neostriatum and the neostriatal control of voluntary movement. Brain Res. Rev., **5:** 109–132.

GUILLEMIN, R. 1980. Beta-lipotrophin and endorphins: Implications of current knowledge. In D. T. KRIEGER AND J. C. HUGHES (Editors), *Neuroendocrinology.* Sinauer Associates, Sunderland, Mass., pp. 67–74.

GUILLERY, R. W. 1956. Degeneration in the posterior commissural fornix and the mammillary peduncle of the rat. J. Anat., **90:** 350–370.

GULLEY, R. L., AND WOOD, R. L. 1971. The fine structure of the neurons in the rat substantia nigra. Tissue Cell, **3:** 675–690.

GWYN, D. G., LESLIE, R. A., AND HOPKINS, D. A. 1979. Gastric afferent to the nucleus of the solitary tract in the cat. Neurosci. Lett., **14:** 13–17.

HA, H., AND LIU, C. N. 1968. Cell origin of the ventral spinocerebellar tract. J. Comp. Neurol., **133:** 185–205.

HABER, S., AND ELDE, R. 1981. Correlation between met-enkephalin and substance P immunoreactivity in the primate globus pallidus. Neuroscience, **6:** 1291–1297.

HABER, S. N., AND NAUTA, W. J. H. 1983. Ramifications of the globus pallidus in the rat as indicated by patterns of immunohistochemistry. Neuroscience, **9:** 243–260.

HAIGLER, H. J., AND AGHAJANIAN, G. K. 1974. Lysergic acid diethylamide and serotonin: A comparison of effects on serotonergic neurons and neurons receiving serotonergic input. J. Pharmacol. Exp. Ther., **188:** 688–699.

HAINES, D. E. 1976. Cerebellar corticonuclear and corticovestibular fibers of the anterior lobe vermis in a prosimian primate (*Galago senegalensis*). J. Comp. Neurol., **170:** 67–96.

HAJDU, F., HASSLER, R., AND BAK, I. J. 1973. Electron microscopic study of the substantia nigra and strionigral projection in the rat. Z. Zellforsch. Mikrosk. Anat., **146:** 207–220.

HALÁSZ, N., LJUNGDAHL, Å., AND HÖKFELT, T. 1978. Transmitter histochemistry of the rat olfactory bulb. II. Fluorescence histochemical, autoradiographic and electron microscopic localization of monoamines. Brain Res., **154:** 253–272.

HALL, E. A. 1963. Efferent connections of the basal and lateral nuclei of the amygdala in the cat. Am. J. Anat., **113:** 139–151.

HAMILTON, W. J., AND MOSSMAN, H. W. 1972. *Human Embryology.* Williams & Wilkins, Baltimore, pp. 478–481.

HAMMOND, C., AND YELNIK, J. 1983. Intracellular labeling of rat subthalamic neurones with horseradish peroxidase: Computer analysis of dentrites and characterization of axon arborization. Neuroscience, **8:** 781–790.

HAMMOND, C., DENIAU, J. M., RIZK, A., AND FÉGER, J. 1978. Electrophysiological demonstration of an excitatory subthalamo-nigral pathway in the rat. Brain Res., **151:** 235–244.

HAMMOND, C., FÉGER, J., BIOULAC, B., AND SOUTEYRAND, J. P. 1979. Experimental hemiballism in the monkey produced by unilateral kainic acid lesion in corpus Luysii. Brain Res., **171:** 577–580.

HAMMOND, C., SHIBAZAKI, T., AND ROUZAIRE-DUBOIS, B. 1983. Branched output neurons of the rat subthalamic nucleus: Electrophysiological study of the synaptic effects on identified cells in the two main target nuclei, the entopeduncular nucleus and the substantia nigra. Neuroscience, **9:** 511–520.

HÁMORI, J., AND SZENTÁGOTHAI, J. 1966. Identification under the electron microscope of climbing fibers and their synaptic contacts. Exp. Brain Res., **1:** 65–81.

HAMPSON, J. L., HARRISON, C. R., AND WOOLSEY, C. N. 1952. Cerebro-cerebellar projections and the somatotopic localization of motor function in the cerebellum. Proc. Assoc. Res. Nerv. Ment. Dis., **30:** 299–316.

HANAWAY, J., AND YOUNG, R. R. 1977. Localization of the pyramidal tract in the internal capsule of man. J. Neurol. Sci., **34:** 63–70.

HANAWAY, J., SCOTT, W. R., AND STROTHER, C. M. 1980. *Atlas of the Human Brain and the Orbit for Computer Tomography,* Ed. 2. Warren H. Green, II, Inc., St. Louis.

HAND, P. J. 1966. Lumbosacral dorsal root terminations in the nucleus gracilis of the cat: Some observations on terminal degeneration in other medullary sensory nuclei. J. Comp. Neurol., **126:** 137–156.

HARA, K., AND FUJINO, Y. 1966. The thalamoperforating artery. Acta Radiol., **5:** 192–200.

HARDY, H., AND HEIMER, L. 1977. A safer and more sensitive substitute for diaminobenzidine in the light microscopic demonstration of retrograde and anterograde axonal transport of HRP. Neurosci. Lett., **5:** 235–240.

HARNOIS, C., AND FILION, M. 1980. Pallidal neurons branching to the thalamus and to the midbrain in the monkey. Brain Res., **186:** 222–225.

HARRIS, F. S., AND RHOTON, A. L., JR. 1976. Anatomy of the cavernous sinus: A microsurgical study. J. Neurosurg., **45:** 169–180.

HARRIS, G. W. 1948. Electrical stimulation of the hypothalamus and the mechanism of neural control of the adenohypophysis. J. Physiol., **107:** 418–429.

Harris, G. W., and George R. 1969. Neurohumoral control of the adenohypophysis and regulation of the secretion of TSH, ACTH and growth hormone. In W. Haymaker *et al.* (Editors), *The Hypothalamus.* Charles C Thomas, Springfield, Ill., Ch. 10, pp. 326–388.

Harris, G. W., and Woods, J. W. 1958. The effects of electrical stimulation of the hypothalamus or pituitary gland on thyroid activity. J. Physiol., **143:** 246–274.

Harrison, J. M., and Howe, M. E. 1974. Anatomy of the afferent auditory nervous system in mammals. In W. D. Keidel and W. D. Neff (Editors), *Handbook of Sensory Physiology,* Vol. III. Springer-Verlag, Berlin, pp. 283–336.

Harting, J. K. 1977. Descending pathways from the superior colliculus: An autoradiographic analysis in the rhesus monkey (*Macaca mulatta*). J. Comp. Neurol., **173:** 583–612.

Harting, K. J., Hall, W. C., Diamond, I. T., and Martin, G. F. 1973. Anterograde degeneration study of the superior colliculus in *Tupaia glis*: Evidence for a subdivision between superficial and deep layers. J. Comp. Neurol., **148:** 361–386.

Harting, J. K., Casagrande, V. A., and Weber, J. T. 1978. The projection of the primate superior colliculus upon the dorsal lateral geniculate nucleus: Autoradiographic demonstration of intralaminar distribution of tectogeniculate axons. Brain Res., **150:** 593–599.

Hartmann-von Monakow, K., Akert, K., and Künzle, H. 1978. Projections of the precentral motor cortex and other cortical areas of the frontal lobe to the subthalamic nucleus in the monkey. Exp. Brain Res., **33:** 395–403.

Hartmann-von Monakow, K., Akert, K., and Künzle, H. 1979. Projections of the precentral and premotor cortex to the red nucleus and other midbrain areas in *Macaca fascicularis.* Exp. Brain Res., **34:** 91–105.

Hassler, O. 1966. Blood supply to the human spinal cord. Arch. Neurol., **15:** 302–307.

Hassler, O. 1967. Arterial pattern of human brain stem. Normal appearance and deformation in expanding supratentorial conditions. Neurology, **17:** 368–375.

Hassler, R. 1939. Zur pathologischen Anatomie des senilen und des parkinsonistischen Tremor. J. Psychol. Neurol., **49:** 193–230.

Hattori, T., and McGeer, E. G. 1977. Fine structural changes in the rat striatum after local injections of kainic acid. Brain Res., **129:** 174–180.

Hattori, T., McGeer, P. L., Fibiger, H. C., and McGeer, E. G. 1973. On the source of GABA-containing terminals of the substantia nigra. Electron microscopic, autotradiographic and biochemical studies. Brain Res., **54:** 103–114.

Hattori, T., Fibiger, H. C., and McGeer, P. L. 1975. Demonstration of a pallido-nigral projection innervating dopaminergic neurons. J. Comp. Neurol., **162:** 487–504.

Hattori, T., McGeer, E. G., and McGeer, P. L. 1979. Fine structural analysis of the cortico-striatal pathway. J. Comp. Neurol., **185:** 347–354.

Hayhow, W. R. 1958. The cytoarchitecture of the lateral geniculate body in the cat in relation to the distribution of crossed and uncrossed optic fibers. J. Comp. Neurol., **110:** 1–64.

Haymaker, W. 1956. *Bing's Local Diagnosis in Neurological Diseases.* C. V. Mosby, St. Louis.

Haymaker, W. 1969. Hypothalamo-pituitary neural pathways and the circulatory system of the pituitary. In W. Haymaker *et al.* (Editors), *The Hypothalamus.* Charles C Thomas, Springfield, Ill., Ch. 6, pp. 219–250.

Haymaker, W., and Woodhall, B. 1945. *Peripheral Nerve Injuries: Principles of Diagnosis.* W. B. Saunders, Philadelphia, 227 pp.

Head, H. 1920. *Studies in Neurology.* Oxford University Press, London, 2 Vols.

Heath, C. J., and Jones, E. G. 1971. An experimental study of ascending connections from the posterior group of thalamic nuclei in the cat. J. Comp. Neurol., **141:** 397–426.

Hedreen, J. C., Struble, R. G., Whitehouse, P. J., and Price, D. L. 1984. Topography of the magnocellular basal forebrain system in human brain. J. Neuropathol. Exp. Neurol., **43:** 1–21.

Heidary, H., and Tomasch, J. 1969. Neuron numbers and perikaryon areas in the human cerebellar nuclei. Acta Anat. (Basel), **74:** 290–296.

Heimer, L., and Nauta, W. J. H. 1967. The hypothalamic distribution of the stria terminalis in the rat. Anat. Rec., **157:** 259.

Heimer, L., and Nauta, W. J. H. 1969. The hypothalamic distribution of the stria terminals in the rat. Brain Res., **13:** 284–297.

Heller, H. 1966. The hormone content of the vertebrate hypothalamo-neurohypophysial system. Br. Med. Bull., **22:** 227–231.

Henderson, Z. 1981. Ultrastructure and acetylcholinesterase content of neurones forming connections between the striatum and substantia nigra of rat. J. Comp. Neurol., **197:** 185–196.

Hendrickson, A. M., Wilson, M. E., and Toyne, M. J. 1970. The distribution of optic nerve fibers in *Macaca mulatta.* Brain Res., **23:** 425–427.

Hendrickson, A. E., Wagoner, N., and Cowan, W. M. 1972. An autoradiographic and electron microscopic study of retino-hypothalamic connections. Z. Zellforsch. Mikrosk. Anat., **135:** 1–26.

Hendry, S. H., Jones, E. G., and Graham, J. 1979. Thalamic relay nuclei for cerebellar and certain related fiber systems in the cat. J. Comp. Neurol., **185:** 679–713.

Herkenham, M., and Nauta, W. J. H. 1977. Afferent connections of the habenular nuclei in the rat: A horseradish peroxidase study, with a note on the fiber-of-passage problem. J. Comp. Neurol., **173:** 123–145.

Herzog, A. G., and van Hoesen, G. W. 1976. Temporal neocortical afferent connections to the amygdala in the rhesus monkey. Brain Res., **115:** 57–70.

Hess, W. R. 1954. *Diencephalon, Autonomic and Extrapyramidal Functions.* Grune & Stratton, New York.

Hickey, T. L., and Guillery, R. W. 1974. An autoradiographic study of retinogeniculate pathways in the cat and the fox. J. Comp. Neurol., **156:** 239–254.

Hickey, T. L., and Guillery, R. W. 1979. Variability of laminar patterns in the human lateral geniculate nucleus. J. Comp. Neurol., **183:** 221–246.

Highstein, S. M. 1977. Abducens and oculomotor internuclear neurons: Relation to gaze. In A. Ber-

THOZ AND R. BAKER (Editors), *Control of Gaze by Brain Stem Neurons* (Developments in Neuroscience, Vol. 1). Elsevier/North-Holland, Amsterdam, pp. 153–162.

HILD, W. 1956. Neurosecretion in the central nervous system. In W. S. FIELDS *et al.* (Editors), *Hypothalamic-Hypophysial Interrelationships.* Charles C Thomas, Springfield, Ill., pp. 17–25.

HILTON, S. M., AND ZBROŻYNA, A. 1963. Defense reaction from the amygdala and its afferent connections. J. Physiol., **165:** 160–173.

HODDEVIK, G. H. 1975. The pontocerebellar projection onto the paramedian lobule in the cat: An experimental study with the use of horseradish peroxidase as a tracer. Brain Res., **95:** 291–307.

HÖKFELT, T. 1967. The possibile ultrastructural identification of tubero-infundibular dopamine-containing nerve endings in the median eminence of the rat. Brain Res., **5:** 121–123.

HÖKFELT, T., AND FUXE, K. 1969. Cerebellar monoamine nerve terminals: A new type of afferent fiber to the cerebellar cortex. Exp. Brain Res., **9:** 63–72.

HÖKFELT, T., AND UNDERSTEDT, U. 1969. Electron and fluorescence microscopical studies on the nucleus caudatus putamen of the rat after unilateral lesions of ascending nigro-neostriatal dopamine neurons. Acta Physiol. Scand., **76:** 415–426.

HÖKFELT, T., KELLERTH, J.-O., NILSSON, G., AND PERNOW, B. 1975. Experimental immunohistochemical studies on the localization and distribution of substance P in cat primary sensory neurons. Brain Res., **100:** 235–252.

HÖKFELT, T., JOHANSSON, O., FUXE, K., GOLDSTEIN, M., AND PARK, D. 1976. Immunohistochemical studies on the localization and distribution of monoamine neuron systems in the rat brain. I. Tyrosine hydroxylase in the mesencephalon and diencephalon. Med. Biol., **54:** 427–453.

HÖKFELT, T., JOHANSSON, O., KELLERTH, J.-O., LJUNGDAHL, Å., NILSSON, G., NYGÅRDS, A., AND PERNOW, B. 1977. Immunohistochemical distribution of substance P. In U. S. VON EULER AND B. PERNOW (Editors), *Substance P.* Raven Press, New York, pp. 117–145.

HÖKFELT, T. A., LJUNGDAHL, A., TERENIUS, L., ELDE, R., AND NILSSON, G. 1977a. Immunohistochemical analysis of peptide pathways possibly related to pain and analgesia: Enkephalin and substance P. Proc. Natl. Acad. Sci. U.S.A., **74:** 3081–3085.

HOLLÄNDER, H. 1974. Projections from the striate cortex of the diencephalon in the squirrel monkey (*Saimiri sciureus*): A light microscopic radioautographic study following intracortical injection of ^{3}H-leucine. J. Comp. Neurol., **155:** 424–440.

HOLLÄNDER, H., AND VANEGAS, H. 1977. The projection from the lateral geniculate nucleus onto the visual cortex in the cat: A quantitative study with horseradish peroxidase. J. Comp. Neurol., **173:** 519–536.

HONG, J. S., YANG, H.-Y. T., RACAGNI, G., AND COSTA, E. 1977. Projections of substance P-containing neurons from neostriatum to substantia nigra. Brain Res., **122:** 541–544.

HOPKINS, D. A., AND NIESSEN, L. W. 1976. Substantia nigra projections to the reticular formation, superior colliculus and central gray in rat, cat, and monkey. Neurosci. Lett., **2:** 253–259.

HORNYKIEWICZ, O. 1966. Metabolism of brain dopamine in human parkinsonism: Neurochemical and clinical aspects. In E. COSTA et al. (Editors), *Biochemistry and Pharmacology.* Raven Press, Hewlett, N.Y., pp. 171–185.

HOSOYA, Y., AND MATSUSHITA, M. 1979. Identification and distribution of the spinal and hypophyseal projection neurons in the paraventricular nucleus of the rat: A light and electron microscopic study with the horseradish peroxidase method. Exp. Brain Res., **35:** 315–331.

HUBBARD, J. I., AND OSCARSSON, O. 1962. Localization of the cell bodies of the ventral spinocerebellar tract in lumbar segments of the cat. J. Comp. Neurol., **118:** 199–204.

HUBEL, D. H. 1963. The visual cortex of the brain. Sci. Am., **209:** 54–62.

HUBEL, D. H., AND WIESEL, T. N. 1959. Receptive fields of single neurons in the cat's striate cortex. J. Physiol., **148:** 574–591.

HUBEL, D. H., AND WIESEL, T. N. 1961. Integrative action in the cat's lateral geniculate body. J. Physiol., **155:** 385–398.

HUBEL, D. H., AND WIESEL, T. N. 1962. Receptive fields, binocular interaction and functional architecture in the cat's visual cortex. J. Physiol., **160:** 106–154.

HUBEL, D. H., AND WIESEL, T. N. 1963. Receptive fields of cells in striate cortex of very young, visually inexperienced kittens. J. Neurophysiol., **26:** 994–1002.

HUBEL, D. H., AND WIESEL, T. N. 1963a. Shape and arrangement of columns in the cat's striate cortex. J. Physiol., **165:** 559–568.

HUBEL, D. H., AND WIESEL, T. N. 1965. Receptive fields and functional architecture in two non-striate visual areas (18 and 19) of the cat. J. Neurophysiol., **28:** 229–289.

HUBEL, D. H., AND WIESEL, T. N. 1967. Cortical and callosal connections concerned with the vertical meridian of visual fields in the cat. J. Neurophysiol., **30:** 1561–1573.

HUBEL, D. H., AND WIESEL, T. N. 1968. Receptive fields and functional architecture of monkey striate cortex. J. Physiol., **195:** 215–243.

HUBEL, D. H., AND WIESEL, T. N. 1970. Stereoscopic vision in macaque monkey. Nature, **225:** 41–42.

HUBEL, D. H., AND WIESEL, T. N. 1972. Laminar and columnar distribution of geniculocortical fibers in the macaque monkey. J. Comp. Neurol., **146:** 421–450.

HUBEL, D. H., AND WIESEL, T. N. 1974. Sequence regularity and geometry of orientation columns in the monkey striate cortex. J. Comp. Neurol., **158:** 267–294.

HUBEL, D. H., AND WIESEL, T. N. 1974a. Uniformity of monkey striate cortex: A parallel relationship between field size, scatter and magnification factor. J. Comp. Neurol., **158:** 295–306.

HUBEL, D. H., LEVAY, S., AND WIESEL, T. N. 1975. Mode of termination of retino-tectal fibers in macaque monkey: An autoradiographic study. Brain Res., **96:** 25–40.

HUBEL, D. H., WIESEL, T. N., AND LEVAY, S. 1977. Plasticity of ocular dominance columns in monkey striate cortex. Philos. Trans. R. Soc. Lond. (Biol.), **278:** 377–409.

HUGHES, J., SMITH, T., KOSTERLITZ, H., FOTHER-

GILL, L., MORGAN, B., AND MORRIS, H. 1975. Identification of two related pentapeptides from the brain with potent opiate agonist activity. Nature, **258:** 577–579.

IBUKA, N., INOUYE, S. T., AND KAWAMURA, H. 1977. Analysis of sleep-wakefulness rhythms in male rats after suprachiasmatic nucleus lesions and ocular enucleations. Brain Res., **122:** 33–47.

IMIG, T. J., AND ADRIAN, H. O. 1977. Binaural columns in the primary field (AI) of cat auditory cortex. Brain Res., **138:** 241–257.

IMIG, T. J., RUGGERO, M. A., KITZES, L. M., JAVEL, E., AND BRUGGE, J. F. 1977. Organization of auditory cortex in the owl monkey (*Aotus trivirgatus*). J. Comp. Neurol., **171:** 111–128.

ITO, M., AND YOSHIDA, M. 1966. The origin of cerebellar-induced inhibition of Deiters' neurones. I. Monosynaptic initiation of the inhibitory postsynaptic potentials. Exp. Brain Res., **2:** 330–349.

ITO, M., YOSHIDA, M., AND OBATA, K. 1964. Monosynaptic inhibition of the intracerebellar nuclei induced from the cerebellar cortex. Experientia, **20:** 575–576.

ITO, M., YOSHIDA, M., OBATA, K., KAWAI, N., AND UDO, M. 1970. Inhibitory control of intracerebellar nuclei by the Purkinje cell axons. Exp. Brain Res., **10:** 64–80.

ITOH, K., AND MIZUNO, N. 1977. Topographical arrangement of thalamocortical neurons in the centrolateral nucleus (CL) of the cat with special reference to a spino-thalamomotor cortical path through CL. Exp. Brain Res., **30:** 471–480.

IVERSEN, L. L. 1972. The uptake, storage, release and metabolism of GABA in inhibitory nerves. In S. H. SYNDER (Editor), Prospectives in Neuropharmacology. Oxford University Press, London, pp. 75–111.

JACKSON, A., AND CROSSMAN, A. R. 1981. Subthalamic projection to nucleus tegmenti pedunculopontinus in the rat. Neurosci. Lett., **22:** 17–22.

JACKSON, I. M. D. 1981. Neural peptides in the cerebrospinal fluid. Adv. Biochem. Psychopharmacol., **28:** 337–356.

JACOBS, B. L., AND TRULSON, M. E. 1979. Mechanisms of action of LSD. Am. Sci., **67:** 396–404.

JANE, J. A., MASTERSON, R. B., AND DIAMOND, I. 1965. The function of the tectum for attention to auditory stimuli in the cat. J. Comp. Neurol., **125:** 165–192.

JANSEN, J., AND BRODAL, A. 1940. Experimental studies on the intrinsic fibers of the cerebellum. II. The corticonuclear projection. J. Comp. Neurol., **73:** 267–321.

JANSEN, J., AND BRODAL, A. 1958. Das Kleinhirn. In W. VON MÖLLENDORFF (Editor), *Handbuch der mikroskopischen Anatomie des Menschen*, Vol. III. J. Springer, Berlin, pp. 1–323.

JASPER, H. H. 1949. Diffuse projection systems: The integrative action of the thalamic reticular system. Electroencephalogr. Clin. Neurophysiol., **1:** 405–420.

JASPER, H. H. 1960. Unspecific thalamocortical relations. In J. FIELD (Editor), *Handbook of Physiology*, Sect. 1, Vol. II. American Physiological Society, Washington, D.C., Ch. 53, pp. 1307–1321.

JAYARAMAN, A., AND UPDYKE, B. V. 1979. Organization of visual cortical projections to the claustrum in the cat. Brain Res., **178:** 107–115.

JAYARAMAN, A., BATTON, R. R., III, AND CARPENTER, M. B. 1977. Nigrotectal projections in the monkey: An autoradiographic study. Brain Res., **135:** 147–152.

JAYATILAKA, A. D. P. 1965. Arachnoid granulations in sheep. J. Anat., **99:** 315–327.

JAYATILAKA, A. D. P. 1965a. An electron microscopic study of sheep arachoid granulations. J. Anat., **99:** 635–649.

JESSELL, T. M. 1981. The role of substance P in sensory transmission and pain perception. In J. B. MARTIN, S. REICHLIN, AND K. L. BICK (Editors), *Neurosecretion and Brain Peptides*. Raven Press, New York, pp. 189–198.

JESSELL, T. M., AND IVERSEN, L. L. 1977. Opiate analgesics inhibit substance P release from rat trigeminal nucleus. Nature, **268:** 549–551.

JESSELL, T. M., EMSON, P. C., PAXINOS, G., AND CUELLO, A. C. 1978. Topographical projections of substance P and GABA pathways in the striato- and pallido-nigral system: A biochemical and immunohistochemical study. Brain Res., **152:** 487–498.

JONES, B. E., AND MOORE, R. Y. 1977. Ascending projections and the locus coerruleus in the rat. II. Autoradiographic study. Brain Res., **127:** 23–53.

JONES, B. E., BOBILLER, P., PIN, C., AND JOUVET, M. 1973. The effects of lesions of catecholamine-containing neurons upon monoamine content of the brain and EEG and behavioral waking in the cat. Brain Res., **58:** 157–177.

JONES, B. E., HARPER, S. T., AND HALARIS, A. E. 1977. Effects of locus coeruleus lesions upon cerebral monoamine content, sleep-wakefulness states and the response to amphetamine in the cat. Brain Res., **124:** 473–496.

JONES, E. G. 1969. Interrelationships of parieto-temporal and frontal cortex in the rhesus monkey. Brain Res., **13:** 412–415.

JONES, E. G. 1975. Some aspects of the organization of the thalamic reticular complex. J. Comp. Neurol., **162:** 285–308.

JONES, E. G. 1981. Anatomy of cerebral cortex: Columnar input-output organization. In F. O. SCHMITT, F. G. WORDEN, G. ADELMAN, AND S. G. DENNIS (Editors), *The Organization of the Cerebral Cortex*. MIT Press, Cambridge, Mass., pp. 199–235.

JONES, E. G. 1983. Distribution patterns of individual medial lemniscus axons in the ventrobasal complex of the monkey thalamus. J. Comp. Neurol., **215:** 1–16.

JONES, E. G., AND BURTON, H. 1974. Cytoarchitecture and somatic sensory connectivity of thalamic nuclei other than the ventrobasal complex in the cat. J. Comp. Neurol., **154:** 395–432.

JONES, E. G., AND HENDRY, S. H. C. 1980. Distribution of callosal fibers around the hand representation in monkey somatic sensory cortex. Neurosci. Lett., **19:** 167–172.

JONES, E. G., AND LEAVITT, R. Y. 1974. Retrograde axonal transport and the demonstration of nonspecific projections to the cerebral cortex and striatum from thalamic intralaminar nuclei in the cat, rat and monkey. J. Comp. Neurol., **154:** 349–378.

JONES, E. G., AND PORTER, R. 1980. What is area 3a? Brain Res. Rev., **2:** 1–43.

JONES, E. G., AND POWELL, T. P. S. 1968. The ipsilateral cortical connexions of the somatic sensory areas in the cat. Brain Res., **9:** 71–94.

JONES, E. G., AND POWELL, T. P. S. 1968a. Projections of the somatic sensory cortex upon the thalamus in the cat. Brain Res., **10:** 369–391.

JONES, E. G., AND POWELL, T. P. S. 1969. Connexions of the somatic sensory cortex of the rhesus monkey. I. Ipsilateral cortical connexions. Brain, **92:** 477–502.

JONES, E. G., AND POWELL, T. P. S. 1969a. Connexions of the somatic sensory cortex of the rhesus monkey. II. Contralateral cortical connexions. Brain, **92:** 717–730.

JONES, E. G., AND POWELL, T. P. S. 1969b. The cortical projections of the ventroposterior nucleus of the thalamus in the cat. Brain Res., **13:** 298–318.

JONES, E. G., AND POWELL, T. P. S. 1970. Connexions of the somatic sensory cortex of the rhesus monkey. III. Thalamic connexions. Brain, **93:** 37–56.

JONES, E. G., AND POWELL, T. P. S. 1970a. An anatomical study of converging sensory pathways within the cerebral cortex of the monkey. Brain, **93:** 793–820.

JONES, E. G., AND POWELL, T. P. S. 1971. An analysis of the posterior group of thalamic nuclei on the basis of its afferent connections. J. Comp. Neurol., **143:** 185–216.

JONES, E. G., AND POWELL, T. P. S. 1973. Anatomical organization of the somatosensory cortex. In A. IGGO (Editor), *Handbook of Sensory Physiology*, Vol. 2. Springer-Verlag, Berlin, pp. 579–620.

JONES, E. G., AND WISE, S. P. 1977. Size, laminar and columnar distribution of efferent cells in the sensory-motor cortex of monkeys. J. Comp. Neurol., **175:** 391–438.

JONES, E. G., COULTER, J. D., BURTON, H., AND PORTER, R. 1977. Cells of origin and terminal distribution of corticostriatal fibers arising in the sensory-motor cortex of monkeys. J. Comp. Neurol., **173:** 53–80.

JONES, E. G., COULTER, J. D., AND HENDRY, S. H. C. 1978. Intracortical connectivity of architectonic fields in the somatic sensory, motor and parietal cortex of monkeys. J. Comp. Neurol., **181:** 291–348.

JONES, E. G., WISE, S. P., AND COULTER, J. D. 1979. Differential thalamic relationships of sensory-motor and parietal cortical fields in monkeys. J. Comp. Neurol., **183:** 833–881.

JOUVET, M. 1967. Neurophysiology of the states of sleep. Physiol. Rev., **47:** 117–177.

JOUVET, M. 1969. Biogenic amines and the states of sleep. Science, **163:** 32–41.

KAADA, B. R. 1951. Somatomotor, autonomic and electrocorticographic responses to electrical stimulation of "rhinencephalic" and other structures in primates, cat and dog. Acta Physiol., Scand., **24:** Suppl. 83, 285 pp.

KAADA, B. R. 1960. Cingulate posterior orbital, anterior insular and temporal pole cortex. In J. FIELD (Editor), *Handbook of Physiology*, Sect. 1, Vol. II. American Physiological Society, Washington, D.C., Ch. 55, pp. 1345–1372.

KAADA, B. R. 1972. Stimulation and regional ablation of the amygdaloid complex with reference to functional representation. In B. E. ELEFTHERIOU (Editor). *The Neurobiology of the Amygdala.* Plenum Press, New York, pp. 205–281.

KAAS, J. H., GUILLERY, R. W., AND ALLMAN, J. M. 1972. Some principles of organization in the dorsal lateral geniculate nucleus. Brain Behav. Evol., **6:** 253–299.

KAAS, J. H., HUERTA, M. F., WEBER, J. T., AND HARTING, J. K. 1977. Patterns of retinal terminations and laminar organization of the lateral geniculate nucleus of primates. J. Comp. Neurol., **182:** 517–554.

KALIA, M. 1977. Neuroanatomical organization of the respiratory centers. Fed. Proc., **36:** 2405–2411.

KALIA, M., AND MESULAM, M.-M. 1980. Brain stem projections of sensory and motor components of the vagus complex in the cat. I. The cervical vagus and nodose ganglion. J. Comp. Neurol., **193:** 435–465.

KALIA, M., AND MESULAM, M.-M. 1980a. Brain stem projections of sensory and motor components of the vagus complex in the cat. II. Laryngeal tracheobronchial, pulmonary, cardiac, and gastrointestinal branches. J. Comp. Neurol., **193:** 467–508.

KALIL, K. 1975. Thalamo-cortical projections of VA and VL in the rhesus monkey. Neurosci. Abstr., Soc. Neurosci., **1:** 171.

KALIL, K. 1978. Patch-like termination of thalamic fibers in the putamen of the rhesus monkey: An autoradiographic study. Brain Res., **140:** 333–339.

KALIL, K. 1979. Projections of the cerebellar and dorsal column nuclei upon inferior olive in the rhesus monkey: An autoradiographic study. J. Comp. Neurol., **188:** 43–62.

KALIL, K. 1981. Projections of the cerebellar and dorsal column nuclei upon the thalamus of the rhesus monkey. J. Comp. Neurol., **195:** 25–50.

KANAZAWA, I., MARSHALL, G. R., AND KELLY, J. S. 1976. Afferents to the rat substantia nigra studied with horseradish peroxidase, with special reference to fibers from the subthalamic nucleus. Brain Res., **115:** 485–491.

KANAZAWA, I., EMSON, P. C., AND CUELLO, A. C. 1977. Evidence for the existence of substance P-containing fibers in striato-nigral and pallido-nigral pathways in rat brain. Brain Res., **119:** 447–453.

KAROL, E. A., AND PANDYA, D. N. 1971. The distribution of the corpus callosum in the rhesus monkey. Brain, **94:** 471–486.

KATZMAN, R. 1976. The prevalence and malignancy of Alzheimer's disease. A major killer. Arch. Neurol., **33:** 217–218.

KAWAMURA, S., SPRAGUE, J. M., AND NIIMI, K. 1974. Corticofugal projections from the visual cortices to the thalamus in the cat. J. Comp. Neurol., **158:** 339–362.

KELLEY, A. E., DOMESICK, V. B., AND NAUTA, W. J. H. 1982. The amygdalostriate projection in the rat: An anatomical study by anterograde and retrograde tracing methods. Neuroscience, **7:** 615–630.

KELLY, J. P., AND GILBERT, C. D. 1975. The projection of different morphological types of ganglion cells in the cat's retina. J. Comp. Neurol., **163:** 65–80.

KELLY, J. P., AND VAN ESSEN, D. C. 1974. Cell structure and function in the visual cortex of the cat. J. Physiol. (Lond.), **238:** 515–547.

KEMEL, M. L., GAUCHY, C., ROMO, R., GLOWINSKI,

J., AND BESSON, M. J. 1983. *In vivo* release of [^{3}H] GABA in cat caudate nucleus and substantia nigra. I. Bilateral changes induced by a unilateral nigral application of muscimol. Brain Res., **272:** 331–340.

KEMP, J. M. 1968. An electron microscopic study of the terminations of afferent fibers in the caudate nucleus. Brain Res., **11:** 464–467.

KEMP, J. M. 1970. The termination of strio-pallidal and strio-nigral fibers. Brain Res., **17:** 125–128.

KEMP, J. M., AND POWELL, T. P. S. 1970. The cortico-striate projection in the monkey. Brain, **93:** 525–546.

KEMP, J. M., AND POWELL, T. P. S. 1971. The structure of the caudate nucleus of the cat: Light and electron microscopy. Philos. Trans. R. Soc. Lond. (Biol.), **262:** 383–401.

KEMP, J. M., AND POWELL, T. P. S. 1971a. The site of termination of afferent fibers in the caudate nucleus. Philos. Trans. R. Soc. Lond. (Biol.), **262:** 413–427.

KEMP, J. M., AND POWELL, T. P. S. 1971b. The connexions of the striatum and globus pallidus: Synthesis and speculation. Philos. Trans. R. Soc. Lond. (Biol.), **262:** 441–457.

KENNEDY, C., DES ROSIERS, M. H., JEHLE, J. W., REIVICH, M., SHARP, F., AND SOKOLOFF, L. 1975. Mapping of functional neural pathways by autoradiographic survey of local metabolic rate with [^{14}C] deoxyglucose. Science, **187:** 850–853.

KENNEDY, C., DES ROSIERS, M. H., SAKURADA, O., SHINOHARA, M., REIVICH, M., JEHLE, J. W., AND SOKOLOFF, L. 1976. Metabolic mapping of the primary visual system of the monkey by means of the autoradiographic [^{14}C]deoxyglucose technique. Proc. Natl. Acad. Sci. U.S.A., **73:** 4230–4234.

KERR, F. W. L. 1961. Structural relation of the trigeminal spinal tract to upper cervical roots and the solitary nucleus in the cat. Exp. Neurol., **4:** 134–148.

KERR, F. W. L. 1963. The divisional organization of afferent fibers of the trigeminal nerve. Brain, **86:** 721–732.

KERR, F. W. L. 1969. Preserved vagal visceromotor function following destruction of the dorsal motor nucleus. J. Physiol. (Lond.), **202:** 755–769.

KERR, F. W. L. 1975. Neuroanatomical substrates of nociception in the spinal cord. Pain, **1:** 325–356.

KERR, F. W. L., AND LIPPMAN, H. H. 1974. The primate spinothalamic tract as demonstrated by anterolateral cordotomy and commissural myelotomy. Adv. Neurol., **4:** 147–156.

KERR, F. W. L., AND PRESHAW, R. M. 1969. Secretomotor function of the dorsal motor nucleus of the vagus. J. Physiol., **205:** 405–415.

KETY, S. S., AND SCHMIDT, C. F. 1948. The nitrous oxide method for the quantitative determination of cerebral blood flow in man. Theory, procedure and normal values. J. Clin. Invest., **27:** 484–492.

KIEVIT, J., AND KUYPERS, H. G. J. M. 1977. Organization of the thalamo-cortical connexions to the frontal lobe in the rhesus monkey. Exp. Brain Res., **29:** 299–322.

KIM, R., NAKANO, K., JAYARAMAN, A., AND CARPENTER, M. B. 1976. Projections of the globus pallidus and adjacent structures: An autoradiographic study in the monkey. J. Comp. Neurol., **169:** 263–289.

KIMURA, H., MCGEER, P. L., PENG, F., AND MCGEER, E. G. 1980. Choline acetyltransferase-containing neurons in rodent brain demonstrated by immunohistochemistry. Science, **208:** 1057–1059.

KITA, H., CHANG, H. T., AND KITAI, S. T. 1983. Pallidal inputs to subthalamus: Intracellular analysis. Brain Res., **264:** 255–265.

KITA, H., CHANG, H. T., AND KITAI, S. T. 1983a. The morphology of intracellularly labeled rat subthalamic neurons: A light microscopic analysis. J. Comp. Neurol., **215:** 245–257.

KITAI, S. T. 1981. Anatomy and physiology of the neostriatum. In G. DICHIARA AND G. L. GESSA (Editors), *GABA and the Basal Ganglia.* Raven Press, New York, pp. 1–21.

KITAI, S. T., AND DENIAU, J. M. 1981. Cortical inputs to the subthalamus: Intracellular analysis. Brain Res., **214:** 411–415.

KITAI, S. T., KOCSIS, J. D., AND WOOD, J. 1976. Origin and characteristics of the cortico-caudate afferents: An anatomical and electrophysiological study. Brain Res., **118:** 137–141.

KLEIN, D. C., AND MOORE, R. Y. 1979. Pineal N-acetyltransferase and hydroxyindole-*o*-methyltransferase: Control by the retinohypothalamic tract and the suprachiasmatic nucleus. Brain Res., **174:** 245–262.

KLEIN, D. C., AND WELLER, J. L. 1970. Indole metabolism in the pineal gland: A circadian rhythm in N-acetyltransferase. Science, **169:** 1093–1095.

KLEIN, D. C., AND WELLER, J. L. 1972. A rapid light-induced decrease in pineal serotonin N-acetyltransferase activity. Science, **177:** 532–533.

KLEIN, D. C., WELLER, J. L., AND MOORE, R. Y. 1971. Melatonin metabolism: Neural regulation of pineal serotonin N-acetyltransferase. Proc. Natl. Acad. Sci. U.S.A., **68:** 3107–3110.

KLEIN, D. C., AUERBACH, D. A., NAMBOOIRI, A. A., AND WHELER, G. H. T. 1981. Indole metabolism in mammalian pineal gland. In R. J. REITER (Editor), *The Pineal Gland.* CRC Press, Boca Raton, Fla., Ch. 8, pp. 199–227.

KLEITMAN, N. 1963. *Sleep and Wakefulness.* University of Chicago Press, Chicago.

KLÜVER, H. 1952. Brain mechanisms and behavior with special reference to the rhinencephalon. Lancet, **72:** 567–574.

KLÜVER, H., AND BUCY, P. 1939. Preliminary analysis of functions of the temporal lobes in monkeys. Arch. Neurol. Psychiatry, **42:** 979–1000.

KNIGGE, K. M., AND SILVERMAN, A. J. 1974. The anatomy of the endocrine hypothalamus. In R. O. GREEP AND E. B. ASTWOOD (Editors), *Handbook of Physiology*, Sect. 7, Vol. IV. American Physiological Society, Washington, D.C., Ch. 1, pp. 1–32.

KNIGHTON, R. S. 1950. Thalamic relay nucleus for the second somatic sensory receiving area in the cerebral cortex of the cat. J. Comp. Neurol., **92:** 183–192.

KOCSIS, J. D., SUGIMORI, M., AND KITAI, S. T. 1977. Convergence of excitatory synaptic inputs to caudate spiny neurons. Brain Res., **124:** 403–413.

KOLATA, G. 1983. Monkey model of Parkinson's disease. A contaminant of illicit drugs has caused Parkinson's disease in humans and monkeys. Science, **230:** 705.

KORNELIUSSEN, H.K. 1972. Histogenesis of the cerebellar cortex and cortical zones. In O. LARSELL AND

J. Jansen (Editors), *The Comparative Anatomy and Histology of the Cerebellum: The Human Cerebellum, Cerebellar Connections and Cerebellar Cortex.* University of Minnesota Press, Minneapolis, pp. 164–174.

Kosel, K. C., Van Hoesen, G. W., and West, J. R. 1981. Olfactory bulb projections to the parahippocampal area of the rat. J. Comp. Neurol., **198:** 467–482.

Kreig, W. J. S. 1953. *Functional Neuroanatomy.* Blakiston Company, New York.

Krettek, J. E., and Price, J. L. 1974. A direct input from the amygdala to the thalamus and the cerebral cortex. Brain Res., **67:** 169–174.

Krettek, J. E., and Price, J. L. 1974a. Projections from the amygdala to the perirhinal and entorhinal cortices and the subiculum. Brain Res., **71:** 150–154.

Krettek, J. E., and Price, J. L. 1978. Amygdaloid projections to subcortical structures within the forebrain and brainstem in the rat and cat. J. Comp. Neurol., **178:** 225–254.

Kruger, L. 1979. Functional subdivision of the brainstem sensory trigeminal nuclear complex. In J. J. Bonica, J. C. Liebeskind, and D. G. Albe-Fessard (Editors), *Proceedings of the Second World Congress on Pain: Advances in Pain Research and Therapy*, Vol. 3. Raven Press, New York, pp. 197–211.

Kudo, M., and Niimi, K. 1978. Ascending projections of the inferior colliculus on the medial geniculate body in the cat studied by anterograde and retrograde tracing techniques. Brain Res., **155:** 113–117.

Kuffler, S. W. 1953. Discharge patterns and functional organization of mammalian retina. J. Neurophysiol., **16:** 37–68.

Kuhar, M. J., Roth, R. H., and Aghajanian, G. K. 1972. Synthesis of catecholamines in the locus ceruleus from H^3-tryrosine *in vivo.* Biochem. Pharmacol., **21:** 2280–2282.

Kuhlenbeck, H. 1948. The derivatives of the thalamus ventralis in the human brain and their relation to the so-called subthalamus. Milit. Surg., **102:** 433–447.

Kuhlenbeck, H. 1969. Derivation and boundaries of the hypothalamus, with atlas of hypothalamic grisea. In W. Haymaker *et al.* (Editors), *The Hypothalamus.* Charles C Thomas, Springfield, Ill., Ch. 2, pp. 13–60.

Kuhlenbeck, H., and Haymaker, W. 1949. The derivatives of the hypothalamus in the human brain; their relation to the extrapyramidal and autonomic systems. Milit. Surg., **105:** 26–52.

Kumazawa, T. E., Perl, E. R. Burgess, P. R., and Whitehorn, D. 1975. Ascending projections from marginal zone (lamina I) neurons of the spinal dorsal horn. J. Comp. Neurol., **162:** 1–12.

Künzle, H. 1973. The topographic organization of spinal afferents to the lateral reticular nucleus of the cat. J. Comp. Neurol., **149:** 103–116.

Künzle, H. 1975. Bilateral projections from precentral motor cortex to the putamen and other parts of the basal ganglia. Brain Res., **88:** 195–210.

Künzle, H. 1975a. Autoradiographic tracing of the cerebellar projections from the lateral reticular nucleus in the cat. Exp. Brain Res., **22:** 255–266.

Künzle, H. 1976. Thalamic projections from the precentral motor cortex in *Macaca fascicularis.* Brain Res., **105:** 253–267.

Künzle, H. 1978. An autoradiographic analysis of the efferent connections from premotor and adjacent prefrontal regions (areas 6 and 9) in *Macaca fascicularis.* Brain Behav. Evol., **15:** 185–234.

Künzle, H., and Akert, K. 1977. Efferent connections of cortical Area 8 (frontal eye field) in *Macaca fascicularis*: A reinvestigation using the autoradiographic technique. J. Comp. Neurol., **173:** 147–164.

Künzle, H., Akert, K., and Wurtz, R. H. 1976. Projections of area 8 (frontal eye field) to superior colliculus in the monkey: An autoradiographic study. Brain Res., **117:** 487–492.

Kuo, D., Pile, E., and Krauthamer, G. M. 1978. Projections of central medianum to caudate nucleus in the cat as demonstrated by retograde transport of horseradish peroxidase. Neurosci. Abstr. Soc. Neurosci., **4:** 45.

Kuo, J.-S., and Carpenter, M. B. 1973. Organization of pallidothalamic projections in the rhesus monkey. J. Comp. Neurol., **151:** 201–236.

Kuriyama, K., Haber, B., Sisken, B., and Roberts, E. 1966. The γ-amino-butyric acid system in rabbit cerebellum. Proc. Natl. Acad. Sci. U.S.A., **55:** 846–852.

Kusama, T., Mabuchi, M., and Sumino, T. 1971. Cerebellar projections to the thalamic nuclei in monkey. Proc. Jpn. Acad., **47:** 505–510.

Kuypers, H. G. J. M. 1958. Corticobulbar connexions to the pons and lower brainstem in man. An anatomical study. Brain, **81:** 364–388.

Kuypers, H. G. J. M. 1960. Central cortical projections to motor and somato-sensory cell groups. Brain, **83:** 161–184.

Kuypers, H. G. J. M., and Brinkman, J. 1970. Precentral projections to different parts of the spinal intermediate zone in the rhesus monkey. Brain Res., **24:** 29–48.

Kuypers, H. G. J. M., and Lawrence, D. G. 1967. Cortical projections to the red nucleus and the brain stem in the rhesus monkey. Brain Res., **4:** 151–188.

Kuypers, H. G. J. M., and Maisky, V. A. 1975. Retrograde axonal transport of horseradish peroxidase from spinal cord to brain stem cell groups in the cat. Neurosci. Lett., **1:** 9–14.

Kuypers, H. G. J. M., and Tuerk, J. D. 1964. The distribution of cortical fibres within the nuclei cuneatus and gracilis in the cat. J. Anat., **98:** 143–162.

Lammers, H. J. 1972. The neural connections of the amygdaloid complex in mammals. In B. E. Eleftheriou (Editor), *The Neurobiology of the Amygdala.* Plenum Press, New York, pp. 123–144.

La Motte, C. C., Pert, C. B., and Snyder, S. H. 1976. Opiate receptor binding in primate spinal cord: Distribution and changes after dorsal root section. Brain Res., **112:** 407–412.

La Motte, C. C., Snowman, A., Pert, C. B., and Snyder, S. H. 1978. Opiate receptor binding in rhesus monkey brain: Association with limbic structures. Brain Res., **155:** 374–379.

Land, L. J. 1973. Localized projection of olfactory nerves to rabbit olfactory bulb. Brain Res., **63:** 153–166.

LANG, W., BÜTTNER-ENNEVER, J. A., AND BÜTTNER, U. 1979. Vestibular projections to the monkey thalamus: An autoradiographic study. Brain Res., **177:** 3–17.

LANGSTON, J. W., BALLARD, P., TETRUD, J. W., AND IRWIN, I. 1983. Chronic parkinsonism in humans due to a product of meperidine-analog synthesis. Science, **249:** 979–980.

LARSELL, O. 1951. *Anatomy of the Nervous System*, Ed. 2. Appleton-Century-Crofts, New York.

LARSELL, O., AND JANSEN, J. 1972. *The Comparative Anatomy and Histology of the Cerebellum: The Human Cerebellum, Cerebellar Connections and Cerebellar Cortex.* University of Minnesota Press, Minneapolis, 264 pp.

LASSEK, A. M. 1940. The human pyramidal tract. II. A numerical investigation of the Betz cells of the motor area. Arch. Neurol. Psychiatry, **44:** 718–724.

LAVAIL, J. H. 1975. Retrograde cell degeneration and retrograde transport techniques. In W. M. COWAN AND M. CUÉNOD (Editors), *The Use of Axonal Transport for Studies of Neuronal Connectivity.* Elsevier, Amsterdam, pp. 217–247.

LAZORTHES, G., AND SALAMON, G. 1971. The arteries of the thalamus: An anatomical and radiological study. J. Neurosurg., **34:** 23–26.

LAZORTHES, G., POULHES, J., BASTIDE, G., ROLLEAU, J., AND CHANCHOLLE, A. R. 1957. Récherches sur las vascularisation artérielle de la moëlle: Application à la pathologie médullaire. Bull. Acad. Natl. Med. (Paris), **141:** 464–477.

LEONARD, C. M., AND SCOTT, J. W. 1971. Origin and distribution of amygdalofugal pathways in the rat: An experimental neuroanatomical study. J. Comp. Neurol., **144:** 313–330.

LEUSEN, I. 1972. Regulation of cerebrospinal fluid composition with reference to breathing. Physiol. Rev., **52:** 1–56.

LEVAY, S., AND SHERK, H. 1981. The visual claustrum of the cat. I. Structure and connections. J. Neurosci., **1:** 956–980.

LEVAY, S., AND SHERK, H. 1981a. The visual claustrum of the cat. II. The visual field map. J. Neurosci., **1:** 981–992.

LEVAY, S., HUBEL, D., AND WIESEL, T. N. 1975. The pattern of ocular dominance columns in macaque visual cortex revealed by reduced silver stain. J. Comp. Neurol., **159:** 559–576.

LEVAY, S., WIESEL, T. N., AND HUBEL, D. H. 1980. The development of ocular dominance columns in normal and visually deprived monkeys. J. Comp. Neurol., **191:** 1–51.

LEVITT, P., AND MOORE, R. Y. 1979. Origin and organization of brainstem catecholamine innervation in the rat. J. Comp. Neurol., **186:** 505–528.

LIDBRINK, P. 1974. The effects of lesions of ascending noradrenaline pathways on sleep and waking in the cat. Brain Res., **74:** 19–40.

LIEDGREN, S. R. C., MILNE, A. C., RUBIN, A. M., SCHWARZ, D. W. F., AND TOMLINSEN, R. D. 1976. Representation of vestibular afferents in somatosensory thalamic nuclei of the squirrel monkey (*Saimiri sciureus*). J. Neurophysiol., **39:** 601–612.

LIGHT, A. R., AND PERL, E. R. 1979. Reexamination of the dorsal root projection to the spinal dorsal horn including observations on the differential termination of course and fine fibers. J. Comp. Neurol., **186:** 117–132.

LIGHT, A. R., AND PERL, E. R. 1979a. Spinal terminations of functionally identified primary afferent neurons with slowly conducting myelinated fibers. J. Comp. Neurol., **186:** 133–150.

LIGHT, A. R., TREVINO, D. L., AND PERL, E. R. 1979. Morphological features of functionally defined neurons in the marginal zone and substantia gelatinosa of the spinal dorsal horn. J. Comp. Neurol., **186:** 151–172.

LIM, R. K. S., KRAUTHAMER, G., GUZMAN, F., AND FULP, R.R. 1969. Central nervous system activity associated with pain evoked by bradykinin and its alteration by morphine and aspirin. Proc. Natl. Acad. Sci. U.S.A., **63:** 705–712.

LINDSLEY, D. B. 1960. Attention, consciousness, sleep and wakefulness. In J. FIELD (Editor), *Handbook of Physiology*, Sect. 1, Vol. III. American Physiological Society, Washington, D.C., pp. 1553–1593.

LINDVALL, O., AND BJÖRKLUND, A. 1974. The glyoxylic acid fluorescence histochemical method: A detailed account of the methodology for the visualization of central catecholamine neurons. Histochemistry, **39:** 97–127.

LINDVALL, O., AND BJÖRKLUND, A. 1978. Organization of catecholamine neurons in the rat central nervous system. In L. L. IVERSEN, S. D. IVERSEN, AND S. H. SNYDER (Editors), *Handbook of Psychopharmacology*, Vol. 9. Plenum Press, New York, pp. 139–231.

LIU, C. N., AND CHAMBERS, W. W. 1964. An experimental study of the corticospinal system in the monkey (*Macaca mulatta*): The spinal pathways and preterminal distribution of degenerating fibers following discrete lesions of the pre-and postcentral gyri and bulbar pyramid. J. Comp. Neurol., **123:** 257–284.

LIVINGSTON, R. B. 1965. Mechanics of cerebrospinal fluid. In T. C. RUCH AND H. D. PATTON (Editors), *Physiology and Biophysics.* W. B. Saunders, Philadelphia, Ch. 47, pp. 935–940.

LJUNGDAHL, A., HOKFELT, T., AND NILSSON, G. 1978. Distribution of substance P-like immunoreactivity in the central nervous system of the rat. I. Cell bodies and nerve terminals. Neuroscience, **3:** 861–943.

LOEWY, A. D., AND BURTON, H. 1978. Nuclei of the solitary tract: Efferent projections to the lower brain stem and spinal cord of the cat. J. Comp. Neurol., **181:** 421–450.

LOEWY, A. D., AND MCKELLAR, S. 1980. The neuroanatomical basis of central cardiovascular control. Fed. Proc., **39:** 2495–2503.

LOEWY, A. D., AND SAPER, C. B. 1978. Edinger-Westphal nucleus: Projections to the brain stem and spinal cord in the cat. Brain Res., **150:** 1–27.

LOEWY, A. D., SAPER, C. B., AND YAMODIS, N. D. 1978. Re-evaluation of the efferent projections of the Edinger-Westphal nucleus. Brain Res., **141:** 153–159.

LORENTE DE NÓ, R. 1934. Studies on the structure of the cerebral cortex. II. Continuation of the study of the ammonic system. J. Psychol. Neurol., **46:** 113–177.

LORENTE DE NÓ, R. 1949. The structure of the cerebral cortex. In J. F. FULTON (Editor), *Physiology of the Nervous System*, Ed. 3. Oxford University Press, New York, pp. 288–330.

LUND, J. S., LUND, R. D., HENDRICKSON, A. E., BUNT, A. H., AND FUCHS, A. F. 1975. The origin of efferent pathways from the primary visual cortex, area 17, of the macaque monkey as shown by retrograde transport of horseradish peroxidase. J. Comp. Neurol., **164:** 287–304.

MACHNE, X., AND SEGUNDO, J. P. 1956. Unitary responses to afferent volleys in amygdaloid complex. J. Neurophysiol., **19:** 232–240.

MACLEAN, P. D. 1958. Contrasting functions of limbic and neocortical systems of the brain and their relevance of psycho-physiological aspects of medicine. Am. J. Med., **25:** 611–626.

MACLEAN, P. D., AND DELGADO, J. M. R. 1953. Electrical and chemical stimulation of fronto-temporal portion of limbic system in the waking animal. Electroencephalogr. Clin. Neurophysiol., **5:** 91–100.

MADIGAN, J. C., JR., AND CARPENTER, M. B. 1971. *Cerebellum of the Rhesus Monkey: Atlas of Lobules, Laminae, and Folia, in Sections*. University Park Press, Baltimore, 137 pp.

MAEDA, T., AND SHIMIZU, N. 1972. Projections ascendantes du locus coeruleus et d'antres neurones aminergiques pontiques au niveau du prosencéphale du rat. Brain Res., **36:** 19–35.

MAFFEL, L., AND POMPEIANO, O. 1962. Cerebellar control of flexor motoneurons. Arch. Ital. Biol., **100:** 476–509.

MAGNIN, M., AND FUCHS, A. F. 1977. Discharge properties of neurons in the monkey thalamus tested with angular acceleration, eye movement and visual stimuli. Exp. Brain Res., **28:** 293–299.

MAGOUN, H. W. 1954. The ascending reticular system and wakefulness. In J. B. DELAFRESNAYE (Editor), *Brain Mechanisms and Consciousness*. Blackwell Scientific Publications, Oxford, pp. 1–20.

MAGOUN, H. W. 1963. *The Waking Brain*, Ed. 2. Charles C Thomas, Springfield, Ill.

MAGOUN, H. W., AND RHINES, R. 1946. An inhibitory mechanism in the bulbar reticular formation. J. Neurophysiol., **9:** 165–171.

MAINS, R. E., AND EIPPER, B. A. 1976. Biosynthesis of adrenocorticotrophic hormone in mouse pituitary tumor cells. J. Biol. Chem., **251:** 4115–4120.

MALONE, E. F. 1910. Über die Kerne des menschlichen Diencephalon. Aus dem Anhang zu den Abhandlungen der königl. preuss. Akademie der Wissenschaften, p. 92.

MALPELI, J. C., AND BAKER, F. H. 1975. The representation of the visual field in the lateral geniculate nucleus of the *Macaca mulatta*. J. Comp. Neurol., **161:** 569–594.

MANNI, E., BORTOLAMI, R., AND DESOLE, C. 1966. Eye muscle proprioception in the semilunar ganglion. Exp. Neurol., **16:** 226–236.

MARKEE, J. E., SAWYER, C. H., AND HOLLINSHEAD, W. H. 1946. Activation of the anterior hypophysis by electrical stimulation in the rabbit. Endocrinology, **38:** 345–357.

MARTIN, G. F., HENKEL, C. K., AND KING, J. S. 1976. Cerebello-olivary fibers: Their origin, course and distribution in the North American opossum. Exp. Brain Res., **24:** 219–236.

MARTIN, J. B., REICHLIN, S., AND BROWN, G. M. 1977. *Clinical Neuroendocrinology*. F. A. Davis, Philadelphia, pp. 229–246.

MARTIN, J. P. 1967. *The Basal Ganglia and Posture*. Pitman, London, 152 pp.

MARTIN, J. P., AND HURWITZ, L. J. 1962. Locomotion and the basal ganglia. Brain, **85:** 261–276.

MARTINEZ-MILLÁN, L., AND HÖLLANDER, H. 1975. Cortico-cortical projections from striate cortex of the squirrel monkey (*Saimiri sciureus*): A radioautoradiographic study. Brain Res., **83:** 405–417.

MASON, S. T., AND FIBIGER, H. C. 1978. Kainic acid lesions of the striatum: Behavior sequelae similar to Huntington's chorea. Brain Res., **155:** 313–329.

MASON S. T., AND FIBIGER, H. C. 1979. Regional topography within noradrenergic locus coeruleus as revealed by retrograde transport of horseradish peroxidase. J. Comp. Neurol., **187:** 703–724.

MASSERMAN, J. H. 1943. *Behavior and Neurosis*. University of Chicago Press, Chicago, Ill.

MASSION, J. 1967. The mammalian red nucleus. Physiol. Rev., **47:** 383–436.

MATSUSHITA, M., AND HOSOYA, Y. 1978. The location of spinal projection neurons in the cerebellar nuclei (cerebellospinal tract neurons) of the cat: A study with the horseradish peroxidase technique. Brain Res., **142:** 237–248.

MATSUSHITA, M., AND IKEDA, M. 1975. The central cervical nucleus as cell origin of a spinocerebellar tract arising from the cervical cord: A study in the cat using horseradish peroxidase. Brain Res., **100:** 412–417.

MATSUSHITA, M., AND IKEDA, M. 1976. Projections from the lateral reticular nucleus to the cerebellar cortex and nuclei in the cat. Exp. Brain Res., **24:** 403–422.

MATSUSHITA, M., AND IWAHORI, N. 1971. Structural organization of the fastigial nucleus. I. Dendrites and axonal pathways. Brain Res., **25:** 597–610.

MATSUSHITA, M., IKEDA, M., AND HOSOYA, Y. 1979. The location of spinal neurons with long descending axons (long descending propriospinal tract neurons) in the cat: A study with the horseradish peroxidase technique. J. Comp. Neurol., **184:** 63–80.

MATSUSHITA, M., HOSOYA, Y., AND IKEDA, M. 1979a. Anatomical organization of the spinocerebellar system in the cat as studied by retrograde transport of horseradish peroxidase. J. Comp. Neurol., **184:** 81–106.

MATSUSHITA, M., IKEDA, M., AND OKADO, N. 1982. The cells of origin of the trigeminothalamic, trigeminospinal and trigeminocerebellar projections in the cat. Neuroscience, *7:* 1439–1454.

MAYNARD, E. A., SCHULTZ, R. L., AND PEASE, D. C. 1957. Electron microscopy of the vascular bed of rat cerebral cortex. Am. J. Anat., **100:** 409–434.

MCBRIDE, R. L., AND SUTIN, J. 1976. Projections of the locus coeruleus and adjacent pontine tegmentum in the cat. J. Comp. Neurol., **165:** 265–284.

MCBRIDE, R. L., AND SUTIN, J. 1977. Amygdaloid and pontine projections to the ventromedial nucleus of the hypothalamus. J. Comp. Neurol., **174:** 377–396.

MCGEER, P. L., MCGEER, E. G., WADA, J. A., AND JUNG, E. 1971. Effects of globus pallidus lesions and Parkinson's disease on brain glutamic acid decarboxylase. Brain Res., **32:** 425–431.

McGuinness, C. M., and Krauthamer, G. M. 1980. The afferent projections to the centrum medianum of the cat as demonstrated by retrograde transport of horseradish peroxidase. Brain Res., **184:** 255–269.

McNeill, T. H., and Sladek, J. R., Jr. 1980. Simultaneous monoamine histofluorescence and neuropeptide immunocytochemistry. II. Correlative distribution of catecholamine varicosities and supraoptic and paraventricular nuclei. J. Comp. Neurol., **193:** 1023–1033.

Mehler, W. R. 1962. The anatomy of the so-called "pain tract" in man: An analysis of the course and distribution of the ascending fibers of the fasciculus anterolateralis. In J. D. French and R. W. Porter (Editors), *Basic Research in Paraplegia.* Charles C Thomas, Springfield, Ill., pp. 26–55.

Mehler, W. R. 1966. The posterior thalamic region. Confin. Neurol., **27:** 18–29.

Mehler, W. R. 1966a. Some observations on secondary ascending afferent systems in the central nervous system. In R. S. Knighton and P. R. Dumke (Editors), *Pain.* Little, Brown, Boston, Ch. 2, pp. 11–21.

Mehler, W. R. 1966b. Further notes on the center median nucleus of Luys. In D. P. Purpura and M. D. Yahr (Editors), *The Thalamus.* Columbia University Press, New York, pp. 109–127.

Mehler, W. R. 1971. Idea of a new anatomy of the thalamus. J. Psychiatr. Res., **8:** 203–217.

Mehler, W. R. 1974. Central pain and the spinothalamic tract. Adv. Neurol., **4:** 127–146.

Mehler, W. R. 1980. Subcortical afferent connections of the amygdala in the monkey. J. Comp. Neurol., **190:** 733–762.

Mehler, W. R., Feferman, M. E., and Nauta, W. J. G. 1956. Ascending axon degeneration following anterolateral chordotomy in the monkey. Anat. Rec., **124:** 332–333.

Mehler, W. R., Feferman, M. E., and Nauta, W. J. H. 1960. Ascending axon degeneration following anterolateral cordotomy: An experimental study in the monkey. Brain, **83:** 718–750.

Meibach, R. C., and Siegel, A. 1977. Efferent connections of the hippocampal formation in the rat. Brain Res., **124:** 197–224.

Mellgren, S. I., Harkmark, W., and Srebro, B. 1977. Some enzyme histochemical characteristics of the human hippocampus. Cell Tissue Res., **181:** 459–471.

Melzack, R., and Wall, P. D. 1965. Pain mechanisms: A new theory. Science, **150:** 971–979.

Merzenich, M. M., and Brugge, J. F. 1973. Representation of the cochlear partition on the superior temporal plane of the macaque monkey. Brain Res., **50:** 275–296.

Merzenich, M. M., and Reid, M. D. 1974. Representation of the cochlea within the inferior colliculus of the cat. Brain Res., **77:** 397–415.

Merzenich, M. M., Knight, P. L., and Roth, G. L. 1973. Cochleotopic organization of primary auditory cortex in the cat. Brain Res., **63:** 343–346.

Merzenich, M. M., Knight, P. L., and Roth, G. L. 1975. Representation of cochlea within the primary auditory cortex in the cat. J. Neurophysiol., **38:** 231–249.

Merzenich, M. M., Kaas, J. H., Sur, M., and Lin, C. S. 1978. Double representation of the body surface within cytoarchitectonic Areas 3b and 1 in "SI" in the owl monkey (*Aotus trivigatus*). J. Comp. Neurol., **181:** 41–74.

Mestres, P. 1978. Old and new concepts about circumventricular organs: An overview. Scan Electron Microsc. **2:** 137–143.

Mesulam, M.-M. 1978. Tetramethylbenzidine for horseradish peroxidase neurohistochemistry: A noncarcinogenic blue reaction-product with superior sensitivity for visualizing neural afferents and efferents. J. Histochem. Cytochem., **26:** 106–117.

Mesulam, M.-M., Mufson, E. J., Levey, A. I., and Wainer, B. H. 1983. Cholinergic innervation of cortex by the basal forebrain: Cytochemistry and cortical connections of the septal area, diagonal band nuclei, nucleus basalis (substantia innominata) and hypothalamus in the rhesus monkey. J. Comp. Neurol., **214:** 170–197.

Mettler, F. A. 1948. *Neuroanatomy*, ed. 2. C. V. Mosby, St. Louis.

Mettler, F. A. 1949. *Selective Partial Ablation of the Frontal Cortex: A Correlative Study of the Effects on Human Psychotic Subjects.* Paul B. Hoeber, New York, 527 pp.

Mettler, F. A., and Lubin, A. J. 1942. Termination of the brachium pontis. J. Comp. Neurol., **77:** 31–397.

Mettler, F. A., Liss, H. R., and Stevens, G. H. 1956. Blood supply of the primate striopallidum. J. Neuropathol. Exp. Neurol., **15:** 377–383.

Meyers, R. E. 1956. Function of corpus callosum in interocular transfer. Brain, **79:** 358–363.

Meynert, T. 1872. Vom Gehirne der Saugethiere. In S. Stricker (Editor), *Handbuch der Lehre von den Geweben des Menschen und der Thiere.* Engelmann, Leipzig, **2:** 694–808.

Millen, J. W., and Woollam, D. H. M. 1961. Observations on the nature of the pia mater. Brain, **84:** 514–520.

Miller, J. J., Richardson, T. L., Fibiger, H. C., and McLennan, H. 1975. Anatomical and electrophysiological identification of a projection from the mesencephalic raphe to the caudate putamen in the rat. Brain Res. **97:** 133–138.

Miller, R. A., and Strominger, N. L. 1973. Efferent connections of the red nucleus in the brainstem and spinal cord of the rhesus monkey. J. Comp. Neurol., **152:** 327–346.

Miller, R. A., and Strominger, N. L. 1977. An experimental study of the efferent connections of the superior peduncle in the rhesus monkey. Brain Res., **133:** 237–250.

Millhouse, O. E. 1979. A Golgi anatomy of the rodent hypothalamus. In P. Morgane and J. Panksepp (Editors), *Handbook of the Hypothalamus; Vol. I. Anatomy of the Hypothalamus.* Marcel Dekker, New York, pp. 221–265.

Miner, L. C., and Reed, D. J. 1972. Composition of fluid obtained from choroid plexus tissue isolated in a chamber in situ. J. Physiol. (Lond.), **227:** 127–139.

Moon Edley, S. L. 1979. *A Neuroanatomical Study of the Nucleus Tegmenti Pedunculopontinus in the*

Cat. Doctoral dissertation, Massachusetts Institute of Technology, Cambridge, Mass.

MOON EDLEY, S., AND GRAYBIEL, A. M. 1983. The afferent and efferent connections of the feline nucleus tegmenti pedunculopontinus, pars compacta. J. Comp. Neurol., **217:** 187–215.

MOORE, R. Y. 1973. Retinohypothalamic projection in mammals: A comparative study. Brain Res., **49:** 403–409.

MOORE, R. Y., AND GOLDBERG, J. M. 1963. Ascending projections of the inferior colliculus in the cat. J. Comp. Neurol., **121:** 109–136.

MOORE, R. Y., AND KLEIN, C. C. 1974. Visual pathways and the central neural control of a circadian rhythm in pineal serotonin *N*-acetyltransferase activity. Brain Res., **71:** 17–33.

MOORE, R. Y., AND LENN, N. J. 1972. A retinohypothalamic projection in the rat. J. Comp. Neurol., **146:** 1–14.

MOORE, R. Y., AND RAPPORT, R. L. 1970. Pineal and gonadal function in the rat following cervical sympathectomy. Neuroendocrinology, **7:** 361–374.

MOORE, R. Y., BHATNAGAR, R. K., AND HELLER, A. 1971. Anatomical and chemical studies of a nigroneostriatal projection in the cat. Brain Res., **30:** 119–135.

MOORE, R. Y., HALARIS, A. E., AND JONES, B. E. 1978. Serotonin neurons of the midbrain raphe: Ascending projections. J. Comp. Neurol., **180:** 417–438.

MOREST, D. K. 1960. A study of the structure of the area postrema with Golgi methods. Am. J. Anat., **107:** 291–303.

MOREST, D. K. 1964. The neuronal architecture of the medial geniculate body of the cat. J. Anat., **98:** 611–638.

MOREST, D. K. 1965. The laminar structure of the medial geniculate body of the cat. J. Anat., **99:** 143–159.

MOREST, D. K. 1965*a*. The lateral tegmental system of the midbrain and the medial geniculate body: Study with Golgi and Nauta methods in the cat. J. Anat., **99:** 611–634.

MOREST, D. K. 1967. Experimental study of the projections of the nucleus of the tractus solitarius and the area postrema in the cat. J. Comp. Neurol., **130:** 277–299.

MORIN, F. 1955. A new spinal pathway for cutaneous impulses. Am. J. Physiol., **183:** 245–252.

MORISON, R. S., AND DEMPSEY, E. W. 1942. A study of thalamocortical relations. Am. J. Physiol., **135:** 281–292.

MORUZZI, G., AND MAGOUN, H. W. 1949. Brain stem reticular formation and activation of the EEG. Electroencephalogr. Clin. Neurophysiol., **1:** 455–473.

MOSKO, S. S., AND MOORE, R. Y. 1979. Neonatal suprachiasmatic nucleus lesions: Effects on the development of circadian rhythms in the rat. Brain Res., **164:** 17–38.

MOSS, M., MAHUT, H., AND ZOLA-MORGAN, S. 1981. Concurrent discrimination learning of monkeys after hippocampal, entorhinal or fornix lesions. J. Neurosci., **1:** 227–240.

MOULTON, D. G., AND BEIDLER, L. M. 1967. Structure and function in the peripheral olfactory system. Physiol. Rev., **47:** 1–52

MOUNTCASTLE, V. B. 1957. Modality and topographic properties of single neurons of cat's somatic sensory cortex. J. Neurophysiol., **20:** 408–434.

MOUNTCASTLE, V. B. 1974. Sensory receptors and neural encoding: Introduction to sensory processes. In V. B. MOUNTCASTLE (Editor), *Medical Physiology*, Vol. I. C. V. Mosby, St. Louis, pp. 285–306 and 348–381.

MOUNTCASTLE, V. B., AND POWELL, T. P. S. 1959. Central nervous mechanisms subserving position sense and kinesthesis. Bull. Johns Hopkins Hosp., **105:** 173–200.

MOUNTCASTLE, V. B., AND POWELL, T. P. S. 1959a. Neural mechanisms subserving cutaneous sensibility with special reference to the role of afferent inhibition in sensory perception and discrimination. Bull. Johns Hopkins Hosp., **105:** 201–232.

MOUNTCASTLE, V. B., LYNCH, J. C., GEORGOPOULOS, A., SAKATA, H., AND ACUNA, C. 1975. Posterior parietal association cortex of the monkey: Command functions for operation within extrapersonal space. J. Neurophysiol., **38:** 871–908.

MUGNAINI, E. 1972. The histology and cytology of the cerebellar cortex. In O. LARSELL AND J. JANSEN (Editors), *The Comparative Anatomy and Histology of the Cerebellum. The Human Cerebellum, Cerebellar Connections, and Cerebellar Cortex.* University of Minnesota Press, Minneapolis, pp. 201–262.

MUGNAINI, E., AND WALBERG, F. 1967. An experimental electron microscopical study on the mode of termination of cerebellar corticovestibular fibres in the cat lateral vestibular nucleus (Deiters' nucleus). Exp. Brain Res., **4:** 212–236.

MULLAN, S., AND PENFIELD, W. 1959. Illusions of comparative interpretation and emotion. Arch. Neurol. Psychiatry, **81:** 269–284.

MURRAY, E. A., AND COULTER, J. D. 1976. Origins of cortical projections to cervical and lumbar spinal cord in monkey. Neurosci. Abstr. Soc. Neurosci., **2:** 917.

MURRAY, E. A., AND COULTER, J. D. 1977. Corticospinal projections from the medial cerebral hemisphere in monkey. Neurosci. Abstr. Soc. Neurosci., **3:** 275.

NAKAI, Y., AND TAKAORI, S. 1974. Influence of norepinephrine-containing neurons derived from the locus coeruleus on lateral geniculate neuronal activities of cats. Brain Res., **71:** 47–60.

NARABAYASHI, H. 1972. Stereotaxic amygdalotomy. In B. E. ELEFTHERIOU (Editor), *The Neurobiology of the Amygdala.* Plenum Press, New York, pp. 459–483.

NARABAYASHI, H., NAGAO, T., SAITO, Y., YOSHIDA, M., AND NAGAHATA, M. 1963. Stereotaxic amygdalotomy for behavior disorders. Arch. Neurol., **9:** 1–16.

NARKIEWICZ, O. 1964. Degenerations in the claustrum after regional neocortical ablations in the cat. J. Comp. Neurol., **123:** 335–356.

NAROTZKY, R. A., AND KERR, F. W. L. 1978. Marginal neurons of the spinal cord. Brain Res., **139:** 1–20.

NAUTA, H. J. W., AND COLE, M. 1978. Efferent projections of the subthalamic nucleus: An autoradiographic study in monkey and cat. J. Comp. Neurol., **180:** 1–16.

NAUTA, H. J. W., AND CUENOD, M. 1982. Perikaryal cell labeling in the subthalamic nucleus following the injection of [^{3}H]-γ-aminobutyric acid into the pallidal complex: An autoradiographic study in cat. Neuroscience, **7:** 2725–2734.

NAUTA, H. J. W., PRITZ, M. B., AND LASEK, R. J. 1974. Afferents to the rat caudoputamen studied with horseradish peroxidase: An evaluation of a retrograde neuroanatomical research method. Brain Res., **67:** 219–238.

NAUTA, H. J. W., KAISERMANN-ABRAMOF, I. R., AND LASEK, R. J. 1975. Electron microscopic observations of horseradish peroxidase transported from the caudoputamen to the substantia nigra in the rat: Possible involvement of the agranular reticulum. Brain Res., **85:** 373–384.

NAUTA, W. J. H. 1956. An experimental study of the fornix in the rat. J. Comp. Neurol., **104:** 247–272.

NAUTA, W. J. H. 1958. Hippocampal projections and related pathways to the midbrain in the cat. Brain, **81:** 319–340.

NAUTA, W. J. H. 1961. Fibre degeneration following lesions of the amygdaloid complex in the monkey. J. Anat., **95:** 515–531.

NAUTA, W. J. H. 1962. Neural associations of the amygdaloid complex in the monkey. Brain, **85:** 505–520.

NAUTA, W. J. H. 1972. The central visceromotor system: A general survey. In C. H. HOCKMAN (Editor), *Limbic System Mechanisms and Autonomic Function.* Charles C Thomas, Springfield, Ill., Ch. 2, pp. 21–33.

NAUTA, W. J. H., AND GYGAX, P. A. 1954. Silver impregnation of degeneration axons in the central nervous system: A modified technic. Stain Technol., **29:** 91–93.

NAUTA, W. J. H., AND HAYMAKER, W. 1969. Hypothalamic nuclei and fiber connections. In W. HAYMAKER *et al.* (Editors), *The Hypothalamus.* Charles C Thomas, Springfield, Ill., Ch. 4, pp. 136–209.

NAUTA, W. J. H., AND KUYPERS, H. G. J. M. 1958. Some ascending pathways in the brain stem reticular formation. In H. H. JASPER *et al.* (Editors), *Reticular Formation of the Brain* (Henry Ford Hospital International Symposium). Little, Brown, Boston, Ch. 1, pp. 3–30.

NAUTA, W. J. H., AND MEHLER, W. R. 1966. Projections of the lentiform nucleus in the monkey. Brian Res., **1:** 3–42.

NAUTA, W. J. H., SMITH, G. P., FAULL, R. L. M., AND DOMESICK, V. B. 1978. Efferent connections and nigral afferents to the nucleus accumbens septi in the rat. Neuroscience, **3:** 385–401.

NIIMI, K., AND INOSHITA, H. 1971. Cortical projections of the lateral thalamic nuclei in the cat. Proc. Jpn. Acad., **47:** 664–669.

NIIMI, K., AND MATSUOKA, H. 1979. Thalamo-cortical organization of the auditory system in the cat studied by retrograde axonal transport of horseradish peroxidase. Adv. Anat. Embryol. Cell Biol., **57:** 1–56.

NIIMI, K., KATAYAMA, K., KANASEKI, T., AND MORIMOTO, K. 1960. Studies on the derivation of the centre median nucleus of Luys. Tokushima J. Exp. Med., **6:** 261–268.

NIIMI, K., NIIMI, M., AND OKADO, Y. 1978. Thalamic afferents to the limbic cortex in the cat studied with the method of retrograde transport of horseradish peroxidase. Brain Res., **145:** 225–238.

NIIMI, M. 1978. Cortical projections of the anterior thalamic nuclei in the cat. Exp. Brain Res., **31:** 403–416.

NOMURA, S., MIZZUNO, N., AND SUGIMOTO, T. 1980. Direct projections from the pedunculopontine tegmental nucleus to the subthalamic nucleus in the cat. Brain Res., **196:** 223–227.

NORGREN, R., AND PFAFFMAN, C. 1975. The pontine taste area in the rat. Brain Res., **91:** 99–117.

NORGREN, R., AND WOLF, G. 1975. Projection of thalamic gustatory and lingual areas in the rat. Brain Res., **92:** 123–129.

NORITA, M. 1977. Demonstration of bilateral claustrocortical connections in the cat with the method of retrograde axonal transport of horseradish peroxidase. Arch. Histol. Jpn., **40:** 1–10.

NYBERG-HANSEN, R. 1966. Functional organization of descending supraspinal fibre systems to the spinal cord: Anatomical observations and physiological correlations. Ergeb. Anat. Entwicklungsgesch., **39:** 1–48.

NYBERG-HANSEN, R., AND BRODAL, A. 1964. Sites and mode of termination of rubrospinal fibres in the cat: An experimental study with silver impregnation methods. J. Anat., **98:** 235–253.

NYGREN, L. G., AND OLSON, L. 1977. A new major projection from the locus coeruleus: The main source of noradrenergic nerve terminals in the ventral and dorsal columns of the spinal cord. Brain Res., **132:** 85–93.

OBATA, K., ITO, M., OCHI, R., AND SATO, N. 1967. Pharmacological properties of the postsynaptic inhibition by Purkinje cell axons and the action of γ-aminobutyric acid on Deiters' neurones. Exp. Brain Res., **4:** 43–57.

OGREN, M. P., AND HENDRICKSON, A. E. 1976. Pathways between the striate cortex and subcortical regions in *Macaca mulatta* and *Saimiri sciureus*: Evidence for a reciprocal pulvinar connection. Exp. Neurol., **53:** 780–800.

OHYE, C., LE GUYADER, C., AND FEGER, J. 1976. Responses of subthalamic and pallidal neurons to striatal stimulation: An extracellular study on awake monkeys. Brain Res., **111:** 241–252.

OKADA, Y. 1976. Role of GABA in the substantia nigra. In E. ROBERTS, T. N. CHASE, AND D. B. TOWE (Editors), *GABA in Nervous System Function.* Raven Press, New York, pp. 235–243.

OKADA, Y., NITCH-HASSLER, C., KIM, J. S., BAK, I. J., AND HASSLER, R. 1971. The role of δ-aminobutyric acid (GABA) in the extrapyramidal motor system. I. Regional distribution of GABA in rabbit, rat and guinea pig brain. Exp. Brain Res., **13:** 514–518.

OLDS, J. 1960. Differentiation of reward systems in the brain by self-stimulation technics. In S. R. RAMEY AND D. S. O'DOHERTY (Editors), *Electrical Studies on the Unanesthetized Brain.* Paul B. Hoeber, New York, Ch. 2, pp. 17–51.

OLDS, J., AND MILNER, P. 1954. Positive reinforcement produced by electrical stimulation of septal area and other regions of the rat brain. J. Comp. Physiol. Psychol., **47:** 419–427.

OLIVECRONA, H. 1957. Paraventricular nucleus and

the pituitary gland. Acta Physiol. Scand., **40**(Suppl. 136): 1–178.

OLIVER, D. L., AND HALL, W. C. 1978. The medial geniculate body of the tree shrew, *Tupaia glis*. I. Cytoarchitecture and midbrain connections. J. Comp. Neurol., **182:** 423–458.

OLIVER, D. L., AND HALL, W. C. 1978a. The medial geniculate body of the tree shrew, *Tupaia glis*. II. Connections with the neocortex. J. Comp. Neurol., **182:** 459–494.

OLPE, H.-R., AND KOELLA, W. P. 1977. The response of striatal cells upon stimulation of the dorsal and median raphe nuclei. Brain Res., **122:** 357–360.

OLSON, C. R., AND GRAYBIEL, A. M. 1980. Sensory maps in the claustrum of the cat. Nature, **288:** 479–481.

OLSON, L., AND FUXE, K. 1971. On the projections from the locus coeruleus noradrenalin neurons: The cerebellar innervation. Brain Res., **28:** 165–171.

OLSSON, Y., AND REESE, T. S. 1971. Permeability of vasa nervorum and perineurium in mouse sciatic nerve studied by fluorescence and electron microscopy. J. Neuropathol. Exp. Neurol., **30:** 105–119.

OLSZEWSKI, J. 1950. On the anatomical and functional organization of the spinal trigeminal nucleus. J. Comp. Neurol., **92:** 401–413.

OLSZEWSKI, J. 1952. *The Thalamus of the Macaca mulatta*. S. Karger, Basel, 93 pp.

OLSZEWSKI, J., AND BAXTER, D. 1954. *Cytoarchitecture of the Human Brain Stem*. J. B. Lippincott, Philadelphia.

ONO, T., NICHINO, H., SASAKA, K., MURAMOTO, K., YANO, I., AND SIMPSON, A. 1978. Paraventricular nucleus connections to spinal cord and pituitary. Neurosci. Lett., **10:** 141–146.

OOMURA, Y., ONO, T., AND OOYAMA, H. 1970. Inhibitory action of the amygdala on the lateral hypothalamic area in rats. Nature, **228:** 1108–1110.

OSCARSSON, O. 1965. Functional organization of the spino- and cuneocerebellar tracts. Physiol. Rev., **45:** 495–522.

OSCARSSON, O. 1967. Termination and functional organization of a dorsal spino-olivocerebellar path. Brain Res., **5:** 531–534.

OSCARSSON, O. 1973. Functional organization of spinocerebellar paths. In *Handbook of Sensory Physiology*, Vol. 2. Springer-Verlag, Berlin, pp. 339–380.

OSCARSSON, O., AND ROSÉN, I. 1966. Short-latency projections to the cat's cerebral cortex from skin and muscle afferents in the contralateral forelimb. J. Physiol., **182:** 164–184.

OSCARSSON, O., AND SJÖLUND, B. 1977. The ventral spino-olivocerebellar system in the cat. I. Identification of five paths and their terminations in the cerebellar anterior lobe. Exp. Brain Res., **28:** 469–486.

OSEN, K. K. 1969. The intrinsic organization of the cochlear nuclei in the cat. Acta Otolaryngol. (Stockh.), **67:** 352–359.

PAGE, R. B., AND BERGLAND, R. M. 1977. The neurohypophysial capillary bed. I. Anatomy and arterial supply. Am. J. Anat., **148:** 345–357.

PALAY, S. L., AND CHAN-PALAY, V. 1974. *Cerebellar Cortex. Cytology and Organization*. Springer-Verlag, Berlin.

PALKOVITS, M. 1981. Catecholamines in the hypothalamus: An anatomical review. Neuroendocrinology, **33:** 123–128.

PALKOVITS, M., AND JACOBOWITZ, D. M. 1974. Topographic atlas of catecholamine and acetylcholinesterase-containing neurons in the rat brain. J. Comp. Neurol., **157:** 29–42.

PALKOVITS, M., BROWNSTEIN, M., AND SAAVEDRA, J. M. 1974. Serotonin content of the brain stem nuclei in the rat. Brain Res., **80:** 237–249.

PALKOVITS, M., BROWNSTEIN, M. J., ARIMURA, A., SATO, H., SCHALLY, A. V., AND KIZER, J. S. 1976. Somatostatin and arcuate nuclei and the circumventricular organs in the rat. Brain Res., **109:** 430–434.

PANDYA, D. N., AND VIGNOLO, L. A. 1971. Intra- and interhemispheric projections of the precentral, premotor and arcuate areas in the rhesus monkey. Brain Res., **26:** 217–233.

PANDYA, D. N., VAN HOESEN, G. W., AND DOMESICK, J. B. 1973. A cinguloamygdaloid projection in the rhesus monkey. Brain Res., **61:** 369–373.

PANNETON, W. M., AND LOEWY, A. D. 1980. Projections of the carotid sinus nerve to the nucleus of the solitary tract in the cat. Brain Res., **191:** 239–244.

PAPEZ, J. W. 1937. A proposed mechanism of emotion. Arch. Neurol. Psychiatry, **38:** 725–743.

PAPPAS, G. D., AND TENNYSON, V. M. 1962. An electron microscopic study of the passage of colloid particles from the blood vessels of the ciliary processes and choroid plexus of the rabbit. J. Cell Biol., **15:** 227–239.

PARDRIDGE, W. M., FRANK, H. J. L., CORNFORD, E. M., BRAUN, L. D. CRANE, P. D., AND OLDENDORF, W. H. 1981. Neuropeptides and the blood brain barrier. Adv. Biochem. Psychopharmacol. **28:** 321–328.

PARENT, A., AND DE BELLEFEUILLE, L. 1982. Organization of efferent projections from the internal segment of the globus pallidus in primate as revealed by fluorescence retrograde labeling method. Brain Res., **245:** 201–213.

PARENT, A., DESCARRIES, L., AND BEAUDET, A. 1981. Organization of ascending serotonin systems in the adult rat brain: A radioautographic study after intraventricular administration of [^{3}H]5-hydroxytryptamine. Neuroscience, **6:** 115–138.

PARK, M. R., FALLS, W. M., AND KITAI, S. T. 1982. An intracellular HRP study of the rat globus pallidus. I. Responses and light microscopic analysis. J. Comp. Neurol., **211:** 284–294.

PARTLOW, G. D., COLONNIER, M., AND SZABO, J. 1977. Thalamic projections of the superior colliculus in the rhesus monkey, *Macaca mulatta*: A light and electron microscopic study. J. Comp. Neurol., **171:** 285–318.

PASIK, P., PASIK, T., AND DI FIGLIA, M. 1976. Quantitative aspects of neuronal organization in the neostriatum of the macaque monkey. In M. D. YAHR (Editor), *The Basal Ganglia*. Raven Press, New York, pp. 57–90.

PASIK, P., PASIK, T., AND DI FIGLIA M. 1979. The internal organization of the neostriatum in mammals. In I. DIVAC (Editor), *The Neostriatum*. Pergamon Press, Oxford, pp. 5–36.

PATTON, H. D., RUCH, T. C., AND WALKER, A. E. 1944. Experimental hypogeusia from Horsley-Clarke lesions of the thalamus in *Macaca mulatta*.

J. Neurophysiol., **7:** 171–184.

PEARSON, R. C., BRODAL, P., AND POWELL, T. P. S. 1978. The projection of the thalamus upon the parietal lobe in the monkey. Brain Res., **144:** 143–148.

PEASE, D. C., AND SCHULTZ, R. L. 1958. Electron microscopy of rat cranial meninges. Am. J. Anat., **102:** 301–313.

PEELE, T. L. 1961. *The Neuroanatomical Basis for Clinical Neurology.* McGraw-Hill, New York.

PENFIELD, W., AND BOLDREY, E. 1937. Somatic motor and sensory representation in the cerebral cortex of man as studied by electrical stimulation. Brain, **60:** 389–443.

PENFIELD, W., AND JASPER, H. H. 1954. *Epilepsy and the Functional Anatomy of the Human Brain.* Little, Brown, Boston.

PENFIELD, W., AND RASMUSSEN, T. 1950. *The Cerebral Cortex of Man: A Clinical Study of Localization of Function.* Macmillan, New York.

PERCHERON, G. 1977. The thalamic territory of cerebellar afferents and the lateral region of the thalamus of the macaque in stereotaxic ventricular coordinates. J. Hirnforsch., **18:** 375–400.

PERLMUTTER, D., AND RHOTON, A. L. 1976. Microsurgical anatomy of the anterior cerebral-anterior communicating-recurrent artery complex. J. Neurosurg., **45:** 259–272.

PERT, C. B. 1978. Opiate receptors and pain pathways. Neurosci. Res. Program Bull., **16:** 133–141.

PERT, C. B., SNOWMAN, A. M., AND SNYDER, S. H. 1974. Localization of opiate receptor binding in synaptic membranes of rat brain. Brain Res., **70:** 184–188.

PETERSON, B. 1979. Reticulo-motor pathways: Their connections and possible roles in motor behavior. In H. ASANUMA AND V. J. WILSON (Editors), *Integration in the Nervous System.* Igaku Shoin, Tokyo, pp. 185–201.

PETERSON, B. 1980. Participation of pontomedullary reticular neurons in specific motor activity. In J. A. HOBSON AND M. A. B. BRAZIER (Editors), *The Reticular Formation Revisited.* Raven Press, New York, pp. 171–192.

PETERSON, B. W., MAUNZ, R. A., PITTS, N. G., AND MACKEL, R. G. 1975. Patterns of projection and branching of reticulospinal neurons. Exp. Brain Res., **23:** 333–351.

PETRAS, J. M. 1964. Some fiber connections of the precentral cortex (areas 4 and 6) with the diencephalon in the monkey (*Macaca mulatta*). Anat. Rec., **148:** 322.

PETRAS, J. M. 1969. Some efferent connections of the motor and somatosensory cortex of simian primates and Felid, Canid and Procyonid carnivores. Ann. N.Y. Acad. Sci., **167:** 469–505.

PETRAS, J. M., AND CUMMINGS, J. F. 1972. Autonomic neurons in the spinal cord of the rhesus monkey: A correlation of the findings of cytoarchitectonics and sympathectomy with fiber degeneration following dorsal rhizotomy. J. Comp. Neurol., **146:** 189–218.

PETRAS, J. M., AND CUMMINGS, J. F. 1977. The origin of spinocerebellar pathways. II. The nucleus centrobasalis of the cervical enlargement and the nucleus dorsalis of the thoracolumbar spinal cord. J. Comp. Neurol., **173:** 693–716.

PFAFF, D. W., AND KEINER, M. 1973. Atlas of estradiol concentrating cells in the central nervous system of the female rat. J. Comp. Neurol., **151:** 121–159.

PHILLIPS, C. G., POWELL, T. P. S., AND WIESENDANGER, M. 1971. Projection from low-threshold muscle afferents of hand and forearm to area 3a of baboons cortex. J. Physiol. (Lond.), **217:** 419–446.

PICKARD G. E., AND SILVERMAN, A. J. 1981. Direct retinal projections to the hypothalamus, piriform cortex, and accessory optic nuclei in the golden hamster as demonstrated by a sensitive anterograde horseradish peroxidase technique. J. Comp. Neurol., **196:** 155–172.

PICKEL, V. M., SEGAL, M., AND BLOOM, F. E. 1974. A radioautographic study of the efferent pathways of the nucleus locus coeruleus. J. Comp. Neurol., **155:** 15–42.

PICKEL, V. M., SUMAI, K. K., BEADY, S. C., MILLER, R. J., AND REIS, D. J. 1980. Immunocytochemical localization of enkephalin in the neostriatum of rat brain: A light and electron microscopic study. J. Comp. Neurol., **189:** 721–740.

PICKFORD, M. 1969. Neurohypophysis-antidiuretic (vasopressor) and oxytocic hormones. In W. HAYMAKER *et al.* (Editors), *The Hypothalamus.* Charles C Thomas, Springfield, Ill., Ch. 13, pp. 463–505.

PIERSON, R. J., AND CARPENTER, M. B. 1974. Anatomical analyis of pupillary reflex pathways in the rhesus monkey. J. Comp. Neurol., **158:** 121–143.

PIN, C., JONES, B., AND JOUVET, M. 1968. Topographie des neurones monoaminerigiques du tronc cérebral du chat: Étude par histofluorescence. C. R. Soc. Biol. (Paris), **162:** 2137–2141.

PLUM, F., GJEDDE, A., AND SAMSON, F. E. 1976. Neuroanatomical functional mapping by the radioactive 2-deoxy-d-glucose method. Neurosci. Res. Program Bull., **14:** 457–518.

POGGIO, G. F., AND MOUNTCASTLE, V. B. 1960. A study of the functional contributions of the lemniscal and spinothalamic systems to somatic sensibility. Bull. Johns Hopkins Hosp., **106:** 266–316.

POIRIER, L. J., AND BOUVIER, G. 1966. The red nucleus and its efferent nervous pathways in the monkey. J. Comp. Neurol., **128:** 223–244.

POIRIER, L. J., AND SOURKES, T. L. 1965. Influence of the substantia nigra on catecholamine content of the striatum. Brain, **88:** 181–192.

POLYAK, S. L. 1957. *The Vertebrate Visual System.* University of Chicago Press, Chicago, 1390 pp.

POMPEIANO, O. 1959. Organizzazione somatotopica delle risposte flessorie alla stimolazione elettrica del nucleo interposito nel gatto decerebrato. Arch. Sci. Biol. (Bologna), **43:** 163–176.

POMPEIANO, O. 1967. The neurophysiological mechanisms of the postural and motor events during desynchronized sleep. Proc. Assoc. Res. Nerv. Ment. Dis., **45:** 351–423.

POMPEIANO, O. 1973. Reticular formation. In A. IGGO (Editor), *Handbook of Sensory Physiology: Somatosensory System,* Vol. 2. Springer-Verlag, Berlin, pp. 381–488.

POMPEIANO, O., AND BRODAL, A. 1957. Experimental demonstration of a somatotopical origin of rubrospinal fibers in the cat. J. Comp. Neurol., **108:** 225–251.

POMPEIANO, O., AND BRODAL, A. 1957a. The origin

of the vestibulospinal fibres in the cat: An experimental-anatomical study, with comments on the descending and medial longitudinal fasciculus. Arch. Ital. Biol., **95:** 166–195.

POMPEIANO, O., AND MORRISON, A. R. 1965. Vestibular influences during sleep. I. Abolition of rapid eye movements of desynchronized sleep following vestibular lesions. Arch. Ital. Biol., **103:** 569–595.

POMPEIANO, O., AND WALBERG, F. 1957. Descending connections to the vestibular nuclei: An experimental study in the cat. J. Comp. Neurol., **108:** 465–502.

POOL, J. L. 1954. Neurophysiological symposium: Visceral brain of man. J. Neurosurg., **11:** 45–63.

PORTER, J. C., AND JONES, J. C. 1956. Effect of plasma from hypophyseal-portal vessel blood on adrenal ascorbic acid. Endocrinology, **58:** 62–67.

PORTER, J. C., ONDON, J. G., AND CRAMER, O. M. 1974. Nervous and vascular supply of the pituitary gland. In R. O. GREEP AND E. B. ASTWOOD (Editors), *Handbook of Physiology*, Sect. 7, Vol. IV. Endocrinology. American Physiological Society, Washington, D.C., Ch. 2, pp. 33–43.

POTTER, H., AND NAUTA, W. J. H. 1979. A note on the problem of olfactory associations of the orbitofrontal cortex in the monkey. Neuroscience, **4:** 361–369.

POWELL, D., LEEMAN, S. E., TREGEAR, G. W., NIALL, H. D., AND POTTS, J. T. 1973. Radioimmunoassay for substance P. Nature, **241:** 252–254.

POWELL, E. W., AND HATTON, J. B. 1969. Projections of the inferior colliculus in the cat. J. Comp. Neurol., **136:** 183–192.

POWELL, T. P. S. 1952. Residual neurons in the human thalamus following hemidecortication. Brain, **75:** 571–584.

POWELL, T. P. S., AND COWAN, W. M. 1956. A study of thalamo-striate relations in the monkey. Brain, **79:** 364–390.

POWELL, T. P. S., AND COWAN, W. M. 1962. An experimental study of the projection of the cochlea. J. Anat., **96:** 269–284.

POWELL, T. P. S., AND COWAN, W. M. 1967. The interpretation of the degenerative changes in the intralaminar nuclei of the thalamus. J. Neurol. Neurosurg. Psychiatry, **30:** 140–153.

POWELL, T. P. S., AND MOUNTCASTLE, V. B. 1959. The cytoarchitecture of the postcentral gyrus of the monkey *Macaca mulatta*. Bull. Johns Hopkins Hosp., **105:** 108–131.

POWELL, T. P. S., AND MOUNTCASTLE, V. B. 1959a. Some aspects of the functional organization of the cortex of the postcentral gyrus of the monkey: A correlation of findings obtained in a single unit analysis with cytoarchitecture. Bull. Johns Hopkins Hosp., **105:** 133–162.

POWELL, T. P. S., GUILLERY, R. W., AND COWAN, W. M. 1957. A quantitative study of the fornix-mammillo-thalamic system. J. Anat., **91:** 419–432.

POWELL, T. P. S., COWAN, W. M., AND RAISMAN, G. 1963. Olfactory relationship of the diencephalon. Nature, **199:** 710–712.

POWELL, T. P. S., COWAN, W. M., AND RAISMAN, G. 1965. The central olfactory connexions. J. Anat., **99:** 791–813.

PRECHT, W. 1978. *Neuronal Operations in the Vestibular System*. Springer-Verlag, Berlin 223 pp.

PRESTON, R. J., BISHOP, G. A., AND KITAI, S. T. 1980. Medium spiny neuron projections from the rat striatum: An intracellular horseradish peroxidase study. Brain Res., **183:** 253–263.

PRICE, D. D., AND MAYER, D. J. 1974. Physiological laminar organization of dorsal horn of *M. mulatta*. Brain Res., **79:** 321–325.

PRICE, J. L., AND POWELL, T. P. S. 1970. The mitral and short axon cells of the olfactory bulb. J. Cell Sci., **7:** 631–652.

PROUDFIT, H. K., AND ANDERSON, E. G. 1975. Morphine analgesia: Blockade by raphe magnus lesions. Brain Res., **98:** 612–618.

PURPURA, D. P. 1970. Operations and processes in thalamic and synaptically related neural subsystems. In F. O. SCHMITT (Editor). *The Neurosciences, Second Study Program*. Rockefeller University Press, New York, Ch 42, pp. 458–470.

PURPURA, D. P. 1972. Intracellular studies of synaptic organization to the mammalian brain. In G. D. PAPPAS AND D. P. PURPURA (Editors), *Structure and Function of Synapses*. Raven Press, New York, pp. 257–302.

PURPURA, D. P., AND SHOFER, R. 1963. Intracellular recordings from thalamic neurons during reticulocortical activation. J. Neurophysiol., **26:** 494–505.

PYCOCK, C., HORTON, R. W., AND MARSDEN, C. D. 1976. The behavioural effects of manipulating GABA function in the globus pallidus. Brain Res., **116:** 353–359.

QUAY, W. B. 1974. *Pineal Chemistry in the Cellular and Physiological Mechanisms*. Charles C Thomas, Springfield, Ill.

RACZKOWSKI, D., DIAMOND, I. T., AND WINER, J., JR. 1976. Organization of thalamocortical auditory system in the cat studied with horseradish peroxidase. Brain Res., **101:** 345–354.

RAISMAN, G. 1966. Neural connexions of hypothalamus. Br. Med. Bull., **22:** 197–201.

RAISMAN, G. 1966a. The connexions of the septum. Brain, **89:** 317–348.

RAISMAN, G., AND FIELD, P. M. 1973. Sexual dimorphism in the neuropil of the preoptic area of the rat and its dependence on neonatal androgen. Brain Res., **54:** 1–29.

RAISMAN, G., COWAN, W. M., AND POWELL, T. P. S. 1965. The extrinsic afferent, commissural and association fibres of the hippocampus. Brain, **88:** 963–996.

RAISMAN, G., COWAN, W. M., AND POWELL, T. P. S. 1966. An experimental analysis of the efferent projections of the hippocampus. Brain, **89:** 83–108.

RANSON, S. W. 1914. The tract of Lissauer and the substantia gelatinosa Rolandi. Am. J. Anat., **16:** 97–126.

RAPOPORT, S. I. 1976. *Blood-Brain Barrier in Physiology and Medicine*. Raven Press, New York, 316 pp.

RASMUSSEN, G. L. 1946. The olivary peduncle and other fiber projections of the superior olivary complex. J. Comp. Neurol., **84:** 141–219.

RASMUSSEN, G. L. 1960. Efferent fibers of the cochlear nerve and cochlear nucleus. In G. L. RASMUS-

SEN AND W. F. WINDLE (Editors), *Neural Mechanisms of the Auditory and Vestibular Systems.* Charles C Thomas, Springfield, Ill., Ch. 8, pp. 105–115.

REESE, T. S., AND KARNOVSKY, M. J. 1967. Fine structural localization of a blood-brain barrier to exogenous peroxidase. J. Cell Biol., **34:** 207–217.

REIS, D. J., AND OLIPHANT, M. C. 1967. Bradycardia and tachycardia following electrical stimulation of the amygdaloid region in the monkey. J. Neurophysiol., **27:** 893–912.

RELKIN, R. 1976. *The Pineal.* Eden Press, Montreal.

REUBI, J. C., AND EMSON, P. C. 1978. Release and distribution of endogenous 5-HT in rat substantia nigra. Brain Res, **139:** 164–168.

REXED, B. 1952. The cytoarchitectonic organization of the spinal cord in the cat. J. Comp. Neurol., **96:** 415–496.

REXED, B. 1954. A cytoarchitectonic atlas of the spinal cord in the cat. J. Comp. Neurol., **100:** 297–400.

REXED, B. 1964. Some aspects of the cytoarchitectonics and synaptology of the spinal cord. In J. C. ECCLES AND J. P. SCHADÉ (Editors), *Progress in Brain Research, Vol. II. Organization of the Spinal Cord.* Elsevier, Amsterdam, pp. 58–92.

REZAK, M., AND BENEVENTO, L. A. 1979. A comparison of the organization of the projections of the dorsal lateral geniculate nucleus, the inferior pulvinar and adjacent lateral pulvinar to primary visual cortex (area 17) in the macaque monkey. Brain Res., **167:** 19–40.

RHOTON, A. L., O'LEARY, J. L., AND FERGUSON, J. P. 1966. The trigeminal, facial, vagal and glossopharyngeal nerves in the monkey. Arch. Neurol., **14:** 530–540.

RIBAK, C. E. 1981. The GABAergic neurons of the extrapyramidal system as revealed by immunocytochemistry. In G. DI CHIARA AND G. L. GESSA (Editors), *GABA and the Basal Ganglia.* Raven Press, New York, pp. 23–26.

RIBAK, C. E., VAUGHN, J. E., SAITO, K., BARBER, R., AND ROBERTS, E. 1976. Immunocytochemical localization of glutamate decarboxylase in rat substantia nigra. Brain Res., **116:** 287–298.

RIBAK, C. E., VAUGHN, J. E., AND ROBERTS, E. 1979. The GABA neurons and their axon terminals in rat corpus striatum as demonstrated by GAD immunocytochemistry. J. Comp. Neurol., **187:** 261–284.

RIBAK, C. E., VAUGHN, J. E., AND ROBERTS, E. 1980. GABAergic nerve terminals decrease in the substantia nigra following hemitransections of the striatonigral and pallidonigral pathways. Brain Res., **192:** 413–420.

RIBAK, C. E., VAUGHAN, J. E., AND BARBER, R. P. 1981. Immunocytochemical localization of GABAergic neurones at the electron microscopical level. Histochem. J., **13:** 555–582.

RICHE, D., AND LANOIR, J. 1978. Some claustro-cortical connections in the cat and baboon as studied by retrograde horseradish peroxidase transport. J. Comp. Neurol., **177:** 434–444.

RICHTER, E. 1965. *Die Entwicklung des Globus Pallidus und des Corpus Subthalamicum.* Springer-Verlag, Berlin.

RINVIK, E. 1968. The corticothalamic projection from the pericruciate and coronal gyri in the cat: An experimental study with silver-impregnation methods. Brain Res., **10:** 79–119.

RINVIK, E. 1975. Demonstration of nigro-thalamic connections in the cat by retrograde axonal transport of horseradish peroxidase. Brain Res., **90:** 313–318.

RINVIK, E., AND GROFOVÁ, I. 1970. Observations on the fine structure of the substantia nigra in the cat. Exp. Brain Res., **11:** 229–248.

RINVIK, E., AND WALBERG, F. 1969. Is there a corticonigral tract? A comment based on experimental electron microscopic observations in the cat. Brain Res., **14:** 742–744.

RINVIK, E., AND WALBERG, F. 1975. Studies on the cerebellar projections from the main and external cuneate nuclei in the cat by means of retrograde axonal transport of horseradish peroxidase. Brain Res., **95:** 371–381.

RINVIK, E., GROFOVÁ, I., AND PETTER OTTERSEN, O. 1976. Demonstration of the nigrotectal and nigroreticular projections in the cat by axonal transport of protein. Brain Res., **112:** 388–394.

RISPAL-PADEL, L., MASSION, J., AND GRANGETTO, A. 1973. Relations between the ventrolateral thalamic nucleus and motor cortex and their possible role in the central organization of motor control. Brain Res., **60:** 1–20.

ROBERTS, T. S., AND AKERT, K. 1963. Insular and opercular cortex and its thalamic projection in *Macaca mulatta.* Schweiz. Arch. Neurol. Neurochir. Psychiatr., **92:** 1–43.

ROBERTSON, R. T., AND RINVIK, E. 1973. The corticothalamic projections from parietal regions of the cerebral cortex: Experimental degeneration studies in the cat. Brain Res., **51:** 61–79.

ROBINSON, B. W., AND MISHKIN, M. 1962. Alimentary responses evoked from forebrain structures in *Macaca mulatta.* Science, **136:** 260–261.

ROBINSON, B. W., AND MISHKIN, M. 1968. Alimentary responses to forebrain stimulation in monkeys. Exp. Brain Res., **4:** 330–366.

ROBINSON, C. J., AND BURTON, H. 1980. Somatotopographic organization in the second somatosensory area of *M. fascicularis.* J. Comp. Neurol., **192:** 43–67.

ROBINSON, C. J., AND BURTON, H. 1980a. The organization of somatosensory receptive fields in cortical area 7b, retroinsular, postauditory and granular insular of *M. fascicularis.* J. Comp. Neurol., **192:** 69–92.

ROBINSON, C. J., AND BURTON, H. 1980b. Somatic submodality distribution within the second somatosensory (S II), 7b, retroinsular, postauditory and granular insular cortical areas of *M. fascicularis.* J. Comp. Neurol., **192:** 93–108.

ROCKEL, A. J., AND JONES, E. G. 1973. The neuronal organization of the inferior colliculus of the adult cat. I. The central nucleus. J. Comp. Neurol., **147:** 11–60.

ROCKEL, A. J., AND JONES, E. G. 1973a. The neuronal organization of the inferior colliculus of the adult cat. II. The pericentral nucleus. J. Comp. Neurol., **149:** 301–334.

ROMANSKY, K. V., USUNOFF, K. G., IVANOV, D. P., AND GALABOV, G. P. 1979. Corticosubthalamic projection in the cat: An electron microscopic study. Brain Res., **163:** 319–322.

ROSE, J. E. 1960. Organization of frequency sensitive

neurons in the cochlear complex of the cat. In G. L. RASMUSSEN AND W. F. WINDLE (Editors), *Neural Mechanisms of the Auditory and Vestibular Systems.* Charles C Thomas, Springfield, Ill., Ch. 9, pp. 116–136.

ROSE, J. E., AND WOOLSEY, C. N. 1958. Cortical connections and functional organization of the thalamic auditory system of the cat. In H. F. HARLOW AND C. N. WOOLSEY (Editors), *Biological and Biochemical Bases of Behavior.* University of Wisconsin Press, Madison, pp. 127–150.

ROSE, J. E., GALAMBOS, R., AND HUGHES, J. R. 1959. Microelectrode studies of the cochlear nuclei of the cat. Bull. Johns Hopkins Hosp., **104:** 211–251.

ROSE, J. E., GREENWOOD, D. B., GOLDBERG, J. M., AND HIND, J. E. 1963. Some discharge characteristics of single neurons in the inferior colliculus of the cat. I. Tonotopical organization, relation of spike-counts to tone intensity, and firing patterns of single elements. J. Neurophysiol., **26:** 293–320.

ROSÉN, I., AND ASANUMA, H. 1972. Peripheral afferent inputs to the forelimb area of the monkey motor cortex: Input-output relations. Exp. Brain Res., **14:** 257–273.

ROSÉN, I., AND SJÖLUND, B. 1973. Organization of group I activated cells in the main and external cuneate nuclei of the cat: Identification of muscle receptors. Exp. Brain Res., **16:** 221–237.

ROSÉN, I., AND SJÖLUND, B. 1973a. Organization of group I activated cells in the main and external cuneate nuclei of the cat: Convergence patterns demonstrated by natural stimulation. Exp. Brain Res., **16:** 238–246.

ROSENE, D. L., AND VAN HOESEN, G. W. 1977. Hippocampal efferents reach widespread areas of cerebral cortex and amygdala in the rhesus monkey. Science, **198:** 315–317.

ROSENQUIST, A. C., EDWARDS, S. B., AND PALMER, L. A. 1974. An autoradiographic study of the projections of the dorsal lateral geniculate nucleus and the posterior nucleus in the cat. Brain Res., **80:** 71–93.

ROSENZWEIG, M. R. 1954. Cortical correlates of auditory localization and of related perceptual phenomena. J. Comp. Physiol. Psychol., **47:** 269–276.

ROSSI, G. F., AND BRODAL, A. 1956. Corticofugal fibers to the brain stem reticular formation: An experimental study in the cat. J. Anat., **90:** 42–62.

ROSSI, G. F., AND BRODAL, A. 1957. Terminal distribution of spinoreticular fibers in the cat. A.M.A. Arch. Neurol. Psychiatry, **78:** 439–453.

ROTH, G. L., AITKIN, L. M., ANDERSON, R. A., AND MERZENICH, M. M. 1978. Some features of the spatial organization of the central nucleus of the inferior colliculus of the cat. J. Comp. Neurol., **182:** 661–680.

ROUDOMIN, P., MALLIANI, A., BARLONE, M., AND ZANCHETTI, A. 1965. Distribution of electrical responses to somatic stimuli in the diencephalon of the cat, with special reference to the hypothalamus. Arch. Ital. Biol., **103:** 60–89.

ROUZAIRE-DUBOIS, B., HAMMOND, C., HAMON, B., AND FÉGER, J. 1980. Pharmacological blockage of the globus pallidus-induced inhibitory response of subthalamic cells in the rat. Brain Res., **200:** 321–329.

ROYCE, G. J. 1978. Centroradiographic evidence for a discontinuous projection to the caudate nucleus from the centromedian nucleus in the cat. Brain Res., **146:** 145–150.

ROYCE, G. J. 1978a. Cells of origin of subcortical afferents to the caudate nucleus: A horseradish peroxidase study in the cat. Brain Res., **153:** 465–475.

ROYCE, G. J. 1982. Laminar origin of cortical neurons which project upon the caudate nucleus: A horseradish peroxidase investigation in the cat. J. Comp. Neurol., **205:** 8–29.

RUGGIERO, D., BATTON, R. R., III, JAYARAMAN, A., AND CARPENTER, M. B. 1977. Brainstem afferents to the fastigial nucleus in the cat demonstrated by transport of horseradish peroxidase. J. Comp. Neurol., **172:** 189–210.

RUGGIERO, D. A., ROSS, C. A., AND REIS, D. J. 1981. Projections from the spinal trigeminal nucleus to the entire length of the spinal cord in the rat. Brain Res., **225:** 225–233.

RUSSELL, J. R., AND DEMYER, W. 1961. The quantitative cortical origin of pyramidal axons of *Macaca rhesus.* Neurology, **11:** 96–108.

SAFFRAN, M. 1959. Activation of ACTH release by neurohypophysial peptides. Can. J. Biochem. Physiol., **37:** 319–329.

SAFFRAN, M. 1974. Chemistry of hypothalamic hypophysiotropic factors. In R. O. GREEP AND E. B. ASTWOOD (Editors), *Handbook of Physiology,* Sect. 7, Vol. IV. Endocrinology, Part 2. American Physiological Society, Washington, D.C., Ch. 43, pp. 563–586.

SAHAR, A. 1972. Choroidal origin of cerebrospinal fluid. Isr. J. Med. Sci., **8:** 594–596.

SAINT-CYR, J. A., AND COURVILLE, J. 1979. Projection from the vestibular nuclei to the inferior olive in the cat: An autoradiographic and horseradish peroxidase study. Brain Res., **165:** 189–201.

SALAMON, G., AND LAZORTHES, G. 1971. *Atlas of the Arteries of the Human Brain.* Sandoz, Paris.

SANIDES, D. 1975. The retinal projection to the ventral lateral geniculate nucleus of the cat. Brain Res., **85:** 313–316.

SAPER, C. B., LOEWY, A. D., SWANSON, L. W., AND COWAN, W. M. 1976. Direct hypothalamo-autonomic connections. Brain Res., **117:** 305–312.

SASA, M., AND TAKAORI, S. 1973. Influence of the locus coeruleus on transmission in the spinal trigeminal nucleus neurons. Brain Res., **55:** 203–208.

SAWYER, C. H. 1959. Nervous control of ovulation. In C. W. LLOYD (Editor), *Endocrinology of Reproduction.* Academic Press, New York, pp. 1–18.

SAWYER, C. H. 1969. Regulatory mechanisms of secretion of gonadotrophic hormones. In W. HAYMAKER *et al.* (Editors), *The Hypothalamus.* Charles C Thomas, Springfield, Ill., Ch. 11, pp. 389–430.

SCALIA, F. 1972. The termination of retinal axons in the pretectal region of mammals. J. Comp. Neurol., **145:** 223–257.

SCARFF, J. E. 1940. Primary cortical centers for movement of upper and lower limbs in man. Arch. Neurol. Psychiatry, **44:** 243–299.

SCHALLY, A. V., KASTIN, A. J., AND ARIMURA, A. 1977. Hypothalamic hormones: The link between brain and body. Am. Sci., **65:** 712–719.

SCHEIBEL, M. E., AND SCHEIBEL, A. B. 1954. Observations on the intracortical relations of the climbing fibers of the cerebellum: A Golgi study. J. Comp.

Neurol., **101:** 733–764.

SCHEIBEL, M. E., AND SCHEIBEL, A. B. 1958. Structural substrates for integrative patterns in the brain stem reticular core. In H. H. JASPERS *et al.* (Editors), *Reticular Formation of the Brain.* Little, Brown, Boston, Ch. 2, pp. 31–55.

SCHEIBEL, M. E., AND SCHEIBEL, A. B. 1966. The organization of the nucleus reticularis thalami: A Golgi study. Brain Res., **1:** 43–62.

SCHEIBEL, M. E., AND SCHEIBEL, A. B. 1966a. The organization of the ventral anterior nucleus of the thalamus: A Golgi study. Brain Res., **1:** 250–268.

SCHELL, G. R., AND STRICK, P. L. 1984. The origin of thalamic inputs to the arcuate premotor and supplementary motor areas. J. Neurosci., **4:** 539–560.

SCHLESINGER, B. 1939. Venous drainage of the brain, with special reference to Galenic system. Brain, **62:** 274–291.

SCHREINER, L. H., AND KLING, A. 1954. Effects of castration on hypersexual behavior induced by rhinencephalic injury in cat. Arch. Neurol. Psychiatry, **72:** 180–186.

SCHRÖDER, K. F., HOPF, A., LANGE, H., AND THÖRNER, G. 1975. Morphometrisch-statische Strukturanalysen des Striatum, Pallidum und Nucleus Subthalamicus beim Menschen. J. Hirnforsch., **16:** 333–350.

SCHÜTZ, H. 1891. Anatomische Untersuchungen über den Faserverlauf im zentralen Höhlengrau und den Nervenfaserschwund in demselben bei der progressiven Paralyse der Irren. Arch. Psychiatr. Nervenkr., **22:** 527–587.

SCHWARCZ, R., AND COYLE, J. T. 1977. Striatal lesions with kainic acid: Neurochemical characteristics. Brain Res., **127:** 235–249.

SCHWARTZ, P., AND FINK, L. 1926. Morphologie und Entstehung der geburtstraumatischen Blutungen im Gehirn und Schädel des Neugeborenen. Z. Kinderheilkd., **40:** 427–474.

SCHWARZ, D. W. F., AND FREDRICKSON, J. M. 1971. Rhesus monkey vestibular cortex: A bimodal primary projection field. Science, **171:** 280–281.

SCHWINDT, P. C. 1981. Control of motoneuron output by pathways descending from the brain stem. In A. L. TOWE AND E. S. LUSCHEI (Editors), *Handbook of Behavioral Neurobiology, Motor Coordination.* Plenum Press, New York, Vol. 5, pp. 139–230.

SCHWYN, R. C., AND FOX, C. A. 1974. The primate substantia nigra: A Golgi and electron microscopic study. J. Hirnforsch., **15:** 95–126.

SCOLLO-LAVIZZARI, G., AND AKERT, K. 1963. Cortical area 8 and its thalamic projection in *Macaca mulatta.* J. Comp. Neurol., **121:** 259–267.

SCOTT, D. E., AND KROBISCH-DUDLEY, G. 1975. Ultrastructural analysis of the mammalian median eminence. In K. M. KNIGGE, D. E. SCOTT, H. KOBAYASHI, AND S. ISHII (Editors), *Brain-Endocrine Interaction,* II. S. Karger, Basel, pp. 29–39.

SCOVILLE, W. B. 1954. Neurophysiological symposium: Limbic lobe in man. J. Neurosurg., **11:** 64–66.

SELZER, M. E., MYERS, R. E., AND HOLSTEIN, S. B. 1972. Maturational changes in brain water and electrolytes in rhesus monkey with some implications for electrogenesis. Brain Res., **45:** 193–204.

SHEALY, C. N., AND PEELE, T. L. 1957. Studies on amygdaloid nucleus of cat. J. Neurophysiol., **20:** 125–139.

SHEARD, M. H. 1969. The effect of PCPA in behavior in rats: Relation to brain serotonin and 5-hydroxyindoleacetic acid. Brain Res., **15:** 524–528.

SHEPARD, G. 1979. *The Synaptic Organization of the Brain.* Oxford University Press, New York, 436 pp.

SHERIDAN, M. N., AND SLADEK, J. R. 1975. Histofluorescence and ultrastructural analysis of hamster and monkey pineal. Cell Tissue Res., **164:** 145–152.

SHERK, H. 1978. Visual response properties and visual field topography in the cat's parabigeminal nucleus. Brain Res., **145:** 375–379.

SHERK, H., AND LEVAY, S. 1981. The visual claustrum of the cat. III. Receptive field properties. J. Neurosci., **1:** 993–1002.

SHERRINGTON, C. S. 1898. Decerebrate rigidity, and reflex co-ordination of movements. J. Physiol. (Lond.), **22:** 319–332.

SHINODA, Y., ZARZECKI, P., AND ASANUMA, H. 1979. Spinal branching of pyramidal tract neurons in the monkey. Exp. Brain Res., **34:** 59–72.

SHRIVER, J. E., STEIN, B. M., AND CARPENTER, M. B. 1968. Central projections of spinal dorsal roots in the monkey. I. Cervical and upper thoracic dorsal roots. Am. J. Anat., **123:** 27–74.

SIDMAN, R. L. 1970. Cell proliferation, migration and interaction in the developing mammalian central nervous system. In F. O. SCHMITT (Editor), *The Neurosciences,* Second Study Program. Rockefeller University Press, New York, pp. 100–116.

SIGGINS, G. F., HOFFER, B. J., BLOOM, F. E., AND UNGERSTEDT. U. 1976. Cytochemical and electrophysiological studies of dopamine in the caudate nucleus. Proc. Assoc. Res. Nerv. Ment. Dis., **55:** 227–248.

SIMANTOV, R., KUHAR, M. J., PASTERNAK, G. W., AND SNYDER, S. H. 1976. The regional distribution of a morphine-like factor enkephalin in monkey brain. Brain Res., **106:** 189–197.

SKINNER, J. E., AND LINDSLEY, D. B. 1967. Electrophysiological and behavior effects of blockage on the nonspecific thalamocortical system. Brain Res., **6:** 95–117.

SMITH, C. A. 1967. Innervation of the organ of Corti. In S. IURATO (Editor), *Submicroscopic Structure of the Inner Ear.* Pergamon, Oxford, pp. 107–131.

SMITH, C. A., AND RASMUSSEN, G. L. 1963. Recent observations on the olivo-cochlear bundle. Ann. Otol. Rhinol. Laryngol., **72:** 489–507.

SMITH, M. C. 1967. Stereotaxic operations for Parkinson's disease—Anatomical observations. In D. WILLIAMS (Editor), *Modern Trends in Neurology,* Vol. 4. Butterworth, London, pp. 21–52.

SNIDER, R. S. 1950. Recent contributions to the anatomy and physiology of the cerebellum. Arch. Neurol. Psychiatry, **64:** 196–219.

SNIDER, R. S., AND ELDRED, E. 1952. Cerebro-cerebellar relationships in the monkey. J. Neurophysiol., **15:** 27–40.

SNIDER, R. S., AND STOWELL, A. 1944. Receiving areas of the tactile, auditory, and visual systems in the cerebellum. J. Neurophysiol., **7:** 331–357.

SOFRONIEW, M. V., AND WEINDL, A. 1980. Identification of parvocellular vasopressin and neurophysin neurons in the suprachiasmatic nucleus of a variety of mammals including primates. J. Comp. Neurol., **193:** 659–676.

SOMANA, R., AND WALBERG, F. 1978. Cerebellar afferents from the paramedian reticular nucleus studied with retrograde transport of horseradish peroxidase. Anat. Embryol. (Berl.), **154:** 353–368.

SOMOGYI, P., BOLAM, J. P., AND SMITH, A. D. 1981. Monosynaptic cortical input and local axon collaterals of identified striatonigral neurons: A light and electron microscopic study using the Golgi-peroxidase transport-degeneration procedure. J. Comp. Neurol., **185:** 567–584.

SPARKS, D. L., HOLLAND, R., AND GUTHRIE, B. L. 1976. Size and distribution of movement fields in the monkey superior colliculus. Brain Res., **113:** 21–34.

SPENCER, H. J. 1976. Antagonism of cortical excitation of striatal neurons by glutamic acid diethyl ester: Evidence for glutamic acid as an excitatory transmitter in the rat striatum. Brain Res., **102:** 91–101.

SPENCER, R. F., AND STERLING, P. 1977. An electron microscope study of motoneurones and interneurones in the cat abducens nucleus identified by retrograde intraaxonal transport of horseradish peroxidase. J. Comp. Neurol., **176:** 65–86.

SPERRY, R. W. 1974. Lateral specialization in the surgically separated hemispheres. In F. O. SCHMITT AND F. G. WORDEN (Editors), *The Neurosciences*, Third Study Program. M.I.T. Press, Cambridge, Mass., pp. 5–19.

SPOENDLIN, H. H. 1972. Innervation densities of the cochlea. Acta Otolaryngol. (Stockh.), **73:** 235–248.

SPRAGUE, J. M. 1972. The superior colliculus and pretectum in visual behavior. Invest. Ophthalmol., **11:** 473–482.

SPRAGUE, J. M., AND MEIKLE, T. H., JR. 1965. The role of the superior colliculus in visually guided behavior. Exp. Neurol., **11:** 115–146.

STARZL, T. E., AND MAGOUN, H. W. 1951. Organization of the diffuse thalamic projection system. J. Neurophysiol., **14:** 133–146.

STEIGER, H.-J., AND BÜTTNER-ENNEVER, J. A. 1978. Relationship between motoneurons and internuclear neurons in the abducens nucleus: A double retrograde tracer study in the cat. Brain Res., **148:** 181–188.

STEIGER, H.-J., AND BÜTTNER-ENNEVER, J. A. 1979. Oculomotor nucleus afferents in the monkey demonstrated with horseradish peroxidase. Brain Res., **160:** 1–15.

STEIN, B. M., AND CARPENTER, M. B. 1967. Central projections of portions of the vestibular ganglia innervating specific parts of the labyrinth in the rhesus monkey. Am. J. Anat., **120:** 281–318.

STEINBUSCH, H. W. M. 1981. Distribution of serotonin-immunoreactivity in the central nervous system of the rat—cell bodies and terminals. Neuroscience, **6:** 577–618.

STEPHENS, R. B., AND STILWELL, D. L. 1969. *Arteries and Veins of the Human Brain.* Charles C Thomas, Springfield, Ill.

STERIADE, M., AND GLENN, L. L. 1982. Neocortical and caudate projections of intralaminar thalamic neurons and their synaptic excitation from midbrain reticular core. J. Neurophysiol., **48:** 352–371.

STERLING, P., AND WICKELGREN, B. G. 1969. Visual receptive fields in the superior colliculus of the cat. J. Neurophysiol., **32:** 1–15.

STEVENSON, J. A. F. 1969. Neural control of food and water intake. In W. HAYMAKER *et al.* (Editors), *The Hypothalamus.* Charles C Thomas, Springfield, Ill., Ch. 15, pp. 524–621.

STONE, J., AND FUKUDA, Y. 1974. Properties of cat retinal ganglion cells: A comparison of W cells with X and Y cells. J. Neurophysiol., **37:** 722–748.

STOPFORD, J. S. B. 1915. The arteries of the pons and medulla oblongata. Part I. J. Anat. Physiol., **50:** 131–164.

STOPFORD, J. S. B. 1916. The arteries of the pons and medulla oblongata. Part II. J. Anat. Physiol., **50:** 255–280.

STRICK, P. L. 1976. Anatomical analysis of ventrolateral thalamic input to primate motor cortex. J. Neurophysiol., **39:** 1020–1031.

STRICK, P. L. 1976a. Activity of ventrolateral thalamic neurons during arm movement. J. Neurophysiol., **39:** 1032–1044.

STRICK, P. L., AND KIM, C. C. 1978. Input to primate motor cortex from posterior parietal cortex (area 5). I. Demonstration by retrograde transport. Brain Res., **157:** 325–330.

STRICK, P. L., AND PRESTON, J. B. 1978. Multiple representation in the primate motor cortex. Brain Res., **154:** 366–370.

STRICK, P. L., AND STERLING, P. 1974. Synaptic terminations of afferents from the ventrolateral nucleus of the thalamus in the cat motor cortex: A light and electron microscope study. J. Comp. Neurol., **153:** 77–106.

STROMINGER, N. L., AND CARPENTER, M. B. 1965. Effects of lesions in the substantia nigra upon subthalamic dyskinesia in the monkey. Neurology, **15:** 587–594.

STRONG, O. S. 1915. A case of unilateral cerebellar agenesia. J. Comp. Neurol., **25:** 361–391.

STUMPF, W. E. 1972. Estrogen, androgen and glucocorticosteroid concentrating neurons in the amygdala, studied by dry autoradiography. In B. E. ELEFTHERIOU (Editor), *The Neurobiology of the Amygdala.* Plenum Press, New York, pp. 763–774.

SUGIMOTO, T., AND HATTORI, T. 1983. Confirmation of thalamosubthalamic projections by electron microscopic autoradiography. Brain Res., **267:** 335–339.

SUGIMOTO, T., HATTORI, T., MIZUNO, N., ITOH, K., AND SATO, M. 1983. Direct projections from the centre median-parafascicular complex to the subthalamic nucleus in the cat and rat. J. Comp. Neurol., **214:** 209–216.

SUH, T. H., AND ALEXANDER, L. 1939. Vascular system of the human spinal cord. Arch. Neurol. Psychiatry, **41:** 659–677.

SWANN, H. G. 1934. The function of the brain in olfaction. II. The results of destruction of olfactory and other nervous structures upon the discrimination of odors. J. Comp. Neurol., **59:** 176–201.

SWANSON, L. W., AND COWAN, W. M. 1975. A note on the connections and development of the nucleus accumbens. Brain Res., **92:** 324–330.

SWANSON, L. W., AND COWAN, W. M. 1975a. The efferent connections of the suprachiasmatic nucleus of the hypothalamus. J. Comp. Neurol., **160:** 1–12.

SWANSON, L. W., AND COWAN, W. M. 1977. An autoradiographic study of the organization of the efferent connections of the hippocampal formation in the rat. J. Comp. Neurol., **172:** 49–84.

SWANSON, L. W., AND KUYPERS, H. G. J. M. 1980. The paraventricular nucleus of the hypothalamus: Cytoarchitectonic subdivisions and organization of projections to the pituitary, dorsal vagal complex, and spinal cord as demonstrated by retrograde fluorescence double-labeling methods. J. Comp. Neurol., **194:** 555–570.

SWANSON, L. W., COWAN, W. M., AND JONES, E. G. 1974. An autoradiographic study of the efferent connections of the ventral lateral geniculate nucleus in the albino rat and the cat. J. Comp. Neurol., **156:** 143–163.

SZABO, J. 1962. Topical distribution of striatal efferents in the monkey. Exper. Neurol., **5:** 21–36.

SZABO, J. 1967. The efferent projections of the putamen in the monkey. Exper. Neurol., **19:** 463–476.

SZABO, J. 1970. Projections from the body of the caudate nucleus in the rhesus monkey. Exp. Neurol., **27:** 1–15.

SZABO, J. 1980. Distribution of striatal afferents from the mesencephalon in the cat. Brain Res., **188:** 3–21.

SZABO, J. 1980a. Organization of the ascending striatal afferents in monkeys. J. Comp. Neurol., **189:** 307–321.

SZENTÁGOTHAI, J. 1964. Neuronal and synaptic arrangement in the substantia gelatinosa Rolandi. J. Comp. Neurol., **122:** 219–239.

SZENTÁGOTHAI, J. 1970. Glomerular synapses, complex synaptic arrangements, and their operational significance. In F. O. SCHMITT (Editor), *The Neurosciences* (Second Study Program). Rockefeller University Press, New York, Ch. 40, pp. 427–443.

SZENTÁGOTHAI, J. 1978. The neuron network of the cerebral cortex: A functional interpretation. Proc. R. Soc. Lond. (Biol.), **201:** 219–248.

SZENTÁGOTHAI, J., AND RAJKOVITS, K. 1959. Über den Ursprung der Kletterfasern des Kleinhirn. Z. Anat. Entwickl.-Gesch., **121:** 130–141.

SZENTÁGOTHAI, J., FLERKÓ, B., MESS, B., AND HALASZ, B. 1968. *Hypothalamic Control of the Anterior Pituitary: An Experimental-Morphological Study.* Akademiai Kiado, Budapest.

TABER, E. 1961. The cytoarchitecture of the brain stem of the cat. I. Brain stem nuclei of cat. J. Comp. Neurol., **116:** 27–70.

TABER, E., BRODAL, A., AND WALBERG, F. 1960. The raphe nuclei of the brain stem in the cat. I. Normal topography and cytoarchitecture and general discussion. J. Comp. Neurol., **114:** 161–187.

TABER-PIERCE, E., HODDEVIK, G. H., AND WALBERG, F. 1977. The cerebellar projection from the raphe nuclei in the cat as studied with the method of retrograde transport of horseradish peroxidase. Anat. Embryol. (Berl.), **152:** 73–87.

TAKAHASHI, T., AND OTSUKA, M. 1975. Regional distribution of substance P in the spinal cord and nerve roots of the cat and the effects of dorsal root section. Brain Res., **87:** 1–11.

TAKEUCHI, Y., UEMURA, M., MATSUDA, K., MATSUSHIMA, R., AND MIZUNO, N. 1980. Parabrachial nucleus neurons projecting to the lower brain stem and the spinal cord: A study in the cat by the Fink-Heimer and the horseradish peroxidase methods. Exp. Neurol., **70:** 403–413.

TANABE, T., YARITA, H., IINO, M., OOSHIMA, Y., AND TAKAGI, S. F. 1975. An olfactory projection area in orbitofrontal cortex of the monkey. J. Neurophysiol., **38:** 1269–1283.

TAVERAS, J. M., AND WOOD, E. H. 1976. *Diagnostic Neuroradiology.* Williams & Wilkins, Baltimore, Ed. 2.

TERNAUX, J. P., HERY, F., BOURGOIN, S., ADRIEN, J., GLOWINSKI, J., AND HAMON, M. 1977. The topographical distribution of serotoninergic terminals in the neostriatum of the rat and the caudate nucleus of the cat. Brain Res., **121:** 311–326.

TERZIAN, H. 1958. Observations on the clinical symptomatology of bilateral partial or total removal of the temporal lobe in man. In M. BALDWIN AND P. BAILEY (Editors), *Temporal Lobe Epilepsy.* Charles C Thomas, Springfield, Ill., pp. 510–529.

TERZIAN, H., AND ORE, G. D. 1955. Syndrome of Klüver and Bucy reproduced in man by bilateral removal of the temporal lobes. Neurology, **5:** 373–380.

THACH, W. T. 1970. The behavior of Purkinje and cerebellar nuclear cells during two types of voluntary arm movement in the monkey. In W. S. FIELDS AND W. D. WILLIS (Editors), *The Cerebellum in Health and Disease.* Warren H. Green, St. Louis, Ch. 8, pp. 217–230.

THACH, W. T., AND JONES, E. G. 1979. The cerebellar dentatothalamic connection: Terminal field, lamellae, rods and somatotopy. Brain Res., **169:** 168–172.

THOMAS, D. M., KAUFMAN, R. P., SPRAGUE, J. M., AND CHAMBERS, W. W. 1956. Experimental studies of the vermal cerebellar projections in the brain stem of the cat (fastigiobulbar tract). J. Anat., **90:** 371–385.

THOMPSON, J. M., WOOLSEY, C. N., AND TALBOT, S. A. 1950. Visual areas I and II of cerebral cortex of rabbit. J. Neurophysiol., **13:** 277–288.

THÖRNER, G., LANGE, H., AND HOPF., A. 1975. Morphometrisch-statistische Strukturanalysen des Striatum, Pallidum und Nucleus Subthalamicus beim Menschen. J. Hirnforsch., **16:** 401–413.

THORNER, M. O., AND LOGIN, I. S. 1981. Prolactin secretion as an index of brain dopaminergic function. In J. B. MARTIN, S. REICHLIN, AND K. L. BICK (Editors), *Neurosecretion and Brain Peptides.* Raven Press, New York, pp. 503–520.

TIGGES, J., AND O'STEEN, W. K. 1974. Terminations of retinofugal fibers in squirrel monkey: A re-investigation using autoradiographic methods. Brain Res., **79:** 489–495.

TOBIAS, T. J. 1975. Afferents to prefrontal cortex from the thalamic mediodorsal nucleus in the rhesus monkey. Brain Res., **83:** 191–212.

TOLBERT, D. L., AND BANTLI, H. 1979. An HRP and autoradiographic study of cerebellar corticonuclear-nucleocortical reciprocity in the monkey. Exp. Brain Res., **36:** 563–571.

TOLBERT, D. L., MASSOPUST, L. C., MURPHY, M. G., AND YOUNG, P. A. 1976. The anatomical organization of the cerebello-olivary projection in the cat. J. Comp. Neurol., **170:** 525–544.

TOLBERT, D. L., BANTLI, H., AND BLOEDEL, J. R. 1976a. Anatomical and physiological evidence for a cerebellar nucleocortical projection in the cat. Neuroscience, **1:** 205–217.

TOLBERT, D. L., BANTLI, H., AND BLOEDEL, J. R. 1977. The intracerebellar nucleocortical projection in a primate. Exp. Brain Res., **30:** 425–434.

TOLBERT, D. L., BANTLI, H., AND BLOEDEL, J. R. 1978. Multiple branching of cerebellar efferent projections in cats. Exp. Brain Res., **31:** 305–316.

TOLBERT, D. L., BANTLI, H., AND BLOEDEL, J. R. 1978a. Organization features of the cat and monkey cerebellar nucleocortical projection. J. Comp. Neurol., **182:** 39–56.

TOMASCH, J. 1969. The numerical capacity of the human cortico-ponto-cerebellar system. Brain Res., **13:** 476–484.

TONCRAY, J. E., AND KRIEG, W. J. S. 1946. The nuclei of the human thalamus: A comparative approach. J. Comp. Neurol., **85:** 421–459.

TORVIK, A. 1956. Afferent connections to the sensory trigeminal nuclei, the nucleus of the solitary tract and adjacent structures: An experimental study in the rat. J. Comp. Neurol., **106:** 51–142.

TRACEY, D. J., ASANUMA, C., JONES, E. G., AND PORTER, R. 1980. Thalamic relay to motor cortex: Afferent pathways from brain stem, cerebellum, and spinal cord in monkeys. J. Neurophysiol., **44:** 532–553.

TRAVIS, A. M. 1955. Neurological deficiencies after ablation of the precentral motor area in *Macaca mulatta*. Brain, **78:** 155–173.

TRAVIS, A. M. 1955a. Neurological deficiencies following supplementary motor area lesions in *Macaca mulatta*. Brain, **78:** 174–198.

TRAVIS, A. M., AND WOOLSEY, C. N. 1956. Motor performance of monkeys after bilateral partial and total cerebral decortications. Am. J. Phys. Med., **35:** 273–303.

TREGEAR, G. W., NIALL, H. D., POTTS, J. T., LEEMAN, S. E., AND CHANG, M. M. 1971. Synthesis of substance P. Nature, **232:** 87–89.

TREVINO, D. L., AND CARSTENS, E. 1975. Confirmation of the location of spinothalamic neurons in the cat and monkey by the retrograde transport of horseradish peroxidase. Brain Res., **98:** 177–182.

TREVINO, D. L., COULTER, J. D., AND WILLIS, W. D. 1973. Location of cells of origin of spinothalamic tract in lumbar enlargement of the monkey. J. Neurophysiol., **36:** 750–761.

TROJANOWSKI, J. Q., AND JACOBSON, S. 1974. Medial pulvinar afferents to frontal eye fields in rhesus monkey demonstrated by horseradish peroxidase. Brain Res., **80:** 395–411.

TROJANOWSKI, J. Q., AND JACOBSON, S. 1975. A combined horseradish peroxidase-autoradiographic investigation of reciprocal connections between superior temporal gyrus and pulvinar in squirrel monkey. Brain Res., **85:** 347–353.

TRUEX, R. C., AND KELLNER, C. E. 1948. *Detailed Atlas of the Head and Neck.* Oxford University Press, New York.

TRUEX, R. C., AND TAYLOR, M. 1968. Gray matter lamination of the human spinal cord. Anat. Rec., **160:** 502.

TSUBOKAWA, T., AND SUTIN, H. 1972. Pallidal and tegmental inhibition of oscillatory slow waves and unit activity in the subthalamic nucleus. Brain Res., **41:** 101–118.

TURNBULL, I. M. 1972. Blood supply of the spinal cord. In P. J. VINKEN AND G. W. BRUYN (Editors), *Handbook of Clinical Neurology.* North-Holland, Amsterdam, **12:** 478–491.

TURNBULL, I. M. 1973. Blood supply of the spinal cord: Normal and pathological considerations. Clin. Neurosurg., **20:** 56–84.

TUSA, R. J., ROSENQUIST, A. C., AND PALMER, L. A. 1979. Retinotopic organization of areas 18 and 19 in the cat. J. Comp. Neurol., **185:** 657–678.

UNGERSTEDT, U. 1971. Stereotaxic mapping of the monoamine pathways in the rat brain. Acta Physiol. Scand. (Suppl.), **367:** 1–48.

UNO, M., AND YOSHIDA, M. 1975. Monosynaptic inhibition of thalamic neurons produced by stimulation of the pallidal nucleus in cats. Brain Res., **99:** 377–380.

URSIN H., AND KAADA, B. R. 1960. Functional localization within the amygdaloid complex in the cat. Electroencephalogr. Clin. Neurophysiol., **12:** 1–20.

VALENSTEIN, E. S., AND NAUTA, W. J. H. 1959. A comparison of the distribution of the fornix system in the rat, guinea pig, cat and monkey. J. Comp. Neurol., **113:** 337–363.

VALVERDE, F. 1965. *Studies on the Piriform Lobe.* Harvard University Press, Cambridge, Mass.

VAN BUREN, J. M., AND BORKE, R. C. 1972. *Variations and Connections of the Human Thalamus.* Springer-Verlag, New York, 2 vols.

VAN DEN POL, A. N., AND POWLEY, T. 1979. A fine-grained anatomical analysis of the role of the rat suprachiasmatic nucleus in circadian rhythms of feeding and drinking. Brain Res., **160:** 307–326.

VAN DER KOOY, D., AND HATTORI, T. 1980. Dorsal raphe cells with collateral projections to the caudate-putamen and substantia nigra: A fluorescent retrograde double labeling study in the rat. Brain Res., **186:** 1–7.

VAN DER KOOY, D., AND HATTORI, T. 1980a. Single subthalamic nucleus neurons project to both the globus pallidus and substantia nigra in rat. J. Comp. Neurol., **192:** 751–768.

VAN DER KOOY, D., KUYPERS, H. G. J. M., AND CATSMAN-BERREVOETS, C. E. 1978. Single mammillary body cells with divergent axon collaterals: Demonstration by a simple fluorescent retrograde double labeling technique in the rat. Brain Res., **158:** 189–196.

VANDESANDE, F., AND DIERICKX, K. 1979. The activated hypothalamic magnocellular neurosecretory system and the one-neuron—one neurohypophysial hormone concept. Cell Tissue Res., **200:** 29–33.

VAN HOESEN, G. W., YETERIAN, E. H., AND LAVIZZO-MOUREY, R. 1981. Widespread corticostriate projections from temporal cortex of the rhesus monkey. J. Comp. Neurol., **199:** 205–219.

VATES, T. S., BONTING, S. L., AND OPPELT, W. W. 1964. Na-K activated adenosine triphosphatase formation of cerebrospinal fluid in the cat. Am. J. Physiol., **206:** 1165–1172.

VELASCO, M., AND LINDSLEY, D. B. 1965. Role of the orbital cortex in regulation of thalamo-cortical electrical activity. Science, **149:** 1375–1377.

VELASCO, M. E., AND TALEISNIK, S. 1969. Release of gonadotropins induced by amygdaloid stimulation in the rat. Endocrinology, **84:** 132–139.

VERNEY, E. B. 1947. The antidiuretic hormone and factors which determine its release. Proc. R. Soc. Lond. (Biol.), **135:** 25–106.

VICTOR, M. 1964. Functions of memory and learning in man and their relationship to lesions in the temporal lobe and diencephalon. In M. A. B. Brazier (Editor), *Brain Function, RNA in Brain Functions: Memory and Learning*, Vol. III. American Institute of Biological Sciences, Washington, D.C.

Victor, M., Angevine, J. B., Jr., Mancall, E. L., and Fisher, C. M. 1961. Memory loss with lesions of hippocampal formation. Arch. Neurol., **5:** 244–263.

Vogt, B. A., and Pandya, D. N. 1978. Cortico-cortical connections of somatic sensory cortex (areas 3, 1, and 2) in the rhesus monkey. J. Comp. Neurol., **177:** 170–192.

Vogt, B. A., Rosene, D. L., and Pandya, D. N. 1979. Thalamic and cortical afferents differentiate anterior from posterior cingulate cortex in the monkey. Science, **204:** 205–207.

Vogt, C., and Vogt, O. 1919. Allgemeine Ergebnisse unserer Hirnforschung. Vierte Mitteilung: die physiologische Bedeutung der architektonischen Rindenreizungen. J. Psychol. Neurol., **25:** 279–462.

von Euler, U. S., and Gaddum, J. H. 1931. An unidentified depressor substance in certain tissue extracts. J. Physiol. (Lond.), **72:** 74–87.

Voogd, J. 1964. *The Cerebellum of the Cat Structure and Fibre Connexions.* Gorcum, The Netherlands.

Walberg, F. 1972. Cerebellovestibular relations: Anatomy. Prog. Brain Res., **37:** 361–376.

Walberg, F. 1974. Crossed reticulo-reticular projections in the medulla, pons and mesencephalon: An autoradiographic study in the cat. Z. Anat. Entwickl.-Gesch., **143:** 127–134.

Walberg, F., and Jansen, J. 1961. Cerebellar corticovestibular fibers in the cat. Exp. Neurol., **3:** 32–52.

Walberg, F., Pompeiano, O., Brodal, A., and Jansen, J. 1962. The fastigiovestibular projection in the cat: An experimental study with silver impregnation methods. J. Comp. Neurol., **118:** 49–75.

Walberg, F., Pompeiano, O., Westrum, L. E., and Hauglie-Hanssen, E. 1962a. Fastigioreticular fibers in the cat: An experimental study with silver methods. J. Comp. Neurol., **119:** 187–199.

Walberg, F., Kotchabhakdi, N., and Hoddevik, G. H. 1979. The olivocerebellar projections to the flocculus and paraflocculus in the cat, compared to the rabbit: A study using horseradish peroxidase as a tracer. Brain Res., **161:** 389–398.

Wald, G. 1968. Molecular basis of visual excitation. Science, **162:** 230–239.

Walker, A. E. 1938. The thalamus of the chimpanzee. IV. Thalamic projections to the cerebral cortex. J. Anat., **73:** 37–93.

Walker, A. E. 1938a. *The Primate Thalamus.* University of Chicago Press, Chicago.

Walker, A. E. 1949. Afferent connections. In P. C. Bucy (Editor), *The Precentral Motor Cortex*, ed. 2. University of Illinois, Urbana, Ch. 4, pp. 112–132.

Walker, A. E. 1959. Normal and pathological physiology of the thalamus. In G. Schaltenbrand and P. Bailey (Editors), *Introduction to Stereotaxis with an Atlas of the Human Brain*, Vol. I. Georg Thieme, Stuttgart, pp. 291–330.

Walker, A. E. 1966. Internal structure and afferent-efferent relations of the thalamus. In D. P. Purpura and M. D. Yahr (Editors), *The Thalamus.* Columbia University Press, New York, pp. 1–12.

Walker, A. E., and Weaver, T. A., Jr. 1940. Ocular movements from the occipital lobe in the monkey. J. Neurophysiol., **3:** 353–357.

Wall, P. D. 1978. The gate control theory of pain mechanisms: A re-examination and re-statement. Brain, **101:** 1–18.

Wall, P. D., and Taub, A. 1962. Four aspects of the trigeminal nucleus and a paradox. J. Neurophysiol., **25:** 110–126.

Wamsley, J. K., Young, W. S., and Kuhar, M. J. 1980. Immunohistochemical localization of enkephalin in rat forebrain. Brain Res., **190:** 153–174.

Wang, H. S. 1977. Dementia of old age. In W. L. Smith and M. Kinsborn (Editors), *Aging and Dementia.* Spectrum, New York, pp. 1–24.

Warwick, R. 1953. Representation of the extraocular muscles in the oculomotor nuclei of the monkey. J. Comp. Neurol., **98:** 449–504.

Watson, S. J., and Akil, H. 1981. Opioid peptides and related substances: Immunocytochemistry. In J. B. Martin, S. Reichlin, and K. L. Bick (Editors), *Neurosecretion and Brain Peptides.* Raven Press, New York, pp. 77–86.

Weinberger, L. M., and Grant, F. C. 1941. Precocious puberty and tumors of the hypothalamus. Arch. Intern. Med., **67:** 762–792.

Weindl, A., and Sofroniew, M. V. 1981. Relation of neuropeptides to mammalian circumventricular organs. Adv. Biochem. Psychopharmacol., **28:** 303–320.

Welch, K. 1963. Secretion of cerebrospinal fluid by choroid plexus of the rabbit. Am. J. Physiol., **205:** 617–624.

Welch, K., and Friedman, J. 1960. The cerebrospinal fluid valves. Brain, **83:** 454–469.

Werner, G. W., and Whitsel, B. L. 1968. The topology of the body representation in somatosensory area I of primates. J. Neurophysiol., **31:** 856–869.

Werner, G. W., and Whitsel, B. L. 1973. Functional organization of the somatosensory cortex. In A. Iggo (Editor), *Handbook of Sensory Physiology*, Vol. 2. Springer-Verlag, Berlin, pp. 621–700.

Wersäll, J. 1960. Electron micrographic studies of vestibular hair cell innervation. In G. L. Rasmussen and W. F. Windle (Editors), *Neural Mechanisms of the Auditory and Vestibular Systems.* Charles C Thomas, Springfield, Ill., pp. 247–257.

Whitehouse, P. J., Price, D. L., Clark, A. W., Coyle, J. T., and DeLong, M. R. 1981. Alzheimer's disease: Evidence for selective loss of cholinergic neurons in the nucleus basalis. Ann. Neurol., **10:** 122–126.

Whitehouse, P. J., Price, D. L., Struble, R. G., Clark, A. W., Coyle, J. T., and DeLong, M. R. 1982. Alzheimer's disease and senile dementia: Loss of neurons in the basal forebrain. Science, **215:** 1237–1239.

Whitlock, D. G., and Nauta, W. J. H. 1956. Subcortical projections from the temporal neocortex in the *Macaca mulatta.* J. Comp. Neurol., **106:** 183–212.

Whitsel, B. L., Petrucelli, L. M., and Werner, G. 1969. Symmetry and connectivity in the map of the body surface in somatosensory area II of primates. J. Neurophysiol., **32:** 170–183.

Whittier, J. R. 1947. Ballism and the subthalamic

nucleus (nucleus hypothalamicus; corpus Luysii). Arch Neurol. Psychiat., **58:** 672–692.

WHITTIER, J. R., AND METTLER, F. A. 1949. Studies on the subthalamus of the rhesus monkey. II. Hyperkinesia and other physiological effects of subthalamic lesions with special reference to the subthalamic nucleus of Luys. J. Comp. Neurol., **90:** 319–372.

WIESEL, T. N., AND HUBEL, D. H. 1974. Ordered arrangement of orientation columns in monkeys lacking visual experience. J. Comp. Neurol., **158:** 307–318.

WIESEL, T. N., HUBEL, D. H., AND LAM, D. M. K. 1974. Autoradiographic demonstration of ocular-dominance columns in the monkey striate cortex by means of transneuronal transport. Brain Res., **79:** 273–279.

WIESENDANGER, M. 1973. Input from muscle and cutaneous nerves of the hand and forearm to neurones of the precentral gyrus of baboons and monkeys. J. Physiol. (Lond.), **228:** 203–219.

WIESENDANGER, M. J., SÉGUIN, J. J., AND KÜNZLE, H. 1974. The supplementary motor area—a control system for posture. Adv. Behav. Biol., **7:** 331–346.

WILLIS, W. D., TREVINO, D. L., COULTER, J. D., AND MAUNZ, R. A. 1974. Responses of primate spinothalamic tract neurons to natural stimulation of hindlimb. J. Neurophysiol., **37:** 358–372.

WILLIS, W. D., HABER, L. H., AND MARTIN, R. F. 1977. Inhibition of spinothalamic tract cells and interneurons by brainstem stimulation in the monkey. J. Neurophysiol., **40:** 968–981.

WILLIS, W. D., LEONARD, R. B., AND KENSHALO, D. R., JR. 1978. Spinothalamic tract neurons in the substantia gelatinosa. Science, **202:** 986–988.

WILSON, C. J., CHANG, H. T., AND KITAI, S. T. 1982. Origins of postsynaptic potentials evoked in identified rat neostriatal neurons by stimulation in substantia nigra. Exp. Brain Res., **45:** 157–167.

WILSON, M. E., AND TOYNE, M. J. 1970. Retino-tectal and cortico-tectal projections in *Macaca mulatta*. Brain Res., **24:** 395–406.

WILSON, S. A. K. 1912. Progressive lenticular degeneration: A familial nervous disease associated with cirrhosis of the liver. Brain, **34:** 295–509.

WILSON, V. J., AND YOSHIDA, M. 1969. Monosynaptic inhibition of neck motoneurons by the medial vestibular nucleus. Exp. Brain Res., **9:** 365–380.

WILSON, V. J., UCHINO, Y., SUSSWEIN, A., AND FUKUSHIMA, K. 1977. Properties of direct fastigiospinal fibers in the cat. Brain Res., **126:** 543–546.

WILSON, V. J., UCHINO, Y., MAUNZ, R. A., SUSSWEIN, A., AND FUKUSHIMA, K. 1978. Properties and connections of cat fastigiospinal neurons. Exp. Brain Res., **32:** 1–17.

WINDLE, W. F. 1926. Non-bifurcating nerve fibers of the trigeminal nerve. J. Comp. Neurol., **40:** 229–240.

WINER, J. A., DIAMOND, I. T., AND RACZKOWSKI, D. 1977. Subdivisions of the auditory cortex in the cat: The retrograde transport of horseradish peroxidase to the medial geniculate body and posterior thalamic nuclei. J. Comp. Neurol., **176:** 387–418.

WISE, S. P., AND TANJI, J. 1981. Supplementary and precentral motor cortex: Contrast in responsiveness to peripheral input in the hindlimb area of the unanesthetized monkey. J. Comp. Neurol., **195:** 433–451.

WONG-RILEY, M. T. T. 1974. Demonstration of geniculocortical and callosal projection neurons in the squirrel monkey by means of retrograde axonal transport of horseradish peroxidase. Brain Res., **79:** 267–272.

WONG-RILEY, M. T. T. 1976. Projections from the dorsal lateral geniculate nucleus to prestriate cortex in the squirrel monkey as demonstrated by retrograde transport of horseradish peroxidase. Brain Res., **109:** 595–600.

WONG-RILEY, M. T. T. 1979. Columnar cortico-cortical interconnections within the visual system of the squirrel and macaque monkeys. Brain Res., **162:** 201–217.

WOODBURY, D. M. 1958. Symposium discussion. In W. F. WINDLE (Editor), *Biology of Neuroglia.* Charles C Thomas, Springfield, Ill., pp. 120–127.

WOOLEY, D. W., AND SHAW, E. 1954. A biochemical and pharmacological suggestion about certain mental disorders. Proc. Natl. Acad. Sci. U.S.A., **40:** 228–231.

WOOLSEY, C. N. 1958. Organization of somatic sensory and motor areas of the cerebral cortex. In H. F. HARLOW AND C. N. WOOLSEY (Editors), *Biological and Biochemical Bases of Behavior.* University of Wisconsin, Madison, pp. 63–81.

WOOLSEY, C. N. 1960. Organization of cortical auditory system: A review and synthesis. In G. L. RASMUSSEN AND W. F. WINDLE (Editors), *Neural Mechanisms of the Auditory and Vestibular Systems.* Charles C Thomas, Springfield, Ill., pp. 165–180.

WOOLSEY, C. N. 1971. Tonotopic organization of the auditory cortex. In M. B. SACHS (Editor), *Physiology of the Auditory System* (A Workshop). National Consultants, Baltimore, pp. 271–282.

WOOLSEY, C. N. 1975. Cortical motor map of *Macaca mulatta* after chronic section of the medullary pyramid. In K. J. ZULCH, O. CREUTZFELDT, AND G. C. GALBRAITH (Editors), *Cerebral Localization.* Springer-Verlag, Berlin, pp. 19–31.

WOOLSEY, C. N., AND WALZL, E. M. 1942. Topical projection of nerve fibers from local regions of the cochlea to the cerebral cortex of the cat. Bull. Johns Hopkins Hosp., **71:** 315–344.

WOOLSEY, C. N., SETTLAGE, P. H., MEYER, D. R., SENCER, W., HAMUY, T. P., AND TRAVIS, A. M. 1951. Patterns of localization in precentral and "supplementary" motor areas and their relation to the concept of a premotor area. Proc. Assoc. Res. Nerv. Ment. Dis., **30:** 238–264.

WURTMAN, R. J. 1971. Brain monoamines and endocrine function. Neurosci. Res. Program Bull., **9:** 177–297.

YELNIK, J., AND PERCHERON, G. 1979. Subthalamic neurons in primates: A quantitative and comparative analysis. Neuroscience, **4:** 1717–1743.

YETERIAN, E. H., AND VAN HOESEN, G. W. 1978. Cortico-striate projections in the rhesus monkey: The organization of certain cortico-caudate connections. Brain Res., **139:** 43–63.

ZACZEK, R., SCHWARCZ, R., AND COYLE, J. T. 1978. Long term sequelae of striatal kainate lesion. Brain Res., **152:** 626–632.

ZANGWILL, O. L. 1960. *Cerebral Dominance and Its*

Relation to Psychological Function. Charles C Thomas, Springfield, Ill.

ZARZECKI, P., STRICK, P. L., AND ASANUMA, H. 1978. Input to primate motor cortex from posterior parietal cortex (area 5). II. Identification by antidromic activation. Brain Res., **157:** 331–335.

ZBROŻYNA, A. W. 1972. The organization of the defense reaction elicited from amygdala and its connections. In B. E. ELEFTHERIOU (Editor), *The Neurobiology of the Amygdala.* Plenum Press, New York, pp. 597–606.

ZEAL, A. A., AND RHOTON, A. L. 1978. Microsurgical anatomy of the posterior cerebral artery. J. Neurosurg., **48:** 534–559.

ZEKI, S. M. 1971. Interhemispheric connections of prestriate cortex in monkeys. Brain Res., **19:** 63–75.

ZIMMERMAN, E. A. 1981. Blood-brain barrier, cerebral fluid and cerebral blood flow. In J. B. MARTIN, S. REICHLIN, AND K. L. BICK (Editors), *Neurosecretion and Brain Peptides.* Raven Press, New York, pp. 299–302.

ZIMMERMAN, E. A., CARMEL, P. W., HUSAIN, M. K., FERIN, M., TANNENBAUM, M., FRANTZ, A. G., AND ROBINSON, A. G. 1973. Vasopressin and neurophysin: High concentrations in monkey hypophyseal portal blood. Science, **182:** 925–927.

ZOLOVICK, A. J. 1972. Effects of lesions and electrical stimulation of the amygdala on hypothalamic-hypophyseal regulation. In B. E. ELEFTHERIOU (Editor), *The Neurobiology of the Amygdala.* Plenum Press, New York, pp. 643–683.

ZÜLCH, K. J. 1954. Mangeldurchblutung an der Grenzzone zweier Gefässgebiete als Ursache bisher ungeklärter Rückenmarksschädigungen. Dtsch. Z. Nervenheilkd., **172:** 81–101.

Index